Improve International Manual of Clinical Small Animal Internal Medicine

Volume 1

Improve
International

Improve International Manual of Clinical Small Animal Internal Medicine

Volume 1

Josep Pastor Milán, James W. Swann, Pippa Elliott, Amalia Agut Giménez, Germán Santamarina Pernas, Josefa Fernández del Palacio, Simón Martí Angulo, Cintia García Echarri, Cristina Pérez Vera

Translated by Gemma Gaitskell-Phillips

Edited by Pippa Elliott

Improve International

First published 2019

Published by
5M Publishing Ltd,
Benchmark House,
8 Smithy Wood Drive,
Sheffield, S35 1QN, UK
Tel: +44 (0) 1234 81 81 80
www.5mpublishing.com

Complementary to Improve International's 2 year modular programme in small animal surgery, this reference manual covers small animal surgery at practitioner level.

Important note
Medicine is an ever-changing science, so the contents of this publication, especially recommendations concerning diagnostic and therapeutic procedures, can only give an account of the knowledge at the time of publication. While utmost care has been taken to ensure that all specifications regarding drug selection and dosage and treatment options are accurate, readers are urged to review the product information sheet and any relevant material supplied by the manufacturer, and, in case of doubt, to consult a specialist. From both an editorial and public interest perspective, the publisher welcomes notification of possible inconsistencies. The ultimate responsibility for any diagnostic or therapeutic application lies with the reader.

A Catalogue record for this book is available from the British Library

ISBN 9781913352097

Book layout by Servis Filmsetting Ltd, Stockport, Cheshire
Printed by Short Run Press Limited, Exeter
Photos by the authors unless otherwise indicated
Illustrations by Elaine Leggett

Contents

Contributors

Simón Martí Angulo Prof. Acred AVEPA Rep
Simón received his DVM from the Complutense University of Madrid in 1983. He has been practising with the ONCE Guide Dog Foundation since 1990, where he manages the Breeding Centre for the Guide Dogs School and is responsible for reproduction, neonatology and paediatrics, in addition to working as a Reproduction Specialist at the Veterinary Clinical Hospital at the Alfonso X el Sabio University and Plutos Veterinary Clinic in Madrid. He is currently Lecturer in Obstetrics and Reproduction at the Alfonso X el Sabio University. He has published papers in numerous national and international journals and received the Scientific Miguel Luera prize in 2003 for the paper "Colposuspensión para prevenir la incontinencia urinaria en perras castradas" (Prevention of urinary incontinence in spayed bitches using colposuspension). He authored the text Feline and Canine Reproduction and Neonatology which was published in 2011 and coordinated and wrote the book Pediatric Medicine in Small Animals which was published in 2012 by Servet Editorial. He is accredited as a specialist in Canine and Feline Reproduction and Neonatology with AVEPA and is a member of EVSSAR and GERPAC. He has also been a member of the Specialist Reproduction Scientific Committee at AVEPA from 2002-2010, treasurer for the Study Group in Companion Animal Reproduction and Paediatrics (GERPAC), board member of AVEPA in Madrid and coordinator of board members for the Board of AVEPA. He works exclusively with small animals and with a special interest in reproduction.

Cintia García Echarri
Cintia was licensed by the University Alfonso X el Sabio in June 2015. She currently works at the Veterinary Hospital Vetersalud INDRA as a veterinarian in emergencies, intensive care and stabilization of critical patients. She also works as a veterinarian in childbirth and reproduction in the ONCE Foundation of the guide dog.

Pippa Elliott BVMS MRCVS
Pippa graduated from the University of Glasgow in 1987 and has worked in first opinion companion animal practice for over three decades. She splits her time between hands on veterinary practice and a second career as a veterinary copywriter and editor.

Amalia Agut Giménez DVM PhD Dip ECVDI
Amalia, DVM and PhD in Veterinary Medicine from the University of Zaragoza, Diplomate of the European College of Veterinary Diagnostic Imaging (ECVDI), is currently a Professor in Radiology in the Department of Small Animal Surgery and Medicine, Head of the Diagnostic Imaging Service at the Clinical Veterinary Hospital at the University of Murcia. She has completed several short stays at various centres in universities in the United Kingdom, in addition to the University of Sydney (Australia). She has been a member of the Board of the ECVDI and is Associate Director of the International Veterinary Radiology Association. She has presented papers, lectures and seminars at national and international congresses and published papers in both national and international journal as well as being author and co-author of books on small animal diagnostic imaging.

Josep Pastor Milán DVM, PhD, Dipl ECVCP
Josep received his DVM from the Veterinary Faculty of the Autonomous University of Barcelona in 1989, subsequently obtaining his PhD in Veterinary Medicine from the same University. Lecturer in Medical Pathology from 1991 where he combines his teaching activities with his role at the Veterinary Clinical Hospital at the Autonomous University of Barcelona. He has completed several short stays at centres in the United States to deepen his knowledge of small animal clinical practice in addition to participating in numerous national and international congresses. He is currently a Diplomate of the European College of Veterinary Clinical Pathology (Dipl ECVCP). His areas of interest are haematology and small animal oncology.

Mª Josefa Fernández del Palacio PhD, Dipl ECVIM-CA
Dr. Mª Josefa Fernández del Palacio is Full Professor of the Department of Medicine and Animal Surgery of the University of Murcia and Responsible for the Cardiorespiratory Service of the Veterinary Hospital of the University of Murcia. She holds a Diploma in Cardiology from the European College of Veterinary Internal Medicine (Dipl ECVIM-CA [Cardiology]). She published numerous articles and book chapters on cardiology in both national and international journals. Her fields of interest are cardiology and nephrology.

Germán Santamarina Pernas DVM PhD
Licenciado en Veterinaria en la Facultad de Veterinaria de Lugo de la Universidad de Santiago de Compostela (USC) en 1989, obtuvo el título de Doctor en Veterinaria en la misma Universidad en 1993. Ha realizado estancias formativas en el campo de la Cardiología y la Medicina Interna en las facultades de Davis (EEUU), Bolonia (Italia), Alfort (Francia) y Lyon (Francia). En la actualidad es Profesor Titular de Patología Médica en el Departamento de Ciencias Clínicas Veterinarias de la Facultad de Veterinaria de Lugo de la USC y desarrolla su actividad clínicoasistencial en el Servicio de Medicina Interna del Hospital Veterinario Universitario Rof Codina.

James W. Swann
James graduated from the University of Cambridge in 2010 and, after working in first opinion practice for 2 years, completed an internship and residency in small animal internal medicine at the Royal Veterinary College, University of London. During this time, he conducted research on immune-mediated haemolytic anaemia in dogs, receiving a Kennel Club International Canine Health Award in 2015. He is currently completing a PhD in immunology and haematology at the University of Oxford.

Cristina Pérez Vera DVM, PhD, Dipl. ACVIM (SAIM) & ECVIM
Cristina received her DVM from the University of Barcelona in 2004. Subsequently undertaking an Internship in Medicine and Surgery and the Autonomous University of Barcelona and after this a second internship and a residency in Internal Medicine at North Carolina State University, in the United States. American Diplomate in Internal Medicine (ACVIM) from 2011. She has worked in the University of Helsinki (Finland), in Leipzig (Germany) and from November 2013 at the University of Bern (Switzerland). Her area of expertise is infectious diseases. In 2015 she completed a PhD at the University of Helsinki looking at Bartonella infections and other tick-borne diseases. From 2013 she has also been a European Diplomate in Internal Medicine (ECVIM).

1

Haematology

Josep Pastor Milán

Chapter summary

The study of haematology at vet school is one of those subjects that polarises students. They either love the subject or alternatively regard it as something to be endured. However, once in practice as a qualified veterinarian, the benefit of a thorough understanding of haematology immediately becomes apparent. For example, the ability to interpret a leukogram or recognise spherocytes in the blood smear of an anaemic patient dramatically narrows down the list of differential diagnoses. In turn, this allows for targeted testing and reaching a rapid diagnosis in the critically ill patient.

Indeed, knowledge of a patient's haematological status is fundamental to a complete and thorough clinical examination. The effects of systemic disease can be far reaching and produce secondary changes in a complete blood count or coagulation tests. While for primary changes, often associated with immune-mediated conditions, spotting such problems in a timely manner and providing prompt treatment can make a material difference to patient outcome.

Key learning points

- Understand the practical benefits of classifying anaemia.
- Develop proficiency in interpreting a blood smear.
- In-house testing for autoagglutination.
- Learn to interpret a leukogram with confidence.
- Clotting disorders, both primary and secondary.

Anaemia

The term 'anaemia' describes a reduction in the **erythrocyte count, haemoglobin concentration and haematocrit value** with respect to the reference ranges (which vary depending on the species, breed, reproductive status and age of the animal). Anaemia is one of the **most frequently occurring haematological alterations** seen in practice.

Aetiology

The causes of anaemia can be divided into **three major categories:**

- **blood loss**
- **destruction** (haemolysis) of erythrocytes or their immature forms
- **decrease** in erythrocyte **production**.

Before initiating treatment, it is important to establish the **underlying cause**.

Clinical history

When taking the animal's clinical history, it is essential to record or rule out the administration of drugs capable of causing bone marrow changes. Those **medications** most closely linked to these alterations (Table 1.1) are:

- antibiotics (especially trimethoprim–sulphadiazine)
- certain hormones such as oestrogen
- anti-inflammatories
- chemotherapeutic or immunosuppressive drugs.

Other fundamental factors to establish include ascertaining whether the animal has **suffered blood loss**, which may be suggested by:

- the presence of dark faeces
- a history of recent trauma
- abdominal distention with hypovolaemic shock

Table 1.1. Medications associated with haematological disorders.

Medication	Comments
Oestrogens	Frequent cause Effects on the bone marrow that can be irreversible
Chemotherapy	Various medications: vincristine, doxorubicin, cyclophosphamide, etc. They usually cause reversible changes which show a delayed effect: • 120 days in **dogs** • 80 days in **cats**
Trimethoprim–sulphadiazine	Frequent cause Reversible changes
Cephalosporins	Few cases described Reversible changes
Phenobarbital	Few cases described Reversible changes
Albendazole	Few cases described Reversible changes
Thiacetarsamide	Few cases described Reversible changes
Immunosuppressants (azathioprine, leflunomide)	Some cases described Changes generally reversible

- possible exposure to rodenticides
- a risk of tick borne disease.

The **presence of vectors** such as ticks can predispose to infections such as *Ehrlichia* spp. or *Babesia* spp. Accurate clinical records, including relevant vaccinations and knowledge of trips outside the local area, help to establish the risk of these conditions.

In **cats**, questions should be asked about the animal with regard to **feline leukaemia virus (FeLV) and feline immunodeficiency virus (FIV)** and the lifestyle of the animal, such as whether it has outside access or is an exclusively indoor cat.

Fundamental questions in animals with anaemia

- Has the animal been given medication or been **in contact with toxic substances** (including onions, garlic) or rodenticides?
- **Has blood been observed** in the stools, urine or have the faeces been dark or black in colour?
- What is the **FeLV or FIV status** of the cat?
- Has the animal been in contact with **ticks**?
- Has the animal been **vaccinated recently** and against what diseases?
- **Has the animal travelled** away from the area where they usually live?

Physical examination

During the physical examination, the clinician should be alert for factors related to **blood loss**, such as:

- hypovolaemic shock
- trauma
- abdominal masses
- hepatosplenomegaly.

Signs associated with anaemia include:

- pale mucous membranes
- tachycardia
- tachypnoea
- exercise intolerance
- weakness.

Diagnosis

The **haematocrit value** is the easiest and most accurate way to confirm the presence of anaemia. However, the use of haematological analysers and supravital stains for reticulocytes, along with **evaluation of a blood smear**, are essential to classify the anaemia and make a specific diagnosis.

Classification

The two classification systems most useful to the clinician are as follows.

1. By **erythrocyte volume** and **haemoglobin concentration.**
2. By the presence or absence of regeneration.

While other classification systems exist, from a clinical standpoint, these two methods (along with a morphological study of erythrocytes) provide the most valuable information.

Classification by erythrocyte volume and haemoglobin concentration

The **mean corpuscular volume** of the erythrocyte (MCV) can be determined by measuring cell size using laser or electrical-impedance-based haematology analysers, by means of the following formula:

$$MCV\ (femtolitres) = \frac{Haematocrit\ value}{Erythrocyte\ count\ (106/\mu l)} \times 10$$

Changes in haemoglobin concentration are described as follows.

- **Normochromic**. Within the normal range.
- **Hypochromic**. There is less haemoglobin per erythrocyte. This may indicate the presence of regenerative anaemia or changes in the haemoglobin within erythrocytes.
- **Hyperchromic**. This is almost always related to **an artefact** (lipaemia, haemolysis, Heinz bodies) or a laboratory error.

When considering the classification of anaemia according to MCV and MCHC, it is important to ensure that the analyser is functioning correctly. A simple way to verify this is to check that the following relationship is true:

$$Haemoglobin\ concentration \times 3 = Haematocrit$$

If this calculation is not correct, this may indicate errors in the erythrocyte count, the measurements of haemoglobin concentration or the haematocrit value.

Various combinations of MCV and MCHC are used for the classification of anaemias, including the following.

- **Hypochromic macrocytic anaemia**. This relates to regenerative anaemias with abundant immature reticulocytes which are large in size.
- **Macrocytic normochromic anaemia**. In cats without polychromasia, this is suggestive of FeLV infections or myelodysplastic syndromes. In some dogs, such as Poodles, it may be normal for the breed, since they normally have macrocytes present in their blood. Variations in vitamin B12 and folate can also lead to this type of anaemia.

Table 1.2. Clinical classification of anaemia according to its severity.

	Normal (0)	Mild (1)	Moderate (2)	Severe (3)
Mucous membrane colour	Normal	Slightly pale	Moderately pale	Very pale
Pulse quality	Normal	Strong	Weak	Weak
Heart rate/min	65–109	110–140	>140	>140
Respiratory rate/min	15–24	25–40	>40	>40
Mental state/exercise tolerance	Alert	Calm, able to walk	Apathy, able to stand	Marked apathy, unable to stand

- **Normochromic normocytic anaemia**. Non-regenerative anaemias with normal residual erythrocytes.
- **Microcytic and hypochromic anaemias**. Usually related to iron deficiencies.

The drawback of this classification system is that the measurements of MCV and MCHC require the majority of the cells to be affected and, therefore, this is not considered very sensitive.

- **Erythrocyte histograms** may be better indicators of regeneration than indices: the **red cell distribution width histogram** (RDW), a measurement of erythrocyte anisocytosis that may indicate the presence of spherocytes and macrocytic cells, is an earlier indicator of regeneration than MCV and MCHC.

Classification according to regeneration

Reticulocytes in peripheral blood are the cells that reflect regeneration. In the dog there is only one type of reticulocyte, while in the cat there are two.

Depending on their characteristics and the time that has elapsed since their release from the bone marrow, feline reticulocytes are classified as follows.

1. **Aggregate**. Those which have been released by the bone marrow in the **48 hours prior** to blood sampling.
2. **Punctate**. Those which have been in circulation for **more than 48 hours**. Before becoming normal erythrocytes, they are visible for about 15 days.

In general, in the face of haemolysis or acute blood loss, an animal needs **3–4 days to show an increase in reticulocyte count** in peripheral blood. During this period, anaemia cannot be correctly classified as regenerative or not, and to narrow the differential diagnosis, the clinical history and the findings of the physical examination must be considered.

Immature erythrocytes (**reticulocytes**) are usually **hypochromic and macrocytic**. On a slide preparation, the large size of these cells gives them a tendency to bend or fold back on themselves. A high percentage of reticulocytes indicate a **regenerative response**. To verify this, **supravital stains** should be used. This is because a characteristic of regenerative anaemias is **polychromasia** (Figure 1.1). Polychromatic cells are reticulocytes that retain a high proportion of RNA, dispersed through the cells to give **bluish appearance** with normal stains. However, not all reticulocytes are polychromatic, which makes this observation less sensitive than specific staining for reticulocytes.

The **most reliable parameter to establish whether an anaemia is regenerative or not** is an **erythrocyte count**. Manual erythrocyte counts are difficult and imprecise, (although they are still used in many laboratories); therefore, new haematological analysers usually include reticulocytes, which are shown **graphically in cytograms**. These analysers do not detect punctate reticulocytes and therefore, in cats, only the aggregate form is counted.

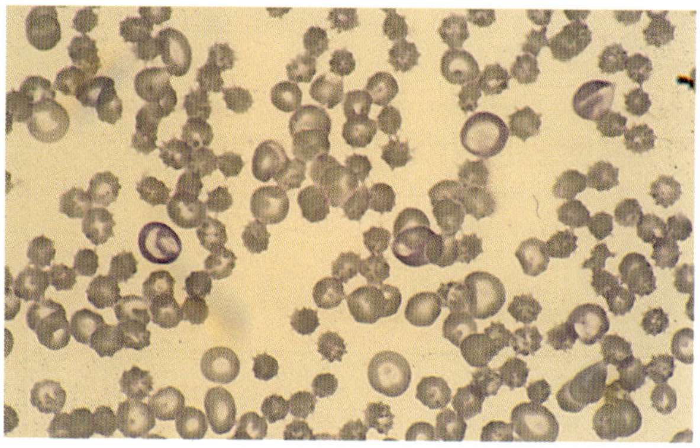

Figure 1.1. Presence of two polychromatic erythrocytes and crenation of erythrocytes. Observe how the erythrocyte on the left-hand side has a fold in the membrane, which is normal in reticulocytes due to their macrocytosis.

Regarding the use of the reticulocyte count to classify anaemia, it is important to note that **regeneration can be seen in animals without anaemia**. It is thought that these animals may have undergone a **splenic contraction** and the count is increased by excitement or exercise. In addition, the reticulocyte count varies throughout the day and some anaesthetic agents can increase or decrease it.

Other considerations include the following.

- The reference range of the analyser for a reticulocyte count can vary.
- With a greater degree of anaemia there is more stimulus for regeneration, and therefore the **reticulocyte count should be interpreted alongside the haematocrit**. For example, if the analyser's normal count is 60,000 reticulocytes/μl and the animal has 75,000 reticulocytes/μl, the haematocrit value should be used to interpret the regeneration: thus, a dog with a haematocrit value of 30% will have a moderately regenerative anaemia, and in an animal with a haematocrit of 15%, anaemia may be non-regenerative.

The **benefit of classifying anaemia** as regenerative or not is that this enables the clinician to draw up a more accurate differential diagnosis list (Figure 1.2). For example, **regenerative anaemias are always due to blood loss or haemolysis**, while **non-regenerative anaemias** are approached differently and require the **investigation of systemic diseases** as a possible cause.

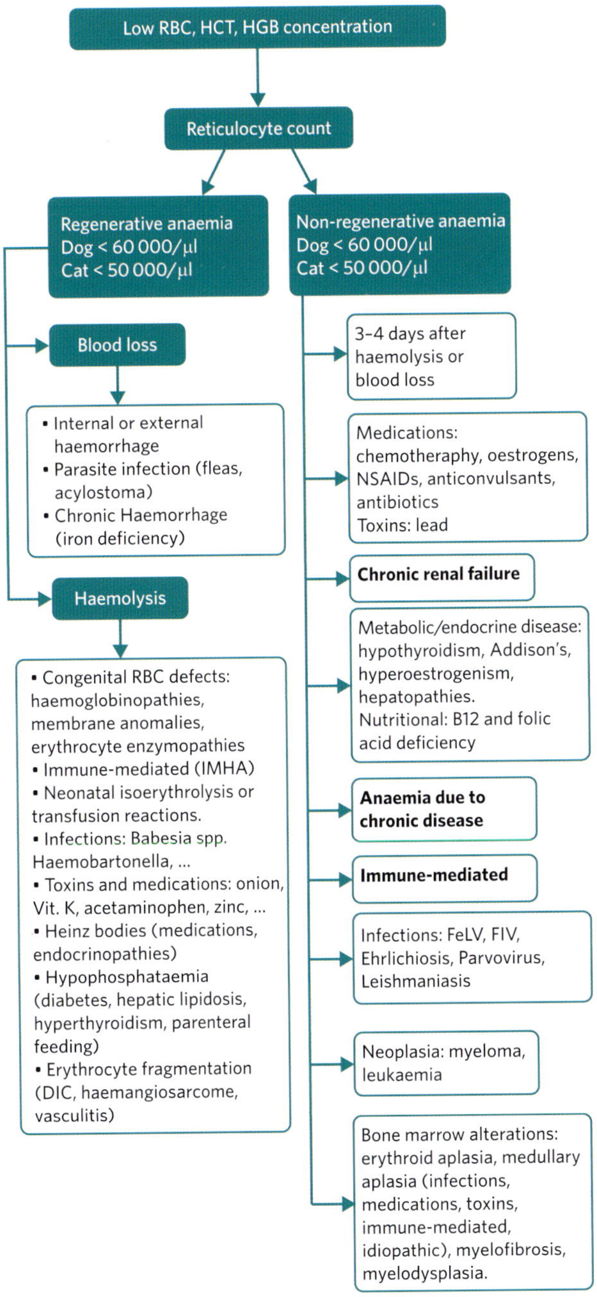

Figure 1.2. Differential diagnosis of regenerative and non-regenerative anaemia.

Blood smear

Erythrocyte morphology is another fundamental part of the approach to these cases. In general, erythrocytes have a biconcave disc shape with a paler central zone that usually represents one third of its diameter.

Morphological changes

Rouleaux or stacks of coins

Description

Rouleaux are formed by the presence of several **erythrocytes in a row**, giving the appearance of a stack of coins (Figure 1.3).

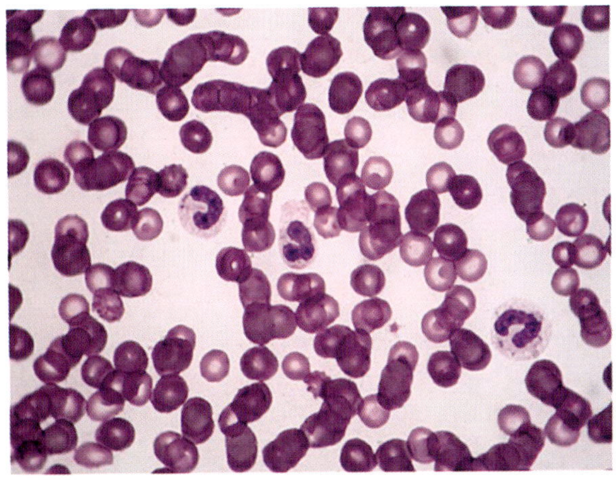

Figure 1.3. Example of the formation of rouleaux. Toxic changes in the neutrophils can also be seen with Döhle bodies.

Causes

Unlike the cat, in which rouleaux formation occurs physiologically, in the dog its presence is usually associated with an **increase in the concentration of proteins** (such as fibrinogen and immunoglobulins) characteristic of **inflammatory conditions**. Therefore, this change can be observed in samples from animals with:

- infectious diseases
- metabolic disorders
- immune-mediated diseases
- neoplastic diseases
- lymphoma or lymphoproliferative conditions
- multiple myeloma.

Agglutination

Description

The presence of **cohesive, disordered groups of erythrocytes**, associated with the existence of immunoglobulins on the erythrocyte surface.

Sometimes agglutination can be confused with aggregates of erythrocytes that are produced in samples with high protein concentrations (rouleaux). One way to **ensure that there is true agglutination** is to perform the **saline dilution test**.

1. A **drop of blood** taken directly from the EDTA K3 tube is placed on a clean slide.
2. **Six drops of saline** are added (using a syringe or a Pasteur pipette).
3. The **blood and saline are mixed** (a micro haematocrit capillary tube can be used) until the mixture is homogenised.
4. A **cover-slip** is placed over the mixture (absorbent paper should be used to remove excess sample that goes over the edges of the slide).

5. The slide is then **observed under the microscope** (since it is a fresh sample, the microscope diaphragm should be partially closed to limit the amount of light).

Interpretation

The test is considered **positive (i.e. presence of agglutination) when cohesive groups of erythrocytes remain**.

If, on the other hand, individual erythrocytes are seen to be separated from one another, the test is considered negative (Figure 1.4).

Cause

Agglutination is associated with **immune-mediated haemolytic anaemia (IMHA)**.

Polychromasia

Description

Polychromatophils are **immature erythrocytes** which are **larger in size than mature erythrocytes**, show a more basic staining pattern (blue or reddish blue) and do not show central pallor. There is a **direct correlation between the percentage of polychromatophilic erythrocytes and the percentage of reticulocytes**. In dogs, polychromasia is considered normal when it constitutes about 1% of the total erythrocyte population (Figures 1.1 and 1.5).

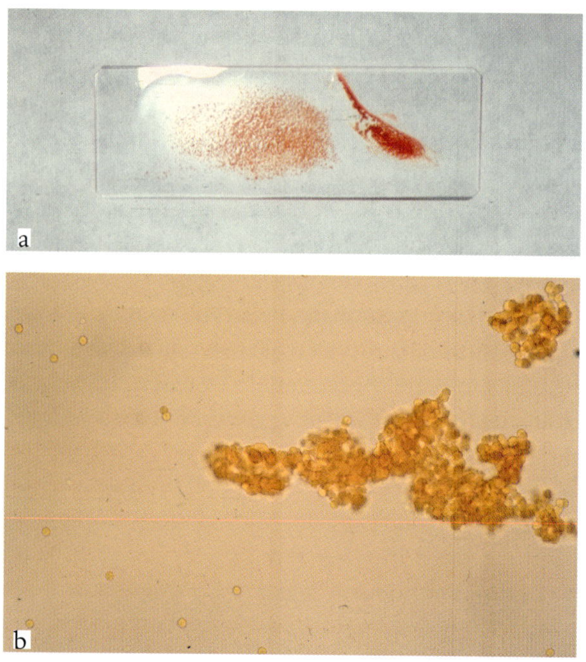

Figure 1.4. (a) Macroscopic blood sample with macroscopic agglutination after dilution with saline. (b) The same sample with aggregation observed under the microscope at × 40 magnification.

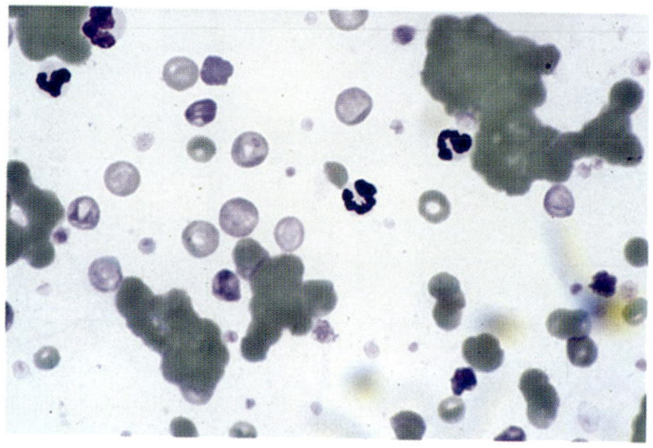

Figure 1.5. Microscopic agglutination suggestive of immune-mediated haemolytic anaemia and obvious polychromasia.

Cause

Regenerative anaemia sees an increase in the number of these cells.

Hypochromasia

Description

Hypochromasia is a **decrease in the haemoglobin concentration** of the erythrocyte which results in an increased area of central pallor and a 'thinning' of the cell (Figure 1.6).

In dogs the pallor should be more marked, since the erythrocytes normally have an area of central pallor, which is why hypochromasia is sometimes difficult to appreciate.

Causes

Hypochromasia can be seen in:

- **regenerative anaemias**, due to the presence of young cells with a lower concentration of haemoglobin

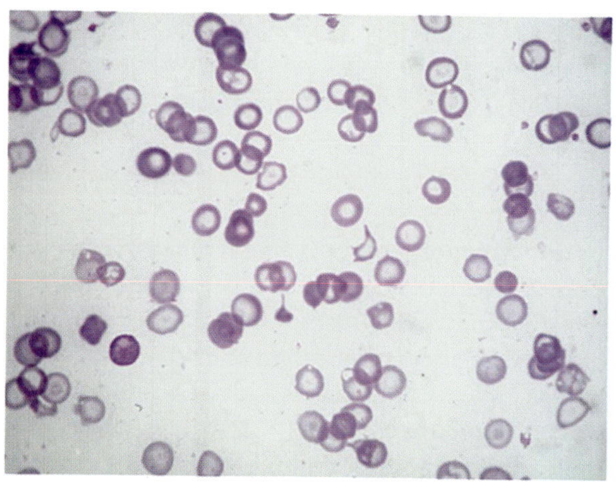

Figure 1.6. Microcytosis and hypochromasia in a dog with an extrahepatic shunt and anaemia due to iron deficiency.

- anaemias caused by **iron deficiency**
- animals with a **portosystemic shunt**.

Anisocytosis

Description

Anisocytosis involves variation in the size (diameter) of erythrocytes. This term is used when erythrocytes of varying sizes, either large or small, are observed in the same sample.

- **Macrocytosis**. A large number of **large erythrocytes** are observed.
- **Microcytosis**. A large number of **small erythrocytes** are observed.

Causes

Anisocytosis/**macrocytosis** is typical of **regenerative anaemias**, due to the presence of large immature cells. Anisocytosis can also be seen in some cases of non-regenerative anaemia, due to dyserythropoiesis.

Microcytosis is usually observed in cases of **iron deficiency anaemia** or in **immune-mediated conditions**. In the Akita and Shiba Inu, it can be **hereditary**.

Burr cells or echinocytes

Description

Burr cells are **erythrocytes with a spiculated border** (Figure 1.7). It is important to differentiate between burr cells and acanthocytes.

Causes

The presence of echinocytes is **usually artefactual** as a result of a poor sample distribution, an excess of EDTA or a prolonged period of time between extraction and performing the smear.

In dogs, echinocytes are associated with:

- glomerulonephritis
- neoplasia
- lymphoma
- haemangiosarcoma
- mastocytoma
- carcinomas.

And occasionally:

- snake bites
- uraemia
- after a blood transfusion
- pyruvate kinase deficiency.

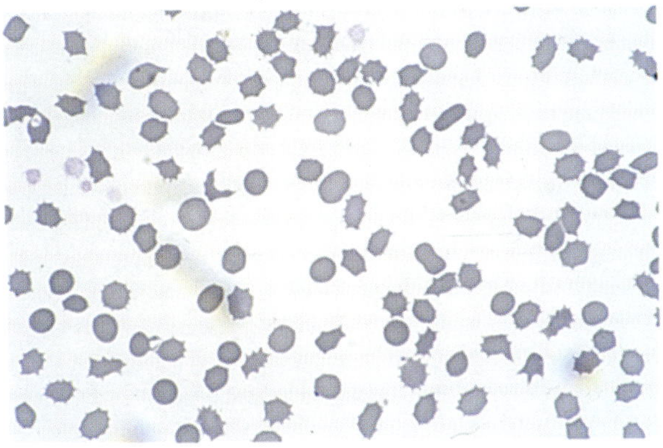

Figure 1.7. Blood sample from a dog with uraemia showing crenation and poikilocytosis.

Acanthocytosis

Description

Acanthocytes are erythrocytes that are similar to echinocytes but with more **rounded spicules**, which are longer and spaced further apart (like the fingers of a glove) (Figure 1.8).

Causes

This change to red blood cell morphology is a **consequence of the physical damage** suffered by the erythrocytes due to vascular changes or turbulent blood flow.

The main causes include:

- disseminated intravascular coagulation (DIC)
- glomerulonephritis
- haemangiosarcoma: **90% of dogs with haemangiosarcoma present with acanthocytes**; therefore in animals where this condition is suspected, blood smears can be of great help in diagnosis
- myelofibrosis
- dyserythropoiesis
- chronic doxorubicin toxicity.

Schistocytes

Description

These are **fragmented erythrocytes that lose their rounded conformation**. It is important to differentiate them from acanthocytes (Figure 1.8).

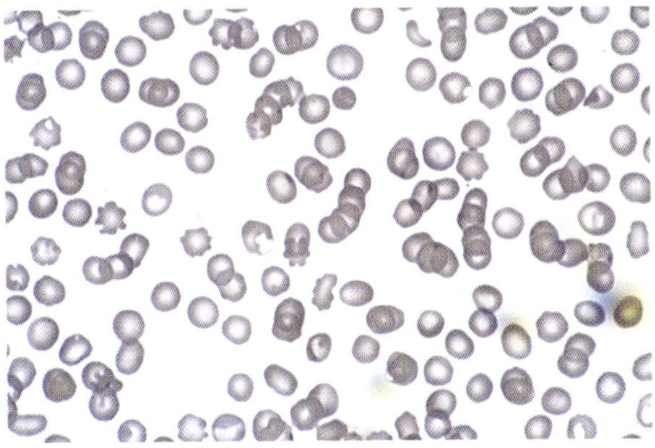

Figure 1.8. Sample from a dog with haemangiosarcoma, showing keratocytes containing vesicles, and acanthocytes.

Causes

The presence of **schistocytes is usually associated with DIC**. They have also been seen in association with:

- severe iron deficiencies
- myelofibrosis
- liver disease
- cardiac failure
- glomerulonephritis
- histiocytic haemophagocytosis
- haemangiosarcoma
- congenital dyserythropoiesis
- splenectomised dogs with pyruvate kinase deficiency.

Keratocytes

Description

These are **erythrocytes that contain one or more intact or broken vesicles** (when the vesicles are intact, they are also called blister cells). The vesicles do not stain and tend to be circular; when they rupture, they give rise to one or two projections (Figure 1.8).

Causes

Keratocytes are seen in samples from dogs undergoing chronic **treatment with doxorubicin** and in **dogs with haemangiosarcoma**. In the latter, there are usually acanthocytes and schistocytes in the same sample.

Codocytes

Description

These are erythrocytes with a fold in the cytoplasmic membrane which gives them a **target-like appearance** (Figure 1.9).

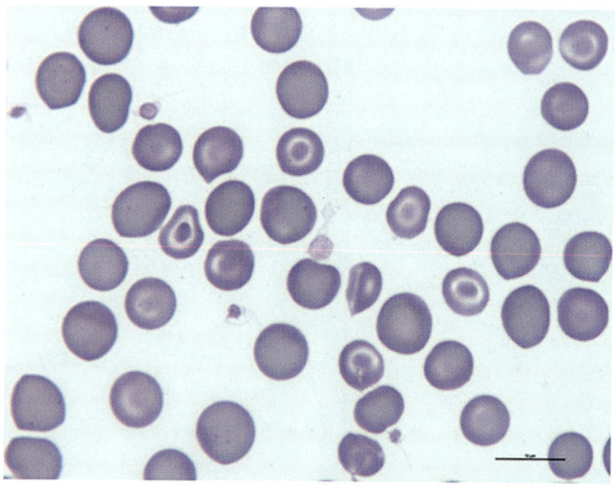

Figure 1.9. Sample from a dog with the presence of codocytes.

Causes

The main causes are:

- **iron deficiency anaemia**
- **hypercholesterolaemia** due to hypothyroidism.

They can also be present in:

- severe liver disease
- cholestasis
- onion poisoning
- splenectomised animals
- congenital dyserythropoiesis.

Spherocytes

Description

Spherocytes are erythrocytes that are smaller than usual, **lack an area of central pallor** and have dense colouring (Figure 1.10).

Causes

The **main cause of spherocyte formation is IMHA**, although they can be found in lower numbers in other conditions such as:

- snake bite poisoning
- zinc toxicity
- blood parasites
- hypophosphataemia.

Nucleated erythrocytes

Description

Nucleated red blood cells are immature erythrocytes that retain a nucleus (usually they are metarubricytes). The presence of a low percentage of nucleated erythrocytes (1–2%) can be considered normal (Figure 1.11).

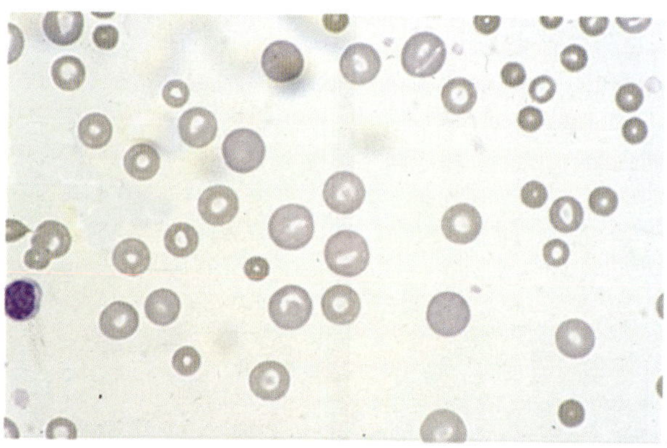

Figure 1.10. Spherocytes in a dog with immune-mediated haemolytic anaemia. Polychromasia can also been seen.

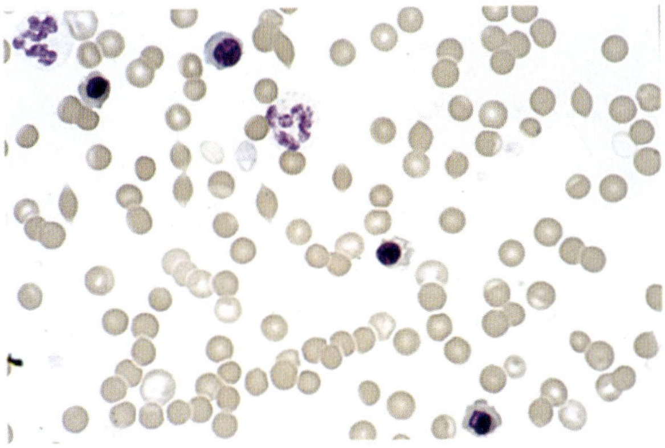

Figure 1.11. Nucleated erythrocytes.

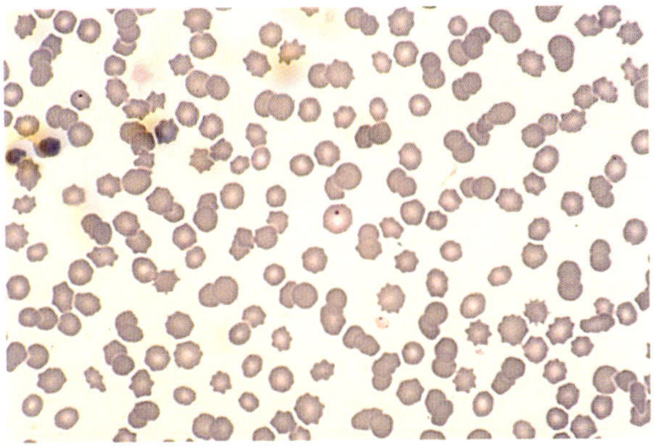

Figure 1.12. A Howell–Jolly body can be seen in the centre of an erythrocyte.

Causes

These erythrocytes are **associated with regenerative anaemias** although they do not necessarily indicate that the anaemia is undergoing a regenerative response. They indicate **regeneration only if they are accompanied by other signs such as the presence of polychromatophils**.

They also occur with:

- lead poisoning (with or without anaemia)
- damage to the bone marrow
- septicaemia
- endotoxic shock
- certain medications, e.g., vincristine.

If there is a non-regenerative anaemia and a marked increase in the number of nucleated erythrocytes, a **bone marrow study is indicated**, and differential diagnoses should include:

- myelodysplasia
- haematopoietic neoplasia
- bone marrow infiltrative disease
- splenic dysfunction
- dyserythropoietic changes.

Cytoplasmic inclusions

Howell–Jolly bodies

Description

These are **rounded structures with a basophilic colour found in the cytoplasm** which are reminiscent of nuclear chromatin (Figure 1.12).

Causes

They tend to be associated with:

- regenerative anaemias
- reduced splenic function
- long-term treatment with corticosteroids
- splenectomy
- macrocytosis in Poodles.

Heinz bodies

Description

Heinz bodies are a product of **haemoglobin oxidation**. They appear as **rounded protrusions in the erythrocyte membrane** and are commonly called 'clown's noses' because of their shape (Figure 1.13). In dogs they may be small and present in large numbers.

Causes

The presence of Heinz bodies is **indicative of an excessive intake** of:

- aspirin
- paracetamol
- propylene glycol
- naphthalene
- onion
- acetaminophen
- vitamin K
- methylene blue.

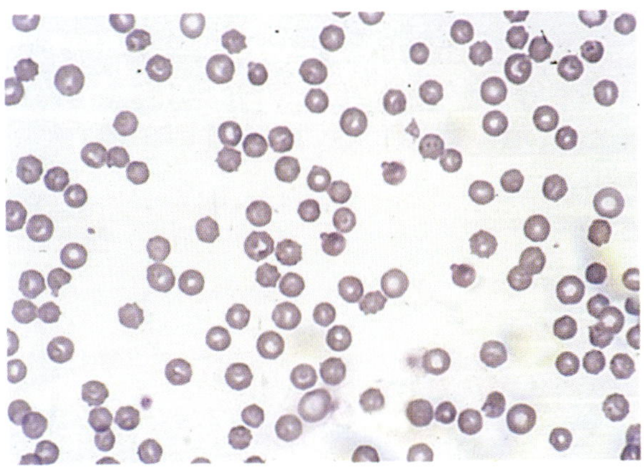

Figure 1.13. Erythrocytes with the characteristic 'clown's nose' which suggests haemoglobin oxidation and the formation of Heinz bodies.

Eccentrocytes

Description

These are erythrocytes with an **eccentric area of empty cytoplasm shaped like a crescent moon** (Figure 1.14).

Causes

This morphological change is related to haemoglobin oxidation and the causes are the same as those described in the section on Heinz bodies.

Intracellular parasites and viruses

When examining a smear for the presence of blood parasites, the entire slide must be checked meticulously, since in some cases there may only be one single infected erythrocyte in the whole smear.

When a suspicious erythrocyte is found at low magnification (×40–60), the oil immersion (×100) lens should be used to zoom in and confirm the object is not an artefact.

The presence of an erythrocyte containing a parasite in the smear confirms the diagnosis. But if no infected cells are seen, this does not rule the disease out and other diagnostic methods should be used, such as polymerase chain reaction (PCR) or serology.

Parasites should be observed in isolated erythrocytes, since the precipitation of proteins or dye that has accumulated among groups of cells can be confusing.

Babesia canis

The **parasites (merozoites) are found within the erythrocyte** and can be piriform, fusiform or have a bacillary or amoeboid shape. Most often, they present a **piriform shape** and appear in pairs within the erythrocyte (Figure 1.15), but one or more than two parasites may also be seen per erythrocyte. The presence of parasites outside red blood cells is a sign of more acute disease.

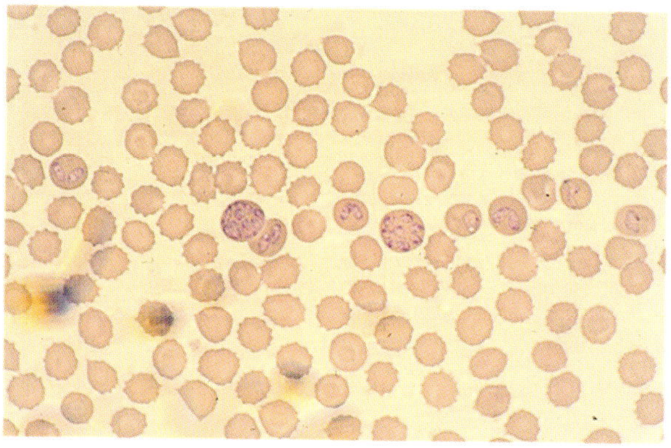

Figure 1.15. Erythrocytes containing numerous *Babesia canis* microorganisms.

Babesia gibsoni

This species is smaller than *Babesia canis*, appears in a ring or small piriform bacillus shape, either isolated or in small groups of two or three individuals (Figure 1.16). It occurs less frequently than *Babesia canis* and is more difficult to identify. Due to its small size, some authors call it *Babesia microti*-like.

Viral inclusions (distemper virus)

These are usually of variable size, shape (rounded, oval or irregular) and colour (pale blue or red carmine). They frequently appear in polychromatophilic erythrocytes and differ from Howell–Jolly bodies because the latter are smaller and much darker.

These inclusions are not specific to the distemper virus (Figure 1.17) and therefore, when they are observed, the differential diagnosis made based on the clinical history of the animal should be taken into consideration.

Artefacts

It is important to note that it is common to find artefacts which can be confused with parasites. An experienced

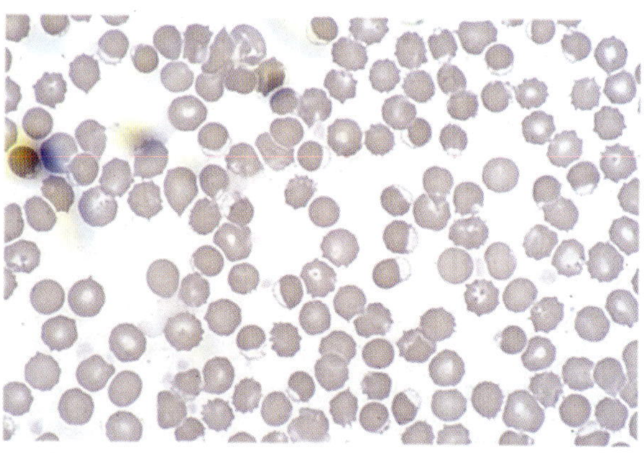

Figure 1.14. Haemoglobin oxidation due to onion poisoning in a dog. The formation of eccentrocytes can be seen.

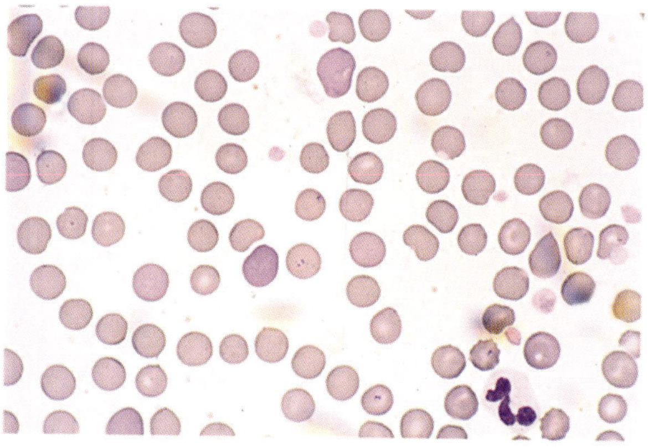

Figure 1.16. Erythrocyte in the centre with a structure compatible with *Babesia gibsoni*. Take note of how difficult it is to detect in comparison with *Babesia canis* (Figure 1.15).

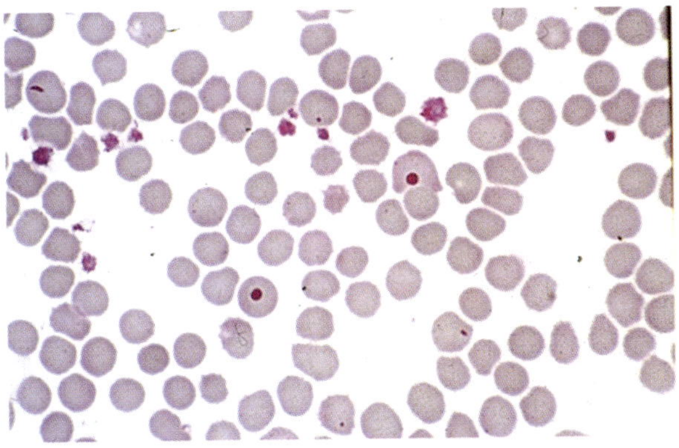

Figure 1.17. Erythrocytes with intracytoplasmic inclusions due to distemper: distemper inclusion bodies.

observer will be able to distinguish an artefact from a parasite, but when starting to read blood smears, it may be helpful to note that **artefacts have the following characteristics**.

- They are **refractile** (they shine when the micrometer moves slightly).
- They **appear in a different plane to the erythrocyte** (when the erythrocyte is focused, the artefact is out of focus).
- Artefacts will appear **more frequently when the stains are used in excess** ('dirty' smears). In these cases, repetition of the smear and staining is recommended.

Immune-mediated haematological disease

Immune-mediated haemolytic anaemia

Epidemiology

IMHA is one of the most commonly occurring and serious haemolytic anaemias in dogs. A genetic predisposition has been described, especially in the Cocker Spaniel.

Aetiopathogenesis

The disease causes anti-erythrocyte antibody production, complement fixation and activation of macrophages, which cause **direct or indirect destruction of erythrocytes** and haemolytic anaemia. There are various trigger factors which can initiate IMHA (infectious agents, medications and neoplasms, and some which are anecdotal such as *Ancylostoma* in young dogs). In most cases the causative factor is unknown, when it is called **idiopathic** or primary IMHA.

Regardless of the cause of IMHA, destruction of erythrocytes is triggered by IgG and IgM binding to the erythrocyte membrane. In most cases the destruction of erythrocytes is an **extravascular process**, where erythrocytes opsonised by IgG or IgM and/or complement are identified by reticuloendothelial cells, mainly macrophages, which phagocytose them. There may also be intravascular destruction if the membranes of the erythrocytes are attacked by the complement system.

In IMHA, in addition to the destruction of erythrocytes, an important **systemic inflammatory response** is triggered that leads to necrosis and the formation of thrombosis in different organs.

Clinical signs and diagnosis

Essential to an accurate diagnosis is confirming immune-mediated erythrocyte destruction and identifying or ruling out any initiating trigger factors. The latter includes infectious agents, such as *Ehrlichia* or *Babesia*, as well as neoplasms.

Initial suspicion of an IMHA lies in the clinical presentation, with symptoms including **jaundice** and a highly **regenerative anaemia** with **bilirubinuria,** with or without **haemoglobinuria**. Although there are exceptions, if the condition is **very acute** or directed against erythroid precursors, the anaemia **may not be regenerative at the time of diagnosis**. Therefore, to establish a diagnosis, immune-mediated destruction of erythrocytes must be documented with one of the following findings:

- persistent autoagglutination
- presence of abundant spherocytes
- positive direct Coombs test.

To follow the evolution and control the IMHA, monitoring of these findings should be carried out. Thus, for example, if autoagglutination does not disappear, it may be that the treatment being used is not effective at that moment in time.

At the same time, **secondary causes** of haemolytic anaemia (diseases transmitted by arthropods such as babesiosis, neoplasms or the action of medications or recent vaccinations) should be ruled out. Therefore, in the diagnosis of IMHA, the following are indicated.

- Complete blood count with observation of the smear.
- Complete biochemistry.
- Urinalysis.
- Abdominal ultrasound.
- Spleen cytology, if affected.
- PCR for *Babesia*.
- Serology for *Ehrlichia* and *Leishmania*. Although these two are not directly related to the IMHA, they have an important impact on the immunosuppressive response.

Autoagglutination

Autoagglutination (Figures 1.4 and 1.5) may be due to the presence of IgM or large amounts of IgG in the erythrocyte membrane. It can be observed with the naked eye in an EDTA tube or on a slide. However, it is important to take into account that agglutination can also be seen in animals due to unknown causes or the presence of cold agglutinins. Therefore, performing a **dilution of the sample in saline solution is recommended**: if the agglutination disappears, it was not due to the presence of immunoglobulins. Some authors also suggest the need to wash the erythrocytes, to confirm the presence of immunoglobulins.

Spherocytosis

When erythrocytes are only partially phagocytosed or lysed by circulating complement, there is a reduction in erythrocyte surface, resulting in what are known as spherocytes (Figure 1.10). **Spherocytes are seen as microcytic erythrocytes, without central pallor**, and are considered more fragile than normal erythrocytes. The existence of a **large number of spherocytes is almost diagnostic of IMHA**. Until recently it was considered that spherocytes were exclusive to IMHA, but they have now been discovered in small quantities in the following conditions:

- DIC
- endotoxaemia or onion poisoning
- oxidative damage to erythrocytes
- zinc poisoning.

In the author's experience, all dogs with a marked spherocytosis show a positive result in a Coombs test.

The erythrocyte osmotic fragility test in specific saline concentrations helps to detect the most fragile erythrocytes, as is the case with spherocytes, which is why it was proposed as a useful test in animals with suspected IMHA. However, there are many other reasons why erythrocytes may have increased fragility (e.g., enzymatic defects).

Direct Coombs test

The direct Coombs test is also known as a direct antiglobulin test. It is **used to detect antibodies and complement on the surface of erythrocytes** when the strength of the anti-erythrocyte antibodies or the concentration of antibodies is too low to cause spontaneous agglutination (subagglutinating titre). There are polyvalent antiglobulins to detect canine IgG, IgM and C3b. These antibodies are added to serial dilutions of washed erythrocytes and incubated at 37°C. The strength of the agglutination in this test does not predict the severity of haemolysis, but monitoring the changes is useful in the follow-up of the disease.

Traditionally, the Coombs test is performed in the laboratory with microtubes or multiwell plates, but there is currently a test available which can be done in the clinic itself (Coombs test, Alvedia, France).

Although many commercial laboratories offer the Coombs test for dogs, its usefulness has been questioned, since **up to 30% of dogs with IMHA can give negative results**. This means that many veterinarians do not perform the test and use the response to treatment with immunosuppressants to diagnose IMHA. However, the negative results in the Coombs test may be due to technical reasons, such as insufficient amounts of antibody bound to erythrocytes, the presence of weakly bound antibodies, or the disease being in remission. It is as unlikely that a short period of immunosuppression will reverse a Coombs test, as it is that a blood transfusion will make it positive.

Prognosis

Although anaemia can be corrected with transfusions, the systemic inflammatory response, with necrosis of various organs and thrombosis, causes significant mortality regardless of the use of aggressive immunosuppressive or antithrombotic treatments.

Bone marrow suppression

In the anaemic patient, if the steps described in the previous sections fail to explain the cause, the possibility of bone marrow suppression should be considered. This is especially pertinent in the case of **mild to moderate, normocytic, normochromic, non-regenerative anaemias**, with haematocrit values of 25–35% (dog) and 20–25% (cat).

Outline of the causes of bone marrow suppression

Anaemia due to inflammatory conditions

The haematocrit value decreases a few days after a condition that triggers inflammation and then stabilises.

The origin is a **sequestration of iron by macrophages** and a subsequent decrease in haematocrit value.

Anaemia associated with neoplasms

These are usually **large or metastatic neoplasms**.

Anaemia associated with renal failure

This type of anaemia has multifactorial elements including:

- a decrease in erythropoietin production
- gastrointestinal ulcers causing blood loss into the gut
- shortening of erythrocyte half-life due to uraemia
- anorexia.

Anaemia associated with liver disease

Involvement of the liver frequently causes animals to present a mild non-regenerative anaemia, due to the low availability of iron transporters and an inflammatory response originating from the organ.

Anaemia associated with hypothyroidism

This is the result of **reduced metabolism** due to a deficiency of thyroid hormones. These animals usually present other biochemical alterations such as **hypercholesterolaemia**.

Anaemia associated with hypoadrenocorticism

To rule out these conditions, a general blood test and specific tests are necessary, which are discussed in the endocrine chapter of this book.

Infectious diseases as a cause of bone marrow suppression

Well-recognised infectious causes include:

- *Ehrlichia*
- *Anaplasma*
- *Leishmania*
- FeLV or FIV
- parvovirus, in young animals.

If ehrlichiosis is suspected, diagnostic tests include PCR (for acute disease) or serological tests (if chronic disease is suspected). The anaemia is more usually linked to the chronic phase of the condition.

The majority of cats affected by FeLV present with macrocytic, normochromic anaemias. PCR of bone marrow is important in cases where FeLV infections are suspected.

Bone marrow study

If at this point no cause for the non-regenerative anaemia has been found, the next step is to perform a **bone marrow biopsy**. For this, a long or flat bone should be used. The conditions that can be identified in this way include:

- immune-mediated non-regenerative anaemias
- aplastic anaemia
- myelonecrosis
- myelofibrosis
- inflammation
- haemophagocytic syndromes
- dysmyelopoiesis
- neoplasms: leukaemias, lymphoma, myeloma or histiocytosis.

Non-regenerative immune-mediated anaemias

Diagnosis

The bone marrow shows evidence of:

- erythroid hyperplasia
- pause in erythroid maturation
- aplasia of the erythroid line.

Prognosis

Approximately 70–75% of these animals respond to immunosuppressive medications, although around 30% may not respond.

Aplastic anaemia

Aetiology

This tends to be secondary to:

- infectious agents
- medications
- chronic renal failure
- or may be idiopathic.

Diagnosis

Aplastic anaemia is seen in young animals with bi- or pancytopenia (i.e. decrease in the count of two or all cell lines) where 95% of the marrow is occupied by adipose tissue.

Prognosis

The response to treatment and long-term prognosis is usually poor, especially if a cause is not identified or the animal does not respond to immunosuppression.

Myelonecrosis

Diagnosis

Abundant areas of focal or diffuse necrosis are seen in the bone marrow.

Aetiology

The causes are similar to those of aplastic anaemia.

Prognosis
With supportive treatment and treatment of the primary cause, animals can recover.

Myelofibrosis
Aetiopathogenesis
This follows the same path as myelonecrosis. The causes are similar, including:

- infectious agents
- immune-mediated
- medications.

Diagnosis
The condition is diagnosed by confirmation of bone marrow occupation by fibroblasts.

Prognosis
With supportive treatment, 50% of animals can recover.

Inflammation
Aetiopathogenesis
Some animals with **sepsis or fungal infections** exhibit intense **inflammation of the bone marrow** which leads to a decrease in division of the erythroid line, with large-scale myeloid activation.

Diagnosis
A marked neutrophilia is observed in blood and bone marrow, with a left shift and possible toxic changes.

Prognosis
The bone marrow response is good if the cause of the inflammation is identified.

Haemophagocytic syndromes
Aetiology
These may be secondary to:

- infectious conditions (e.g., ehrlichiosis)
- proliferative diseases.

Histiocytic conditions are also included in the group of haemophagocytic syndromes.

Diagnosis
In these syndromes an intense phagocytosis of erythrocytes by the macrophages in the bone marrow can be observed.

Animals with these syndromes usually present with **multiple cytopenias** and it is rare to see only anaemia.

Prognosis
If the disease is not histiocytic, 20% of animals respond to immunosuppression.

Condition secondary to dysmyelopoiesis
Aetiopathogenesis
Dysmyelopoiesis is common in cats and frequently associated with FeLV or FIV infections. It is characterised by the presence of morphological changes in cell maturation and some animals may have bi/pancytopenia.

Neoplasia
The bone marrow biopsy may detect evidence of:

- leukaemia
- lymphoma
- myeloma
- histiocytosis.

Aetiopathogenesis
There is proliferation of neoplastic cells in the bone marrow.

Diagnosis
To diagnose leukaemia, immunophenotyping is necessary. **Myeloid leukaemias have a very poor prognosis** and do not respond to treatment, with a life expectancy after diagnosis of less than 4 weeks.

Prognosis
Lymphoid leukaemias may have a better prognosis.

- 40% partially respond to chemotherapy.
- 20% completely respond to chemotherapy.
- 40% die in just a few weeks (less than 8).

Polycythaemia

Polycythaemia is a **relative or absolute increase in the erythroid mass** (erythrocyte count, haematocrit value and haemoglobin concentration).

The measurement of **serum erythropoietin values can help to differentiate between primary and secondary absolute polycythaemia**, with increased values due to secondary causes (Figure 1.18).

Relative polycythaemia

Aetiopathogenesis
Relative polycythaemia is the result of a **reduction in the animal's plasma volume**. It is generally accompanied by an **increase in total protein**. The most

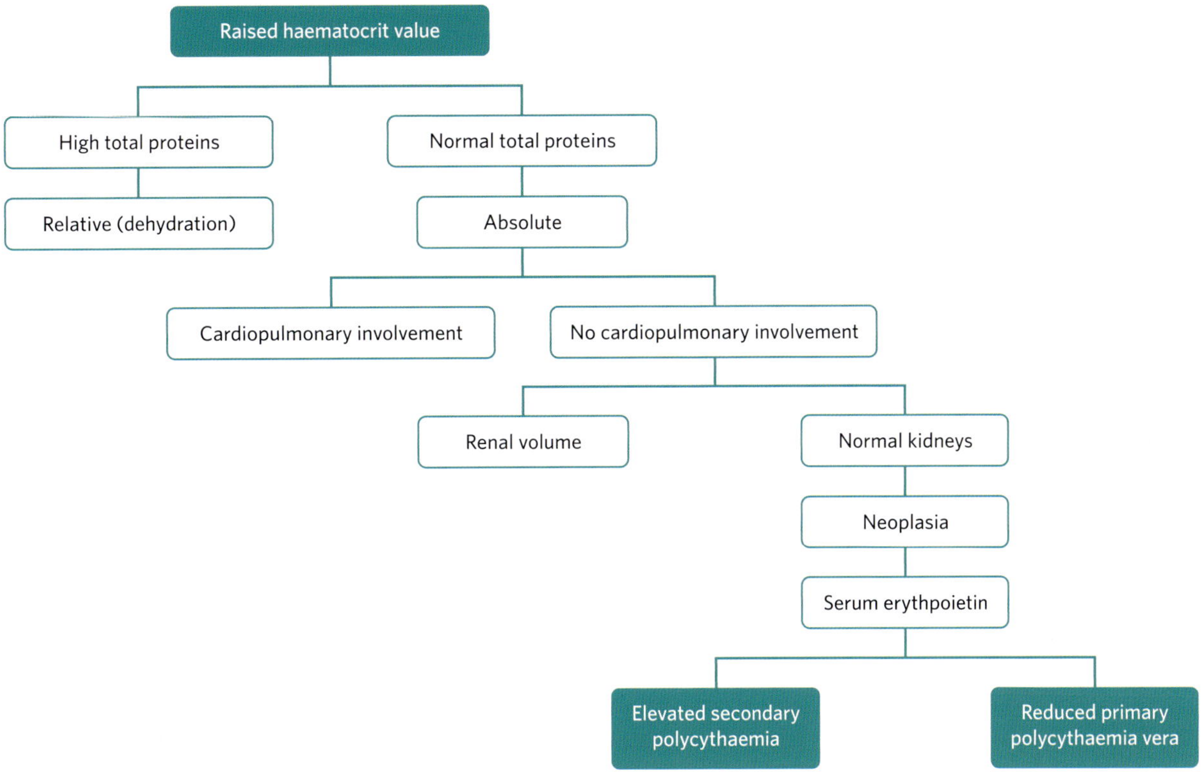

Figure 1.18. Diagnostic algorithm in animals with polycythaemia.

frequent cause is an external loss of fluids (**dehydration** and haemoconcentration). It can also be observed in some animals secondary to **splenic contraction** due to excitement or fear, but in this case it is usually transient.

Clinical signs

In the case of relative polycythaemia **due to dehydration**, physical examination of the animal reveals dry mucous membranes of intense colour and with prolonged capillary refill times, along with signs of dehydration such as reduced skin elasticity, depending on the degree of dehydration.

Diagnosis

The organic cause of dehydration should be identified and treated.

Absolute polycythaemia

Aetiopathogenesis

Absolute polycythaemia is due to **an increase of the erythroid mass without the presence of dehydration**. It may be **primary** or **secondary**.

Primary absolute polycythaemia is due to **an increase in erythropoiesis without increased erythropoietin** and is considered a **chronic myeloproliferative process of mature erythrocytes**.

Clinical signs

The clinical symptoms are caused by blood **hyperviscosity** and may include:

- functional changes to the central nervous system:
  - behavioural changes
  - seizures.
- erythematous mucous membranes and skin
- abdominal organomegalies:
  - splenomegaly
  - renomegaly.

Secondary polycythaemia

Aetiopathogenesis

Secondary polycythaemia is due to the **overproduction of erythropoietin** or substances similar to it. The cause can be any condition that generates hypoxia.

- Chronic pulmonary disease.
- Cardiac changes with right to left communications, which do not usually occur with heart murmurs, so specific tests should be used to rule them out.

In these animals, the measurement of blood gases, diagnostic studies using thoracic imaging and an echocardiogram are usually sufficient to determine the cause.

- Paraneoplastic syndrome, described in:
  - renal lymphomas
  - renal carcinomas
  - renal fibrosarcoma
  - pyelonephritis (uncommon).

Non-neoplastic leukocyte changes

A leukogram consists of a tabulation of all the white cells circulating in peripheral blood.

Reference values for the total number of leukocytes are:

- in dogs, 5000 to 17,000/µl
- in cats, 5000 to 15,000/µl.

These values correspond to **95% of the healthy population**. Approximately 5% of animals lie outside the reference range; this is especially true with cats, which are also much more resistant to septic processes than dogs.

Neutrophils are the predominant cell type in both species. However, lymphocytes, mature and immature neutrophils, monocytes, eosinophils and basophils can all be identified in a leukogram (Figure 1.19).

Neutrophils are characterised by a very short circulating lifespan of 7 hours, after which they migrate into the tissues. **Selectins** mediate the interaction between neutrophils and the endothelium, so that in response to chemotactic agents, **neutrophils adhere to the endothelium** (through the interaction of integrins) and migrate to the tissues where they perform **phagocytic functions**. Subsequently, they are eliminated by macrophages.

Neutrophils are the initial defence against any microorganism invasion: their function is to eliminate bacteria and participate in the destruction of fungal and viral agents, which is why they accumulate in areas of inflammation as a result of chemotaxis. This migration is unidirectional.

An important feature of neutrophils is their **presence in several compartments**: maturation, marginal, circulating and tissues. In the circulating compartment, neutrophils spend an average of 7 hours, and then migrate according to chemotaxis to tissues where they perform their defensive functions (Figure 1.20).

Neutrophils **mature in approximately 4–6 days** and move to the circulating, peripheral blood, where they are in equilibrium with the marginal compartment (formed by small vessels and capillaries) and usually remain for approximately 5 days (in dogs the marginal cell/circulating cell ratio is 1:1; in cats it is 3:1).

Before interpreting changes in the leukogram, it is essential to perform a thorough study of the leukocyte population and identify the different types of leukocyte in a blood smear.

Neutrophils

The majority of circulating neutrophils (95–100%) in healthy dogs are segmented or mature, with few band neutrophils.

Description

Neutrophil size is **2–2.5 times the size of a normal erythrocyte**. The nucleus is lobed (3–5 lobes) or partially segmented with dense chromatin, which is dark purple in colour. The cytoplasm is usually light blue or pink with granulation ranging from negligible to slightly eosinophilic (Figure 1.21).

Morphological changes

Band neutrophils

Also considered immature neutrophils, these can occur normally as a small percentage in peripheral blood.

It is important to take into account that **automatic counters do not differentiate between mature and band neutrophils**. Therefore it is essential to examine a blood smear to assess whether there is a left shift and its severity.

Band neutrophils have a curved nucleus (in the form of a C) and an absence of lobulations. The condensation of chromatin is evident, and the cytoplasm is usually the same as that of the mature neutrophil (Figure 1.22).

Toxic neutrophils

Toxic neutrophils show characteristic morphological changes. They are observed in cats suffering from severe inflammatory diseases or toxaemias.

The **toxic changes are classified from 1+ to 4+** according to the individual changes to the neutrophils (Figures 1.23 and 1.24).

- 1+. **Döhle bodies**, grey spots that appear in the cytoplasm of neutrophils and represent aberrant aggregations of the endoplasmic reticulum. They are the mildest form of toxic change.
- 2+. Döhle bodies and diffuse **cytoplasmic basophilia**.
- 3+. Döhle bodies, diffuse cytoplasmic basophilia and **cytoplasmic vacuolisation**.
- 4+. The changes described above together with nuclear alterations or ring-shaped nucleoli, swelling and **nuclear lysis**.

The severity of the morphological alterations is **proportional to the intensity of the disease**.

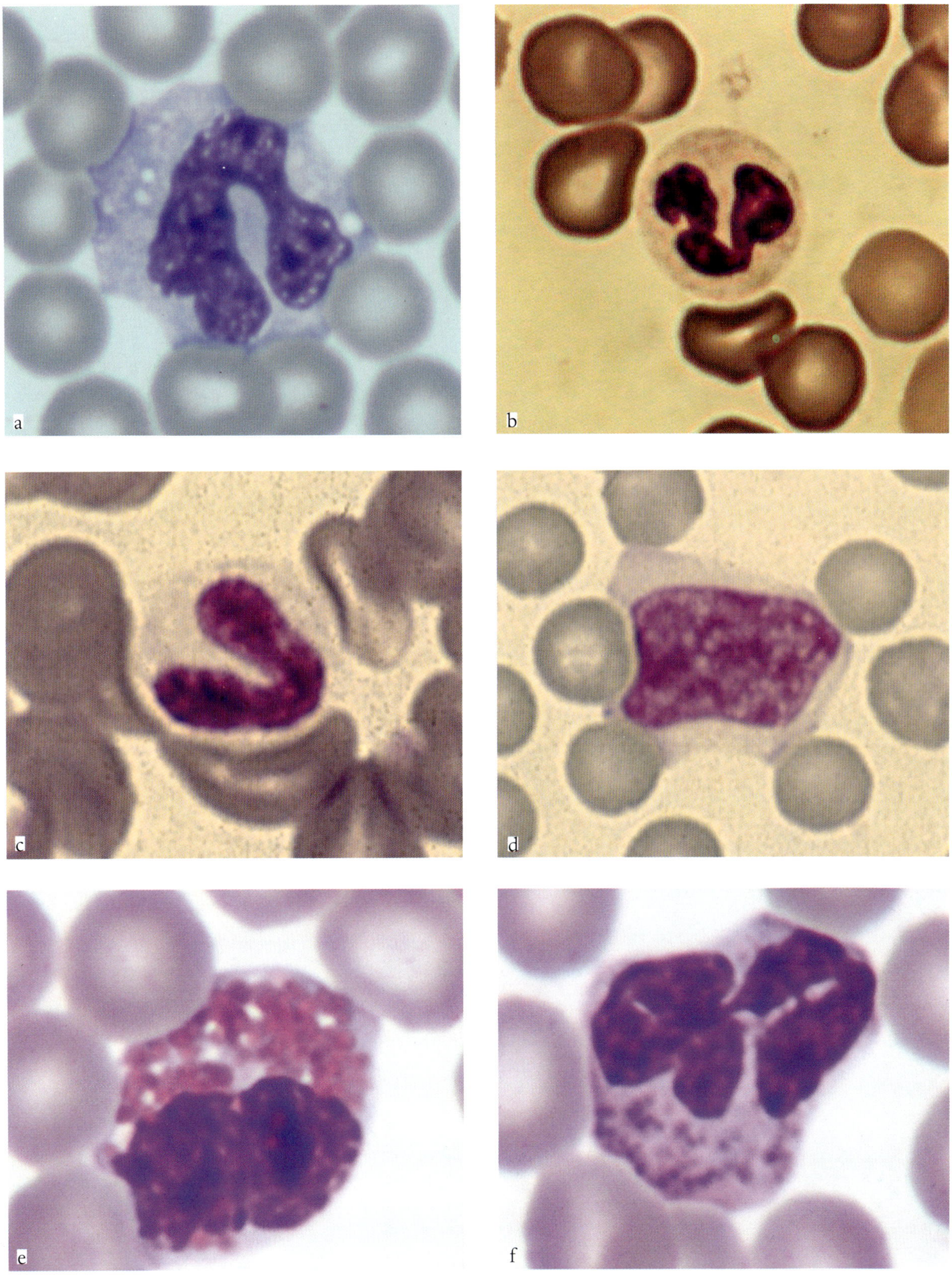

Figure 1.19. Cells which should be identified in a leukocyte count: (a) monocyte, (b) segmented neutrophil, (c) band neutrophil, (d) lymphocyte, (e) eosinophil and (f) basophil.

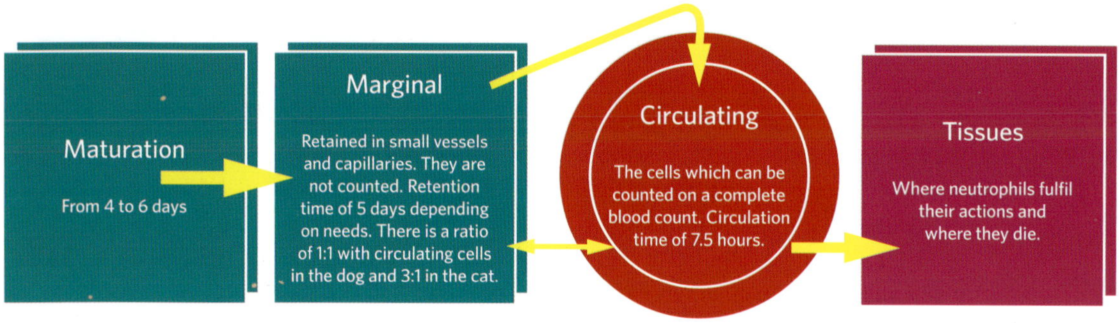

Figure 1.20. Diagram showing the distribution of neutrophils in different cellular compartments.

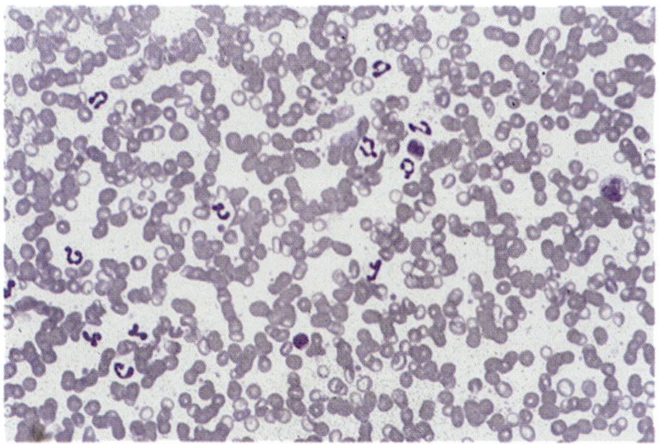

Figure 1.21. Normal segmented neutrophils in a dog (×40 objective). This objective is also used to estimate the leukocyte count; in this case there are 11 segmented neutrophils, 1 lymphocyte and 2 monocytes.

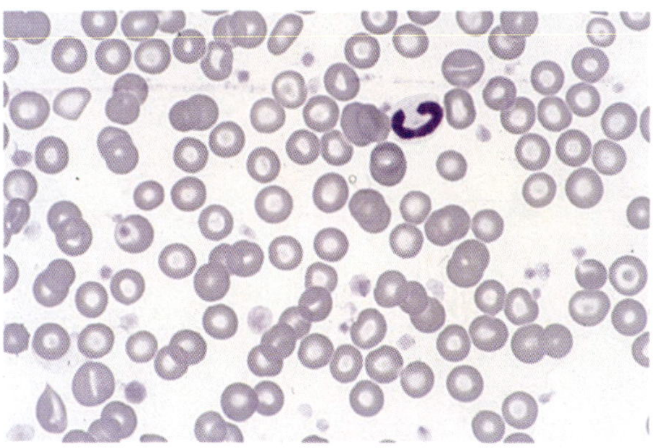

Figure 1.22. Band neutrophil.

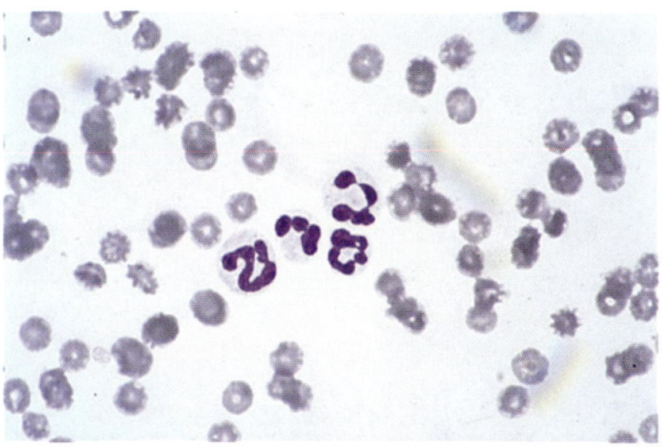

Figure 1.23. Neutrophils with toxic changes, showing basophilia and vacuolisation of the cytoplasm.

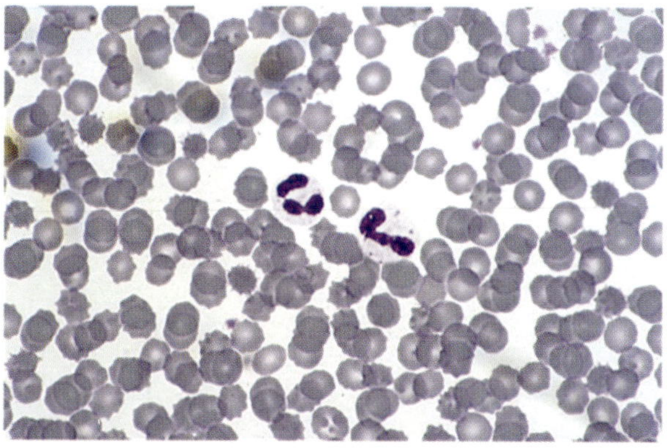

Figure 1.24. Döhle bodies in a neutrophil.

The presence of toxicity is associated with the systemic effect of inflammation; in severe cases (3+ or 4+) it can be attributed to **severe bacterial infections or toxaemias produced by drugs, poisons or intoxications**.

Toxic change is also evaluated according to the number of affected neutrophils, as follows:

- mild: <10% of neutrophils
- moderate: 20–30%
- severe: >30%.

Hypersegmented neutrophils

These are neutrophils with five or more nuclear lobes.

If there is a high percentage of hypersegmented neutrophils, this is termed a **right shift**. This process is caused by the **normal ageing of circulating neutrophils** and reflects the fact that they have been in circulation for a prolonged period. It is usually attributed to:

- chronic inflammatory conditions
- an increase in endogenous glucocorticoids (hyperadrenocorticism) or exogenous glucocorticoids
- myeloproliferative disorders
- dogs with inherent defects in cobalamin absorption
- blood left in the collection tube for more than 24 hours.

Parasites and intracytoplasmic inclusions

Viral inclusions (distemper virus)

These cytoplasmic inclusions, as in the erythrocyte, can be found in **acute phases of viraemia**. With Diff-Quik staining, round, oval or even irregular structures, similar to those seen in the red blood cell, are easily visualised (Figure 1.25).

Ehrlichia canis

Ehrlichia morulae appear as **small groups of rounded and basophilic organisms** found within neutrophils. They are usually seen during the acute phases of the infection (Figure 1.26).

Hepatozoon canis

Gametocytes are **pale blue oval (capsule-shaped) parasites**, although they do not normally stain clearly. Their large size is characteristic and they can even displace the neutrophil's nucleus. They are easily observed without the immersion objective (×40–60) (Figure 1.26).

Leishmania canis

The presence of a *Leishmania* amastigote is indicative of a defect in neutrophilic function or of an advanced disease state.

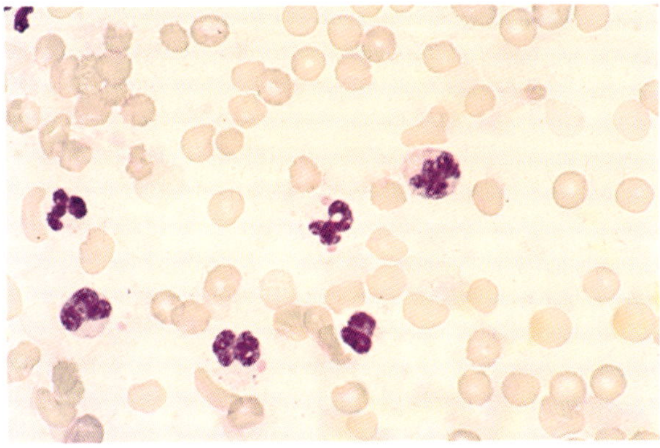

Figure 1.25. Inclusion bodies inside neutrophils from a 6-month-old dog with distemper.

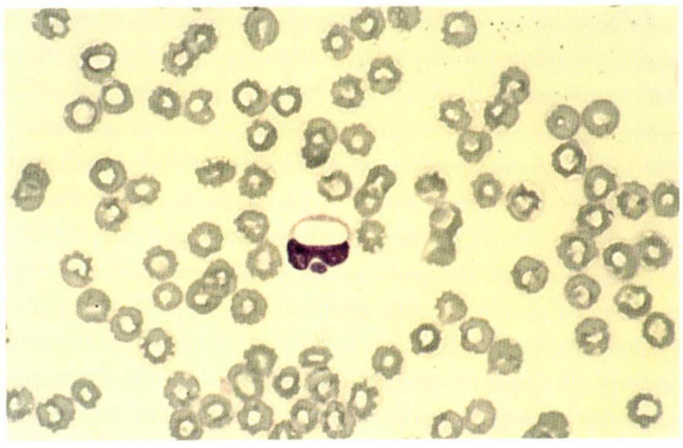

Figure 1.26. *Ehrlichia* spp. morula and *Hepatozoon canis* in the same neutrophil.

Other changes

There are hereditary changes, which are **rare in dogs**, such as **lysosomal storage disease** or mucopolysaccharidosis, which are characterised by the presence of **purple granules in the cytoplasm of neutrophils**.

Eosinophils

Description

Eosinophils are similar in size or slightly larger than neutrophils. Each eosinophil has a lobed or segmented nucleus with dense dark chromatin. The cytoplasm stains pale blue and contains **reddish-orange granules**, which are highly variable, and can be rod or bacillus-shaped (Figure 1.19).

Morphological changes

Immature eosinophils have a band nucleus, as do band neutrophils, but in healthy animals these represent only a **low percentage** of the white cell count. An **increase in the number** of these cells usually indicates a **hypersensitivity reaction**. The presence of a large number of these immature eosinophils can be attributed to **eosinophilic leukaemia**, a variant of chronic myeloid leukaemia.

Basophils

Description

Basophils are similar in size or larger than a neutrophil. Their cytoplasm is greyish blue. The granules that they contain vary in size, number and colour intensity (dark brown), and they are located both in the cytoplasm and nucleus. These granules do not always stain well with fast Diff-Quik type stains.

Count

It is unusual for basophils to be found in the peripheral blood of healthy dogs.

An increase in their numbers can be attributed to or seen in:

- allergic reactions
- parasites
- hyperlipidaemia
- inflammatory conditions such as gastroenteritis
- mastocytoma
- thrombocytopenia
- chronic granulocytic leukaemia
- basophilic leukaemia (very rare)
- the Basenji Hound, from 2 to 4 months of age.

Morphological changes

They have been described in *Ehrlichia canis* morulae.

Monocytes

Description

Monocytes are larger than neutrophils, and of a similar size to eosinophils. The nucleus is very pleomorphic, with a **kidney shape** being the most common, although rounded forms also occur and are typical of the most immature monocytes, as well as indented or coiled forms.

A key factor which can be used to differentiate them from other cells is that they have **blue-grey cytoplasm** with or without vacuoles. When there are vacuoles, these are located in the periphery of the cytoplasm.

Monocytes can be easily confused with band neutrophils or more immature phases such as metamyelocytes, and this is particularly likely to occur when the nucleus of the monocyte is kidney shaped.

To differentiate these cells, the chromatin should be observed: in neutrophils it is more condensed. The presence of cytoplasmic vacuolisation in monocytes is also very helpful (Figure 1.21).

When there is neutrophil toxicity, differentiation from monocytes is complicated, but, significantly, toxic neutrophils present with Döhle bodies.

Morphological changes

Changes in morphology are uncommon, the following being the principle examples.

- Haemosiderin inclusions, which are usually associated with inflammatory conditions or haemolytic anaemias.
- Iron inclusions associated with severe inflammatory conditions.
- In cases of malignant melanomas, monocytes may contain melanin granules.

Lymphocytes

Description

In dogs, it is normal to find lymphocytes of varying sizes, with the small and intermediate forms dominating.

- **Small**. These have a round or slightly indented eccentric nucleus, with aggregated chromatin, and have good uptake of the stain. The cytoplasm is sparse and pale blue (Figure 1.21).
- **Large**. The nuclear chromatin is less condensed, the cytoplasm is more abundant and there is a slight basophilia.
- **Medium.** These present with intermediate characteristics.

Morphological changes

Reactive or activated lymphocytes

Description

These are larger than normal lymphocytes and of variable morphology. Reactive lymphocytes may have a nucleolus, the chromatin is less dense than in a normal lymphocyte, and the cytoplasm is larger and basophilic. They can be confused with monocytes, although this is unlikely, since lymphocytes have scant and more basophilic cytoplasm and monocytes may also present with vacuolisation in the cytoplasm.

Causes

Lymphocytes become activated in response to antigenic stimulation.

Atypical lymphocytes

Description

Atypical lymphocyte morphology is similar to that of reactive lymphocytes, although they have a dentate or divided nucleus and irregular large purple or bluish granules in the cytoplasm. Like reactive lymphocytes, they are much larger than an erythrocyte.

Causes

These lymphocytes can be found in both **infectious and neoplastic conditions**, and are considered non-specific.

When present in large numbers, a lymphoproliferative process should be suspected.

Lymphoblasts

Description

Lymphoblasts are large lymphocytes with a round or indented nucleus. Their nuclear chromatin is usually thin and dotted with an evident nucleolus, and the cytoplasm is usually more basophilic than a normal lymphocyte and may contain vacuoles.

Causes

A blood count that has a **significant number of lymphoblasts is suggestive of a lymphoproliferative disorder**. They are a rare finding in peripheral blood following antigenic stimulation.

Leukogram interpretation

An important part of leukogram interpretation is the correct identification and classification of changes in the counts of different cell populations (Figure 1.27). In general, the clinician should define whether it is a **non-inflammatory or inflammatory leukogram**, as well as

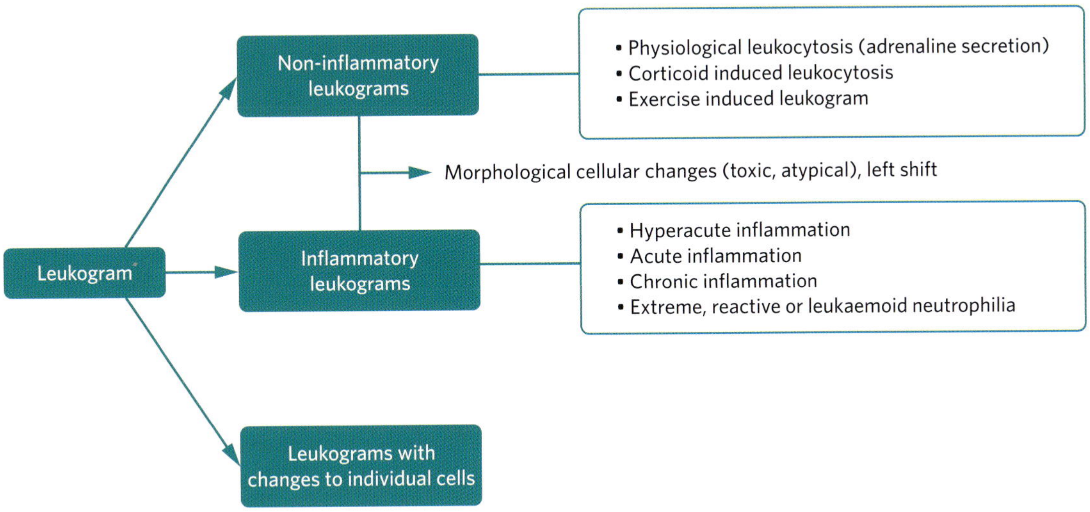

Figure 1.27. Leukogram classification in dogs and cats.

noting individual changes in different cell populations according to the clinical history, laboratory findings and complementary tests.

Non-inflammatory leukograms

Physiological leukocytosis

Definition

Physiological leukocytosis is characterised by **lymphocytosis with mature neutrophilia**. It occurs as a consequence of **adrenaline release**, which causes the movement of neutrophils from the marginal compartment to the circulatory system. The total number of circulating and marginal neutrophils does not change, which is why some authors call it **pseudoneutrophilia**.

The **lymphocytes are blocked by adrenaline** when trying to enter lymphoid tissues and are mobilised from the thoracic duct and lymphoid organs into the circulation.

Epidemiology

In general, this type of leukogram is **common in puppies** and very unusual in adult animals. Cats are more predisposed to this response than dogs.

Aetiopathogenesis

Physiological leukocytosis is usually caused by a **state of nervousness** (because of excitement or subjection to blood sampling, for example) or intense fear that induces momentary adrenaline secretion.

Diagnosis

The response in the leukogram is immediate and **lasts approximately 20–30 minutes**. This characteristic can be important in differentiating this condition from persistent lymphocytosis due to lymphoma, leukaemia or response to immune stimulation.

The **total lymphocyte count should not exceed 20,000/µl**. It must be remembered that young animals tend to have a higher number of circulating lymphocytes than adults, or in other words, numbers of circulating lymphocytes tend to decrease with age.

In dogs, this leukogram can be observed after brief periods of intense exercise. In cats, transient hyperglycaemia associated with adrenaline secretion can be seen.

Corticosteroid-induced leukocytosis

Definition

The typical pattern of a leukocytosis induced by corticoids, or stress leukogram, is a **leukocytosis with mild to moderate mature neutrophilia, monocytosis, lymphopenia and eosinopenia**. This response is less frequent in cats than in dogs, and when it occurs, monocytosis is not usually seen and eosinopenia is difficult to measure accurately.

The white blood cell count can vary between 15,000 and 25,000 cells/µl (sometimes 30,000 cells/µl). It is rare to find band neutrophils.

Aetiopathogenesis

Factors linked to a stress leukogram include:

- acute pain
- chronic pain
- low body temperature
- acute and chronic diseases
- exogenous or endogenous presence of corticoid.

The mechanisms responsible for the **neutrophilia** include the following.

- A decrease in the migration of neutrophils from the peripheral blood to the tissues.
- An increase in the transit time of neutrophil circulation.
- The mobilisation of neutrophils from the marginal compartment to the circulation.
- The stimulation of granulopoiesis.
- Increased release of neutrophils from the bone marrow.

The route of administration and the dose of corticosteroids can affect the magnitude of the leukocyte response.

The response to short-acting exogenous corticosteroids, such as an injection of prednisolone, occurs immediately with a peak at 4–8 hours, and the total leukocyte count returns to normal at 24 hours after administration.

In long-term treatments, the leukogram takes 48 to 86 hours to return to normal once treatment has finished.

Lymphopenia is caused by redistribution and/or destruction of circulating lymphocytes. The decrease in the number of lymphocytes can occur due to transient sequestration in lymphoid tissue or bone marrow, or destruction caused by a high dose of exogenous corticosteroids.

Eosinopenia associated with a stress response is disputed in cats because it is difficult to identify. The following are some of the causes of eosinopenia associated with stress.

- Marginalisation or sequestration of eosinophils within the microcirculation or tissues.
- Inhibition of the release of eosinophils from the bone marrow.
- Inhibition of the production of cytokines that control eosinophil development.

Exercise-induced leukogram

Epidemiology

This mainly affects dog breeds with a **high level of activity** or in training.

Definition

It is characterised by **mild leukocytosis with mature neutrophilia**, moderate lymphopenia and mild monocytosis. There may also be a **slight decrease in haematocrit** after strenuous exercise.

Aetiopathogenesis

This pattern is due to the **release of catecholamines** at the start of exercise and intermittent release of corticosteroids during exercise. It follows a mixed physiological pattern and is induced by corticosteroids, with great variability between individuals and possibly breeds.

Inflammatory leukograms

The leukogram is a useful method to evaluate the inflammatory response in dogs and cats, which may be induced by:

- bacteria (including rickettsia), viruses, fungi and parasites
- immune-mediated diseases
- tissue necrosis
- neoplasms.

In general, based on the clinical history and other findings in the animal, as well as the presence of **toxic neutrophils or a left shift** (presence of immature neutrophils), inflammatory leukocytosis is classified as one of the following leukograms:

- **hyperacute** inflammation (Figure 1.28a)
- **acute** inflammation (Figure 1.28b)
- **chronic** inflammation (Figure 1.28c)
- **severe neutrophilia**, reactive or leukaemoid reaction.

Hyperacute inflammatory leukogram

Definition

Some authors define this as a **leukogram that surpasses or exceeds the body's defence possibilities**. It is characterised by the acute appearance of a very intense inflammatory response, and is usually accompanied by **severe neutropenia**.

Aetiopathogenesis

The following are possible causes.

- **Sepsis** due to infection in the lungs, thorax, uterus or peritoneum caused by Gram-negative bacteria.
- **Severe inflammatory conditions** (large-scale tissue necrosis, hypotension with bacterial translocation).

As the name suggests, this leukogram picture occurs quickly, within 1–3 hours, and changes persist in the leukogram for more than 2–3 hours. Neutropenia is caused by the marginalisation of neutrophils, mediated by endotoxins, towards the focus of inflammation/infection.

This leukogram is less frequent in the cat than in the dog, possibly due to the importance of the marginal compartment in this species, with a 3:1 ratio of marginal to circulating neutrophils.

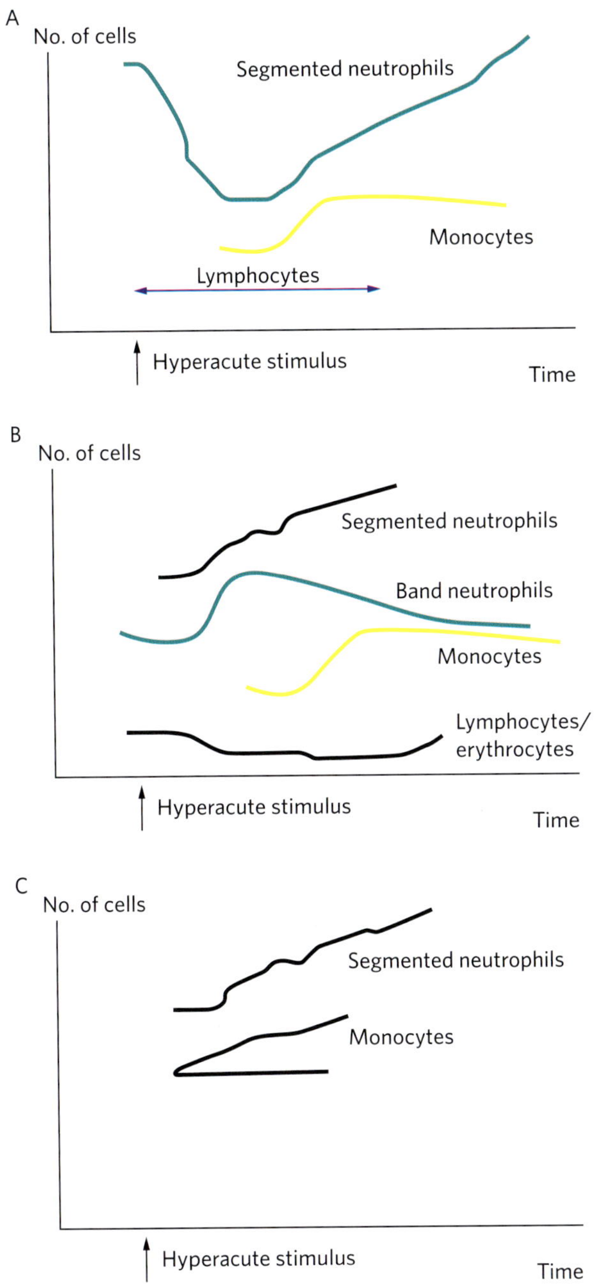

Figure 1.28. Predicted evolution of different leukocyte populations. (a) Hyperacute inflammatory leukogram. (b) Acute inflammatory leukogram. (c) Chronic inflammatory leukogram.

Acute inflammatory leukogram

Definition

An acute inflammatory leukogram occurs at 6–8 hours after an inflammatory stimulus. This leukogram is characterised by **neutrophilia with a left shift** (presence of band neutrophils >300/µl). The release of immature forms is ordered (first bands, then metamyelocytes and lastly myelocytes). There may be toxic changes in neutrophils, in addition to lymphopenia and eosinopenia due to the release of endogenous corticosteroids.

Monocytosis is inconsistent, depending on the presence of endogenous corticosteroids.

Aetiopathogenesis

The bone marrow responds by releasing neutrophils, mobilised from the marginal compartment, so a neutrophilia occurs in peripheral blood. In parallel, the bone marrow releases and produces neutrophils in a higher number than normal, so these immature forms are usually seen in the peripheral blood (left shift).

Chronic inflammatory leukogram

Definition

This occurs **days or weeks after an inflammatory stimulus**, and is characterised by neutrophilia, which is usually mature and with scarce band forms. Monocyte numbers may be normal or high, depending on whether the process is granulomatous or requires phagocytosis of necrotic material (tissue necrosis).

Leukogram with severe neutrophilia

Definition

This is characterised by a **marked neutrophil response with a left shift**. The animals usually show evident clinical symptoms and leukocytosis is between 50,000 and 100,000 neutrophils/µl. It can be difficult to differentiate from a chronic granulocytic leukaemia.

Aetiology

A leukogram with severe neutrophilia, also called a leukaemoid reaction, may be due to:

- infectious agents and infections:
  - peritonitis
  - *Hepatozoon canis* infections
  - abscesses in internal organs.
- neoplasia:
  - renal carcinoma
  - fibrosarcoma
  - pulmonary adenocarcinomas
  - rectal adenomas
  - hepatocellular carcinomas
  - inflammatory mammary carcinoma
  - mammary carcinoma.
- immune-mediated conditions:
  - immune-mediated haemolytic anaemia (rare in the cat).
- other causes:
  - adhesion defects in neutrophils (CD11/CD18)
  - feline eosinophilic syndromes.

Individual changes in leukocyte populations

The most common causes of change in leukocyte populations are listed in Table 1.3.

Table 1.3. Frequent causes of changes in eosinophil, lymphocyte and monocyte counts.

Leukocyte population	Changes observed	Causes
Eosinophils	Increase	Hypersensitivity (eosinophilic pneumonia, allergic dermatitis) Parasites that invade tissues Neoplasms (especially lymphoma) Eosinophilic complex in the **cat**
	Decrease	Generally related to the use or presence of glucocorticoids
Lymphocytes	Increase	Reactive lymphocytosis to infectious agents (ehrlichiosis, babesiosis), generally <20,000/µl Lymphoproliferative processes (lymphoma, thymoma, leukaemia), usually >20,000/µl Secondary to endocrinopathies (Addison's) Physiological response
Monocytes	Decrease	Glucocorticoids Chemotherapy Sequestration or blockage of normal lymphatic flow (protein losing enteropathies, lymphangiectasia or chylothorax)
	Increase	Tissue necrosis Inflammatory, infectious or immune-mediated processes with increased phagocytosis

Platelet disorders: thrombocytopenia and thrombocytosis

Platelet production

Platelets are the **second most numerous cell type** in the blood circulation and are essential for **coagulation, maintenance of vascular integrity and haemostasis**. They play a fundamental role both in **primary haemostasis** (where they are the predominant component) and in **secondary haemostasis** (providing soluble factors for the stabilisation of the clot).

Platelets **originate in the bone marrow** from a line of pluripotent cells and subsequently differentiate into myeloid progenitor cells, which give rise **to erythroid and megakaryocytic lines** (megakaryocytes give rise to platelets by cytoplasm fragmentation). The first morphologically recognisable cell in the bone marrow is the promegakaryoblast, which has a high nucleus/cytoplasm ratio and dark blue cytoplasm and is about 15–50 µm in diameter.

Platelet production is controlled by several hormones and cytokines.

- **Thrombopoietin**. This growth factor is produced by hepatocytes, the stromal cells of bone marrow and renal epithelium cells, where the concentration is inversely proportional to platelet mass rather than number. It plays a determining role in megakaryopoiesis and thrombocytopoiesis. In states of thrombocytopenia, high levels of free thrombopoietin may be administered to stimulate platelet production.
- Other cytokines: **IL-3, IL-6, IL-11, IL-12**.
- Granulocyte and monocyte colony stimulating factor (**GM-CSF**).
- **Erythropoietin**.

In healthy animals the number of platelets is relatively constant, but when there is increased demand for platelets their **production can increase up to 20 times**.

When **damage to the vascular endothelium** is recorded, platelets bind to the defect in a manner which is **dependent on von Willebrand factor (vWF)**. After adhesion, components that promote the binding and activation of new platelets are simultaneously activated and released, playing a fundamental role in coagulation (e.g., fibrinogen activation) and repair of vessels. Finally, platelets facilitate wound closure by promoting contraction processes that induce clot retraction.

Circulation and useful lifespan

Approximately **30% of circulating platelets** are retained in the **splenic compartment** for a short period of time. In healthy patients there is a balance between the numbers of platelets which are destroyed and those which are produced.

Platelets circulate in the bloodstream for:

- about **5 days in the dog**
- about **30 hours in the cat**.

At the end of their useful life, platelets are removed from the bloodstream by macrophages in the liver or spleen.

Thrombocytopenia

Thrombocytopenia is a **decrease in the number of non-circulating platelets** and causes the most frequent acquired **alteration to haemostasis** in veterinary and human medicine. Physiologically, non-circulating platelets are found in the spleen (30–40%) and, to a much lesser extent, in the liver and bone marrow.

Aetiopathogenesis

This is usually an acquired process that **accompanies an underlying disease** (Table 1.4).

Decreased or defective production of platelets

Factors that cause thrombocytopenia **may only affect the megakaryocytes** in the bone marrow, but it is more common to see an additional involvement of other cell lines. The existence of **bicytopenia or pancytopenia suggests generalised bone marrow disease.** Megakaryocytic selective hypoplasia is not common, but acquired immune-mediated amegakaryocytic thrombocytopenias in dogs and cats have been described.

The following can all lead to bone marrow hypoplasia.

- Some **medications**, chemical substances and **toxins** with cytotoxic effects or those that produce **idiosyncratic** reactions.
- **Irradiation** with bone marrow suppression and cell death.
- Infection with certain **viruses** (canine parvovirus, FeLV, FIV) or rickettsial agents.
- Myelophthisis due to **primary or metastatic neoplasia**.
- **Myelofibrosis** and myelonecrosis.

Platelet loss

Thrombocytopenia due to a **rapid loss of platelets** occurs in the following situations.

- Large-scale **trauma**.
- **Severe external haemorrhage**. Normally, when thrombocytopenia is accompanied by haemorrhage it is more likely the haemorrhage is due to thrombocytopenia than the other way round.
- **Blood transfusion**.

In the case of external trauma or haemorrhage, thrombocytopenia is usually mild to moderate, transient and usually reversible with specific treatment. Dogs intoxicated with rodenticides usually have moderate but almost never severe thrombocytopenia, due to the loss of platelets associated with bleeding and their consumption during the formation of blood clots in the locations of the haemorrhages.

Increase in platelet consumption

An accelerated increase in platelet consumption can occur when there is a **generalised activation of coagulation or endothelial damage**.

Several complex syndromes are characterised by widespread use of platelets.

- Intravascular coagulation (**DIC**).
- Thrombocytopenic purpura.
- Haemolytic-uremic syndrome.

The first of these three conditions is a common complication in veterinary and human medicine, while the other two are rare in domestic animals.

Platelet destruction

Immune-mediated

The **immune-mediated destruction of platelets** can be:

- **primary**: the immune response is directly against autoantigens, without an underlying cause.

Or it may be associated with other conditions such as:

- **systemic immune-mediated diseases** (e.g., immune-mediated haemolytic anaemia)

Table 1.4. Causes of thrombocytopenia in the dog.

Main categories	Examples
Infectious	Viruses: distemper, herpesvirus, infectious hepatitis, parvovirus Bacteria: septicaemia, endotoxaemia, *Anaplasma phagocytophilum, A. platys, Ehrlichia canis, Rickettsia rickettsii*, leptospirosis, salmonellosis, bartonellosis, borreliosis
Neoplasia	Haemangiosarcoma, lymphoproliferative and myeloproliferative neoplasms, various soft tissue neoplasms
Medications/toxins	Antibiotics (sulphonamides, cephalosporins), chemotherapeutic drugs (cyclophosphamide, doxorubicin), anti-inflammatory drugs (phenylbutazone, carprofen), phenobarbital, thiacetarsamide, oestrogens, snake venoms
Miscellaneous	Immune-mediated thrombocytopenia, DIC, distribution disorders

- **neoplasia** (lymphoma, leukaemia or various solid tumours)
- administration of **medications**
- **infections**.

Diagnosis of primary or idiopathic immune-mediated thrombocytopenia is made by exclusion and by the response to immunosuppressive treatment.

The **destruction of platelets** by the immune system occurs when circulating platelets bound to antibodies, antigen–antibody complexes or complement are destroyed or **phagocytosed by macrophages** in the spleen, liver and bone marrow, resulting in a decrease in the half-life of platelets.

This is one of the **most frequent causes of thrombocytopenia** in domestic animals.

Non-immune-mediated

This type of platelet destruction occurs in the following situations.

- **Acute viral** infections.
- **Acute bacterial** infections. Platelet destruction can occur as a result of platelet adhesion or aggregation of platelets to monocytes or activated neutrophils. In Gram-negative infections, **monocytes stimulated by endotoxins** express a tissue factor on their surface and **generate thrombin**, a potent platelet agonist, producing **platelet activation and aggregation**. Platelets adhere to monocytes and are phagocytosed. The role of neutrophils is much less important in these processes. Exotoxins produced by Gram-positive bacteria can directly damage platelets, contributing to thrombocytopenia.
- **Cardiovascular** diseases.
- **Snake bites**, where thrombocytopenia may be secondary to DIC or occur by direct aggregation of platelets.
- Severe and **extensive burns**.

The pathogenesis of thrombocytopenia associated with viral infections is usually multifactorial, although one of the mechanisms predominates. One of the ways in which viruses can destroy platelets is by replacing the sialic acid in the membrane with viral neuraminidase, thus decreasing their half-life.

Abnormal platelet distribution

The **total platelet mass is not affected**, so an increase in thrombocytopoiesis is not expected.

Hypersplenism is a pathological state in which up to 90% of circulating platelets are sequestered, predominantly in the spleen.

Clinical signs

Animals with low platelet levels can be **asymptomatic or present weakness**, lethargy, fever or other signs of the underlying cause. Clinical signs that suggest thrombocytopenia include:

- petechiae or ecchymosis in the mucous membranes
- epistaxis
- melena
- haematochezia
- haematuria
- prolongation of bleeding time after venepuncture
- retinal haemorrhage
- hyphaema.

Even though there may be no signs of bleeding, animals with thrombocytopenia are at a **high risk of bleeding**. Haemorrhage caused solely by thrombocytopenia does not usually occur until the **number of platelets falls below 50,000/µl**. The risk of bleeding increases if it drops by 10,000 platelets/µl, or if there is impaired platelet functionality or vascular damage.

Diagnosis

Thrombocytopenia is most commonly identified in **routine blood tests** (Figure 1.29).

Evaluation of platelet function

Platelet function tests are used to **diagnose haemostatic disorders** and to **predict the risk of bleeding** associated with invasive procedures. At present, their application in detecting platelet hyperactivation in conditions where there is a risk of thrombosis is gaining ground.

Bleeding time of the oral mucosa

This is one of the oldest tests that is still used today. It consists of performing a **standardised cut in the oral mucosa of the upper lip** using a single-use scalpel blade. This system is used to:

- perform a preoperative assessment
- find the cause of active bleeding
- determine the existence of a hereditary haemostasis defect (such as von Willebrand's disease)
- assess the effects of certain medications.

The oral mucosa **bleeding time is increased in cases** of thrombocytopenia and severe azotaemia and remains normal in some dogs which are deficient in coagulation factors.

There is no good correlation between the results of this test and surgical bleeding in the dog. Clotting times

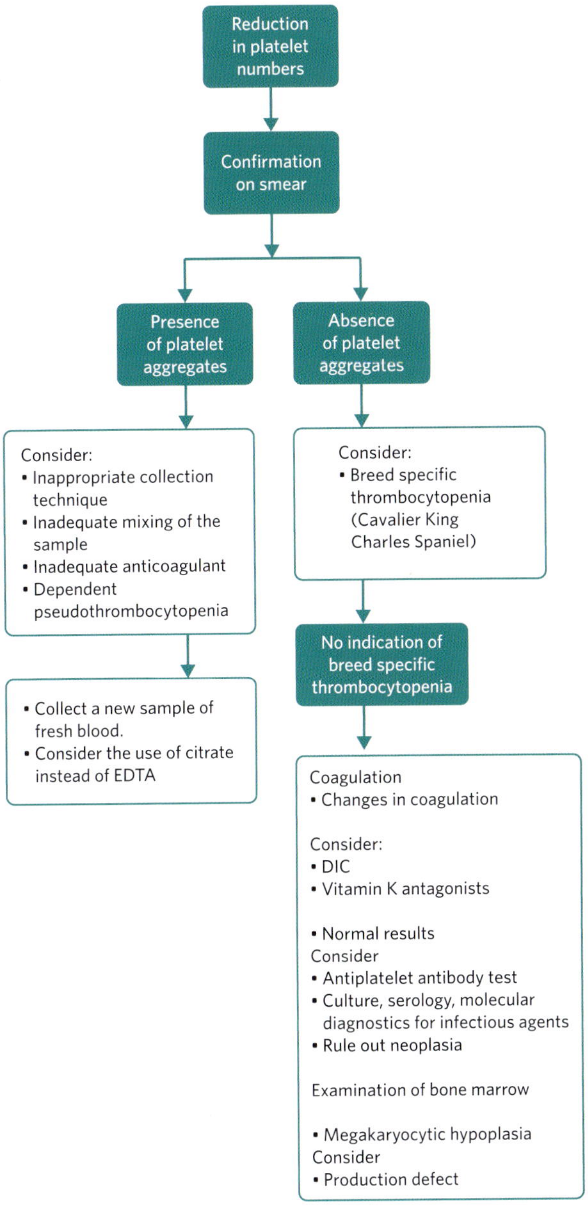

Figure 1.29. Algorithm for evaluation of thrombocytopenia.

under 4 minutes are considered normal. In the case of the Greyhound the results can vary by ±2 minutes.

Although there are more sensitive tests, these are not available to all clinicians, so this test may still be used as a first approach to the diagnosis of alterations in primary haemostasis (Table 1.5).

Clot-retraction time

This is a test which is **not very sensitive** for the evaluation of platelet function, so if more reliable methods are available, it is **not recommended**. It consists of maintaining a tube of coagulated blood at 37°C for 1 hour. After this time, the clot should be observed separating from the serum in the sample, which remains between the retracted clot and the wall of the tube. If the sample is incubated for a further 24 hours and lysis of the clot

Table 1.5. Normal bleeding times in dogs and cats.

Species	Normal bleeding time (seconds)	Technique
Dog	157 ± 29	Buccal mucosa
Dog (Greyhound)	129.5 ± 44.2	Buccal mucosa
Cat	114 ± 30	Oral mucosa

occurs, it is suggestive of an abnormal increase in fibrinolytic activity.

Other platelet functionality tests are described in the following sections.

Platelet function analyser

The **PFA-100®** is the most widespread automatic platelet function analyser in veterinary medicine. It involves measuring the bleeding time and evaluates the three stages of platelet activity: adhesion, aggregation and secretion. It **emulates a damaged endothelium**, presenting a small hole with a membrane composed of platelet agonists (collagen and epinephrine or collagen and adenosine diphosphate (ADP), depending on the cartridge used) and **measures the time it takes for a clot to form** and stop the blood flow through a capillary. As a result, the capillary closure time is obtained, which is proportional to platelet functionality.

The established reference intervals for **dogs are 53–98 seconds** with the ADP cartridge and from 92 to over 300 with the epinephrine cartridge.

It is advisable to carry out parallel studies for platelet aggregation and to **measure von Willebrand factor activity**.

Some factors that can cause an increase in capillary closure time in dogs are:

- haematocrit less than 30–40%
- low levels of vWF
- excessive citrate concentrations in the sample
- storage of the sample for more than 2 hours.

Flow cytometry

This involves passing a blood sample with the cells aligned, one by one, in front of a focused laser beam that, upon impact with each cell, emits scatter and fluorescence signals that are collected and converted into electrical signals. These are subsequently digitised and interpreted based on different cellular parameters.

Flow cytometry allows each **cell to be characterised** by both its antigenic characteristics and **its morphology** (size and complexity).

Whole blood, platelet rich plasma or washed platelets can be used to assess platelets.

The uses of flow cytometry include the following.

- Measuring the activation and reactivity of circulating platelets.
- Diagnosis of specific platelet function defects.
- **Monitoring thrombopoiesis** by quantifying reticulated platelets.
- Performing a **platelet count**.
- Monitoring the antiplatelet effects of some drugs.
- Obtaining platelet parameters for research.

Hypersplenism

Definition

Hypersplenism is characterised by the presence of **one or more cytopenias with corresponding bone marrow hyperplasia and significant splenomegaly**.

Epidemiology

It is a **rare phenomenon** in animals.

Diagnosis

The size of the spleen is possibly the most important factor determining the degree of thrombocytopenia. However, while hypersplenism is **characterised by splenomegaly**, the presence of an enlarged spleen is not necessarily indicative of hypersplenism.

The diagnosis is made by ruling out all other possible causes of splenomegaly. Hypersplenism differs from other causes of spleen enlargement in the following ways.

- The condition is **reversible**.
- The total **number of platelets is not altered** (although the circulating platelet count is).
- The production and **half-life of platelets are normal**.

Treatment

Splenectomy is the **treatment of choice**.

Thrombocytopenia associated with infectious conditions

Aetiopathogenesis

Thrombocytopenia can be associated with infectious agents, which can affect the production of platelets in the bone marrow in the following ways.

- Direct infection of megakaryocytes.
- Induction of an immune response against megakaryocytes.
- Induction of an inflammatory reaction in the bone marrow with production of immunosuppressive cytokines.

The **half-life of platelets is reduced** by different pathophysiological mechanisms including the following.

- Increase in consumption due to platelet activation and associated DIC.
- Direct infection of platelets causing their destruction.
- Removal of platelets by the mononuclear phagocyte system.
- Sequestration of platelets in the spleen or other tissues.

Rickettsial diseases are often associated with thrombocytopenia.

- Acute infection with *Ehrlichia canis* is usually accompanied by immune-mediated and non-immune-mediated platelet destruction in dogs, and a chronic infection by bone marrow hypoplasia.
- *Anaplasma platys* and *Rickettsia rickettsii* in **dogs**.
- *Anaplasma phagocytophilum* produces granulocytic anaplasmosis (granulocytic ehrlichiosis). Although it is described as infecting megakaryocytes, it does not affect platelet production.

Other bacterial infections sporadically associated with thrombocytopenia are:

- leptospirosis
- salmonellosis
- Lyme disease
- bartonellosis.

Viral infections that occur with thrombocytopenia are listed below.

In the **dog**:

- Canine distemper, due to viral damage of platelets, secondary immune-mediated thrombocytopenia and decreased production due to direct infection of megakaryocytes.
- Infectious canine hepatitis or herpes viruses, due to endothelial damage and DIC.
- Parvovirus infection.

In the **cat**:

- Feline infectious peritonitis, resulting from vasculitis, secondary immune-mediated thrombocytopenia, direct damage to platelets and DIC.
- Feline leukaemia virus.
- Feline immunodeficiency.
- Parvovirus.

Other agents related to thrombocytopenia are:

- protozoa (e.g., babesiosis, cytauxzoonosis, leishmaniasis, theileriosis and toxoplasmosis)
- fungi (e.g., disseminated candidiasis, histoplasmosis)
- metazoan parasites (e.g., heartworm).

Diagnosis

The history and clinical examination may suggest an infectious origin, with the resulting thrombocytopenia usually being moderate to severe.

The infectious agent should be identified by:

- microscopic examination of blood or bone marrow
- serology, culture and molecular diagnostic techniques.

Thrombocytopenia induced by drugs or toxins

Aetiopathogenesis

The mechanisms causing the thrombocytopenia differ depending on the causative agent.

- **Chemotherapy** induces **dose-dependent** and predictable thrombocytopenia, which is usually transient and resolves when the drug is metabolised.
- **Sulphonamides** produce an **idiosyncratic** thrombocytopenia with unpredictable results.
- Some **medications** (heparins, sulphonamides, cimetidine) can cause **immune-mediated thrombocytopenia**, against platelets or megakaryocytes. In most cases the immune response only occurs while the drug or its metabolites are present. When the response is independent of the dose and persists once the drug is eliminated, it can be difficult to diagnose.
- Some **medications** (cyclosporin A) directly **activate platelets**, causing an increase in their consumption, or damage to them, which leads to their withdrawal by the mononuclear phagocyte system.
- **Snake venoms** can also **activate platelets directly** or can promote the production of substances such as thrombin that produce platelet aggregation.

Diagnosis

A diagnosis of drug-associated thrombocytopenia is generally identified through the clinical history, including administration of a specific drug, the development of thrombocytopenia, and normalisation of the platelet concentration once the pharmacological treatment has ceased.

Thrombocytopenia associated with neoplasia

Epidemiology

Thrombocytopenia has been detected in **10–36% of animals** with neoplasia, especially those undergoing chemotherapy. The majority of cases correspond to lymphoma, carcinoma, haemangiosarcoma or haematopoietic tumours.

Aetiopathogenesis

Thrombocytopenia is mainly caused by **chemotherapy treatment** (decreased platelet production or DIC). It may also result from a decrease in platelet production due to **myelophthisis**, the **production of oestrogen** by some tumours or the administration of chemotherapeutic immunosuppressant drugs.

DIC is a frequent complication of neoplasia, with a higher risk when it comes to haemangiosarcoma, mammary carcinomas or adenocarcinomas of the lung. Neoplasms are the main recognised cause of DIC in cats.

In the majority of cases, secondary immune-mediated thrombocytopenia occurs, although other mechanisms causing thrombocytopenia may be a change in platelet distribution (especially in large vascular neoplasms), the loss of platelets due to tumour-associated haemorrhage or the destruction of platelets by neoplastic cells.

Clinical signs

Clinical signs are usually related to the underlying neoplasia, and thrombocytopenia may or may not be severe enough to produce a deficit in primary haemostasis.

Diagnosis

The diagnosis is made on cytology or histopathological identification of neoplastic cells. If the neoplasm is of haematological origin, there may be abnormal blood cells.

Breed-associated thrombocytopenia

Thrombocytopenia can be an **accidental finding in certain dog breeds**, and even in healthy animals that do not have any haemostatic disorders.

Greyhounds usually have thrombocytopenia when their values are compared with the established reference intervals, but in any case they are usually above 100,000/μl.

Thrombocytopenia is also present in **50% of Cavalier King Charles Spaniels** (CKCS), which have a **macrothrombocytopenia** that can lead to errors when an automated platelet count is performed. In this breed, the concentration is usually between 30,000 and 100,000/μl and is not associated with bleeding.

In some cases, prolongation of coagulation times has been seen, but this may be due to **von Willebrand disease**, caused by a **concomitant mitral valve regurgitation** to which CKCS are predisposed, rather than macrothrombocytopenia. Changes in von Willebrand factor associated with valvar pathology are caused by mechanical damage (from the turbulent blood flow) to part of the molecule and its **consequent inactivation**.

Pseudothrombocytopenia

This occurs when for some reason platelets are excluded from automatic counting. A decrease in platelet concentration detected automatically should always be **confirmed by observing the blood smear** to identify the formation of platelet aggregates that escape detection by analysers.

Pseudothrombocytopenia is a phenomenon that occurs *in vitro* secondary to a poor or complicated venepuncture, with consequent platelet activation, or by the exposure of blood to certain anticoagulants, as occurs occasionally when EDTA is used and platelet aggregates are formed. It is believed that this **EDTA-dependent pseudothrombocytopenia** is influenced by numerous factors. However, the main mechanism involves platelet agglutination mediated by autoantibodies, as occurs in humans, although the mechanism by which it occurs in animals is not completely understood. The phenomenon has been described in various species including the dog.

Feline platelets are especially sensitive to aggregation during blood collection. To avoid this phenomenon, a clean venepuncture or the addition of platelet inhibitors to the sample is essential.

Pseudothrombocytopenia can also occur when macroplatelets are present, since these are excluded from the count by some automatic analysers, and also when there is excessive filling of the sample tubes or inadequate mixing with the anticoagulant.

Thrombocytosis or thrombocythaemia

Definition

An elevated platelet count or, more specifically, a count above the established reference range for each species.

One consequence of thrombocytosis is the **pseudohyperkalaemia** which occurs in serum samples due to the release of intracellular potassium during clot formation. This effect is more pronounced the greater the thrombocytosis. To avoid this, it is preferable to measure potassium in samples of **heparinised plasma**.

Aetiopathogenesis

The causes and mechanisms of thrombocytosis are varied (Table 1.6).

Pseudothrombocytosis

Thrombocytosis can be **an artefact** (pseudothrombocytosis) caused by a **change in platelet circulation** (e.g., release from storage sites) or by **increased production**, sometimes secondary to medications, cytokines (reactive pseudothrombocytosis), haematopoietic disorders or hereditary alterations to megakaryocytes.

It can occur when small fragments of haemolysed erythrocytes, leukocytes (mostly with leukaemia) or **cellular debris are counted erroneously as platelets**. This artefact depends on the analyser, so it is important to confirm thrombocytosis through inspection of a stained blood smear. This also allows cell morphology to be assessed, and alterations in platelets and other cellular abnormalities to be identified.

Physiological thrombocytosis

More than a third of platelets are sequestered in the red pulp of the spleen and can be released by **splenic contraction mediated by adrenaline**. In human medicine, a transient or persistent thrombocytosis occurs, but this finding does not normally occur in the dog. Although there is no definitive evidence, some authors describe the presence of a pool of platelets in the lungs that are released in response to adrenaline.

Drug-induced thrombocytosis

Aetiopathogenesis

The mechanisms by which this occurs are not fully understood, but include:

- underlying disease in treated animals
- rebound effect after thrombocytopenia
- the drug itself:
  - **vincristine**: believed to act by stimulating megakaryopoiesis
  - **adrenaline**: produces a rapid but transient increase in the number of platelets by splenic contraction.

Although thrombocytosis is **common in animals with hyperadrenocorticism**, no consistent increase in

Table 1.6. Causes and mechanisms of thrombocytosis.

Cause	Mechanism
Pseudothrombocytosis	Elements that are not platelets but are counted as such
Fragments of fragile erythrocytes and leukocytes	
Physiological	
Adrenaline (trauma, exercise, excitement)	Splenic contraction
Post splenectomy	Lack of sequestration
Drug induced	
Adrenaline	Splenic contraction
Vincristine	Stimulation of megakaryopoiesis
Reactive	
Inflammation, infection, neoplasia (haematopoietic and non-haematopoietic), trauma, rebound post-thrombocytopenia	Cytokine mediated (directly or indirectly through the production of thrombopoietin), stimulation of megakaryopoiesis
Related to iron deficiency	Unknown
Neoplastic type megakaryocytes	Hereditary or acquired genetic mutations that produce thrombopoietin-dependent megakaryocyte proliferation
Chronic myeloproliferative disease: essential thrombocythaemia, chronic myeloid leukaemia, chronic basophilic leukaemia, polycythaemia vera, chronic idiopathic myelofibrosis	
Acute megakaryocytic leukaemia	Hereditary or acquired genetic mutations
Hereditary/familial	Hereditary genetic mutations

the number of platelets has been demonstrated with the administration of exogenous glucocorticoids.

Reactive or secondary thrombocytosis

Aetiopathogenesis

This is the **most frequent cause of thrombocytosis**, both in human and veterinary medicine.

The most common causes of reactive thrombocytosis are **inflammation and neoplasia**, which can cause thrombocytosis as marked as 1,000,000 platelets/µl up to 2 months after the onset of the trigger for reactivity. The reaction is produced as a result of the **stimulation of thrombopoiesis by cytokines**, which can be secreted directly by the tumour or by the host cells, affected by the presence of inflammation or neoplasia. The most relevant inflammatory mediator seems to be **IL-6**, whose levels are persistently high in patients with thrombocytosis due to inflammation or neoplasia. Initiation of thrombocytosis is **indirect** and produced by stimulation of liver cells to produce thrombopoietin.

In other conditions typically associated with thrombocytosis (e.g., iron deficiency), the mechanisms by which it is produced are not completely understood.

Essential thrombocytosis

Definition

A clonal alteration of haematopoiesis with a primary effect on megakaryocytes.

Aetiopathogenesis

In human medicine it appears asymptomatically, or patients have microvascular thrombosis (often in the brain, heart and extremities) or skin and mucosal haemorrhage.

Diagnosis

It is difficult to differentiate cases of essential thrombocytosis from those of reactive thrombocytosis, since **many parameters overlap**. The degree of increase in platelet count is not useful when distinguishing between these two conditions, so some cases of essential thrombocytosis reported in veterinary medicine may possibly be due to reactive thrombocytosis.

The diagnosis is made by exclusion, and the following criteria should be met.

- A marked or persistent thrombocytosis (> 600,000 platelets/µl for more than 1 month).
- Megakaryocytic hyperplasia.
- Normal levels of thrombopoietin.
- Absence of signs of dysplasia (normal number of erythrocytes and lymphocytes with normal morphology).
- A lack of iron deficiency or underlying inflammation/neoplasia.

Treatment

Treatment includes:

- apheresis (separation of blood components)
- hydroxyurea

- anagrelide (phospholipase A2 inhibitor that also inhibits the proliferation and differentiation of megakaryocytes)
- interferon α
- aspirin, to try and reduce the risk of thrombosis.

Familial/hereditary thrombocytosis

Aetiopathogenesis

Familial thrombocytosis is attributed to mutations in genes that code for the germ lines involved in thrombopoiesis, to produce a **non-neoplastic polyclonal thrombopoiesis**.

Diagnosis

High platelet counts are observed at birth or at an early age, and may be asymptomatic throughout the animal's life or may cause thrombohaemorrhagic complications, although the latter is very rare.

Coagulation

Haemostasis is a complex process in which proteins and cells interact in a coordinated and orderly manner. The **objective is to form a fibrin clot** that will later be dissolved to allow normal recovery of the blood vessels (Figure 1.30). Clinically, it is important to identify alterations in coagulation in animals with haemorrhages and situations where there is hypercoagulability, although the latter are less frequent.

Traditionally, haemostasis is divided into **three stages**. These stages are not activated sequentially but can be **activated simultaneously and coexist** at the same time. Viscoelastic testing (thromboelastography) can be performed and allows all stages to be assessed in a single test.

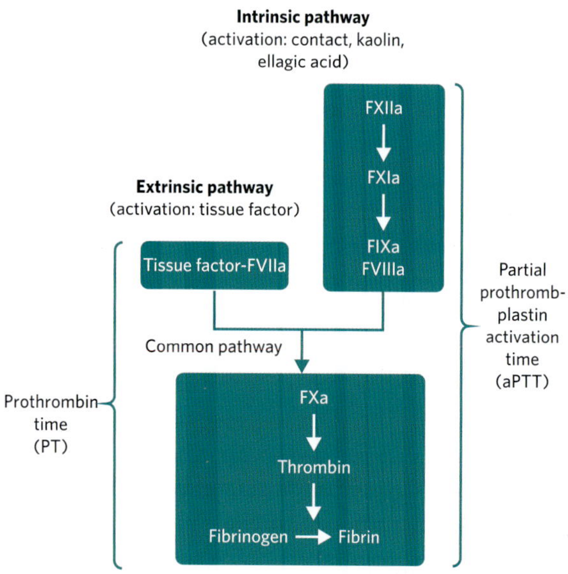

Figure 1.30. Classic pathways which are evaluated for secondary haemostasis.

The **ideal sample** to determine changes in haemostasis is blood collected in the following ways.

- **EDTA** tubes for:
  - platelet count
  - genetic tests.
- **Citrate** for the evaluation of:
  - the von Willebrand antigen
  - platelet functionality
  - classic secondary coagulation tests
  - presence of inhibitors
  - measurement of D-dimer or fibrin degradation products
  - thromboelastographic tests.

Knowing the citrate to blood ratio (e.g., 1:10, 0.1 ml with 0.9 ml of blood) or the correct proportion of citrate (3.2 to 3.8%) is essential for correct interpretation of coagulation tests. Table 1.7 shows the most widely used tests to detect changes in each stage of coagulation.

Changes in primary haemostasis

Aetiopathogenesis

Alterations in primary haemostasis can affect:

- platelets
- endothelial cells
- von Willebrand factor.

This leads to defective formation of the primary clot.

Clinical signs

The clinical manifestations are **haemorrhages of small blood vessels**, especially those that can suffer minor daily trauma (those in the nasal mucosa [epistaxis], urinary [haematuria] or digestive [melena, haematochezia] systems).

Spontaneous haemorrhages may occur if there is severe thrombocytopenia (less than 50,000 platelets/µl) or if trauma or surgery occur.

If there is **very severe thrombocytopenia**, **petechiae** are often present, which are not evident in animals with vWF deficiency.

An increase in platelet count may lead to an increased risk of thrombosis, but in practice this is unlikely on its own and is therefore not usually considered a cause of thrombosis.

Table 1.7. Most widely used tests for the detection of changes in each of the different stages of coagulation.

Coagulation stage	Cells involved	Facilitating proteins	Inhibitory proteins	Final result	Evaluation tests
Primary haemostasis	Platelets	von Willebrand factor, collagen, fibrinogen	ADPase, prostacyclin, nitric oxide	Platelet clot	**Trace:** • Buccal bleeding time • Platelet count **Specific:** • Platelet functionality • von Willebrand: factor, antigen, breed genetic tests • Biopsy: vascular integrity
Secondary haemostasis	Initiators: fibroblasts	Initiators: tissue factor, FVII	Initiators: tissue factor pathway inhibitors	Fibrin clot	**Extrinsic pathway** (factor VII and common pathway): • **Trace:** prothrombin time • **Specific:** factor VII activity
	Progression: platelets	Progression: thrombin, factor XII, factor X	Progression: antithrombin, C protein, S protein, non-specific proteinase inhibitors (alpha-2-macroglobulin)		**Intrinsic pathway** (factors XII, XI, IX and VIII, and common pathway): • **Trace**: partial activated thromboplastin time • **Specific**: activity of factors XIIa, XIa, IXa and VIIIa, and genetic tests **Common pathway** • **Trace**: fibrinogen, thrombin time • **Specific**: factor Xa, Va and XIIIa activity **Study of inhibitors:** • Antithrombin activity, C protein activity, S protein, thrombin–antithrombin complexes
Fibrinolysis	Endothelial cells	Plasminogen, plasminogen tissue activator	Inhibitors of fibrinolysis activated by thrombin, antiplasmin, plastinogen-1 inhibitor	Vascular permeability	**Trace:** • Fibrinogen degradation products (FDP), D-dimers **Specific:** • Plasminogen, activated tissue plasminogen, plasmin

Thrombocytopenia

Aetiopathogenesis

See Table 1.8 and the previous section on thrombocytopenia in 'Platelet disorders: thrombocytopenia and thrombocytosis' for the common causes of reduced platelet numbers. However, it is pertinent to remember that thrombocytopenia of genetic origin is often asymptomatic, for example in:

- macrothrombocytopenia of the Cavalier King Charles or the Akita Inu
- thrombocytopenia in the Cairn Terrier.

Platelet dysfunctions and thrombopathies

Aetiopathogenesis

Thrombopathies can be **congenital** (Table 1.9) or acquired. The latter are more frequent and are secondary to:

- hepatic and renal disease
- neoplasms
- infectious agents
- DIC
- medications (aspirin).

Von Willebrand disease

Epidemiology

Von Willebrand disease is the **most frequently diagnosed genetic alteration in dogs** but is very rare in cats.

Aetiopathogenesis

The cause of this disease is an **autosomal dominant gene**.

Clinical signs

The clinical symptoms include **excessive bleeding in young animals** when teething or at the time of surgery for neutering.

Classification

There are three types of von Willebrand disease.

- **Type I.** Decrease in vWF with a normal multimeric structure. This type has a high prevalence in Dobermans (60%), Airedale Terriers and Rottweilers. Animals with a concentration of the vWF antigen lower than 35% may show bleeding, and increased bleeding times if the value is below 20%.
- **Type II.** Decrease in vWF with changes in its structure. Seen in short-haired Pointers. Clinically it is more serious than type I.
- **Type III.** Absolute deficiency of the vWF (less than 1%). Described in the Scottish Terrier, Shetland Sheepdog, Chesapeake Bay Retriever and Dutch Kooikerhondje dog.

Changes in secondary haemostasis

Clinical signs

Defects linked to compromised function of a component of secondary haemostasis tend to manifest as bleeds from large vessels and present as:

- **haematomas** (skin, muscle or subcutaneous tissue)
- **haemorrhages in body cavities** (haemothorax, haemoperitoneum, haemarthrosis).

Aetiopathogenesis

Hypercoagulability in secondary haemostasis results from excessive thrombin production or the loss or **reduction in production of inhibitors** (such as antithrombin or protein C). Excessive production of thrombin occurs in situations of large-scale endothelial damage and aberrant tissue factor expression by monocytes or cancer cells.

Hypercoagulability leads to the formation of **microthrombi in the microvasculature**, which can lead to the dysfunction of some organs as a result of the hypoxic

Table 1.8. Pathophysiological mechanisms and frequent causes of thrombocytopenia.

Mechanism of thrombocytopenia	Causes
Decrease in production	Immune-mediated Infectious agents: FeLV, parvovirus, distemper Cytotoxic or immunosuppressive drugs Neoplasms Infiltration or necrosis of bone marrow
Destruction and consumption	Immune-mediated (both primary and secondary to infectious agents) Activation of coagulation
Sequestration and redistribution	Splenomegaly Pulmonary sequestration due to sepsis or endotoxaemia
Loss	Severe haemorrhage from serious trauma or rodenticide poisoning

Table 1.9. Known types of congenital thrombopathy in small animals.

Disease	Defect	Affected breeds
Glanzmann thrombasthaenia	GPIIb/IIa (fibrinogen receptor)	Pyrenean Mountain Dog
Thrombopathy	CalDAG-GEF1 of the catalytic domain	Basset Hound, Eskimo Spitz
	ADP receptor signal defect (P2Y12)	Swiss Pyrenean Mountain Dog
Storage deficiency	Defect in dense granules	American Cocker Spaniel
Chediak–Higashi syndrome	Defect in dense granules	Persians
Scott syndrome	Defect in phosphatidylserine exposure	German Shepherd
Non-specific thrombopathy	Transcription defects	Boxer, cross-breeds

Table 1.10. Most frequent changes observed in secondary haemostasis in small animals.

Pathology	Platelet count	Bleeding time	Prothrombin time (PT)	Activated partial thromboplastin time (aPTT)	Fibrinogen	D-dimers
Platelets ↓	↓	↑	N	N	N	–
Hepatic	N	N	↑	↑↑	N ↓	–
Rodenticide poisoning	N	N	↑↑↑	↑↑↑	N	N
DIC	↓	↑	↑↑	↑↑	↓	+
Haemophilia A	N	N	N	↓	N	–
Factor VII deficit	N	N	↑	N	N	–

Note: DIC, disseminated intravascular coagulation; N, normal or within the normal reference range

damage generated. However, these changes are usually masked by the initial disease causing hypercoagulation (e.g., the presence of pulmonary thrombosis in animals with severe protein-losing enteropathies).

Haemophilia A and B

Epidemiology and aetiopathogenesis

Haemophilia A and B are **linked to sex**, with **males clinically affected**, and females are carriers. **Haemophilia A (defect in factor VIII)** is most common, and mainly affects the German Shepherd, although many other breeds are also affected. **Haemophilia B** is due to a defect in **factor IX**.

Clinical signs

Symptoms in young animals include:

- haematomas
- bleeding after surgery
- lameness due to haemarthrosis.

Diagnosis

A combination of **specific genetic tests** and measurement of certain clotting factors allow for the correct diagnosis of this condition. In screening tests, the activated partial thromboplastin time is usually prolonged, although there are several degrees of deficiency.

Rodenticide poisoning

Aetiopathogenesis

Rodenticides inhibit epoxide reductase and block vitamin K recycling, which is essential for the synthesis of factors II, VII, IX and X. The factors that are produced in vitamin K deficiency are not functional.

Clinical signs

Animals intoxicated with rodenticides show **bleeding into body cavities**.

Diagnosis

An increase in coagulation time is frequently seen: as factor V has a shorter half-life, prothrombin time usually increases first and then activated partial thromboplastin time becomes prolonged. The presence of coagulation factors affected by vitamin K deficiency can be measured in the laboratory and is usually a confirmatory test for rodenticide poisoning.

Treatment

The duration of the intoxication, and consequently the treatment, depends on the type of rodenticide ingested.

- First generation rodenticides (warfarin) have a short half-life of 15 hours, and the treatment for poisoning is carried out over 1 week.

- Second generation (brodifacoum) have a longer half-life and the treatment is usually extended for 4 weeks.
- Third generation rodenticides need longer treatments, of at least 6 weeks.

The treatment of choice is the administration of fresh plasma or fresh blood, and **vitamin K1** (initially at a dose of 5 mg/kg/d SC which is later reduced to 2.5 mg/kg/d).

Before discontinuing treatment completely, it is recommended **to verify clotting times remain normal 24–48 hours after stopping treatment** with vitamin K1 supplementation.

Vitamin K deficiency

Aetiopathogenesis

Vitamin K deficiency has several causes.

- **Liver diseases with cholestasis** (vitamin K is fat soluble and bile acids are essential for its absorption).
- **Malabsorption of fats** (e.g., in the case of exocrine pancreatic insufficiency).
- Some drugs (e.g., sulphaquinoxaline).

In the Devon Rex cat, deficiency of an alpha-carboxylase enzyme has been described, so supplementation in these animals should be higher than for other breeds.

Changes in fibrinolysis

Aetiopathogenesis and clinical signs

Defects in fibrinolysis are mainly caused by **an excess of the plasminogen-1 inhibitor**, and to a lesser extent by low concentrations of tissue plasminogen or plasmin.

In dogs and cats, fibrinolysis defects are seen in animals with:

- diseases associated with thrombosis
- systemic inflammation
- protein-losing nephropathies
- hyperadrenocorticism
- diabetes mellitus
- disseminated intravascular coagulation (DIC) associated with sepsis (mainly described in humans).

Excess fibrinolysis is usually the consequence of DIC and is associated with an excess of plasmin production, which results in rapid **destruction of fibrin clots and haemorrhages**. Therefore, the most frequent clinical manifestation of excess fibrinolysis is the presence of **haemorrhage**.

Overall changes in haemostasis

Disseminated intravascular coagulation

Aetiopathogenesis

DIC is never a primary disease: **it is always initiated by another condition**. The most frequent causes are:

- injury to the vascular endothelium
- stasis of the blood
- hypercoagulability due to trauma or a septic process, either systemic inflammatory or neoplastic.

Clinical signs and diagnosis

It is essential to correctly diagnose the initial cause to establish a suitable treatment. There is no single test that allows a correct diagnosis; therefore, the correct diagnosis depends on investigating the changes to coagulation and a clinical suspicion of DIC.

Two phases of DIC are considered to exist.

- **Thrombotic DIC**. In this phase there is an **excess of thrombin production**. D-dimers are usually high, but they are not specific to DIC. Classic DIC tests are normal or even shortened, leading to a prothrombotic study, where **platelets are usually slightly diminished**. In this phase, there are signs of **generalised congestion** and initial shock. If the animal is not treated correctly, it usually evolves into a thrombohaemorrhagic DIC in 48–72 hours. Treatment is focused on preventing thrombosis and solving the precipitating primary cause.
- **Thrombohaemorrhagic DIC**. In this phase the animal presents an evident **haemorrhagic syndrome**. Coagulation tests are affected, with a low platelet count and prolonged coagulation times. D-dimers are high and there is usually a deficiency of antithrombin and protein C inhibitors, in addition to schistocytes formed by fragmentation of erythrocytes due to the formation of microcoagulates. In this situation, treatment is complex and requires coagulation factors and proteins, as well as an effective approach to the primary cause.

Bibliography

Anaemia and polycythaemia

Balch, A. and Mackin, A. (2007) Canine immune-mediated haemolytic anaemia: pathophysiology, clinical signs, and diagnosis. *Compendium: Continuing Education for Veterinarians* 29, 217–225.

Harvey, J.W. (2012) *Veterinary Hematology: A Diagnostic Guide and Color Atlas*. Elsevier, St Louis, Missouri, pp. 234–359.

Paes, G., Paepe, D., Meyer, E., Kristensen, A.T., Duchateau, L., Campos, M. and Daminet, S. (2013) The use of the rapid osmotic fragility test as an additional test to diagnose canine immune-mediated haemolytic anaemia. *Acta Veterinaria Scandinavica* 55, 74.

Piek, C.J., Teske, E., Van Leeuwen, M.W. and Day, M.J. (2012) Good agreement of conventional and gel-based direct agglutination test in immune-mediated haemolytic anaemia. *Acta Veterinaria Scandinavica* 54, 10.

Piek, C.J. (2011) Canine idiopathic immune-mediated haemolytic anaemia: a review with recommendations for future research. *Veterinary Quarterly* 31(3), 129–141.

Quigley, K.A., Chelack, B.J., Haines, D.M. and Jackson, M.L. (2001) Application of a direct flow cytometric erythrocyte immunofluorescence assay in dogs with immune-mediated haemolytic anaemia and comparison to the direct antiglobulin test. *Journal of Veterinary Diagnostic Investigation* 13(4), 297–300.

Wardrop, K.J. (2012) Coombs' testing and its diagnostic significance in dogs and cats. *Veterinary Clinics of North America. Small Animal Practice* 42(1), 43–51.

Warman, S.M., Murray, J.K., Ridyard, A., Eastwood, J., Silva, S. and Day, M.J. (2008) Pattern of Coombs' test reactivity has diagnostic significance in dogs with immune-mediated haemolytic anaemia. *Journal of Small Animal Practice* 49(10), 525–530.

Non-neoplastic leukocyte changes

Harvey, J.W. (2012) *Veterinary Hematology: A Diagnostic Guide and Color Atlas*. Elsevier, St Louis, Missouri, pp. 234–359.

Latimer, K.S. and Rakich, P.M. (1989) Clinical interpretation of leukocyte responses. *Veterinary Clinics of North America. Small Animal Practice* 19(4), 637–668.

Platelet disorders: thrombocytopenia and thrombocytosis

Abrams-Ogg, A.C., Kruth, S.A., Carter, R.F., Valli, V.E., Kamel-Reid, S. and Dubé, I.D. (1993) Preparation and transfusion of canine platelet concentrates. *American Journal of Veterinary Research* 54(4), 635–642.

Bass, M.C. and Schultze, A.E. (1998) Essential thrombocythemia in a dog: case report and literature review. *Journal of the American Animal Hospital Association* 34(3), 197–203.

Bianco, D., Armstrong, P.J. and Washabau, R.J. (2007) Treatment of severe immune-mediated thrombocytopenia with human IV immunoglobulin in 5 dogs. *Journal of Veterinary Internal Medicine* 21(4), 694–699.

Cortese, L., Sica, M., Piantedosi, D., Ruggiero, G., Pero, M.E., Terrazzano, G., Mastellone, V. and Ciaramella, P. (2009) Secondary immune-mediated thrombocytopenia in dogs naturally infected by Leishmania infantum. *Veterinary Record* 164(25), 778–782.

Dircks, B.H., Schuberth, H.J. and Mischke, R. (2009) Underlying diseases and clinicopathologic variables of thrombocytopenic dogs with and without platelet-bound antibodies detected by use of a flow cytometric assay: 83 cases (2004–2006). *Journal of the American Veterinary Medical Association* 235(8), 960–966.

Jacobs, G., Calvert, C. and Kaufman, A. (1998) Neutropenia and thrombocytopenia in three dogs treated with anticonvulsants. *Journal of the American Veterinary Medical Association* 212(5), 681–684.

Kristensen, A.T., Weiss, D.J., Klausner, J.S., Laber, J. and Christie, D.J. (1994) Comparison of microscopic and flow cytometric detection of platelet antibody in dogs suspected of having immune-mediated thrombocytopenia. *American Journal of Veterinary Research* 55(8), 1111–1114.

Northern, J. Jr and Tvedten, H.W. (1992) Diagnosis of microthrombocytosis and immune-mediated thrombocytopenia in dogs with thrombocytopenia: 68 cases (1987–1989). *Journal of the American Veterinary Medical Association* 200(3), 368–372.

Putsche, J.C. and Kohn, B. (2008) Primary immune-mediated thrombocytopenia in 30 dogs (1997–2003). *Journal of the American Animal Hospital Association* 44(5), 250–257.

Ridyard, A.E., Shaw, D.J. and Milne, E.M. (2010) Evaluation of platelet activation in canine immune-mediated haemolytic anaemia. *Journal of Small Animal Practice* 51(6), 296–304.

Singh, M.K. and Lamb, W.A. (2005) Idiopathic thrombocytopenia in Cavalier King Charles Spaniels. *Australian Veterinary Journal* 83(11), 700–703.

Smedile, L.E., Houston, D.M., Taylor, S.M., Post, K. and Searcy, G.P. (1997) Idiopathic, asymptomatic thrombocytopenia in Cavalier King Charles Spaniels: 11 cases (1983–1993). *Journal of the American Animal Hospital Association* 33(5), 411–415.

Weiss, P.J. and Wardrop, K.J. (2010) *Schalm's Veterinary Hematology*, 6th edn. Wiley-Blackwell, Ames, Iowa.

Coagulation

Koi, A. and Borjesson, D.L. (2012) Application of thromboelastography/thromboelastometry in veterinary medicine. *Veterinary Clinical Pathology* 39, 405–416.

Ralph, A.G. and Brainard, B.M. (2012) Update on disseminated intravascular coagulation: when to consider it, when to expect it and when to treat it. *Topics in Companion Animal Medicine* 27, 65–72.

Stokol, T. (2016) Disorders of haemostasis. In: Villiers, E. and Ristic, J. (eds) *BSAVA Manual of Canine and Feline Clinical Pathology*, 3rd edn. BSAVA, Gloucester, UK, pp. 94–122.

Waddell, L.S., Poppenga, R.H. and Drobatz, K.J. (2012) Anticoagulant rodenticide screening in dogs: 123 cases (1996–2003). *Journal of the American Veterinary Medical Association* 242, 516–521.

Test

1. **Which of the following is true of the reticulocyte count?**
   A) It stabilises with time.
   B) It varies according to the animal's state of excitement.
   C) It varies due to numerous factors such as, for example, anaesthetics.
   D) B and C are both correct.
2. **Regenerative anaemias due to blood loss can be:**
   A) Regenerative
   B) Non-regenerative
   C) Hypochromic and microcytic
   D) All of the above.
3. **Thrombocytopenia may manifest clinically with:**
   A) Epistaxis
   B) Petechiae
   C) Haematuria
   D) All of these are correct.
4. **In cats with FeLV infection, the anaemia which occurs is classified as:**
   A) Regenerative
   B) Non-regenerative microcytic hypochromic
   C) Non-regenerative macrocytic normochromic
   D) Non-regenerative macrocytic hypochromic.
5. **For diagnosis of an immune-mediated haemolytic anaemia, some indication of auto-immune involvement should be seen as well as:**
   A) Agglutination
   B) Rouleaux
   C) Positive Coombs test
   D) Spherocytes.
6. **Which of the following factors are involved in the intrinsic coagulation pathway?**
   A) X
   B) XII
   C) VIII
   D) All of these are correct.
7. **Which of the following factors is principally involved in the extrinsic coagulation pathway?**
   A) VII
   B) X
   C) XII
   D) VIII.
8. **In the initial stages when compensating for a DIC, which of the following can be seen?**
   A) Decrease in platelets.
   B) Very significant increases in PT.
   C) Very significant increases in PTT.
   D) Absence of fibrinogen.
9. **Thromboelastography allows evaluation of:**
   A) Primary haemostasis
   B) Secondary haemostasis
   C) Neither of the above
   D) Both A and B.
10. **Which of the following artefacts in a sample can produce an increase in MCHC?**
    A) Haemolysis
    B) Lipaemia
    C) Jaundice
    D) Both A and B are correct.

11. **If lymphopenia, eosinopenia, monocytosis and mature neutropenia are seen in a leukogram, it can be classified as a:**
    A) Stress leukogram
    B) Physiological leukogram
    C) Acute inflammatory leukogram
    D) Normal leukogram.
12. **The presence of a left shift in a leukogram is due to:**
    A) Acute inflammation
    B) Chronic inflammation
    C) Lymphoid leukaemia
    D) All of these.
13. **Leukograms with extreme neutrophilia can be caused by:**
    A) Severe infections
    B) Paraneoplastic syndromes
    C) Immune-mediated conditions
    D) All these answers are correct.
14. **Which coagulation factor is dependent on vitamin K?**
    A) FVII
    B) FVII
    C) FXII
    D) vWF.
15. **Which of the following situations can lead to thrombosis?**
    A) Venous stasis
    B) Cushing's syndrome
    C) Some neoplasms
    D) All of these are correct.
16. **Haemolytic anaemias can be caused by:**
    A) Immune-mediated conditions
    B) Parasitic diseases (babesiosis etc.)
    C) Paraneoplastic syndromes
    D) All of these are correct.

Answers on page 41

Clinical case 1

Signalment: A 4-year-old Chihuahua with a history of generalised weakness lasting 24 hours is brought is for a consultation.

Physical examination: Pale mucous membranes are seen. Tachycardia (100 bpm). Tachypnoea (40 bpm). Possible splenomegaly. T 38.9°C.

Differential diagnosis: Anaemia or hypoperfusion (due to the pale mucous membranes).

Diagnostic plan initially includes a blood count, biochemical profile, urinalysis and abdominal ultrasound.

Urinalysis: Reddish colour. Density 1030. Negative urinalysis strip to everything except bilirubin 1+. Inactive sediment.

Complete blood count.

Haematology	Results	Reference values
Red blood cell count (10^6/µl)	0.9	5.5–8.5
Haemoglobin (g/dl)	5.1	12–18
Haematocrit (%)	13	35–55
MCV (fl)	69.2	60–77
MCHC (g/dl)	56.6	30–36
Leukocyte count (10^3/µl)	28,500	6000–17,500
Lymphocytes	1000	1000–4800

Haematology	Results	Reference values
Monocytes	1700	200–1500
Segmented neutrophils	25,350	3000–11,500
Band neutrophils	400	<300
Eosinophils	50	50–800
Basophils	0	Rare
Platelet count (10^3/µl)	150	200–500
Total protein (g/dl)	9	6–8
Reticulocyte count (10^6/µl)	65,000	<60,000
Cellular morphology	Presence of autoagglutination and spherocytes. Neutrophils with toxic changes 1+. Haemolytic plasma	

Biochemistry	Results	Reference values
Sodium (meq/l)	146	141–152
Potassium (meq/l)	3.8	3.5–5.3
Glucose (mg/dl)	100	65–118
Urea (mg/dl)	23	21–64
Creatinine (mg/dl)	1.5	<1.5
Calcium (mg/dl)	10	9–11.3
Total protein (g/dl)	7	6–8
Albumin (g/dl)	3.2	2.6–3.3
Alanine aminotransferase (IU/l)	5450	21–102
Alkaline phosphatase (IU/l)	560	20–156
Bilirubin (mg/dl)	2.4	0.1–0.5

1. How should changes in the blood count be interpreted?

2. And the changes in serum biochemistry?

Answers on page 41

Clinical case 2

1. How should changes in the blood count be interpreted?

The blood count shows a very severe anaemia.

The MCHC is higher than normal; this is not possible and is usually associated with a laboratory error or the presence of an artefact, which in this case could be due to haemolysis and haemoglobinuria/haemoglobinaemia.

A non-regenerative anaemia is also seen. However, changes in cell morphology (autoagglutination and spherocytes) make the diagnosis more likely to be an immune-mediated haemolytic anaemia. Additional tests should be performed to rule out infectious causes of haemolysis, independent of the presence of signs of immune-mediated haemolytic anaemia, as well as a Coombs test. Anaemia is non-regenerative, possibly because it is a hyperacute process, and the animal will regenerate within 4–5 days.

On the leukogram a neutrophilia is observed with a slight left shift, with monocytosis: an acute inflammatory leukogram. The most likely cause is the inflammatory effect of the destruction of red blood cells, but hypoxia cannot be ruled out in other tissues such as the liver.

2. And the changes in serum biochemistry?

On serum biochemistry an increase in transaminases is observed, possibly due to hypoxic changes, although the presence of thrombi cannot be ruled out, so it would be advisable to perform coagulation tests to rule out disseminated intravascular coagulation.

Case follow-up

Abdominal ultrasound revealed generalised splenomegaly and fine-needle aspiration was consistent with reactive splenitis with extramedullary haematopoiesis. The rest of the examination was normal. Laboratory tests (PCR) to rule out diseases transmitted by vectors were negative for *Babesia*, *Ehrlichia* and *Anaplasma* spp. The Coombs test was positive but can be negative in up to 30–40% of cases. As leishmaniasis is endemic in the area, serology for leishmaniasis and ehrlichiosis was performed but was negative for both. The animal was treated with prednisone at immunosuppressive doses and showed an improvement.

Correct answers

Test

1: D	7: A	13: D
2: D	8: A	14: A
3: D	9: D	15: D
4: C	10: D	16: D
5: B	11: A	
6: D	12: A	

2

Immunology

James Swann and Pippa Elliott

Chapter summary

The main evolutionary impetus for the development of the immune system was to protect the body from infectious pathogens. However, it is now recognized that the immune system has other important functions, such as removing senescent cells and debris in the blood and central nervous system, along with protection against the development of certain cancers.

This chapter covers many practical aspects of immunology that are pertinent to clinicians. Understanding how the immune system works and what triggers inappropriate reactions will allow the clinician to prescribe effective treatment. An example of this is recognizing how immune-mediated haemolytic anaemia is often associated with a hypercoagulable state. The clinician can then supply an adjunctive medication, clopidogrel, to reduce the risk of complications and improve the outcome. With the insight provided by this chapter, the clinician will feel confident investigating patients that fail to respond to treatment and provide treatment to those that relapse.

Key learning points

- Describe the difference between the innate and adaptive immune system, and the implications of this distinction.
- Understand the pathophysiology of autoinflammatory diseases (such as Shar Pei fever), which involve the innate immune system, and how this differs from autoimmune disease (such as immune-mediated haemolytic anaemia).
- When a diagnosis of autoimmune disease is made, understand the importance of identifying trigger factors, such as infection, neoplasia or medications.
- Describe the treatment of specific immune-mediated diseases, including the pharmacological options, combination therapies and management of relapses.
- List the major autoimmune diseases in cats and their treatment options.

Introduction to the immune system

The immune system can be defined by:

- Its **structural components**, meaning the cells and tissues of the immune system. This is the traditional approach and is briefly considered here.
- Its **functional elements and actions**, regardless of which cells and tissues actually perform these actions. This is a modern concept where the same outcome is achieved differently in different individuals through a combination of varying immune responses.

Functional immunity

Barriers to infection

The normal mammalian body provides **several barriers** to establishment of infection, at the **skin** and **internal mucous membranes**. These surfaces physically separate exogenous organisms from critical internal organs and also prevent colonization of bacteria and other pathogens by virtue of their physical and chemical properties.

For example, the skin is cooler than the internal body core and maintains a slightly acidic pH, which does not support the growth of many types of bacteria. Additionally, the outer cells of the skin and mucous membranes are constantly shed and replaced by new cells produced by the division of basal stem cells. When the outer cells are shed, this also removes any adherent bacteria, reducing the total numbers of organisms present on the body surfaces.

Innate immunity

The immune system is often discussed in terms of innate and adaptive responses. **Innate immune** responses are not specific to a single antigen but are **activated by molecular signatures** shared by many different pathogens, such as lipopolysaccharide in the cell wall of bacteria. Innate responses occur rapidly and consistently because they are initiated by cells that are already resident in the tissue. Innate responses cause inflammation, which can be detected clinically.

Inflammatory responses are initiated by **cells that are already resident in the tissue**, such as tissue macrophages, mast cells and endothelial cells. These cells express **pattern recognition receptors (PRRs)** that are able to recognize molecular patterns shared by infectious agents, collectively called **pathogen-associated molecular patterns (PAMPs)**, or molecules released when tissues are subject to physical, chemical, or thermal damage (damage-associated molecular patterns, DAMPs).

Activation of resident cells via PRRs results in production of **inflammatory mediators**, such as histamine, prostaglandins and the cytokine tumour necrosis factor-alpha (TNF-α).

These mediators cause **vasodilation** and **increased permeability** of the local endothelium and also recruit inflammatory cells to the tissue.

In a typical inflammatory response, listed below is the sequence of events resulting in the development of the clinical features described in Table 2.1.

1. Entry of bacteria into a wound following an injury or other defect in the normal tissue barrier.
2. Recognition of (bacterial) PAMPs by PRRs expressed on tissue macrophages, or other tissue resident cells.
3. Production of prostaglandins, histamine and inflammatory cytokines by cells that become activated after PRR ligation.
4. Local vasodilation of blood vessels, causing redness and heat.
5. Increased permeability of blood vessels, allowing effusion of proteins into the inflamed tissue. Some of these proteins, such as the complement components, may have antibacterial effects.
6. Recruitment of inflammatory cells from the blood into the inflamed tissue, as a result of changes in

Table 2.1. *Inflammation*: the typical clinical features of inflammation are described using a set of Latin terms.

Feature	Clinical Description
Dolor	Pain caused when inflammatory mediators activate receptors on neurones in the tissue
Calor	Feeling of heat caused by increased blood flow to the region of inflammatory mediators due to vasodilation of local blood vessels
Rubor	Redness of the tissue that occurs when inflammatory mediators cause vasodilation of local blood vessels
Tumour	Swelling of the tissue caused by leakage of fluid and protein across blood vessel walls, as inflammatory mediators cause increased permeability
Functio laeso	Loss of normal function caused by altered blood flow, infiltration of inflammatory cells or damage to tissue cells

the endothelium of the blood vessels induced by vasoactive mediators and cytokines.

The above reflects inflammation and innate immunity in the context of pathogenic infections, but a similar response also occurs when tissue is damaged under sterile conditions. This is because some endogenous molecules, **DAMPs**, may act as ligands for PRRs on inflammatory cells, producing the same inflammatory response. This phenomenon has produced the '**danger hypothesis**', which suggests that the immune system does not respond only to pathogens, but to any stimulus associated with damage to normal host tissues, whatever the cause.

Inflammatory cells

Inflammatory cells are recruited from the blood to the site of inflammation by the production of **chemoattractants**, such as interleukin-8 (IL-8), and **changes in the endothelium** that allow them to move through the vessel wall.

The principal inflammatory cells are all myeloid cells produced in the bone marrow:

- Neutrophils: the **predominant inflammatory cell** found in inflamed tissues within the **first 12–24 hours**. These cells phagocytose bacteria and other debris and produce inflammatory cytokines.
- Monocytes: are **recruited after 24–48 hours** if the inflammatory response persists. Once they enter tissues, they **become macrophages** and play an important role in determining the outcome of the inflammatory response. They are capable of phagocytosis and production of cytokines, but they can also stimulate tissue repair and fibrosis.
- Eosinophils: are recruited to sites of **parasitic infection**, where they release the contents of their (eosinophilic) granules. These contain proteins and vasoactive mediators that interfere with parasite feeding, movement or reproduction.

Acute phase response

Most of the changes observed with inflammation are highly localized and affect only the tissue where the response is initiated. However, some cytokines, such as interleukin-1β (IL-1β), TNF-α and interleukin-6 (IL-6), may be released into the blood in large quantities, where they produce the acute phase response.

The **acute phase response** is **a systemic response to tissue inflammation**, which is probably intended to direct the body's resources towards fighting infection and to create an environment hostile to pathogen replication.

The **typical features** of the acute phase response are outlined in Table 2.2.

Additionally, **inflammatory leukograms**, consisting of **neutrophilia with monocytosis**, are often observed in dogs with **tissue inflammation**. This effect is probably mediated by the effect of inflammatory cytokines on myeloid progenitors in the bone marrow, increasing the production of mature myeloid cells, which are released into the circulation.

Inflammation also causes neutrophils to move from a marginated state (where they move slowly along the periphery of blood vessels) into a circulating state, which produces a relative increase in the number of neutrophils measured in blood samples.

Finding increased **concentrations of neutrophils and monocytes** in a patient with a reason to have tissue inflammation, such as a dog shortly **after surgery**, does not therefore demonstrate that an animal has an infection, and is **not an indication for antimicrobials** unless a positive bacterial culture is obtained from an inflamed tissue or it shows signs of systemic illness.

Adaptive immunity

Innate immune responses occur quickly and reliably in any tissue that is damaged or infected. However, this inflammatory response is often insufficient to clear pathogens and it does not produce any 'memory' to allow the immune system to respond more effectively if exposed to the same pathogen again.

These problems are solved by the **adaptive immune system**, an evolutionarily younger system that is able to mount powerful responses against specific antigens. Development of an adaptive immune response also results in **immunological memory**, facilitating a more

Table 2.2. Typical features of the acute phase response.

Clinical feature	Underlying pathogenesis
Pyrexia	Cytokines increase the homeostatic set point for body temperature by altering prostaglandin production in the hypothalamus
Increased serum c-reactive protein (CRP)	Cytokines alter the proteins produced in the liver by hepatocytes, causing the production of 'acute phase proteins' and decreasing production of albumin
Mild, non-regenerative anaemia	Cytokines decrease the activity of bone marrow erythroid progenitors and limit the absorption and accessibility of iron

rapid and effective response in the event of exposure to pathogens bearing the same antigen; this forms the **basis for vaccination** in people and animals.

Role of lymphocytes in adaptive immunity

Adaptive immune responses are largely **mediated by lymphocytes**. These are produced from common lymphoid progenitors in the bone marrow, but their subsequent development is variable:

- T cells migrate to the **thymus**, where they undergo rounds of selection to ensure they are functional but not likely to respond to normal host tissues. Once this is completed, they circulate in the blood, enter peripheral lymph nodes and other lymphoid tissues, and then return to the blood in the lymphatic fluid.
- B cells undergo similar selection in the **bone marrow**, and then recirculate in the same way as T cells.

Resident innate immune cells can respond to groups of pathogens expressing the same PAMPs, using their PRRs. The genes encoding PRRs are inherited from the parents, so the range of pathogens that can be recognized by innate immune cells is fixed before birth and does not change during life. By definition, PAMPs are shared by many different types of pathogen, so the specificity of the PRRs is low.

In contrast, immature **T and B cells** undergo a process of rearrangement where the genes encoding the T- and B-cell receptors are altered in each individual cell by randomly shuffling numerous small gene segments. This produces a large number of T- and B-cell clones with the ability to respond to a single, unique antigen, meaning that adaptive immune responses are much **more specific** to the inciting cause than innate responses.

Initiation of adaptive immune responses begins with **activation of CD4$^+$ T cells**. Because this process may cause harm if the wrong antigens are targeted, it must be tightly controlled and is usually confined to specialized lymphoid organs.

In inflamed or damaged tissues, **resident dendritic cells (DCs)** collect proteins and migrate to local lymph nodes. Here, they display digested fragments of the proteins collected in conjunction with molecules called **major histocompatibility complexes (MHC, class II)**.

Helper T cells in the lymph node survey the arriving DCs to determine whether they recognize any of the peptide/MHC complexes, using their T-cell receptors. If they do **recognize the antigen**, a strong interaction is formed between DC and T cell and the DC stimulates the **T cell to proliferate** and differentiate.

Following activation, helper T cells may interact with a number of other cell types (see below) that recognize the same antigen to produce the **adaptive immune response**:

- B cells: If a B cell clone recognizes the same antigen as an activated helper T cell in a lymph node, it will be stimulated to proliferate. Some of these B cells will differentiate into **plasma cells**, which produce large quantities of antibodies, and some will become memory B cells, which will be able to produce the same antibodies more easily in the event of future exposure to the antigen.
- Cytotoxic (CD8$^+$) T cells: These cells may be activated to destroy cells that are infected with viruses and other intracellular pathogens.
- Macrophages and other inflammatory cells: Helper T cells produce cytokines and other mediators that can recruit or activate inflammatory cells, sustaining an inflammatory response.
- Some helper T cells will also differentiate into memory T cells, which can persist for the lifetime of the animal.

Antibodies

Antibodies are produced by plasma cells, which are a terminally differentiated type of B cell. Antibodies are composed of two regions:

- The **constant (Fc) region**, that determines which receptors can recognize the antibody. There are several different types of Fc region, producing different isotypes of antibody.
- The variable region that binds to **antigen (Fab)**, which contains hypervariable regions at its tips that differ between different antibodies. It is the variation in this region that gives the adaptive immune response its specificity to individual antigens.

The genes encoding antibodies undergo a process of rearrangement in immature B cells, where different sections of the gene are shuffled to create millions of different variants, each with unique specificity for a particular antigen.

Before activation, B cells are able to make only one isotype of antibody, IgM. After receiving help from a T cell, they can produce different isotypes, a process called '**class switching**'. The major types of antibody in mammals include:

- IgG: This is the most common isotype in the serum, and is able to opsonize and neutralize. This is the only class of antibody to cross the placenta during gestation.

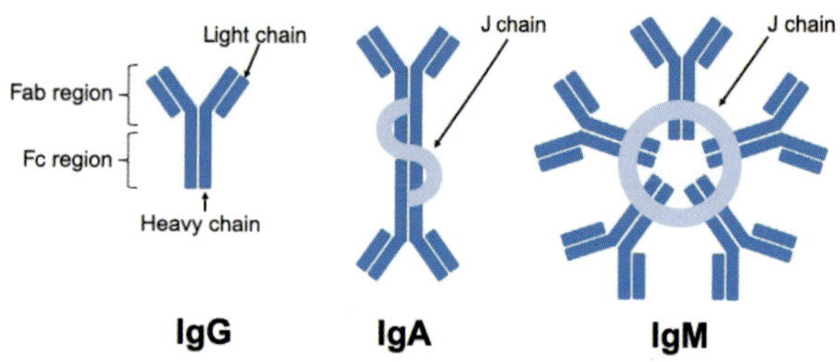

Figure 2.1. Diagram of the structural organisation of antibody isotypes. Antibodies consist of two heavy chains and two light chains joined by disulphide bonds. The end of one light and one heavy chain form the 'fragment antigen binding' (Fab), which recognises specific antigens. The other ends of the two heavy chains form the 'fragment constant' (Fc), which binds to receptors expressed on phagocytes and other cells. IgA antibodies form dimers and IgM antibodies form pentamers joined by the separate J chain proteins.

- IgA: These antibodies form pairs (dimers) joined by a protein called the secretory component. They are present at low concentrations in serum because most are transported onto mucosal surfaces in the gut, respiratory tract, urinary tract and on the skin, where they modulate populations of commensal bacteria, viruses and fungi.
- IgM: This is the first isotype expressed on the surface of B cells. In the serum, IgM antibodies can combine in groups of five (called pentamers), which are more efficient for activation of the complement cascade.
- IgE: After production, most of these antibodies bind to receptors (FcεRI) on the surface of mast cells in tissues. If they bind to their ligand, they cause immediate degranulation of the mast cell, which can produce a localized inflammatory response or, if systemic, an anaphylactic response.

Antibodies have a number of diverse functions in immune responses. The major mechanisms of action include:

- **Neutralization of viruses and toxins**. This is the basis for tetanus vaccination and administration of tetanus antitoxin, which neutralizes the toxin.
- **Marking of bacteria for phagocytosis** by neutrophils. This process is called opsonization.
- **Marking of infected cells for destruction** by cytotoxic ($CD8^+$) T cells. This process is called antibody-dependent cell cytotoxicity (ADCC).
- **Activation of the complement cascade to cause lysis** of bacterial cells. IgM antibodies are particularly effective in activating the complement cascade.

Passive transfer of immunity

Dogs and cats have an endotheliochorial placenta, which largely prevent transfer of large proteins from the dam to the fetus during gestation. In contrast, humans have a haemochorial placenta in which large proteins, including IgG, are transferred directly from the placenta into the fetal bloodstream. Consequently, neonatal dogs and cats obtain only **5–10% of maternal antibodies through the placenta**; the remainder are **absorbed across the gastrointestinal tract after ingestion of colostrum** within the first 24 hours of life. Puppies also produce small amounts of their own antibodies, but these do not reach adult concentrations until approximately ten months of age.

The **half-life of maternal antibodies** in neonatal dogs is **approximately 8–9 days** and approximately 4 days in cats, which means that maternal antibodies persist at significant concentrations for 8–16 weeks after birth. Since one of the major functions of antibodies is to neutralize bacterial toxins and viral particles, these antibodies may prevent the neonate from mounting a complete immune response against vaccines administered in this period, explaining why most vaccines are licensed for administration from at least 7–8 weeks of age in dogs, with the last dose administered at 16 weeks.

Changes in the immune system with age

Over the first six months of life, the cellular composition of the immune system also changes rapidly. The **thymus is functional at birth in dogs and cats** but produces more $CD4^+$ T cells than $CD8^+$ T cells in neonatal dogs and cats. The number of $CD8^+$ T cells produced increases over the first 6–12 months, so the ratio of $CD4^+$:$CD8^+$ T cells changes from approximately 4:1 to 1.5–2:1, and then remains stable during adulthood.

The number of B cells in the blood of neonatal animals is actually slightly higher than in adults, but this decreases considerably from birth to 10–12 months of age. A larger proportion of the B cells present at birth are of a primitive type called B1 B cells, which are capable of producing IgM antibodies with a limited range of specificities, without always requiring T-cell help. With increasing age, these are largely replaced by B2 B cells, which can mount more advanced antibody responses of any class and with a much wider range of specificities.

With age, there is a general trend for animals to mount less effective immune responses, which is sometimes described as '**immunosenescence**'. This may reduce the effectiveness of vaccination and make older animals more susceptible to infectious diseases.

This topic has been the subject of research in colonies of dogs kept for nutrition studies. When tested every year throughout adulthood, the following changes were observed:

- a general reduction in the numbers of B and T cells
- decreased responsiveness of T cells to various stimuli
- no major change in the total amount of antibody in the serum.

Breed differences in the immune system

Owing to their different genetic backgrounds, the immune system also differs between dogs of different breeds. This topic has not been investigated fully, but there are some important examples, including German shepherd dogs (GSD).

It has been proposed that **GSDs have a selective deficiency** in the production of **IgA antibodies** (but not in other classes of antibody), which is made at mucosal surfaces and modulates the interaction between the immune system and commensal bacteria. The concentration of IgA is lower in the GSD in blood and bile than in other breeds, but it is disputed as to whether there is less antibody in faeces. GSDs also have fewer B cells in their blood than other breeds. It has been suggested that this deficiency in IgA may **increase the risk of inflammatory bowel disease**, which is seen with increased frequency in this breed. However, it is unclear whether the relatively lower concentrations of IgA observed in the GSD are of any pathological importance.

Principles of vaccination

Vaccination, or immunization, involves **administration of an attenuated version** or part of a pathogen to **stimulate an immune response** that will protect the host against clinical disease in the event of exposure to the pathogen.

It is important to note that most vaccines do not 'prevent' infection by pathogens; instead they are intended to **limit the extent of disease**, or to clear the pathogen more quickly than would otherwise occur. This means that a vaccinated animal could still carry a pathogen or develop some clinical signs if exposed to it, even if it was previously vaccinated.

Vaccines usually consist of the **attenuated pathogen** (or part of the pathogen), which provides the antigens to which the immune response will mount a response, and **an adjuvant**, which stimulates the innate immune system to ensure an immune response develops.

Adjuvants provide ligands for PRRs, facilitating activation of DCs and presentation of vaccine antigens to T cells. Development of this **adaptive immune response takes several days**, so there is a **lag period** from administration of the vaccine to development of protective immunity.

The following events are expected after injection of a viral vaccine in a healthy animal:

1. Virus infects host cells, causing lysis of some cells.
2. Viral proteins are taken up by resident DCs and processed for presentation on MHC molecules.
3. Dendritic cells are activated when their PRRs recognize typical viral structures or DAMPs released from dying cells.

Table 2.3. Vaccines commonly used in practice.

Vaccine type	Mechanism of action	Example(s)
Live, attenuated	Contains a live variant of the pathogen that has been modified, to decrease its virulence. For example, this could include a bacterium that does not contain certain critical virulence genes that would normally allow it to cause severe disease	In dogs: canine distemper virus, parvovirus 2, adenovirus 1 and 2 and parainfluenza virus 2 In cats: herpes virus 1, calicivirus and panleucopenia virus
Killed	Contains bacterial or viral particles that have been killed by thermal or chemical methods. These vaccines may require adjuvants to ensure that the immune system mounts a response	Vaccines against *Leptospira* spp. in dogs. This explains why these need to be administered more frequently to maintain immunity
Subunit	Contains a purified or recombinant protein derived from the pathogen. These are frequently 'immunodominant' proteins, which refers to the protein(s) to which the immune system is most likely to respond during a real infection. Again, these vaccines require adjuvants to ensure the immune system responds to them	Some feline leukaemia virus (FeLV) vaccines are subunit vaccines, consisting of purified p45 protein from the virus delivered with adjuvants
Recombinant	Consists of a harmless virus (usually canarypox) that has been modified to produce a protein derived from a pathogen. These vaccines act as their own adjuvant because the immune system responds to PAMPs produced by the replicating virus, but will make specific responses against the pathogen-derived protein it expresses	Some FeLV vaccines include recombinant products, consisting of a canarypox vector that expresses the *env* and *gag/pro* genes from FeLV

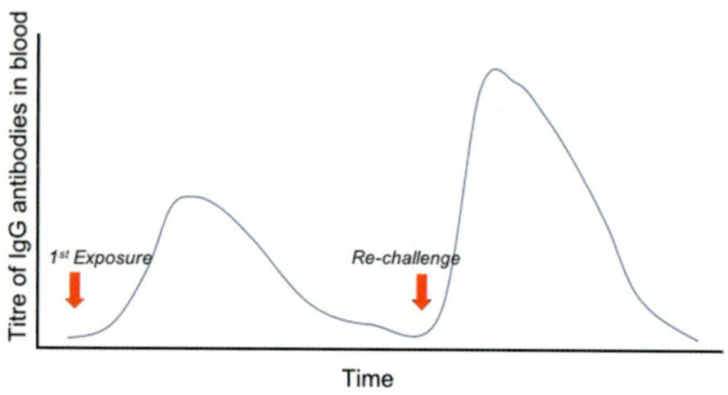

Figure 2.2. Changes in IgG concentration in serum following initial vaccination and re-challenge with the same antigen. Note that the production of antibodies is more rapid and reaches greater concentrations than on initial exposure due to the development of a memory response.

4. Dendritic cells carrying viral antigens migrate to local lymph nodes.
5. Dendritic cells interact with naïve T cells in the lymph node, activating any T cells that recognize the viral antigens on their MHC molecules.
6. Activated T cells provide help in the lymph node to B cells, which also recognize viral antigens.
7. Activated B cells differentiate into plasma cells and produce antibodies specific for the virus.
8. Antibodies and activated T cells clear the virus from infected tissues.

Vaccination makes use of the memory response of the immune system, because immune responses develop more quickly and effectively after repeated exposure to the same antigens.

These responses are dependent on **memory T and B cells**. These are long-lived cells produced during immune responses that are able to respond directly to their antigen, permitting more rapid production of antibodies by B cells, production of cytokines by $CD4^+$ T cells or generation of activated cytotoxic ($CD8^+$) T cells.

Routes of vaccination

Most vaccines used in veterinary practice are administered by **subcutaneous injection**, where they will be absorbed systemically to generate an immune response in the lymph nodes and spleen. However, some vaccines, such as live attenuated strains of *Bordetella bronchiseptica*, are administered directly to the site of anticipated infection in the respiratory mucosa.

For pathogens that normally infect mucosal surfaces, such as *B. bronchiseptica* in the nasal cavity and respiratory tract, protective immunity depends on **stimulation of local, mucosal immunity**. This occurs because some immune responses can be generated in **mucosa-associated lymphoid tissue** (**MALT**), rather than in the lymph nodes or spleen.

Like lymph nodes, MALT usually contains T and B cells but these are situated directly in the tissue, which means that DCs and other antigen-presenting cells are usually in constant contact with lymphocytes and do not need to migrate.

Mucosa-associated lymphoid tissues are typically found in regions where the body comes into **contact with commensal organisms** and occasionally pathogens, including in the mucosal tissues of the respiratory, gastrointestinal and urogenital tracts. Normally, this MALT tissue prevents immune responses against harmless commensals, but it is capable of responding to pathogens if the mucosa is damaged.

Autoimmune and autoinflammatory disease

Nomenclature

Autoinflammatory diseases are caused by **inappropriate activity of the innate immune system**, without activation of T cells or other components of the adaptive immune system. Innate immune cells are normally regulated to stop inflammation from happening all of the time. In autoinflammatory diseases this regulation fails, which permits the development of **uncontrolled inflammation**. **Autoimmune diseases** occur when the adaptive immune system mounts an immune response against specific normal antigen(s) in the host.

In veterinary medicine, diseases are frequently described as '**immune-mediated'** because it is not clear whether they are autoimmune or autoinflammatory. Such diseases may have clear features suggesting they are caused by the immune system, such as responsiveness to immunosuppressive drugs, but detailed research studies are lacking to establish whether this is caused by an adaptive immune response specific for a normal self-antigen, or inappropriate activity of the innate immune system. Hence, we traditionally describe haemolytic anaemia as immune-mediated (IMHA) in dogs and cats, whereas this disease is described as autoimmune (AIHA) in people, in whom it is known to be caused by an autoimmune response.

Clinical features

Owing to the different causes of autoimmune and autoinflammatory diseases, the clinical features may be different.

The clinical signs of **autoimmune disease** depend on **where** the particular self-antigen is expressed. In some cases, such as autoimmune (lymphocytic) thyroiditis, the antigen is expressed in a **single location** (the thyroid gland), producing an autoimmune response that causes targeted destruction of the glandular tissue without affecting the rest of the body.

In other cases, the immune response is directed against antigens that are expressed in **multiple locations** or all over the body. This occurs with systemic lupus erythematosus, a rare autoimmune disease of dogs, where immune responses are specific for nuclear proteins produced in practically every cell in the body. This produces a very broad range of clinical signs, including blood disorders, polyarthritis, dermatitis and the formation of immune complexes. Therefore, the **clinical signs** of an autoimmune disease can largely be predicted by knowledge of **the location of the target antigen**.

The **innate immune system** does not mount specific responses against single antigens. Instead, it produces inflammatory reactions and the **systemic acute phase response**. Therefore, autoinflammatory diseases typically display the same features as an acute phase response, including (intermittent) fever, lethargy and malaise, generalized lymph node enlargement, and occasionally joint pain and arthritis.

Some diseases involve a **combination of these mechanisms**, with some perhaps beginning as an **autoinflammatory disease that progresses to an autoimmune response** if T cells become activated.

We can consider two examples to illustrate these principles:

- **Shar Pei fever** is an **autoinflammatory disease**. This disease is associated with the typical features of an acute phase response, including pyrexia, joint pain, swelling and inflammation. It also causes production of acute phase proteins, particularly serum amyloid A, which can be deposited in multiple tissues to cause amyloidosis. Some people now call this disease 'Shar Pei Autoinflammatory Disease', SPAID.
- **Addison's disease** is an **autoimmune disease**. Most cases of primary hypoadrenocorticism are related to an autoimmune response directed against antigens that are found only in the adrenal glands, producing a lymphocytic infiltrate of the glands on histological examination. In humans and dogs with hypoadrenocorticism, it is possible to detect antibodies against enzymes involved in the production of aldosterone, proving that T cells have been activated and provided help to B cells to make antibodies, a defining event for an autoimmune response.

Clinical signs of autoimmune diseases

The clinical signs of an **autoimmune disease** depend on the expression of the particular antigen targeted. In addition, some autoimmune diseases are mediated by distinct mechanisms.

Antibodies bind to antigens on cell surfaces

The clinical signs of IMHA and thrombocytopenia (IMTP) are caused by destruction of red blood cells and platelets, respectively, by antibodies. These **antibodies bind to target antigens on the surface of the cell** and either activate the complement cascade (causing intravascular haemolysis in IMHA) or opsonize the cells for phagocytosis by macrophages in the spleen (causing extravascular haemolysis). In other autoimmune diseases, such as rheumatoid arthritis, antibodies are produced which are diagnostic, but do not cause tissue damage.

Autoantibodies form immune complexes

In other cases, **autoantibodies form immune complexes** by binding to soluble self-antigens. This can produce large, complex **aggregates composed of antibodies and antigens**, which can activate the complement cascade. These immune complexes are preferentially deposited in the glomerular capillaries and synovial membranes. After deposition, local activation of the complement cascade and infiltration of immune cells may cause glomerulonephritis or immune-mediated polyarthritis, respectively.

Activation of cytotoxic T cells

Finally, some autoimmune diseases cause clinical features due to **activation of CD8$^+$ (cytotoxic) T cells**. These cells normally destroy cells infected by viruses. If they become activated in an autoimmune response, they will destroy cells bearing the antigen that stimulated the autoimmune response. This is thought to be the explanation for the destruction of pancreatic cells seen in pancreatic acinar atrophy (PAA), the most common cause of exocrine pancreatic insufficiency (EPI), particularly in GSDs.

Risk factors

Genetic background

Some autoimmune diseases occur with increased frequency in particular breeds but rarely in others. For example, autoimmune diseases are classically seen with increased frequency in the **Cocker spaniel**. This provides strong evidence the disease is at least partially attributable to the genetic background of the animal, but there are differences in how this might occur.

Single-gene mutations

In some cases, the disease may be caused by a **single mutation** in a gene governing the immune system.

This may be the cause of Shar Pei fever, with the recent discovery of a mutation in the gene encoding for an anti-inflammatory protein (MDM2)-binding protein, MTBP. In dogs with the mutation, the protein does not function normally, allowing systemic inflammatory responses to develop. This mutation has been identified in only a single research study but appears to be strongly associated with the risk of developing clinical signs of SPAID.

Multiple-gene mutations

In most cases, however, the genetic risk is likely to be caused by **variations in the sequence of many different genes** that regulate the activity of the immune system. In many breeds, variations in the sequence of the MHC molecules, which present peptides to T cells to initiate an adaptive immune response, have been associated with the risk of developing autoimmune diseases. For example, some genetic variants of the MHC complex are associated with an increased risk of developing hypoadrenocorticism.

Environmental exposure

Not all individuals in high-risk breeds develop autoimmune diseases, suggesting that environmental risk factors may also play a part. Among the known or suspected environmental risk factors are **gender** and **neutering status**, **infections**, **neoplasia**, ingestion of **certain drugs** and exposure to **ultra-violet light**.

Gender

For many autoimmune diseases, **female animals have a higher risk** of disease compared to males. There are several proposed reasons for this difference, particularly the suggestion that **oestrogen may enhance inflammatory responses**. In addition, normal cells of female animals inactivate one X chromosome but this process may fail in some individuals, increasing the expression of the genes of the X chromosome, which includes many related to the regulation of the immune system.

Infections

Infections may increase the risk of an autoimmune response, which is why tests are often recommended to search for any evidence of infection in animals presenting with an immune-mediated disease. Again, the reasons for this are likely to be numerous, but include **molecular mimicry** or the development of an **inflammatory response** causing non-specific T-cell activation. Some bacteria, including *Streptococcus equi* ssp. *zooepidemicus*, also produce **toxins that activate T cells** directly, producing a form of haemorrhagic pneumonia in dogs due to inappropriate activation of the immune system.

Neoplasia

Autoimmune responses are frequently observed with some forms of cancer in people. For example, there is a strong association between the development of autoimmune haemolytic anaemia and underlying chronic lymphocytic leukaemia. Indeed, the **malignant B cells** appear to **produce the autoantibodies** that cause red blood cell destruction. Another well-known association exists in people and animals with thymoma, who frequently develop myasthenia gravis due to inappropriate production of antibodies directed against the acetylcholine-gated ion channels in the neuromuscular junction.

Drugs

Some drugs are known to increase the risk of autoimmune reactions, possibly by **changing the expression of genes** regulating the immune system or by altering the structure of normal proteins so the immune system identifies them as foreign. Such drugs include **penicillins**, which can cause an antibody-mediated hypersensitivity reaction, and **propylthiouracil and methimazole (thiamazole)**, used for treatment of hyperthyroidism in cats, which may cause the production of antibodies against nuclear components, occasionally causing vasculitis lesions around the face. There is no proven association between vaccination and autoimmune disease in dogs and cats, but this is frequently reported anecdotally and is included as a warning in the datasheet of some vaccine products.

Molecular mimicry

In some cases, **bacteria** or other pathogens may have **molecular structures very similar** or identical to normal host molecules. In this situation, an appropriate immune response against the pathogen may **'cross-react' with host tissues**, resulting in immune-mediated damage. This was a popular theory to explain autoimmune diseases in the past but it is difficult to reproduce this phenomenon in laboratory animals, and most animals and people with autoimmune disease do not have evidence of any concurrent or pre-existing infection. Hence, this theory seems **too simplistic** to explain the development of autoimmunity.

Microbiome

Mammals harbour **communities of bacteria**, **viruses and fungi** in the gut, upper respiratory tract and on the skin. Collectively, these micro-organisms **outnumber** the cells that make up the mammalian body, containing more genes than the host. From birth onwards there is constant interaction between these microbial communities and the immune system at mucosal sites. It is increasingly clear that this interaction shapes the

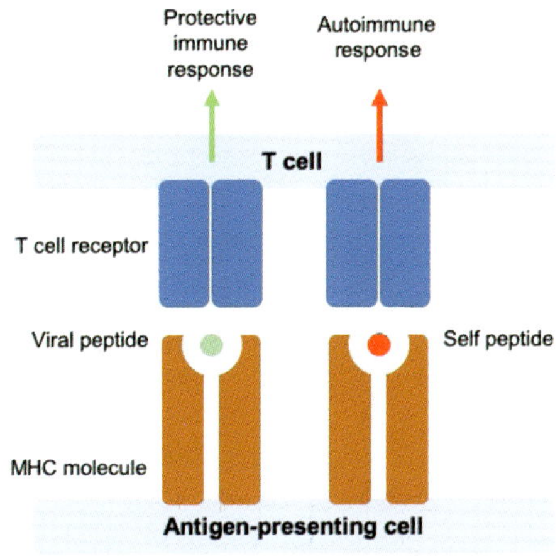

Figure 2.3. Proposed mechanism for molecular mimicry. In this example, a viral peptide is presented by an MHC molecule to a T cell receptor that recognises the combined structure of the MHC-peptide complex. The same T cell receptor is able to recognise a combined complex of MHC molecule and self-peptide, which has a similar structure to the viral peptide. The potential for molecular mimicry arises from the ability of MHC molecules to bind many different peptides and from the limited ability of T cell receptors to recognise structures that have slight differences in peptide sequence.

development of the immune system and immune responses.

For example, mice raised under **sterile conditions**, with no microbial community, have a **decreased risk of many autoimmune diseases**. Conversely, some strains of bacteria present in the gastrointestinal tract are associated with particular autoimmune diseases, though it is not clear whether they cause these diseases or accumulate after the disease has started to develop.

This area is still poorly understood, especially in dogs and cats, and it is likely there will be extensive discussion of this topic in the next 10–20 years; and the development of interventions to improve health by modulating the microbial communities that exist in the gastrointestinal tract. Currently, there is **insufficient evidence to recommend probiotics**, **antibiotics** or any other intervention targeted at the microbiome in dogs and cats diagnosed with an immune-mediated disease.

Underlying causes

Some dogs with autoimmune disease may have **an underlying cause** for their disease, which informs the clinical approach to cases in practice. As a result, when presented with a dog or cat with signs indicative of an autoimmune disease, consider performing some or all of the following diagnostic tests:

- Thorough **history**, including exposure to any drugs and toxins, or medications that the owners may be taking. This should also include information about tick exposure and any history of travel abroad.
- Thorough **physical examination**, including checking all the peripheral lymph nodes in case of gross enlargement, which could be a sign of lymphoproliferative disease.
- **Imaging of the thorax and abdomen** (e.g. thoracic radiographs and abdominal ultrasonography) to check for masses or internal lymph node enlargement.
- **Testing for infectious agents**, particularly if there is a travel history. Recently, there have been reports of *Babesia canis* and *Ehrlichia canis* in dogs in the UK that have not travelled abroad, so tests for these diseases could be considered even in dogs exclusively resident in the UK.
- **Urinalysis with culture** to check for urinary tract infection. However, it is difficult to establish whether UTIs are the cause of autoimmune diseases or simply concurrent.

Immune-mediated diseases

Immune-mediated haemolytic anaemia (IMHA)

It is important to determine whether an anaemic patient has **regenerative or non-regenerative anaemia**. This can be established by counting the **number of reticulocytes** circulating in the blood, which is most reliably expressed as the absolute reticulocyte count (ARC). If the haematology analyser gives a reticulocyte percentage (of the total number of red blood cells), multiply this percentage by the red blood cell count and divide by 100 to obtain the ARC. **An ARC greater than 6×10^9/l (=60,000/µl) is indicative of an appropriate regenerative response** in an anaemic dog. Without access to a haematology analyser that can quantify reticulocytes, examine a blood smear for polychromatophils, which are larger red blood cells with a blue/purple cytoplasm. If these are plentiful, the anaemia is likely to be regenerative.

Regenerative anaemia may be caused by **haemorrhage or haemolysis**. However, a regenerative response may take several **days to develop**, so acute haemorrhage or haemolysis may occur before any reticulocytes/polychromatophils can be detected in the circulation, a situation that is often described as 'pre-regenerative anaemia'. **Non-regenerative anaemia** is normally associated with **defects in the production** of new red blood cells in the bone marrow.

A diagnosis of haemolytic anaemia in a dog may be attributable to IMHA, but this is not diagnostic because there are other possible causes of haemolysis.

It is important to **exclude these other causes** before beginning therapy.

Babesiosis

In dogs that have **travelled outside the UK**, and now perhaps also in some parts of South-East England, infection with *B. canis* should be considered. This is a protozoal parasite that reproduces inside red blood cells. The presence of the **parasite may cause direct lysis** of the red blood cells or stimulate an immune response against the red blood cells that results in further damage. Consequently, babesiosis may produce a clinical presentation that closely resembles IMHA. However, *B, canis* organisms can often be **detected within red blood** cells in fresh blood smears by a trained pathologist. If the dog has a travel history to (southern) Europe or has come from an area where other cases have been reported in the UK, it is worthwhile to have a blood sample examined at an external laboratory and to request **polymerase chain reaction (PCR)** for *B. canis*.

PFK deficiency

Dogs of certain breeds are born with **defects in enzymes required for normal metabolism within red blood cells**, increasing the risk of haemolysis. Of these, the most common is **phosphofructokinase (PFK) deficiency**, which was diagnosed occasionally in **English Springer spaniels** but now seems to be extremely rare in the UK. This disease causes **severe haemolysis after exercise** or excitement, because the red blood cells are particularly fragile in an alkaline environment, which occurs when dogs pant or breathe very rapidly. Following a bout of haemolysis, affected dogs have a strong regenerative response and return to normal without any treatment, so owners may report **intermittent haemoglobinuria**.

The other reported disease, **pyruvate kinase (PK) deficiency**, has been described uncommonly in several breeds, including **West Highland white terriers** (in the UK), Basenjis, Cairn terriers, miniature Poodles and Pugs. This disease causes mild, **chronic haemolytic anaemia with a regenerative response** and, rarely, liver failure due to iron overload (haemosiderosis). The anaemia is so mild in some cases that it may only be detected incidentally if blood samples are collected for another reason. **Genetic tests are available** for both diseases if suspected in a dog of a reported breed.

Other causes of haemolysis

Haemolysis may be caused uncommonly by a few other diseases, including:

- **Severe acute leptospirosis**. In this situation, the disease is usually accompanied by severe azotaemia and signs of hepatic dysfunction, a combination strongly suggestive of leptospirosis.
- **Oxidizing toxins**, including zinc (included in some Euro coins), onions and paracetamol in cats.
- **Mycoplasma haemocanis**, transmitted by tick bites, may cause haemolytic anaemia that resembles IMHA, but this occurs almost exclusively in dogs that have previously undergone splenectomy and are therefore unable to clear the bacterium from the blood.

Signalment of dogs with IMHA

Several breeds are predisposed to development of IMHA, particularly the **Cocker spaniel**, which is approximately 4–6 times more likely to develop the disease compared to cross-breeds. Other known breed associations include:

- English Springer spaniel
- Irish setter
- Maltese terrier
- Bichon frise
- Old English sheepdog.

There is some dispute as to whether female dogs are more likely to develop IMHA than males. Some studies have shown that IMHA is more likely to develop in females (entire or neutered), but this is not supported by all investigations.

Similarly, there have been suggestions that the incidence of IMHA may vary with time of year or season, though this has never been demonstrated in the UK. In the USA, it does appear to have a seasonal incidence in some areas, but this may be related to the life cycle of vector-borne pathogens that may induce immune-mediated disease in exposed dogs.

Clinical features of IMHA in the dog

Immune-mediated haemolytic anaemia usually has an **acute onset** in dogs, causing signs related to anaemia. Anaemia decreases the carriage of oxygen in blood, causing circulatory changes that try to maintain oxygen delivery to the tissues (**tachycardia** at rest or, when relaxed, **increased respiratory rate**).

The **decreased viscosity** of the blood decreases the resistance to flow, causing a more rapid increase and decrease in the arterial pressure. This produces a **hyperdynamic pulse**, sometimes described as a 'water-hammer pulse' when palpated over the femoral artery. The decreased viscosity of the blood also increases the likelihood of turbulent flow, particularly as blood flows through the heart. This may produce a **'haemic' cardiac murmur**, which is usually a mild, systolic murmur not recorded previously in the same patient.

Reduced haemoglobin concentration in the blood causes **pallor**, and severe haemolysis may cause **prehepatic icterus**. In dogs with pigmented oral mucosae, this can be appreciated in the sclera and on the concave surface of the pinnae. The serum bilirubin concentration must be more than approximately 50 μmol/l for icterus to be apparent, and this will normally be accompanied by bilirubinuria. **Discoloured urine** may also be noted due to haemoglobinuria, as excess quantities of free haemoglobin released from lysed red blood cells are excreted in urine.

For the owner, the most frequent signs include **non-specific and progressive lethargy**, and reduced exercise tolerance. **Episodes of syncope** are common, particularly when dogs try to run or become excited. Dogs with IMHA often have a history of having **vomited** in the last few days before they are presented for investigation, possibly related to **hypoxia of the gastrointestinal tract**, or to the effect of excess bilirubin, which causes a feeling of nausea in people.

Pathogenesis of IMHA

Immune-mediated haemolytic anaemia is an **autoimmune disease**. This means that the immune system has mounted an adaptive immune response against one or more normal antigens within the body. In the case of IMHA, the most common target for the immune response is **glycophorin molecules on the surface of red blood cells**, though this appears to vary considerably among individual dogs with the disease. As a consequence of the immune response, antibodies are produced against these surface molecules, which may have two major outcomes:

1. The **antibodies may activate the complement cascade**, which is a system of proteins within the blood that may cause lysis of the red blood cell as it circulates. Only some types of antibody are capable of activating the complement cascade (particularly IgM antibodies), so this direct, 'intravascular', haemolysis does not occur in most dogs.
2. The **antibodies may mark ('opsonize') the red blood cells as targets for destruction** for macrophages in the spleen. Macrophages are capable of phagocytosis, but this process is highly dependent on the presence of opsonins, which mark the targets for engulfment and destruction. The presence of antibodies bound to red blood cells allows them to be removed efficiently from the circulation by splenic macrophages, causing anaemia due to 'extravascular' haemolysis.

IMHA is therefore an example of an autoimmune disease that is **dependent on production of antibodies**, though other parts of the immune system are also required, including complement components, macrophages and T cells, which provide help to B cells to enable them to produce antibodies.

Intravascular and extravascular haemolysis

The autoimmune response in dogs with IMHA may cause **intravascular haemolysis, extravascular haemolysis or both**. These terms have also been used clinically but without any consistency. For example, authors of some studies and books indicate that intravascular haemolysis can be diagnosed if an animal has haemoglobinuria or haemolysed plasma. However, in reality it is difficult to differentiate haemoglobinuria from bilirubinuria or haemolysed plasma from icteric plasma. In people, the serum haemoglobin concentration (NOT the blood haemoglobin concentration included on the complete blood count) is measured to determine whether there is a large amount of free haemoglobin in the circulation, which would be suggestive for intravascular haemolysis, but this test is not routinely offered in veterinary laboratories.

It is **unclear whether this distinction matters** in clinical cases. It was suggested historically that dogs with signs of intravascular haemolysis (i.e. urine with a red colour, or plasma with a red colour) might carry a poorer prognosis than dogs without these features, but this has not been confirmed in studies examining many different prognostic factors in dogs with IMHA.

Thromboembolism in IMHA

Dogs with IMHA are also at **high risk of thromboembolic complications**, which may include pulmonary thromboembolism (PTE) or formation of thromboemboli in the liver, spleen, kidneys or brain. Of the dogs that die from IMHA, it is estimated that **half succumb to thromboembolic complications** rather than the anaemia itself, so this is an important target for both further understanding of the disease and treatment.

The cause of the **hypercoagulable state** in dogs with IMHA is probably multifactorial, with possible risk factors including release of pro-thrombotic substances from lysed red blood cells, the effects of inflammatory cytokines on the coagulation cascade, activation of platelets and vascular endothelial cells due to the inflammatory disease, and development of a disseminated intravascular coagulation (DIC)-like state in affected dogs.

Clinicopathological features of IMHA

Regenerative anaemia

IMHA typically causes **strongly regenerative anaemia**. This occurs because decreased oxygen carriage in blood results in hypoxia in the kidneys, causing

release of the hormone erythropoietin (EPO) which stimulates the bone marrow to produce large numbers of new red blood cells. If the disease has a very acute onset, the regenerative response may be poorly developed or even absent at the point when the dog is presented for care, so absence of a regenerative response does not 'rule out' IMHA. Some dogs with IMHA have **persistently non-regenerative anaemia**, which may indicate that the **autoimmune response** is directed against antigens that are expressed only on the surface of erythroid progenitor cells in the **bone marrow**.

Inflammatory leukogram

In addition to the anaemia, most dogs with IMHA have an inflammatory leukogram, consisting of **neutrophilia and monocytosis**, which is probably related to the release of large amounts of pro-inflammatory cytokines as the disease develops.

Thrombocytopenia

Approximately **half of dogs with IMHA will have concurrent thrombocytopenia**, though this varies considerably in its severity. Dogs with immune-mediated thrombocytopenia usually have extremely low platelet counts ($0–10 \times 10^9/l$), so dogs with IMHA with such low counts are likely to have concurrent ITP and IMHA, a syndrome described as **Evans syndrome** in people. However, more commonly, dogs with IMHA have mild or moderate thrombocytopenia ($50–100 \times 10^9/l$), which may be caused by many different factors, particularly the DIC-like state and thrombo-emboli that often develop concurrently.

Organ dysfunction

Decreased oxygen carriage in the blood will often result in **hypoxia** and reduced function of multiple organs. This may cause mild azotaemia and increased hepatocellular enzyme activities. Dogs with IMHA may also develop azotaemia due to the excretion of large amounts of haemoglobin through the kidneys, though this complication is actually rarely encountered in dogs and it is likely that this idea has entered the veterinary literature because it is common in people with haemolysis.

Raised serum bilirubin

The **serum bilirubin concentration is likely to be increased**, even if this is not sufficiently severe to cause clinical icterus. Most of this bilirubin in circulation is unconjugated bilirubin, which is a breakdown product of haem. Unconjugated bilirubin is conjugated in the liver and then excreted in bile. Bilirubin has a very low renal threshold in dogs, so increased concentrations in serum will always result in discoloured urine due to bilirubinuria.

Specific tests for IMHA

With so many other possible causes of haemolytic anaemia, it is important to reach a definitive diagnosis of IMHA. This relies on tests that can **demonstrate the presence of antibodies** directed against red blood cells, which is the defining feature of the disease. There are several tests available, though these vary in their reliability and availability:

1. The direct antiglobulin test (DAT, Coombs' test) is used to detect **antibodies bound to red blood cells**. In the traditional version of the test, red blood cells were washed (to remove the serum) and then mixed with a solution of antibodies raised against other antibodies (the Coombs' reagent or antiserum). If there were red blood cells already bound to the surface of red blood cells, the Coombs' reagent could bind to them and cause the **red blood cells to clump or agglutinate**, which could be observed visually. The amount of Coombs' reagent needed to cause this agglutination could then be titrated to determine the lowest concentration needed to produce a positive result. Consequently, the result of the test is expressed as a titre, with a 'high' titre (e.g. 1/256) indicating that only a small amount of the antiserum is needed to cause agglutination. In most tests, **a titre of 1/16** or higher is considered to be consistent with IMHA because it indicates that a large number of antibodies are bound on the surface of the red blood cells, but titres less than this could be caused by non-specific binding of the antiserum so low titres (e.g. ½) are less convincing in dogs with IMHA. The DAT is **not affected by blood transfusions**, so it is possible to administer a transfusion and then submit a test within the next few days. It is unclear what effect immunosuppressive drugs have on the DAT, so it is best to submit samples before starting treatment. The DAT is probably the single best test for IMHA, with a **sensitivity of approximately 66%** (i.e. 66% of tested dogs with IMHA will have a positive result) and **specificity of approximately 90%** (i.e. 10% of tested dogs that do NOT have IMHA will have a positive result). The test has been out of favour for a long time, because results used to take several days to come back from diagnostic laboratories. However, there are now **'point of care' DATs**, which can be run 'in house' in a few minutes with a very small amount of blood. These simply report a positive or negative result at a particular cut-off, rather than a quantitative titre result. One could argue that DATs are not necessary for diagnosis of IMHA if other test results are supportive, but it is

recommended to submit the test if possible because it represents 'due diligence' in making the diagnosis and committing the patient (and owner) to several months' treatment with immunosuppressive drugs.

2. Saline agglutination of blood can be appreciated in some dogs with IMHA, particularly after diluting a drop of blood in saline to prevent rouleaux formation. There are many different ways to perform this test – some authors advocate washing the red blood cells three times beforehand (i.e. centrifuging the sample, removing the serum, adding saline and repeating three times), whereas others perform the test directly by **mixing one drop of fresh blood with one drop of (unheparinized) saline on a slide**. Either way, the slide should be examined macroscopically and microscopically for evidence of agglutination. Ideally, blood should not be cooled or refrigerated because this may cause non-pathological agglutination in some dogs, or the blood should be warmed to 37°C again before performing the test. Agglutination is a less specific test than the DAT (i.e. there is a higher likelihood of false-positives) because it may occur in dogs with other diseases. There is also some subjectivity in interpreting this test, particularly for macroscopic agglutination.
3. Observation of spherocytes on a blood smear is also used to support the diagnosis of IMHA. These are **small red blood cells that lack normal central pallor**, and they are thought to develop when a macrophage in the spleen partially phagocytoses the cell, causing changes in its structure. There is no accepted cut-off for how many spherocytes are needed to make a diagnosis of IMHA, but these **should be plentiful**, with several cells seen in each microscopic high-power field. If a haematology report simply states 'spherocytes', call and ask how many were seen. **Spherocytes cannot be reliably detected in cats** because their red blood cells are smaller and often lack central pallor anyway when observed microscopically.

Exclusion of underlying causes of IMHA

Autoimmune diseases can be induced or stimulated by other inflammatory insults, including infectious agents, cancer or changes in the oestrous cycle. So, even after establishing that a dog has IMHA, it is recommended to perform additional tests to determine whether there is any underlying cause of the disease, **present in approximately 20–25%** of cases.

There are many factors that have been described as possible underlying causes for IMHA.

- **Cancer,** particularly **lymphoma** or other forms of lymphoproliferative disease. A syndrome resembling IMHA also occurs in some dogs with histiocytic sarcoma, but this is probably related to phagocytosis of red blood cells by the neoplastic cells themselves.
- **Drugs** have been associated with IMHA, particularly antimicrobials of the **beta-lactam** and **sulphonamide** classes. In people, penicillin molecules may bind to antigens on the surface of the red blood cell to create a novel antigen, which becomes a target for the immune response. Strictly, this is a hypersensitivity reaction rather than an autoimmune response because the immune system is responding to an innocuous, but external, antigen.
- **Infectious agents**, particularly **vector-borne parasites**, have been associated with IMHA, though a causative relationship has not been established definitively.

IMHA in the cat

Immune-mediated haemolytic anaemia also occurs in the cat but is much **less common** than in the dog. It causes very similar clinical signs and pathological changes, though there may be a longer gap between onset of clinical signs and presentation for investigation because lethargy may be difficult to appreciate in some cats. Furthermore, cats more often have non-regenerative anaemia at presentation but then develop a satisfactory regenerative response after they start to receive treatment.

As with dogs, other **causes of anaemia should be excluded**, particularly infection with feline FeLV and/or haemotropic *Mycoplasma* spp. These bacteria replicate within red blood cells, causing direct lysis of cells or prompting an immune response that causes destruction of the red blood cells (i.e. secondary IMHA). There are three species/subspecies of haemotropic *Mycoplasma* in cats: *M. haemofelis*, *Candidatus M. turicensis* and *Candidatus M. haemominutum*. Of these, only *M. haemofelis* is thought to cause anaemia that is sufficiently severe to be detected clinically. These bacteria can be detected using **PCR of whole blood**; a quantitative PCR assay can be used to indicate whether there is a high bacterial load in the blood, which is more likely to be associated with clinical signs. Feline immunodeficiency virus (FIV) has been reported to cause immunological complications, but more often this causes chronic, non-regenerative anaemia due to bone marrow dysfunction.

Spherocytes cannot be reliably detected in cats, so diagnosis is based on a **positive DAT** and/or **in-saline agglutination.** Presence of 'ghost cells', red blood cell remnants that persist after haemolysis, may also be associated with IMHA in cats, but this is not specific to immune-mediated disease and may also be observed with oxidizing toxins, such as paracetamol.

Traditionally, it was suggested that IMHA in cats was more likely to be associated with an underlying disease compared to dogs, but this does not appear to be true in larger studies of cats with the disease. Indeed, in approximately **60–75% of dogs or cats with IMHA, no underlying cause can be detected** after excluding endemic infectious agents, toxin and drug exposure, and after imaging the thorax and abdomen.

Non-regenerative forms of IMHA in the dog and cat

Immune-mediated haemolytic anaemia is considered a classical cause of regenerative anaemia, but some cases present with **non-regenerative anaemia** even after a sufficiently long time has elapsed to allow bone marrow regeneration to occur. In these cases, it is thought that the **autoimmune response may be directed against erythroid progenitors in the bone marrow**, preventing normal regeneration. In the majority of cases, these dogs and cats still have evidence of peripheral haemolysis, including hyperbilirubinaemia, haemoglobinuria, in-saline agglutination and spherocytosis (in the dog), so the diagnosis can still be reached without needing further tests. In most of these cases, the anaemia will become regenerative shortly after treatment has commenced.

In some cases, there are no signs of peripheral destruction of red blood cells, in which case **sampling of the bone marrow** is required. This tends to reveal one of three possible patterns:

- Strongly regenerative response (**'erythroid hyperplasia'**) in the bone marrow, with peripheral non-regenerative anaemia. This suggests that red blood cells are being destroyed just before they mature and enter the circulation. This form of disease often has features of peripheral haemolysis.
- Lack of a regenerative response in the bone marrow (**'erythroid hypoplasia'**), with peripheral non-regenerative anaemia. It is difficult to prove that these dogs definitely have an autoimmune disease as they often don't have features of peripheral haemolysis. These dogs also appear to have a poorer outcome when treated.
- Complete absence of erythroid stem cells in the bone marrow, also described as pure **red cell aplasia** (**PRCA**). These dogs often have signs of peripheral destruction as well, and they respond well to treatment.

Immediate care of the dog and cat with IMHA

Development of acute anaemia may cause **cardiovascular compromise**, resulting in life-threatening disease. Various measures can be instituted, even while diagnostic tests are pending.

Since most of the clinical signs caused by IMHA are related to decreased carriage of oxygen in the blood, **blood transfusion** is indicated in dogs with signs of compromise. There is no standard threshold for transfusion because this will depend on the **speed of onset of anaemia** (and the extent to which the dog has compensated), the **severity of the anaemia** and the **severity of the clinical signs**. Even dogs with relatively mild anaemia (e.g. haematocrit of 25%) may therefore benefit from transfusion if it has developed very acutely and if they show signs of cardiovascular instability (tachycardia, tachypnoea, obtundation/inability to stand or move). It is preferable to **administer packed red blood cells** to dogs with IMHA, rather than fresh whole blood, because affected animals do not require volume expansion, so the plasma included with fresh whole blood is not needed.

There is **little benefit to providing supplemental oxygen** to dogs with IMHA, unless pulmonary thromboembolism is suspected and/or the dog has respiratory distress, because the amount of oxygen dissolved in blood is a tiny fraction of the amount carried on haemoglobin molecules. The priority should therefore be to restore the ability of the blood to carry oxygen by administering a blood transfusion.

Immune-mediated thrombocytopenia (IMTP)

Investigating problems of primary haemostasis

Defects of primary haemostasis caused by platelet deficiencies are characterized by **haemorrhages**. Because the secondary coagulation system (consisting of the coagulation factors and fibrin) is usually still intact, this produces relatively mild haemorrhages from surface capillaries in the skin and mucous membranes. Nevertheless, this haemorrhage can result in severe anaemia because the gastrointestinal tract has an extremely large surface area, creating the potential for major blood loss into the gastrointestinal lumen. **Petechiae** are usually considered to be surface haemorrhages **less than 1 cm in diameter**, whereas **ecchymotic haemorrhages** have a similar appearance but are usually **>1 cm in diameter**. Common sites for these surface haemorrhages on the skin include the oral mucous membranes, inguinae and axillae, and on the concave surface (the inside) of the pinnae. These haemorrhages will frequently resolve and re-form rapidly, so owners sometimes notice these lesions for some time, sometimes weeks, but are not concerned because they always seem to resolve.

These haemorrhages may be related to **thrombocytopenia**, or a platelet function defect (**thrombocytopathia**). Thrombocytopenia is far more common and can be readily diagnosed by complete blood cell count, or even examination of a **fresh blood smear**. If the platelet count is normal, further investigations for thrombocytopathia are indicated. This can be confirmed in the first instance by performing a **buccal mucosal bleeding test (BMBT)**, which consists of making a shallow cut on a mucosal surface and then measuring the time for the haemorrhage to stop. This test is imprecise because the depth of the cut is difficult to standardize and because it is easy for the dog or veterinary surgeon to disturb the platelet plug as it forms. A **normal value of 4 minutes** is often stated for bleeding to cease, though patients with genuine defects will usually have values >10 minutes, and normal canine values <2 minutes. There is no need to perform a BMBT if the platelet count is decreased, because you have already identified a cause for the signs and the BMBT will be prolonged due to this.

In an emergency, an approximate platelet count can be obtained by examining a fresh blood smear. Count the **average number of platelets in ten different high-power fields** of the blood smear monolayer and then **multiply by 20** to obtain the estimate, expressed as $\times 10^9/l$. Take care to check for the presence of platelet clumps on the feathered edge of the smear, which will artificially decrease this estimate if present.

Thrombocytopenia

Thrombocytopenia refers to a **reduction in the normal platelet count**. The lower reference limit provided by most laboratories and analysers is approximately **$150 \times 10^9/l$**, but spontaneous haemorrhage is unlikely unless the platelet count drops below $30–50 \times 10^9/l$. It is common to see **artefactual thrombocytopenia** on complete blood cell counts due to **clumping during sampling** or in the collection tube. It is therefore essential that unexpectedly low platelet counts are confirmed by examining a blood smear to check for platelet clumps and to estimate the number of platelets per high power field. If artefacts occur repeatedly, it may be worth collecting the **blood sample into a citrate tube**, as platelet clumping is less likely with this anticoagulant and the blood sample is still suitable for all haematology analysers.

These are the major **causes of thrombocytopenia** in animals:

1. Platelet destruction: Destruction of platelets may be caused by an autoimmune response directed against **normal antigens on their surfaces.** This is the most common cause of confirmed (i.e. non-artefactual) severe thrombocytopenia in dogs. Increased consumption of platelets may also occur with thromboembolic diseases, either with formation of a single large thrombus (as with arterial or portal vein thrombi) or with disseminated intravascular coagulation (DIC), where platelets and coagulation factors are consumed. Platelet destruction may also occur with some **infectious agents**, including *Anaplasma platys*, a tick-borne organism that replicates inside platelets and causes cyclic thrombocytopenia. Many other infectious diseases are often associated with mild thrombocytopenia, including leptospirosis, *Angiostrongylus vasorum*, *Ehrlichia cani*, *Anaplasma phagocytophilum*, and *B. canis*, probably related to **increased destruction** or consumption.
2. Reduced platelet production: Reduced production of platelets implies a problem with the **bone marrow**, where platelets are released as fragments from megakaryocytes. It is unusual to see thrombocytopenia alone in animals with bone marrow diseases; instead, most patients have **multiple cytopenias**.
3. Platelet sequestration: Finally, platelets may become **sequestered inside large, blood-filled spaces**. This occurs with splenic enlargement, or with **splenic tumours**. This process is almost never sufficiently severe to result in clinical signs of defective primary haemostasis.

Diagnosing IMTP

In a dog or cat presented with thrombocytopenia and signs of defective primary haemostasis, it is important to establish whether or not this is due to immune-mediated disease.

For dogs with IMHA, this can be ascertained by testing for the presence of anti-RBC antibodies, a critical part of the pathogenesis. Similarly, IMTP is dependent on **production of antibodies** directed **against platelets**, but there are no clinical tests available to detect these in the UK. In a research setting and at some centres in Europe and the USA, it has been possible to do flow cytometry to detect antibodies bound to the surface of platelets, though these tests require careful validation because it appears some normal dogs have anti-platelet antibodies without having thrombocytopenia.

One helpful feature noted in dogs with **IMTP** is that the **platelet count is extremely low** (**$<20 \times 10^9/l$**), whereas other causes of thrombocytopenia rarely cause such severe reductions. Also, IMTP may be associated with **microplatelets**, probably for similar reasons that IMHA is associated with spherocytosis, because the cells may be partially destroyed or phagocytosed as they pass through the spleen. However, this is not a particularly sensitive finding, with many dogs with IMTP lacking this feature, and detection is highly subjective.

As with IMHA, even in a dog or cat suspected of having IMTP, it is important to determine whether there could be an **underlying cause for the disease**. Again, the number and nature of the tests performed will vary depending on the characteristics of the individual case.

The more common **underlying causes** for IMTP include **cancer** (particularly lymphoma and other lymphoproliferative diseases), **infectious diseases** (especially *A. phagocytophilum*, *E. canis* and *B. canis*), and exposure to **drugs and toxins**.

Consequently, **tests** that should be considered in dogs with suspected IMTP include **imaging** of the thorax and abdomen, and **serology or PCR** for the various infectious agents described above. Consider, however, that even if an abdominal mass were identified, it would probably not be possible to sample it by fine-needle aspiration/biopsy due to the risk of subsequent haemorrhage. If taking a urine sample from a dog with IMTP, it should not be collected by cystocentesis due to the risk of haemorrhage.

Variants of IMTP

Angiostrongylus vasorum has become increasingly prevalent in the UK. Clinically, lungworm infestation is often associated with **mild thrombocytopenia** but it appears that it may cause **IMTP in a small proportion of cases**. In cases like this, however, it is difficult to establish whether the lungworm caused the disease or simply whether it was present at the same time. Many clinicians now perform a test (either SNAP test on blood or Baermann flotation of a faecal sample) to exclude the possibility of lungworm infestation in dogs with suspected IMTP.

A recent study suggested that some dogs with IMTP have a **'non-regenerative' form**, where the **megakaryocytes in the bone marrow** are also targeted and **destroyed**. These dogs had a **poorer prognosis**, were more likely to require blood transfusion and were more likely to be anaemic at the time of presentation, compared to dogs that had normal numbers of megakaryocytes in the bone marrow. The authors of the study suggested that bone marrow aspirates could be used to categorize dogs into regenerative and non-regenerative forms, but this is clearly associated with some risk in collecting the sample in a dog that may be, or is at risk of, anaemia. Additionally, it is unclear whether different types of treatment could or should be used in dogs with these two different forms of disease, so the diagnostic testing may not change the therapeutic approach.

IMTP in the cat

Primary IMTP is rarely reported in the cat and is **much less common** than in the dog. A recent study of cats with thrombocytopenia at a single hospital in the UK revealed that 19% of cases with a final diagnosis were attributed to immune-mediated disease, but several of these cats had evidence of concurrent immune-mediated haemolysis. However, similar to dogs, cats with IMTP were more likely to have **severe thrombocytopenia**, with an average value of **19×10^9/l,** compared to cats with other causes of thrombocytopenia.

Other underlying causes of thrombocytopenia should be considered in cats, particularly FeLV and feline immunodeficiency virus infections, even though the prevalence of both viruses has been declining in the UK.

Immediate treatment of IMTP

Dogs with confirmed thrombocytopenia should be handled carefully, and **jugular venepuncture avoided**. When blood samples are obtained, it is usually necessary to apply pressure for longer to prevent haemorrhage from the site.

Since most **blood loss occurs through the gastrointestinal tract** in dogs with IMTP (as melaena), it is advisable to administer a gastric acid suppressant, such as omeprazole at 1 mg/kg IV BID.

Dogs with IMTP and anaemia will often require **blood transfusion** to replace the red blood cells that are lost. Indeed, if there is severe melaena, dogs with IMTP may be transfusion-dependent for several days, requiring three or more units of blood, until a response to immunosuppressive treatment is seen.

There are currently no viable options to administer platelets to thrombocytopenic dogs. **Platelets** have a very short half-life and are **easily damaged** or activated by contact with artificial surfaces, so the platelets present in fresh whole blood are usually damaged as they are administered, or lost within a few hours of the transfusion. Similarly, packed red blood cell units contain very few platelets. In some specialist centres, it is possible to produce **platelet-rich plasma** (PRP, which is different from fresh frozen plasma [FFP], which does not contain platelets), or a **lyophilized platelet concentrate**, but these are not currently being produced in the UK.

In a dog with a strong suspicion of underlying **vector-borne disease**, it would be appropriate to administer **doxycycline** until test results are available.

Immune-mediated neutropenia (IMNP)

Investigation of neutropenia

As with thrombocytopenia and anaemia, neutropenia may be caused by either **decreased production** of neutrophils in the bone marrow or **increased consumption** or **destruction of neutrophils** in the periphery. If the neutropenia is caused by peripheral destruction, the bone marrow responds by increasing production and by releasing **immature (band) neutrophils** into the circulation, producing the typical appearance of a '**left shift**'.

Perhaps the most common cause of neutropenia is related to severe **bacterial infections** and **sepsis**, where neutrophils are consumed rapidly in trying to control the infection. This clearly complicates the diagnostic process, because it is often difficult to establish whether an **infection is the cause or result** of the neutropenia. It is important to collect diagnostic samples prior to starting antimicrobials.

Investigation of sepsis

To exclude sepsis or a septic focus in a dog with neutropenia, it is common to try to consider the following investigations:

- **Imaging of the thorax and abdomen** to look for particular foci, such as an abscess, foreign body, developing pyothorax or discospondylitis (including collection of a sterile urine sample by cystocentesis for culture).
- Collection of **sterile samples** from any other **site that appears abnormal**, such as any swollen joints, which could indicate septic arthritis, or CSF if the dog has neck/spinal pain.
- **Echocardiography** to look for vegetative lesions on the heart valves, which would be indicative of endocarditis.
- Collection of three or more blood samples in a sterile fashion for **blood culture**. The sensitivity of blood cultures is relatively low, so it is important to collect a relatively large volume of blood (5–10 ml per sample) and to place this into a blood culture bottle. The sample is usually collected by sterile technique, with clipping and preparation of the skin over the vein and with the phlebotomist wearing sterile gloves.

Diagnosing IMNP

The **pathogenesis** of immune-mediated neutropenia (IMNP) is **similar to that of IMTP and IMHA**–an autoimmune response is mounted against normal antigens on the surface of neutrophils, resulting in production of antibodies that opsonize the cells, facilitating their phagocytosis and removal by phagocytes in the spleen. However, just as with thrombocytopenia, there are **no specific diagnostic tests** available in the UK for detection of anti-neutrophil antibodies. This test has been described and validated in dogs at a centre in the USA (using flow cytometry), and this is the test that would be performed in a person with suspected IMNP.

Diagnosis of IMNP therefore relies on **exclusion of other causes** of neutropenia. Aside from the investigations described, this would include testing for vector-borne pathogens, of which the most likely to cause neutropenia would be chronic infection with *E. canis*. In addition, most clinicians would recommend **sampling the bone marrow** to exclude bone marrow pathology and/or neoplasia. As for IMTP and IMHA, investigations would also be indicated to exclude any underlying cause for IMNP, though these largely overlap with the tests used to rule out a septic focus (especially imaging of the thorax and abdomen). Finally, approximately **25% of dogs** with IMNP are reported to have **concurrent thrombocytopenia** that also seems to be immune-mediated, so observing concurrent neutropenia and thrombocytopenia may increase suspicion for immune-mediated disease.

Combinations of immune-mediated haematological diseases

It is not uncommon to see dogs with combinations of immune-mediated haemolytic anaemia, thrombocytopenia and neutropenia, possibly due to an autoimmune response directed against antigens expressed by several types of blood cell. In a dog where this is suspected, the clinical approach is similar to that described for the individual diseases, with tests used to confirm the presence of pathogenic antibodies (if possible), followed by exclusion of underlying causes.

Immune-mediated polyarthritis (IMPA)

The most useful test for the investigation of **joint effusions** is to **sample the synovial fluid**, which will usually provide a definitive diagnosis on cytological examination. Samples of synovial fluid can be obtained easily from all of the more distal joints (carpi, tarsi and stifles). In dogs where immune-mediated polyarthritis (IMPA) is suspected, it is recommended to **sample at least three different** joints to prove that the dog really has similar inflammation in multiple joints. Because immune-mediated arthritis typically causes more severe changes in the more distal joints, **sampling both carpi and both tarsi** is recommended even though the stifles are easier to sample.

After collection, the fluid should be analysed. Its gross appearance is helpful in estimating whether the fluid is normal or not. **Normal synovial fluid should be colourless or a light straw colour, and it should be viscous**, forming a tendril if you press it between two fingers and then separate them. Most normal joints

Table 2.4. Results for the major parameters measured in synovial fluid in dogs with various diseases.

Parameter	Normal synovial fluid	Osteoarthritis	Septic arthritis	Immune-mediated arthritis
Colour, consistency	Clear/pale straw	Clear/pale straw	Dark yellow/red, turbid	Pale or dark straw, turbid
Viscosity	Viscous	Viscous	Watery	Watery
Volume	Minimal (0.1–0.3 ml)	Possibly slightly increased	Greatly increased (0.5–1 ml)	Increased (0.5 ml or more)
Nucleated cell count (cells/ml)	<2500	2000–4000	>10,000 (usually >100,000)	>5000
Protein concentration (g/l)	0.2–0.25	0.2–0.25	Increased	Increased

will also typically yield a very small volume of fluid, certainly <0.5 ml.

If there is only a small amount of fluid, small drops should be put on several **microscope slides, smeared and allowed to dry**. If there is more fluid available, this should be put into an **EDTA tube** for measurement of the total cell count and protein concentration. Finally, a small amount of fluid should be submitted for **bacterial culture** if septic arthritis is considered possible. This can be done by placing a drop of the fluid onto a **charcoal swab**, or by injecting some fluid into a blood culture bottle. A detailed description of the clinical presentation will aid the pathologist making their interpretation.

Analysis of synovial fluid

Table 2.4 provides results for the major parameters measured in synovial fluid in dogs with various diseases.

Types of IMPA

Immune-mediated polyarthritis is commonly divided into **erosive** and **non-erosive types**. Erosive arthritis causes **lytic damage** to the subchondral bone in the joint, and this is usually associated with **more severe clinical signs** and deformity of the affected joints if left untreated. It is unclear whether non-erosive cases of IMPA would develop into erosive lesions if left untreated, or whether this genuinely reflects a difference in the underlying (auto)immune response. Erosive lesions can usually be readily detected on plain radiographs of the joints, particularly the carpi and tarsi.

Historically, **erosive IMPA** has been considered a similar disease to rheumatoid arthritis (RhA) in people, but it does not closely resemble the human disease and is not associated with the systemic complications that are frequently observed in the human. Consequently, it is preferable to describe this syndrome as '**erosive polyarthritis**' in dogs, rather than RhA. In dogs suspected of erosive polyarthritis, it is possible to submit serum samples for measurement of **rheumatoid factor** (**RF**). Rheumatoid factor refers to IgM antibodies in the serum that are specific for other antibodies; these antibodies are probably not particularly important in development of the disease, but they can be used as **markers of the disease**. As with the direct antiglobulin test for IMHA, the test is reported as a titre, with **high titres** indicating **large amounts of rheumatoid factor** are present, and low titres indicating only small amounts. Unlike most DAT tests available at commercial laboratories, the validity of tests for rheumatoid factor is questionable because some healthy dogs may have these antibodies and because the cut-off for diagnosis of disease has not been established. Furthermore, a positive RF factor result does not appear to prompt any change in treatment compared to non-erosive IMPA.

If the arthritis is **non-erosive**, which is **more common**, the disease may be classified in several ways according to its possible cause. Because there may be underlying causes for IMPA, as with other types of immune-mediated disease, the following classification system was suggested in the 1980s for dogs with IMPA:

- Type 1: **No underlying cause detected**. This is the most common type.
- Type 2: Related to underlying **bacterial infection**, including pyometra, bacterial prostatitis, pyelonephritis or severe pyoderma. This is sometimes called 'reactive arthritis'.
- Type 3: Related to underlying **gastrointestinal disease**, particularly pancreatitis or inflammatory bowel disease. This is sometimes called 'enteropathic arthritis'.
- Type 4: Related to underlying **neoplasia**.

This is primarily a descriptive classification system, and the critical point is that many different diseases may increase the risk of developing IMPA by causing the production of immune complexes, which may then become deposited in the joints and stimulate an inflammatory reaction.

It is important to exclude the underlying causes of IMPA by performing additional tests. The exact tests should be based on the individual case, and its risk factors but would often include **complete blood count** and **biochemical profile** (to look for other organ dysfunction), **imaging** of the thorax and abdomen (to exclude mass lesions) and **infectious disease testing** (see next section).

If there is a strong suspicion of IMPA and if costs allow, these investigations can be combined with the initial diagnostics to reduce the number of episodes of sedation or anaesthesia. For example, the dog could be sedated or anaesthetized for concurrent synovial fluid sampling, imaging of the thorax and abdomen and radiography of a peripheral joint to look for erosive lesions. As discussed later, a CSF tap could be performed at the same time in dogs suspected of having both steroid-responsive meningitis arteritis (SRMA) and IMPA.

Up to **10% of dogs with IMPA** may have **concurrent proteinuria**, which may be related to concurrent immune-mediated **glomerulonephritis**. Consider obtaining a urine sample at the same time as the initial investigations to determine whether there is significant proteinuria that may require treatment beyond that needed for IMPA alone.

Infectious causes of IMPA

There is a clear association between some infectious agents and development of IMPA. In particular, this is a common feature of clinical **leishmaniosis in dogs** that have travelled to, or been imported from, southern Europe. Indeed, *Leishmania* organisms can often be seen on cytological examination of synovial fluid samples from dogs with this disease.

IMPA can also be observed with *E. canis* and *A. phagocytophilum*, and dogs with a history of travel to Europe or exposure to ticks in the UK should be tested for these agents.

IMPA in the cat

Immune-mediated polyarthritis may occur in the cat, but appears to be much **less common** than in the dog. A particular clinical syndrome, called **periosteal proliferative polyarthritis (PPP)**, has been reported to occur most commonly in young adult male neutered cats. This disease causes erosive lesions, particularly affecting the **distal joints (carpi and tarsi)** and also causes formation of new periosteal bone around these joints, which is not a common feature of rheumatoid arthritis or IMPA.

Polyarthritis may occur occasionally in cats with virulent **calicivirus infection**, and may also occur as a reaction to **calicivirus vaccines** in a small proportion of kittens after the first vaccine course.

Polyarthritis in association with other immune-mediated diseases

Inflammation of the peripheral joints may be a feature in up to **30% of dogs with SRMA**. This is also an immune-mediated disease that causes inflammation of the meninges, resulting in stiffness, neck and spinal pain and pyrexia. These signs are evidently very similar to those seen with IMPA, particularly since IMPA can also affect the joints of the spine, also causing neck and spinal pain, but the neck pain observed with SRMA is usually much more severe than with IMPA alone. In dogs presented with joint effusions and neck/spinal pain, it is therefore common to consider **sampling the CSF** to determine whether there is concurrent inflammation in the subarachnoid space.

Immediate treatment of IMPA in the dog and cat

After collection of synovial fluid and other diagnostic samples, there is often some delay in awaiting the results of synovial fluid analysis and other tests. In this time, the dog usually has clear signs of illness but it is **not recommended to administer immunosuppressive medications** in case the dog does turn out to have septic arthritis or an infectious cause for the polyarthritis. However, it is possible to give some treatment that would be safe and improve quality of life.

Paracetamol can be administered as an effective analgesic and antipyretic. This is a good choice for analgesia because it can be used at the same time as corticosteroids, whereas conventional NSAIDs should not be used concurrently with corticosteroids due to the risk of gastrointestinal side effects. Additional analgesia can be administered using opioids if required. If there is a strong suspicion of septic arthritis, it would also be appropriate to administer antimicrobials while awaiting the results of the culture samples.

In dogs where there is a strong suspicion of IMPA, it is possible to administer an **anti-inflammatory dose of a corticosteroid**. This will not resolve all of the clinical signs but should still be safe even if an infectious agent is present because it will not result in marked immunosuppression. Suitable doses would be 0.05 mg/kg dexamethasone IV once daily, OR 0.5 mg/kg prednisolone orally once daily.

Systemic immune-mediated disease

Immune-mediated diseases may be characterized by autoimmune responses directed against several different antigens, or against **antigens shared by several different tissues**. This results in immune-mediated diseases that affect multiple different tissues, often referred to as **multi-systemic immune-mediated diseases**. Examples include the combination of IMHA and IMTP, producing a condition sometimes called Evans syndrome. IMNP may also occur with IMTP.

Endocrine polyglandular autoimmune diseases

Several endocrine diseases are caused by autoimmune responses directed against single **antigens exclusively expressed within an endocrine organ**, including most cases of **hypothyroidism** in dogs (caused by lymphocytic thyroiditis and often accompanied by production of anti-thyroglobulin antibodies), **hypoadrenocorticism** (caused by lymphocytic adrenalitis), **hypoparathyroidism** (caused by lymphocytic parathyroiditis) and (insulin-dependent) **diabetes mellitus** (associated with an immune response that causes destruction of the beta cells of the islets of Langerhans). In some cases, combinations of endocrine diseases may occur in the same individual, producing an autoimmune polyglandular syndrome.

In people, these syndromes are related to variants or mutations in genes that regulate the immune system, producing distinct clinical syndromes described as type 1 and type 2 autoimmune polyglandular syndromes (APS).

- Type 1 APS is characterized by concurrent adrenal insufficiency, hypoparathyroidism and decreased gonadal function. This syndrome is related to mutations in the AIRE gene, which regulates the expression of self-antigens in the thymus during selection of immature T cells, and a similar disease has not been described in dogs.
- Type 2 APS is characterized by concurrent hypoadrenocorticism and hypothyroidism, and this has been reported a number of times in dogs of several breeds, including individual Dobermann pinschers and Boxers. The causative mutation is not known for this syndrome in people or dogs, and it is not known whether the pathogenesis of the disease is similar in the two species.

Systemic lupus erythematosus

Systemic lupus erythematosus (SLE) is a complex disease of people and animals associated with **autoimmune responses directed against multiple tissues within the body**. The autoimmune response is typically directed **against nuclear antigens** that are shared by all cells in the body, explaining the extremely wide range of clinical syndromes observed with this disease. This may also make the disease difficult to diagnose because it produces clinical signs associated with many other (autoimmune) diseases. Indeed, in people, the diagnosis is made only if a certain number of key criteria associated with the disease are present.

Immunologically, SLE is associated with production of antibodies against cellular components, formation of immune complexes that may be deposited in the glomeruli and joints, and with T-cell reactions to normal antigens. The disease therefore demonstrates all of the major immunological effector mechanisms that can be implicated in causing tissue damage.

A syndrome resembling human SLE has been reported sporadically in dogs, but it is not clear whether the immunological processes occurring in dogs are similar to those in people, or whether this is a different form of multi-systemic disease. Using the criteria specified in human medicine for diagnosis of SLE, the disease would appear to be extremely rare in dogs, though many more cases are described as 'SLE-like' because they have clinical features that are suggestive. In particular, a form of 'SLE-like' disease appears to affect Nova Scotia duck tolling retrievers in Scandinavia.

The **common clinical features** observed in people with SLE include:

- **Fever** (which may be intermittent) and generalized lymph node enlargement.
- **Haemolytic anaemia and/or thrombocytopenia**, related to production of anti-red blood cell and/or platelet antibodies, respectively.
- **Polyarthritis**, related to formation of immune complexes that becomes deposited in the synovial capillaries.
- **Glomerulonephritis**, resulting in significant proteinuria related to the deposition of immune complexes in the glomeruli.
- **Ulcerative skin lesions**, or ulcers within the mouth, especially on the tongue. This may be accompanied by diffuse, oedematous swelling of the limbs, which is suggestive for concurrent vasculitis.
- Other rare features include inflammation of **multiple muscles** (polymyositis) or of body cavities (serositis), and neurological signs, including seizures.

SLE should therefore be suspected in any dog that is presented with a combination of these signs, though the most common abnormalities are polyarthritis with concurrent skin lesions.

Diagnosis of SLE

Establishing a diagnosis of SLE relies on **confirming the presence of more than one immunological syndrome**, in addition to a **positive titre** in an antinuclear antibody (ANA) test or detection of lupus erythematosus (LE) cells.

ANA test: Like the direct antiglobulin (DAT, Coombs') test for IMHA, the ANA test provides evidence of **antibodies directed against nuclear antigens**, which is a central part of the pathogenesis of SLE. However, as with other immunological tests available in veterinary medicine, the method used differs between laboratories and cut-off values to define a positive result have **not been established definitively** because the disease is so rare.

The test is performed by adding the patient's serum to cells (usually sections of normal rat liver) and then washing and staining the sections for any canine antibodies that have bound to the tissue. The detection of antibodies binding to nuclei of the hepatocytes is diagnostic for SLE, and this may occur with either a homogenous pattern (where the whole nucleus is stained uniformly) or a speckled pattern (where only certain parts of the nucleus are stained). The **pattern of staining** may have **diagnostic significance**, as the homogenous pattern is apparently associated with more severe, multi-systemic signs whereas the speckled pattern is associated with fever and musculoskeletal signs.

The ANA test result is **reported as a titre**, with increasing dilutions of the patient's serum used to run the test to determine whether the positive result is still obtained at low concentrations. As with the DAT, **high titre results (i.e. >1/640) indicate that more antibodies** are present and provide a more robust diagnosis of SLE. Low titres (<1/100) may be observed in normal dogs or those with other inflammatory diseases, so the diagnosis should not be based on a low titre in the absence of the other clinical features.

LE test: **LE cells are phagocytes** (neutrophils or macrophages) that have ingested entire nuclei and which can be **observed within the cytoplasm by cytology**. These cells are most readily detected in phagocytes on cytological examination of **synovial fluid** samples. As with the ANA test, the presence of LE cells confirms the presence of an immune response directed against nuclear antigens and which is resulting in phagocytosis of entire nuclei. In human medicine, the ANA test is considered to be much more sensitive than detection of LE cells in sampled fluids and has largely superseded this test. However, synovial fluid would usually be sampled in the dog with evidence of multiple joint effusions, and it is worthwhile to let the pathologist know if there are other features suggestive for SLE so that they can examine the submitted slides carefully.

Underlying causes of SLE

In dogs with features suggestive for SLE, it is worthwhile pursuing investigations to **assess the severity** of disease and to determine whether there could be any **underlying cause.** This is important because **SLE is associated with a relatively poor prognosis** compared to other immune-mediated diseases, so it is important to determine how many body systems are affected because this may lead to a decision for euthanasia rather than attempting treatment.

Recommended investigations for dogs with suspected SLE include:

- Tests to confirm the diagnosis
  - **Complete blood count** (to determine whether the red blood cell and platelet counts are normal).
  - Examination of a **blood smear**, or DAT or detection of agglutination in saline (to determine whether any anaemia is immune-mediated).
  - **Aspirates from effused joints** (for cytological examination as described for IMPA, but with particular emphasis on searching for LE cells).
  - Submission of blood for **ANA titre**.
  - It is recommended to perform **urinalysis** to determine whether the dog does have proteinuria and, if so, the severity using a **urine protein/ creatinine ratio**.
- **Imaging** of the thorax and abdomen.
- Testing for relevant **infectious disease agents** to determine whether there is an underlying cause for the immune-mediated disease.

Occasionally, a syndrome resembling SLE has been reported in dogs treated with penicillamine, and in cats that have received propylthiouracil for the treatment of hyperthyroidism. Both drugs are now rarely used, and an SLE-like syndrome is therefore rarely encountered with either product.

Shar-Pei fever: an autoinflammatory disease

Some immune-mediated diseases are caused by inappropriate activity of the innate immune system, without activation of the adaptive immune response. Shar Pei fever, now also called Shar Pei autoinflammatory disease (SPAID), is a good example of the latter group in veterinary medicine.

The exact aetiopathogenesis of SPAID is still the subject of debate. A recent genetic linkage study suggested that it is associated with a mutation in a gene encoding for an anti-inflammatory protein (MTBP, which stands for MDM2-binding protein). It is suggested that the absence of this anti-inflammatory activity predisposes Shar Pei dogs to development of bouts of systemic inflammation, causing the typical signs. Previously, it was suggested that the disease could be related to dysregulation of the genes encoding hyaluronic acid, a component of the normal dermal matrix. This theory seemed to explain why Shar Pei dogs with particularly marked skin folds (the 'meat mouth' appearance) had more severe inflammatory disease.

Whatever the underlying cause or mutation, SPAID results in **increased concentrations of the pro-inflammatory cytokine interleukin-6 (IL-6)** in the blood, which drives the acute phase response. This happens **episodically**, so affected dogs may have long periods where they appear clinically normal, followed by bouts of inflammation. These may also be subclinical and cause only **transient lethargy** or other vague signs.

One of the acute phase proteins induced by IL-6 is **serum amyloid A**, which may form insoluble deposits because the protein has a beta pleated sheet structure. These amyloid deposits may accumulate in multiple organs, ultimately causing **organ dysfunction**. In the Shar Pei, the most important outcome of this process is **renal amyloidosis**, characterized by deposits of amyloid in the medulla of the kidneys. This causes **severe proteinuria** and, ultimately, azotaemia and renal failure. When such dogs are examined post-mortem, however, amyloid deposits are usually found in multiple organs, particularly the gastrointestinal tract, liver, adrenal glands and skin.

It is possible to measure the serum concentration of serum amyloid A (SAA) in dogs, but because this does not correspond to tissue amyloid deposits, this **test has limited usefulness** to predict whether dogs with SPAID will ultimately develop renal failure or other forms of amyloid-related disease.

Treatment of SPAID

There is **no specific treatment** available for SPAID in dogs. Similar diseases are treated in people using therapeutic antibodies directed against IL-6, neutralizing the cytokine and halting the inflammation. Monoclonal antibody therapies are just starting to be produced in dogs, but there is no similar treatment available for SPAID. Human products rarely work in different species due to the high specificity of antibodies, which recognize a very small region of their target molecules that may differ between species.

Instead, treatment of SPAID largely consists of **supportive care** using **non-steroidal anti-inflammatory drugs** to control pyrexia when required. Treatment with corticosteroids is not recommended. Some authors have suggested that affected dogs should receive **colchicine**, which is a drug intended to slow the development of fibrosis, but there is currently no evidence to suggest that this slows the development of amyloidosis. Affected dogs should be **monitored for development of proteinuria**, and appropriate therapies should be introduced as soon as this is detected, including **ACE inhibitors** or angiotensin receptor antagonists, a moderately **protein-restricted diet** and **control of hypertension** if this develops concurrently.

Treatment of immune-mediated disease

Glucocorticoids

Introduction to corticosteroids

Endogenous corticosteroids with glucocorticoid action (particularly cortisol) are **produced** in the zona fasciculata of the **adrenal cortex**. Their major physiological role is in **adaptation to stress**, which includes modulation of the immune system.

Endogenous and exogenous corticosteroids bind to the glucococorticoid receptor, which is present in the cytoplasm of most cells. After binding to the corticosteroid, the receptor complex translocates into the nucleus of the cell, where it interacts with particular sequences of DNA called **glucocorticoid response elements (GREs)**. Binding of the receptor to these GREs causes widespread changes in gene expression, producing **many effects on cellular metabolism, hormonal regulation and the immune system**.

Different corticosteroids have **different ratios of glucocorticoid action** (meaning their ability to bind to the glucocorticoid receptor) and **mineralocorticoid action** (meaning their ability to bind to the mineralocorticoid receptor). For example, for **dexamethasone**, the ratio of glucocorticoid to mineralocorticoid activity is 30/1, explaining why it is used as an immunomodulatory drug, whereas **fludrocortisone** has a ratio of approximately 1/12, explaining why it was traditionally used for treatment of hypoadrenocorticism.

Glucocorticoids exert the following immunomodulatory effects:

- **Decreased production of inflammatory cytokines**: The production of many pro-inflammatory cytokines is decreased by glucocorticoids, particularly TNF-α and IL-2.
- **Decreased expression of Fc receptors on macrophages**: Fc receptors are used by macrophages and other cells to phagocytose cells marked by antibodies, increasing the efficiency of phagocytosis. Decreased expression of these receptors therefore decreases the likelihood of phagocytosis, even if the target is opsonized by antibodies.
- **Decreased production of inflammatory mediators**: Glucocorticoids inhibit the activity of phospholipase A2, which catalyses the first step in the production of prostaglandins and leukotrienes from the fatty acid arachidonic acid.

Problems associated with use of glucocorticoids in animals

Glucocorticoids suppress the endogenous adrenocortical axis, reducing production of cortisol and related hormones. Consequently, if glucocorticoids are withdrawn rapidly, there is a risk of causing **iatrogenic hypoadrenocorticism**, which may resemble the spontaneous disease. This is one of the reasons why the dose of glucocorticoid drugs is usually gradually tapered before stopping, to ensure that endogenous production of cortisol is restored.

The **adverse effects** of glucocorticoids are well known and include polyuria, polydipsia, polyphagia, excessive panting, muscle wastage, weakness, lethargy, anxiety and changes to the skin. Dermatological changes include thinning of the skin, formation of visible striae, development of symmetrical alopecia of the flanks, increased risk of pyoderma and, rarely, calcinosis cutis.

When treating dogs with immune-mediated diseases, it is essential to **strike a sensible balance** between control of the underlying disease and glucocorticoid-related side effects, because side effects of treatment are a frequently cited reason for euthanasia among owners of dogs with immune-mediated diseases.

Glucocorticoid resistance

Approximately 30% of human patients are said to be '**glucocorticoid resistant**', meaning that the typical immunomodulatory effects of the drugs are not seen at standard dosages. There appear to be several different reasons for this phenomenon, including polymorphisms in the glucocorticoid receptor gene, altering the affinity of the drugs for the receptor. There may also be variations in the expression of efflux pumps, such as P glycoprotein, which remove the drugs from particular tissues. It is known that P glycoprotein is expressed at higher levels in the small intestine of dogs with inflammatory bowel disease compared to healthy dogs, suggesting that the intestine may become less sensitive in some affected dogs to the effects of glucocorticoids.

There are no tests available in veterinary medicine to determine whether dogs are 'glucocorticoid resistant', but this might be suspected in cases that fail to show typical biochemical or haematological changes after administration of the drugs at standard dose rates.

Use of glucocorticoids for immune-mediated disease

After diagnosis of IMHA, ITP, IMNP, IMPA, erosive arthritis, SRMA and SLE, and exclusion of underlying causes, **primary treatment is normally started with glucocorticoids**. For all of these diseases an initial dose rate of **2–3 mg/kg of prednisolone per day is appropriate**, either administered as a single daily dose or divided into two doses. Traditionally, higher doses of prednisolone have been reported (even up to 8 mg/kg/day), but there is no evidence to suggest that such high doses are more effective, whereas they will produce more severe adverse effects.

In **larger dogs (greater than 25 kg bodyweight)**, many clinicians prefer to calculate a dose rate according to the **body surface area** rather than the bodyweight, because this may give a more accurate reflection of the rate of metabolism. With this approach, an appropriate starting dose would be 50–60 mg/m^2/day. A bodyweight/surface area conversion is available in the back of most formularies.

As with other indications, it is recommended that **prednisolone is administered with food**. If the dog is inappetant, a starting dose of 0.2–0.4 mg/kg dexamethasone IV once daily (usually the sodium phosphate preparation) may be administered. Again, there is no evidence to suggest that a higher dose or more frequent administration of this drug will result in a better outcome or faster response for any of the diseases listed above.

This starting dose of prednisolone (or dexamethasone) is usually **maintained until the dog shows signs of a response**, which will vary depending on the disease being treated. For example, with IMHA or ITP, this would mean that the red blood cell or platelet counts were stable or increasing, and other features, such as agglutination, spherocytosis and hyperbilirubinaemia, were also improving. Irrespective of this, many clinicians would not use a dose of prednisolone above 2 mg/kg/day for more than 1 week, due to the risk of incurring severe side effects.

Following confirmation of a response to treatment, the dose of the glucocorticoid drug is gradually decreased until it can be stopped. With most of the immune-mediated diseases of dogs, a total course of **4–8 months of treatment** with a glucocorticoid agent would be expected, but more prolonged or lifelong treatment may be expected with some diseases, particularly SLE and erosive arthritis.

Typically, if the dog continues to make good progress the dose of prednisolone would be **decreased by 25–33% every 3 weeks**. Before each dose reduction, it is important to confirm that the disease is continuing to respond. For IMHA or ITP, this means that a **complete blood cell count should be checked before the dose reduction**, or, for IMPA, the joints should be carefully palpated at these intervals. In the later stages of treatment, it is advisable to increase the **dosing interval to every other day** when making further reductions, because this allows endogenous adrenocortical hormone production to recover more quickly.

Once the prednisolone dose has been decreased to **0.25 mg/kg every other day or lower**, it is **safe to stop treatment** provided there has been no recurrence of disease while treating at this low dose, and providing the dose has been decreased incrementally as described above.

The most important component of the monitoring of this drug therapy consists of owner observations of the side effects observed, and changes noted on physical examination. Beyond this, it is also advisable to consider **periodic urine sampling** (by cystocentesis) to check for possible urinary tract infection. With glucocorticoid treatment, such infections are often occult and may progress to cause pyelonephritis without clinical signs. Although bacteriuria in the absence of clinical signs would not typically necessitate antimicrobial therapy, many clinicians would introduce this in dogs receiving immunosuppressive drugs.

Glucocorticoids in the cat

Cats are **relatively more resistant to the effects** and adverse effects of glucocorticoids compared to dogs or people, so starting doses are typically higher in this species. For prednisolone, a **starting dose of 4 mg/kg per day** would be appropriate, with the intention to decrease this gradually as described for dogs.

Cats are more prone to **volume overload** than dogs, and this can become a problem because most corticosteroids have some **mineralocorticoid activity**. For example, administration of large doses of prednisolone to cats may cause some **sodium retention**, expanding the **extracellular fluid volume** and causing volume overload. If there is an underlying cardiomyopathy, or concurrent anaemia, administration of glucocorticoids may therefore be a risk factor for development of **fulminant heart failure**, which typically occurs within a few days of starting the drugs. Particular care should therefore be taken in cats with known or suspected cardiac disease, and it may be possible to treat such patients with **dexamethasone in preference to prednisolone** because it has a higher ratio of glucocorticoid: mineralocorticoid activity.

Among the side effects displayed by cats receiving glucocorticoids, **diabetes mellitus** occurs more commonly in this species than in dogs. This is diagnosed by finding concurrent hyperglycaemia and glycosuria, with consistent clinical signs. This complication is still rare in the population of cats receiving glucocorticoids. Glucocorticoid-related diabetes mellitus often requires treatment with insulin, but it may be possible to achieve diabetic remission when the dose of prednisolone is decreased. For the same reason, there is also a risk of inducing hypoglycaemic episodes when the dose of prednisolone is decreased, because this ameliorates the insulin resistant state.

Polypharmacy

In an effort to decrease the occurrence of adverse effects and their impact on quality of life, many clinicians will **start another immunosuppressive drug** at the same time as prednisolone in a patient diagnosed with an immune-mediated disease. For all of these diseases, there is **no evidence** to suggest that introducing a second drug from the outset will improve the outcome or result in a faster response to treatment, but this approach is adopted so that a lower dose of prednisolone can be used from the outset, or so that the dose of prednisolone can be decreased more quickly or in larger increments than would otherwise be possible.

Although this approach seems sensible, combining immunosuppressive drugs with different mechanisms of action may **increase the risk of opportunistic infections**, or result in unpredictable drug interactions that alter the efficacy of the therapy.

Ciclosporin

Within target cells, ciclosporin binds to proteins called cyclophilins in the cytoplasm, and the complex of cyclophilin/ciclosporin then inhibits a calcium-dependent phosphatase called calcineurin. Ciclosporin and its related drugs are therefore often described as '**calcineurin inhibitors**'. Calcineurin normally activates a transcription factor, NFAT, which promotes the expression of pro-inflammatory cytokines, particularly IL-2. By inhibiting calcineurin, ciclosporin therefore decreases the activation of NFAT and **decreases the production of IL-2 and other cytokines**.

This process is particularly important in T cells because they are dependent on IL-2 for survival and proliferation after they recognize their MHC-peptide complex. **Ciclosporin has a lesser effect on B cells**, but it still decreases the production of antibodies when administered because B cells require T-cell help for optimal antibody production.

Ciclosporin is poorly absorbed across the gastrointestinal tract, and its absorption is further impaired if it is administered with food. It is therefore preferable to **administer it on an empty stomach** providing this does not cause unacceptable adverse effects.

Administration

There is preliminary evidence to suggest that ciclosporin is more effective if given twice daily, at a dose of

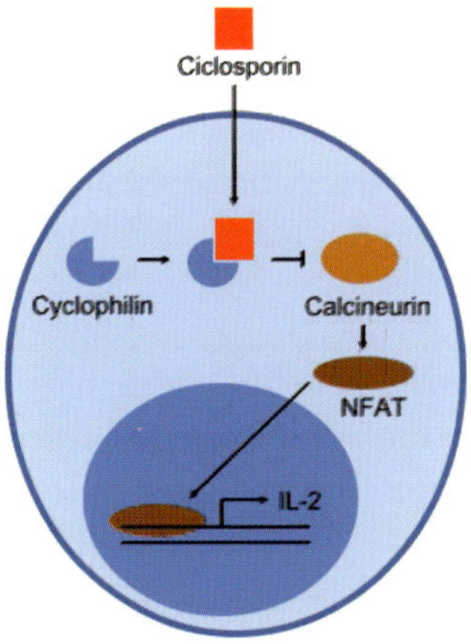

Figure 2.4. Schematic diagram of the mechanism of action of the drug ciclosporin. Ciclosporin binds to cyclophilin molecules in the cytoplasm; this complex inhibits the signalling molecule calcineurin, which normally activates T cells via the transcription factor NFAT. The inability to produce interleukin (IL)-2 prevents T cells from dividing and differentiating into effector cells.

5 mg/kg PO BID. However, due to its poor absorption and variable effect among individual animals, it is possible to consider two forms of monitoring to ensure that a therapeutic dose is achieved.

Pharmacokinetic monitoring involves measuring the **trough concentration** of the drug in serum, **immediately before the next dose** is due. This can reveal whether a dog has problems with absorbing the drug if the concentration is extremely low. However, this type of monitoring has fallen out of favour because it is clear that the same serum concentrations have very different effects in different individual dogs.

As a result, it is more useful to consider pharmacodynamic monitoring for the effects of ciclosporin. This refers to measuring an effect of the drug and increasing its concentration until the desired effect is achieved. For ciclosporin, it is possible to measure the expression of the IL-2 gene in blood of treated dogs and determine whether this is being suppressed. If not, the concentration can be increased until this is achieved. Conversely, if excessive suppression is seen, the dose may be decreased. This test is currently available through Mississippi State University in the USA.

Side effects

The most common adverse effects of ciclosporin are **vomiting and diarrhoea**, which are usually acute and self-limiting. Development of these complications does not usually necessitate withdrawal of the drug, but it may be administered with food to try to decrease the likelihood of this problem. However, as mentioned previously, this may interfere with the absorption of the drug and result in unpredictable effects. Alternatively, the drug can be **frozen before administration**, which reduces the likelihood of side effects but does not interfere with its pharmacokinetic parameters.

Occasionally, prolonged administration of ciclosporin may cause **gingival overgrowth** and **reactivation of papilloma virus**, resulting in multiple oral or cutaneous papillomas. In extremely rare cases, ciclosporin may cause hepatotoxicity and/or nephrotoxicity.

Ciclosporin is **metabolized in the liver** by P450 enzymes. These enzymes may be inhibited by concurrent use of other drugs, particularly ketoconazole. For this reason, some clinicians previously administered ketoconazole so that they could use a lower dose of ciclosporin to save costs. This approach is no longer recommended because it may result in unpredictable pharmacokinetics for ciclosporin, and because ketoconazole is associated with a number of other side effects.

Ciclosporin and opportunistic infections

Unlike several other immunosuppressive drugs, **ciclosporin is not myelosuppressive** but it does increase the risk of opportunistic infections. In particular, **cutaneous fungal infections** have been reported in dogs receiving ciclosporin with glucocorticoids, and this should be considered if a patient receiving this combination of drugs develops new skin lesions.

In cats, ciclosporin has been identified as a risk factor for **reactivation of *Toxoplasma gondii***. Normally, following infection, this parasite spreads through the body and forms latent cysts, containing bradyzoites, in multiple tissues. If it becomes reactivated because the immune system is no longer able to suppress it, it may produce active parasite stages (tachyzoites) that spread around the body again, potentially causing meningitis, hepatitis, pancreatitis and interstitial pneumonia. For this reason, many clinicians recommend submitting a blood sample for **measurement of anti-*Toxoplasma* antibodies in serum before considering treatment with ciclosporin**. Others would argue that this approach is illogical because the prevalence of *Toxoplasma* seropositivity is very high in all cats, and the occurrence of clinical toxoplasmosis in cats treated with ciclosporin is still relatively rare.

Long-term treatment

Ciclosporin is normally used in combination with glucocorticoids, but its sole use could be considered in patients that might not tolerate prednisolone, such as dogs and cats with diabetes mellitus. When used in combination with prednisolone, the **dose of ciclosporin is usually maintained at a constant level while the dose of the prednisolone is tapered**. When the prednisolone has been stopped, the dose of ciclosporin may also be tapered over several weeks or months, though some clinicians would also continue at the same dose for a fixed period of time (normally 6–8 weeks), then stop without tapering. Neither approach is proven to reduce the risk of relapse or result in a better outcome, and both may be considered in patients with immune-mediated diseases.

Purine analogues

Both azathioprine and mycophenolate mofetil **interfere with the production of purines**, including the nucleotides adenine and guanine that are **required for synthesis of DNA and RNA**. However, the two drugs achieve this through different mechanisms:

- **Azathioprine** is metabolized into 6-mercaptopurine. This metabolite competes with adenine and guanine for incorporation into nucleotide strands, producing abnormal sequences that prevent replication of cells during mitosis and interfere with cellular metabolism.
- **Mycophenolate** is metabolized into mycophenolic acid, which inhibits the enzyme inosine monophosphate dehydrogenase (IMPDH) required for synthesis of new purines.

The **onset of the effects of azathioprine appears to be delayed**, with little effect on serum antibody concentrations even after administration to healthy dogs for **two weeks**. However, the drug does have a measurable effect on T-cell proliferation in response to stimulation within one week of the start of treatment, suggesting that its clinical effects will be apparent before reductions in serum antibody concentrations are detectable.

One important step in the **metabolism of azathioprine** is catalysed by the enzyme **thiopurine methyltransferase (TPMT)**. This enzyme is present at different levels in different individuals and in different breeds of dog, which may explain the **variation observed in the efficacy of the drug** or in the development of side effects.

Azathioprine

Azathioprine is usually administered at 2 mg/kg PO SID, but some clinicians also prefer to calculate the dose rate according to the **body surface area**, in which case the starting dose would be 50 mg/m^2 PO SID. Due to the risk of adverse effects, some clinicians would also increase the dosing interval to every other day after the first 2–3 weeks of treatment, but there is no evidence to suggest that this will reduce the likelihood of **side effects because many of these are idiosyncratic**. As with ciclosporin, if it is used alongside prednisolone the dose of azathioprine is usually maintained at the same level until the prednisolone has been tapered and stopped, after which the azathioprine may be continued at the same dose for a fixed period of time (**normally 6–8 weeks**) before stopping, or it can be tapered further before stopping. There is no evidence to suggest that either of these approaches will produce a better outcome or reduce the risk of relapses.

Mycophenolate mofetil

Mycophenolate mofetil is normally dosed at 10 mg/kg PO BID, though more recent evidence suggests that doses of 7–8 mg/kg PO BID may be just as effective but associated with fewer adverse effects. This dose is normally maintained at the same level throughout treatment and is not normally decreased or tapered.

Adverse effects

Both drugs above are associated with a number of important adverse effects. Azathioprine may cause idiosyncratic hepatotoxicity, pancreatitis and myelosuppression. Due to its mechanism of action, high doses of azathioprine may cause myelosuppression because it suppresses the replication of stem and progenitor cells in the bone marrow. However, in most dogs that develop myelosuppression when receiving azathioprine, this occurs at lower doses and seems to be an unpredictable, idiosyncratic reaction. Most of these adverse effects appear to be reversible if the drug is withdrawn. As a result of these possible side effects, it is usually recommended to monitor complete blood cell counts and biochemical profiles regularly in dogs receiving azathioprine.

The most common side effect associated with mycophenolate mofetil is acute gastrointestinal disease (vomiting and diarrhoea). This is more likely to occur with the higher doses of mycophenolate that were originally reported (15–20 mg/kg PO BID), but is less likely to be observed when a dose of 8–10 mg/kg PO BID is used. The gastrointestinal effects are usually self-limiting, but they may progress to cause ulcerative enterocolitis in some dogs and may be sufficiently severe to cause euthanasia. In people, mycophenolate may cause severe, idiosyncratic myelosuppression but this is rarely reported in the dog. In people, it also may cause fatal neurological disease, but neither has this been reported in the dog. As a result of these possible complications, it is usually recommended to monitor complete blood cell counts in dogs receiving mycophenolate, though myelosuppression is much less likely than with azathioprine.

Use in immune-mediated diseases

Either drug may be combined with prednisolone, but it is not recommended to use them together because they have such a similar mechanism of action. The use of azathioprine is not recommended for cats because they develop severe myelosuppression and other side effects at very low doses. There is some evidence to suggest that mycophenolate mofetil may be safe to use in cats, at a dose of 10–15 mg/kg PO BID, but this is difficult to achieve in the UK because the drug is not available in a sufficiently small capsule size, and capsules should not be split due to the risk of exposure to the owner. As with dogs, the major side effect for cats appears to be acute vomiting and diarrhoea, which also appears to be dose dependent in the cat.

Azathioprine is a cytotoxic drug, and mycophenolate has the potential to cause myelosuppression and other adverse effects in people. It is therefore extremely important to warn owners about the possible risks associated with handling the tablets during administration, and to select a dose and size that does not require breaking tablets or opening capsules.

Pyrimidine biosynthesis inhibitors

Leflunomide inhibits the synthesis of the pyrimidine molecules (thymine and cytosine) by inhibiting the enzyme dihydro-orotate reductase. As for the purine synthesis inhibitors, this **limits the replication of dividing cells**, including activated lymphocytes, because these cells are unable to obtain pyrimidine molecules through other molecular pathways. Leflunomide was used historically as an anti-rejection drug in dogs that had undergone kidney transplantation, but it was also used more frequently for treatment of immune-mediated disease in dogs because it is relatively well tolerated.

Previously, an initial dose rate of 3–4 mg/kg PO SID was recommended for leflunomide, but recent evidence suggests that a dose of 2 mg/kg PO SID is just as effective in the treatment of immune-mediated diseases.

There are few reported side effects of leflunomide in the dog, but this may reflect its less widespread use in relation to other immunosuppressive drugs. In a recent study in dogs, it was reported to cause lethargy, inappetence, vomiting, diarrhoea and hepatotoxicity. In people, it may also cause cutaneous drug reactions and lung pathology. As a result of these possible side effects, **periodic biochemistry panels** are recommended for dogs receiving this drug.

Alkylating agents

Chlorambucil and cyclophosphamide are both alkylating agents, which means they donate alkyl groups to nucleotides of DNA, resulting in breakage of the DNA strand and **impaired DNA replication**. These effects result in selective death of cells undergoing mitosis, explaining why both drugs form part of chemotherapy protocols for some types of cancer. As a consequence, the **major side effect of these drugs is myelosuppression** caused by death or impaired replication of progenitors in the bone marrow.

Chlorambucil has been **used extensively in cats** with immune-mediated diseases, particularly IMHA, alongside prednisolone. Chlorambucil is the least myelosuppressive of the alkylating agents in clinical use, meaning that it is generally well tolerated, and it is typically administered to cats at a fixed dose of 2 mg PO every other day, or every third day for cats <3 kg.

Traditionally, **cyclophosphamide** was used in the treatment of dogs with IMHA but this is **no longer recommended** because it offered no additional advantage over prednisone alone in one clinical trial and was later shown to be associated with a poorer outcome in a further study. Additionally, cyclophosphamide is associated with more severe and long-lasting adverse effects.

Adverse effects

As discussed, the major concern with the use of alkylating agents is **myelosuppression**. It is therefore important to check a **complete blood cell count** regularly in cats receiving chlorambucil for treatment of immune-mediated disease, with particular attention to the neutrophil count. **Neutrophils have the shortest circulating half-life**, so the first sign of bone marrow suppression is typically a reduction in their numbers in the blood. If myelosuppression is observed with this drug, it may be managed by reducing the dose because the effect is usually dose dependent and will resolve within 2 weeks of this change. Chlorambucil may also occasionally cause gastrointestinal toxicity (vomiting, diarrhoea), which is also related to its effects on the dividing cells of the gastrointestinal tract.

As with azathioprine, chlorambucil is a **cytotoxic drug**, so owners should be warned of the possible complications, and **capsules should not be split, opened or crushed** for administration.

Intravenous immunoglobulin

Human intravenous immunoglobulin (or **gamma globulin, IVIG**) is a product made by isolating the antibodies from thousands of units of donated human blood, followed by various purification and quality control steps. The final product contains a mixture of antibodies with specificity to many different antigens. In people, this product is used for treatment of various immune-mediated and autoimmune diseases, including myasthenia gravis, immune thrombocytopenia and some neurological diseases.

This product has been used widely in dogs with immune-mediated diseases, particularly those that appear to be refractory to 'conventional' immunosuppressive treatment, but there is little evidence to suggest that it will alter the outcome for its recipients. Its exact **mechanism of action**, in either people or dogs, **is not known**, but it is suggested to occupy the Fc receptors on the surface of macrophages and neutrophils, preventing the phagocytosis of targets that have been opsonized by antibodies. This may be important for IMHA and ITP, where red blood cells and platelets are coated with autoantibodies that normally facilitate phagocytosis by these cells. In addition, it is suggested that IVIG may neutralize harmful autoantibodies, and activate anti-inflammatory Fc receptors on some cells.

Intravenous immunoglobulin is a preparation for intravenous injection, which is administered at 0.5–1 g/kg, as a single infusion over 4–6 hours. Because this product contains foreign proteins, there is a **risk of allergic reactions** and the dog should be monitored carefully in a hospital as for a blood transfusion. Some clinicians would also administer a dose of an **antihistamine**, such as chlorphenamine, before starting the IVIG infusion, to reduce the risk of these reactions. For the same reason, some clinicians would not recommend administering IVIG more than once (because the dog may have produced antibodies against the product that would cause a reaction when administered a second time).

The effects of IVIG are expected to be rapid, so a response should be expected within 1–2 days if the treatment has been successful. In many cases, the cost of this product limits its use and some human hospitals will not supply it to veterinary practices because its **availability is limited**.

Treatment with multiple immunosuppressive drugs

For all immune-mediated diseases, the **initial treatment of choice is prednisolone** (or dexamethasone if the patient is not able to tolerate oral medications) because this is licensed for use in dogs and cats, seems to act more rapidly than other drugs and is supported by the largest volume of published evidence. However, glucocorticoids may be combined with another immunosuppressive drug so that the dose of the glucocorticoid product may be started at a lower level or tapered more quickly. Possible combinations include:

- prednisolone + azathioprine or mycophenolate mofetil
- prednisolone + ciclosporin
- prednisolone + leflunomide.

If starting two different drugs from the outset, the dose of prednisolone should ideally be limited to 2 mg/kg per day.

In some cases of particularly severe disease it may seem reasonable to add a third drug, but this approach is generally not recommended because the risk of opportunistic infections appears to be particularly high when three different agents, all suppressing particular parts of the immune system, are used concurrently. This increases the risk of opportunistic fungal and bacterial infections in the dog and cat, and clinical toxoplasmosis in the cat.

Treatment of specific conditions

IMHA

The **major drugs** used for management of IMHA and other immune-mediated diseases are **glucocorticoids**, which may be introduced after a diagnosis has been confirmed. In addition, many clinicians would consider starting another immunosuppressive drug at the same time, so the initial dose of prednisolone is lower and its dose tapered more quickly over the following months.

A rational starting protocol would therefore include:

- **Glucocorticoid**: Prednisolone at 2–3 mg/kg PO per day (all as one dose, or split into two doses), or dexamethasone at 0.2–0.4 mg/kg IV SID if inappetant. If introducing a second drug, the selected dose of prednisolone should be at the lower end of the range described above (i.e. 2 mg/kg per day).
  - ± either azathioprine 2 mg/kg PO SID or 50 mg/m^2 PO SID or
  - ciclosporin 5 mg/kg PO BID or
  - mycophenolate mofetil 8–10 mg/kg PO BID.

All of these 'second-line' drugs have been used for dogs with IMHA, but there is no published evidence that one is more effective than another. Most clinicians would therefore consider any of them to be suitable, provided there are no specific contraindications with that particular patient.

This starting protocol would typically be continued until there were signs the dog was responding to treatment. It should be expected the animal might require further blood transfusions or other **supportive care within the first 3–5 days** after starting this treatment, because the effects of glucocorticoids take this long to become apparent. Therefore, even if there is no apparent response to treatment within 3–5 days, there is unlikely to be any benefit in increasing the dose rates or adding another drug.

Establishing response to treatment

There are several aspects to consider when determining whether dogs with IMHA are responding to treatment. In a disease that causes anaemia, **the key clinical index to monitor is the red blood cell count**, usually by packed cell volume (PCV) or haematocrit (Hct). If this is stable or increasing, then the dog is making a clear response to treatment, particularly if there is evidence of a progressive increase over several days. However, even a dog with an abnormal but stable PCV is showing some form of response, because a severely affected animal would have a continued reduction in the PCV if it were not responding to treatment.

Similar to the PCV/Hct, the **total bilirubin concentration will decrease** in animals responding to treatment because this indicates that fewer free haem molecules are being released into the blood. Serum bilirubin has a relatively short half-life, so this parameter will often decrease as the PCV/Hct increases. However, in animals that have had icterus for some time, bilirubin molecules may bind to proteins in tissues, producing the appearance of mild icterus even after the bilirubin concentration has returned to normal. It is therefore worthwhile to **assess the bilirubin concentration by biochemical measurement**, rather than relying on the clinical appearance of the animal.

Response to treatment can also be assessed by looking at the other tests that indicate that the anaemia had an immune-mediated cause. It is expected that the agglutination (after saline dilution) will resolve and the **number of spherocytes decrease** as an animal responds to treatment. However, there are some preliminary data to suggest that agglutination, and positive DAT results, may persist for some time after initial diagnosis, even in dogs responding well to treatment. Therefore, if the PCV/Hct is increasing and other parameters (such as bilirubin) are improving, continued agglutination would not a be a major concern and would not warrant an increase in dose rates.

Dogs refractory to treatment

There are several options to consider in dogs that fail to respond to the initial treatment described above, in this order:

- **Has enough time elapsed to see a response?** This is a common source of frustration in dogs with IMHA, and it is important to warn the owners that it may **take 5 days or more to see a response to treatment**, even when the selected treatment is appropriate and administered correctly. In severely affected dogs, it should be expected that further blood transfusions will be needed during this period to ensure that cardiovascular parameters remain stable, and to give enough time for the immunosuppressive drugs to work.
- **Are the drugs given at the correct doses and by an appropriate route?** This is a basic concern, but such mistakes are relatively common. Dogs severely affected with IMHA are often recumbent and inappetant, so drugs may need to be administered intravenously to ensure they reach a therapeutic concentration. For drugs that are available only orally, these should be tableted, rather than put into food, to make sure they are swallowed.
- If **after 5–7 days** the dog is refractory to treatment, then **consider giving IVIG** or adding a second/third immunosuppressive drug temporarily to try to achieve a response.

Thromboprophylaxis

Dogs with IMHA are at high risk of **thromboembolic complications** because the disease causes a **hypercoagulable state**. It is therefore sensible to administer a thromboprophylactic drug from the outset of treatment, and to continue this while the dog is receiving prednisolone. Some preliminary data suggest that only around 10% of veterinary surgeons in first-opinion practice administer a thromboprophylactic drug in dogs with IMHA, so this is an area that could result in improved outcomes.

In larger hospitals, this thromboprophylactic treatment is delivered by administering unfractionated or **low-molecular weight heparins**. However, these drugs should be used only if **appropriate monitoring** is available to ensure that a therapeutic dose is being achieved without inducing haemorrhage.

Instead, it may be more realistic to administer an antiplatelet drug, such as clopidogrel (1.1–4 mg/kg PO SID) and/or aspirin (1 mg/kg PO SID or BID), which rarely cause complications. Administration of low-dose aspirin has been associated with improved outcome in dogs with IMHA, even though up to a third of dogs appear to be 'non-responders' to aspirin at anti-inflammatory doses.

Long-term treatment

Once the initial response is established, the **starting doses are maintained for 2–3 weeks**. If the dog is improved or stable, with a normal or increasing PCV/Hct and improved agglutination, spherocytosis and hyperbilirubinaemia, the dose of **prednisolone may be decreased by 25–33%** after this time. **Further reductions** may then be made **approximately every 3 weeks** if the dog continues to make good progress, which should be assessed before each dose reduction by measuring the PCV/Hct as a minimum, with additional tests if there are concerns about relapse or poor response.

Once the prednisolone is decreased to 0.25 mg/kg PO SID or less, it may be stopped. After this, any second immunosuppressive drug may either be continued for a fixed period and then stopped without tapering, or tapered gradually and stopped. The thromboprophylactic may be stopped when the prednisolone is stopped.

It is important to monitor for the side effects associated with the drugs used. For example, if azathioprine has been combined with prednisolone, periodic biochemical profiles should be assessed to make sure that hepatotoxicity is not developing.

Approach to relapses

Relapses occur in approximately 12–15% of dogs with IMHA, usually while the prednisolone dose is being decreased. This may be detected by the return of clinical signs, or by a reduction in the PCV/Hct at re-examination, following a previous reduction in the dose of prednisolone. If this occurs while the dog is still receiving treatment, then **the dose of prednisolone may be increased to the initial dose** used to achieve the response to treatment. After this, the dose should be **tapered more gradually** and in smaller increments than previously. In a very small number of dogs, it may be necessary to continue with lifelong immunosuppressive treatment at a low dose if there are repeated relapses when trying to taper the treatment.

In dogs with an **acute relapse**, **IVIG may be administered** to produce a response to treatment again, though this should be used with caution if it was administered previously, because there may be a risk of allergic reactions. In dogs with repeated relapses, it may also be reasonable to **consider splenectomy**, removing the macrophages that are principally responsible for the destruction of the red blood cells. This should ideally be conducted after all other options have been exhausted, and when the dog is not receiving immunosuppressive or thromboprophylactic drugs.

IMHA in the cat

Treatment of the cat follows principles similar to those in the dog but with a few important differences. The **starting dose of the glucocorticoid should be higher** because cats are more resistant to the effects of these drugs. This would typically mean a starting dose of 4 mg/kg per day of prednisolone, or 0.4–0.6 mg/kg dexamethasone IV SID. After this, the tapering process and assessment of response to treatment is comparable to those for dogs, but the rate of relapse seems to be greater in cats, with **more cats needing to receive lifelong treatment** compared to dogs.

The most commonly used **'second-line' immunosuppressive drugs in cats** are **ciclosporin** and **chlorambucil**, though there are reports of the safe use of mycophenolate mofetil. As for dogs, either of these drugs may be introduced from the outset to limit the side effects of glucocorticoid treatment, or introduced later if there is a poor response to glucocorticoid treatment alone.

IMTP

The same approach described for IMHA is appropriate for dogs with IMTP, starting with a **high dose of prednisolone** ± one of the same **additional drugs** (ciclosporin, azathioprine or mycophenolate mofetil).

A randomized, controlled trial of dogs with ITP showed that administration of a single dose of IVIG shortly after diagnosis resulted in a faster improvement in the platelet count, but no difference in survival. This suggested that IVIG might be an appropriate initial therapy for dogs with IMTP to achieve a response to treatment.

Some clinicians administer a single dose of vincristine to dogs with IMTP at the start of treatment. This is because vincristine is thought to increase the release of platelets from megakaryocytes in the bone marrow, and may produce a transient rise in the platelet count. In a trial comparing administration of a single dose of either IVIG or vincristine in dogs with IMTP, there was no difference in survival to discharge from the hospital, indicating that either treatment may be suitable. If vincristine is used for this purpose, it should be used at a lower dose than for cancer chemotherapy (usually 0.02 mg/kg IV), using all of the same precautions as for cancer treatment.

Response to treatment

The most appropriate parameter to assess response to treatment in dogs with IMTP is the **platelet count**, which should be checked by **examination of a blood smear every 1–2 days** after starting treatment. As for IMHA, it is important to make the owner aware there may be a **lag of 5 days** or more before an effect of treatment is seen, and advanced supportive care, **including blood transfusion**, may be needed during this period.

When response to treatment begins there is often a sudden and dramatic increase in the platelet count. This may be heralded by seeing a **small number of very large macroplatelets** on a blood smear. Once the platelet count improves **above 50 × 10^9/l**, there is a much **lower risk of spontaneous haemorrhage** and any cutaneous haemorrhages would typically resolve in the few days after this.

Long-term treatment

Long-term treatment of IMTP is the same as for IMHA, but with **regular measurements of the platelet count** rather than the erythroid parameters. The approach to relapse is also the same, though the rate of relapse of IMTP is not known in dogs.

Interestingly, in people and dogs with IMTP, a hypercoagulable state develops once the platelet count starts to return to normal. At this time, thromboprophylactic treatment is not administered because clinical thromboembolic disease seems to be very rare, and this treatment would be contraindicated while the platelet count is low as it would increase the risk of spontaneous bleeding.

IMPA

Initial immunosuppressive treatment of dogs with IMPA is as described for IMHA and IMTP.

Initial treatment usually produces a rapid improvement in the clinical signs of IMPA, including increased alertness and activity and **resolution of the joint stiffness and pain**. This is a very fulfilling process to observe, but continued response to treatment can be difficult to assess, particularly in dogs that start to develop muscle weakness related to prednisolone causing similar signs to the original IMPA.

Differentiation of these two problems may be achieved by repeated sampling of the joints for analysis of the synovial fluid, but this would require repeated sedation and is therefore not indicated in the majority of dogs. This procedure is indicated in dogs that develop **acute swelling of a single joint** during treatment, because they could be developing **septic arthritis** as a complication of the immunosuppressive treatment.

More recently, the **acute phase CRP** has been used to monitor the severity of inflammation in dogs with IMPA and SRMA. This protein is produced by the liver under stimulation from pro-inflammatory cytokines as part of the abnormal immune response, and is a good marker of the severity of inflammation. However, the CRP levels vary considerably between individual patients, so it is most helpful to collect an initial sample at the time of diagnosis to act as a baseline, and then measure it after resolution of clinical signs to check that it has decreased. If the dog then develops signs suggestive of a relapse or chronic inflammation, you will have upper and lower values for the individual dog when the CRP is measured again.

Emerging treatments

Recently, a small study described treatment of dogs with IMPA with **ciclosporin alone**, without prednisolone or another glucocorticoid. The authors concluded that the two drugs produced a similarly good outcome, but very few dogs were recruited to the trial. Nevertheless, this could be a suitable approach for dogs that would not tolerate high doses of glucocorticoids.

Similarly, there has been a short report of treating dogs with IMPA with leflunomide alone, at 3–4 mg/kg PO SID, a higher dose than currently recommended, without glucocorticoids. In this study, there was no comparison to a group of dogs receiving prednisolone, so it is difficult to determine whether this treatment was similar, better or worse than would be expected with the 'standard' treatment approach. However, as for ciclosporin, this could be an option for dogs that would not tolerate prednisolone.

Management of erosive arthritis

Unlike (non-erosive) IMPA, erosive arthritis will often cause destabilization and laxity of joints, contributing to lameness and poor mobility. In such cases, after control of the immune response it is often necessary to consider **surgical stabilization procedures**, such as pancarpal arthrodesis, to permit a return to acceptable mobility.

Although rarely diagnosed, **erosive arthritis** appears to require more aggressive immunosuppressive treatment than IMPA, with most dogs requiring **lifelong treatment**.

SLE

A similar approach should be adopted for treatment of SLE as outlined for IMHA, but it is appropriate to use a second immunosuppressive drug from the outset because such cases are relatively refractory to treatment. As for erosive arthritis, these patients are also likely to require lifelong immunosuppressive treatment to maintain remission, if this can be achieved.

Complications of immune-mediated therapy

Relapse may occur at any stage during treatment as the intensity of the immunosuppressive regimen is decreased, or even months or years after finishing all treatment. Before increasing or re-starting treatment, it is important to ask whether this **relapse could be occurring because an underlying cause of immune-mediated disease was overlooked** when the diagnosis was first made. For example, if the immune-mediated disease is related to occult cancer, the disease will keep relapsing every time treatment is withdrawn and until the underlying problem is addressed.

Side effects

Side effects of immunosuppressive drugs, particularly glucocorticoids, may be more severe than the signs of the disease being treated, and may be a reason for euthanasia of some cases. It is important to take a **pragmatic approach** when using and decreasing the dose of glucocorticoids during treatment. For example, if a dog with IMHA has a stable PCV of 30% and no signs of continued agglutination or active disease, it would still be appropriate to try decreasing the dose of prednisolone after 2–3 weeks to avoid excessive side effects, even though this is not a normal value. This approach clearly requires careful monitoring and discussion with the owners.

In some cases, side effects of treatment may be confused with the disease itself, such as when dogs with IMPA develop severe muscle weakness and lethargy related to administration of prednisolone. In this situation, it is important not simply to increase the dose of prednisolone without asking whether the disease is under control – for example, by measuring the CRP concentration or sampling the synovial fluid.

Recommended reading

Balog, K. et al. (2013) A prospective randomized clinical trial of vincristine versus human intravenous immunoglobulin for acute adjunctive management of presumptive primary immune-mediated thrombocytopenia in dogs. *Journal of Veterinary Internal Medicine* 27, 536–541.

Ellis, J. et al. (2018) Prevalence and disease associations of feline thrombocytopenia: a retrospective study of 194 cases. *Journal of Small Animal Practice* 59, 531–538.

Felsburg, P.J. (2002) Overview of immune system development in the dog: comparison with humans. *Human Experimental Toxicology* 21, 487–492.

Foster, J.D. et al. (2014) Serum biomarkers of clinical and cytologic response in dogs with idiopathic immune-mediated polyarthropathy. *Journal of Veterinary Internal Medicine* 28, 905–911.

Gershwin, L.J. (2018) Adverse reactions to vaccination: from anaphylaxis to autoimmunity. *Veterinary Clinics of North America Small Animal Practice* 48, 279–290.

Naor, A.W. et al. (2017) Pathology in practice. Systemic lupus erythematosus (SLE) in a dog. *Journal of the American Veterinary Medical Association* 250, 627–629.

Riggs, C. et al. (2013) Analytical validation of a quantitative reverse transcriptase polymerase chain reaction assay for evaluation of T-cell targeted immunosuppressive therapy in dogs. *Veterinary Immunology and Immunopathology* 156, 229–234.

Swann, J.W. and Skelly, B.J. (2013) Systematic review of evidence relating to the treatment of immune-mediated hemolytic anemia in dogs. *Journal of Veterinary Internal Medicine* 27, 1–9.

Swann, J.W. and Skelly, B.J. (2015) Systematic review of prognostic factors for mortality in dogs with immune-mediated hemolytic anemia. *Journal of Veterinary Internal Medicine* 29, 7–13.

Case study 1: Meet Stanley

Stanley is a 6-year-old, male, neutered Rottweiler.

- He has no previous medical problems, but once travelled to Spain 2 years ago.
- He is fully vaccinated, with the last dose administered 8 months ago.
- He is up to date with routine anthelmintic and flea treatment.

History

For the last week, his owners have noted that he has been quieter than usual at home and less willing to go for walks. When he does go out for walks, he seems slower than usual and wants to sit down about half-way through. He has been eating and drinking normally.

Clinical examination

Stanley has pale mucous membranes, but no signs of petechiae.
His femoral pulse quality is slightly hyperdynamic, but synchronous with the cardiac beat.
His heart rate is 136 beats per minute at rest in the consultation room.
In the appointment, after initial excitement, he lies down in the corner of the room.

What are the problems identified and their differential diagnoses?

The following problems can be identified from the history and physical examination:

- lethargy
- reduced exercise tolerance
- hyperdynamic peripheral pulse
- relative tachycardia at rest
- pallor.

Differential diagnoses

Lethargy

It is extremely difficult to provide a meaningful differential list for this problem because it is associated with so many different conditions.

Reduced exercise tolerance

This could be related to cardiorespiratory disease, particularly with the concurrent tachycardia and pallor (which could be related to peripheral vasoconstriction). However, cardiac disease causing signs of this magnitude would normally be associated with a hypodynamic peripheral pulse.

This could be related to musculoskeletal or neurological disease, but would not explain the other problems.

This could be related to anaemia, which would also explain the pallor, tachycardia and pulse changes.

Pallor

This could be related to peripheral vasoconstriction, which may occur with some forms of shock (particularly cardiogenic shock), associated with a prolonged capillary refill time (CRT). Septic shock typically results in peripheral vasodilation, with a rapid CRT.

Pallor may also be associated with anaemia.

Tachycardia at rest

It is important to relate the heart rate to the status of the animal. This heart rate would not be abnormal in an excited or nervous dog, but is worrying in a dog at rest or that appears very lethargic.

This tachycardia could be related to pain, stress or shock, as outlined above.

Tachycardia may be associated with primary cardiac disease, as the heart tries to maintain cardiac output.

Tachycardia may be related to anaemia, as the body tries to maintain normal oxygen delivery to the peripheral tissues despite reduced oxygen carriage in the blood.

What investigations would you like to consider for this patient?

Initial investigations

Sensible investigations at this stage would include:

- Complete blood count, since there is a high suspicion of anaemia from the clinical problems.
- A basic electrolyte/metabolite panel – for example, with an 'iStat' machine. This should provide us with a lactate measurement, which would help us to see if peripheral perfusion is adequate.
- Further investigations for cardiac disease, such as echocardiography, NT-proBNP or cardiac troponin I, are probably not indicated until the results above have been reviewed.

Complete blood cell count

Table 2.5.

Parameter	Result	Reference interval
Red blood cell count	3.8 x 10^{12}/l	5.5–8.5
Haematocrit	25.3%	37–55
Reticulocytes	78,000/µl	
White blood cell count	19.2 x 10^9/l	6–17
Neutrophils	17.2 x 10^9/l	3–11.5
Bands	1.4 x 10^9/l	
Monocytes	1.7 x 10^9/l	0.15–1.5
Lymphocytes	0.1 x 10^9/l	1–4.5
Eosinophils	0.1 x 10^9/l	0–1.2
Platelets	78 x 10^9/l	150–800
Smear examination	Platelet count appears genuine, no platelet clumps seen. Occasional macroplatelets observed. Marked anisocytosis and polychromasia. Moderate number of spherocytes (4–5 per high power field)	
Plasma colour	Red (haemolysed)	

Emergency profile

Table 2.6.

Parameter	Result	Reference interval
Haematocrit	25.6%	37–55
Urea	8.2 mmol/l	2.5–9.6
Creatinine	65 μmol/l	45–160
Lactate	08 mmol/l	0.6–2.5

What abnormalities are identified in the laboratory results?

Laboratory results

- The CBC reveals moderate, regenerative anaemia.
- There is an inflammatory or stress leukogram, characterized by mild–moderate neutrophilia (with left shift), monocytosis and lymphopenia.
- There is moderate thrombocytopenia, confirmed by examination of a blood smear.
- There is moderate spherocytosis.
- Results of the emergency panel are within normal limits, suggesting that peripheral perfusion is currently maintaining vital organ function.

How would you like to proceed with this clinical case?

Next steps

Stanley has regenerative anaemia, with some indication that this could be immune-mediated, due to the spherocytes.

Ideally, we would gather additional evidence of a possible immune-mediated cause before pursuing any invasive diagnostic tests.

This could be achieved by submitting blood for a direct antiglobulin (Coombs') test or with saline agglutination. In this case, the latter test was performed.

Saline agglutination test

Result: positive macroscopic agglutination.

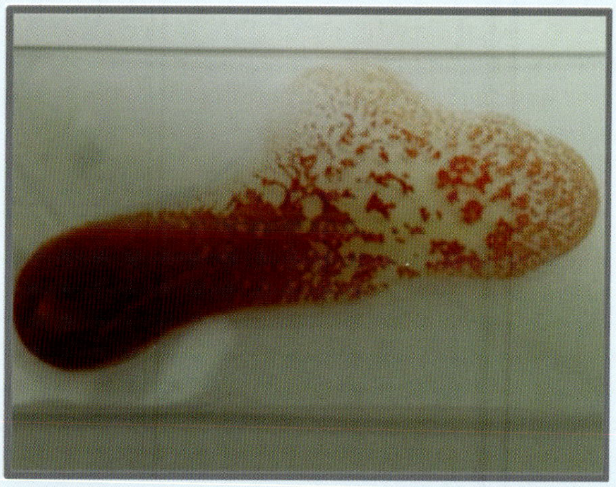

Figure 2.5.

Further investigations

Stanley has regenerative anaemia that appears to be immune-mediated. It would be sensible to undertake further investigations at this point to exclude any underlying cause for the IMHA, particularly in a middle-aged dog with a travel history. Investigations at this point should include:

- Imaging of the thorax (radiographs) and abdomen (ultrasound).
- Serum biochemistry.
- Serology for *E. canis* and *Anaplasma* spp., antigen testing for *Dirofilaria immitis* and PCR for *B. canis*.

- Urinalysis, ideally collected by cystocentesis, for dipstick, sediment examination and culture. The diagnostic utility of this test is questionable, as urinary tract infection is not clearly associated with IMHA.

Diagnostic imaging

The following results were obtained:

- thoracic radiographs: no abnormalities detected
- abdominal ultrasonography:
  - mild hyperechogenicity of the liver
  - marked enlargement of the spleen, with increased echogenicity
  - mild enlargement of the mesenteric lymph nodes.

Serum biochemistry

Table 2.7.

Parameter	Result	Reference interval
Total protein	62 g/l	53–75
Albumin	36 g/l	28–40
Globulin	26 g/l	25–45
Urea	4.6 mmol/l	2.5–9.6
Creatinine	72 μmol/l	45–160
ALT	163 U/l	10–125
AST	48 U/l	0–50
ALP	178 U/l	25–250
Total bilirubin	23.6 μmol/l	0–0.5
Cholesterol	2.8 mmol/l	3–8.5

Infectious disease testing

The following results were obtained:

- *Ehrlichia* spp. serology: negative
- *Anaplasma* spp. serology: negative
- *D. immitis* antigen: negative
- *B. canis* PCR: negative.

Urinalysis

Table 2.8.

Parameter	Result
Protein	–/+
Blood	–
Haemoglobin	++
Bilirubin	+++
Urobilinogen	–
pH	7.4
Specific gravity (refractometer)	1.037
Sediment examination	Some acellular debris
Bacterial culture	Negative

What is your interpretation of these results? Would you recommend any additional tests before starting treatment?

Case summary

We can refine our clinical problem list to the following areas:

- lethargy, reduced exercise tolerance
- IMHA, resulting in moderate regenerative anaemia
- moderate thrombocytopenia

- inflammatory leukogram
- splenomegaly
- increased bilirubin and ALT, probably related to haemolysis and hypoxia, respectively.

Let's now examine some of the problems in more detail.

What are the possible causes of the thrombocytopenia?

- This could be attributable to an immune response against platelets (as well as red blood cells), but the platelet count is typically much lower in such cases (<20 × 10^9/l).
- This is most likely to be related to consumption of platelets, such as with formation of thromboemboli, which occur relatively commonly in dogs with IMHA.
- The decreased count could also be related to sequestration of platelets in the enlarged spleen.
- In any case, Stanley should not be at risk of spontaneous haemorrhage with a platelet count of 78, so this abnormality does not warrant any further tests or changes in treatment.

What are the possible causes of the splenomegaly?

Possible causes include:

- Extramedullary haematopoiesis, which refers to compensatory production of new red blood cells in the spleen to replace those destroyed due to the disease process.
- (Diffuse) neoplasia, which is usually related to a round cell tumour.
- Congestion of the spleen, possibly related to splenic vein thrombus, though this should be evident by ultrasound.

Would you recommend any further investigations for this problem?

Splenic FNA

Cytology interpretation:

Good cellular yield and preservation, with moderate blood contamination. There are large numbers of erythroid progenitors, consistent with extramedullary erythropoiesis. There are large numbers of large mononuclear cells phagocytosing red blood cells, consistent with erythrophagocytosis.

Diagnosis

Extramedullary haematopoiesis; erythrophagocytosis, related to IMHA.

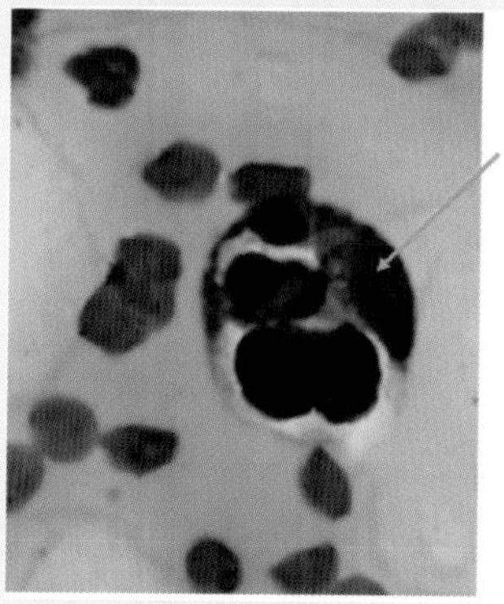

Figure 2.6.

What is your final diagnosis?

IMHA with no apparent underlying cause.

What treatment plan would you recommend? (Stanley weighs 36.2 kg)

Treatment plan

Packed RBC transfusion

This decision is equivocal at this stage. The anaemia is not particularly severe, but Stanley clearly has clinical signs that could have occurred if this anaemia has developed very quickly. It would be appropriate to transfuse now, or to monitor carefully and begin transfusing if his heart rate, respiratory rate, demeanour or ability to stand and walk deteriorate.

It would be sensible to obtain his blood type now, however, to speed up the process of transfusion if needed.

Immunosuppressive treatment

Stanley has been eating normally, so he can start to receive prednisolone immediately. In such a large dog, it would be more sensible to calculate the dose based on surface area, at 50 mg/m^2. His surface area is 1.1 m^2, so his starting dose will be 55 mg prednisolone, either as a single dose or 27.5 mg twice daily.

It would be reasonable to start a second drug at the same time to allow faster reduction of the prednisolone dose. In this case, azathioprine was also started at 50 mg/m^2 (= 50 mg) daily. This is a slight under-dose, but it is not advisable to split the tablets because they are cytotoxic.

Antithrombotic treatment

Due to the high risk of thromboembolic disease in dogs with IMHA, clopidogrel was also started at this stage, at a dose of 2 mg/kg (= 75 mg) daily.

This treatment is generally continued for as long as the prednisolone is administered.

Stanley initially made a good response to treatment, with his PCV increasing to 29% within 4 days. He was discharged but re-presented 4 days later, collapsed, with a PCV of 12%.

What would you recommend next?

Stanley urgently requires transfusion of packed red blood cells now (or fresh whole blood if pRBCs are not available) to stabilize his condition.

We should then consider the following areas:

- Have his medications been administered at home?
- Has he been receiving the correct dose of his medications?
- If no problems are identified, Stanley can be considered refractory to 'standard' treatment.

After he has received his blood transfusion, would you make any adjustments to Stanley's treatment?

Possible options include:

- Increasing the prednisolone dose (to 60 mg/m^2), although there is no evidence to suggest that higher doses will produce a better outcome.
- Giving more time with the existing regimen. Azathioprine may take 2 weeks to exert its maximal effect, so it may be reasonable to wait for longer now that he is stable again.
- Administer intravenous immunoglobulin (IVIG, 1 g/kg as an infusion over 6 hours), though there is no evidence to show that this will improve survival. This is the option that was chosen for Stanley.

Following IVIG, Stanley's PCV improved again to 31%. After 2 weeks, his dose of prednisolone was decreased to 50 mg PO SID and azathioprine and clopidogrel were continued.

Five days later, Stanley re-presented collapsed, with a PCV of 14%. He had also become icteric.

What would you recommend at this point?

Stanley now gives serious cause for concern because he has suffered two relapses despite appropriate treatment.

Due to continued concerns about the severity of his disease and a possible underlying cause, it was recommended that he underwent a splenectomy after stopping the clopidogrel for several days.

Histological examination of the spleen revealed histiocytic sarcoma, a type of neoplasia that has been associated with erythrophagocytosis and secondary IMHA. Rottweilers are predisposed to this type of cancer. In hindsight, the erythrophagocytic cells observed in the splenic aspirates were actually cancer cells, not normal splenic macrophages.

Sadly, Stanley developed disseminated intravascular coagulation 24 hours after surgery and developed haemorrhagic complications, resulting in euthanasia.

Prognosis and discussion

Histiocytic sarcoma causing erythrophagocytic syndrome has a particularly poor prognosis in dogs, so the initial diagnosis of primary IMHA probably only slightly delayed the same outcome.

In hindsight, this abnormality might have been suspected more quickly due to the concurrent hypocholesterolaemia, which is a typical feature of this syndrome.

If Stanley's spleen had been normal histologically, removal of the spleen would have been an appropriate, though fairly drastic, option to try to manage the IMHA.

Continued poor response to treatment with an immune-mediated disease is an indication to look for an underlying cause that might have been missed.

Case study 2: Meet Jasper

- Jasper is a 4-year-old, male, neutered Springer spaniel.
- He had previous surgery for patellar luxation of his right stifle 2 years ago.
- He was last vaccinated 18 months ago.
- He does not receive routine anthelmintic and flea treatment.

History

- Jasper has been very reluctant to get out of bed in the morning for the last 2 days.
- When standing and walking, he is very stiff and has been crying frequently when walking and when picked up.
- He vomited twice yesterday and has not eaten for 2 days, though he is drinking water.

Clinical examination

- Jasper is very painful when flexing any of the distal joints of all four limbs.
- There are moderate effusions of both carpi, and questionable effusions of the tarsi and stifles.
- His rectal temperature is 39.5°C.
- General examination is otherwise unremarkable.

What are the problems identified and their differential diagnoses?

The following problems can be identified from the history and physical examination:

- effusions of multiple joints
- pain and stiffness
- acute vomiting.

Which do you think is the most helpful problem for further investigation?

Differential diagnoses

Pain and stiffness

This problem is very probably related to the joint effusions and underlying disease process.

Effusions of multiple joints

This could be related to inflammatory disease, including erosive or non-erosive immune-mediated polyarthritis.

This could also be caused by infective arthritis, though this is less likely to affect multiple joints. Occasionally, bacteria may spread to multiple joints via the haematogenous route, though affected dogs are typically extremely unwell.

Multiple effusions may occasionally be related to haemorrhage, and are sometimes seen with (severe) secondary coagulopathy, such as congenital haemophilia or rodenticide intoxication.

Vomiting

Clearly, there are a large number of possible causes for acute vomiting and this is not a particularly useful problem to follow to lead to a diagnosis.

Pertinent possible causes include:

- systemic inflammatory disease, including immune-mediated or infectious diseases, which may affect normal gastric mucosal barrier function

- prolonged inappetence
- dietary indiscretion
- pain or stress.

What investigations would you like to consider for this patient?

Initial investigations

Sensible investigations at this stage would include:

- Sampling of the effused joints – this will require sedation or general anaesthesia so it would be sensible to consider performing any other major investigations at the same time.
- Complete blood cell count and serum biochemistry – to look for possible underlying causes or concurrent haematological abnormalities (that could suggest SLE, for example).
- Imaging of the thorax and abdomen – to look for possible underlying causes. In this breed, it will be particularly relevant to look for any evidence of foreign body tracts, unexplained abscess lesions or pyothorax.
- Imaging of one or more joints – to look for erosive lesions. Note that it is only necessary to image one or two affected joints as the same process is assumed to be occurring in all.
- Testing for endemic infectious agents – to look for possible underlying causes.
- Measurement of CRP. This will not be particularly helpful for diagnosing the cause of the effusions, but will help to establish a baseline for future treatment.

Complete blood cell count

Table 2.9.

Parameter	Result	Reference interval
Red blood cell count	5.8 x 10^{12}/l	5.5–8.5
Haematocrit	39.3%	37–55
White blood cell count	25.1 x 10^9/l	6–17
Neutrophils	21.6 x 10^9/l	3–11.5
Bands	1.2 x 10^9/l	
Monocytes	2.4 x 10^9/l	0.15–1.5
Lymphocytes	0.1 x 10^9/l	1–4.5
Eosinophils	0.1 x 10^9/l	0–1.2
Platelets	356 x 10^9/l	150–800
Smear examination	No platelet clumps seen. Moderate to marked neutrophilia, of which the majority are mature neutrophils, with a small but appropriate number of band neutrophils.	
Plasma colour	Straw coloured (normal)	

Serum biochemistry

Table 2.10.

Parameter	Result	Reference interval
Total protein	68 g/l	53–75
Albumin	29 g/l	28–40
Globulin	39 g/l	25–45
Urea	2.3 mmol/l	2.5–9.6
Creatinine	68 µmol/l	45–160
ALT	112 U/l	10–125
AST	45 U/l	0–50
ALP	102 U/l	25–250
Total bilirubin	1.2 µmol/l	0–0.5
Cholesterol	4.1 mmol/l	3–8.5
C reactive protein	240 mg/l	<20

What abnormalities are identified in the laboratory results? How would you explain these results?

Blood sample results

- The CBC shows a moderate to marked mature neutrophilia, with mild left shift and monocytosis. This is consistent with an inflammatory leukogram, suggesting there is an ongoing inflammatory process. This is NOT the same as an infection: remember that sterile inflammation will produce this pattern as part of the acute phase response.
- There are borderline low albumin concentration and red blood cell count, which are also probably associated with inflammation. Remember that albumin is a negative acute phase protein (its production is decreased in the presence of inflammation so that other proteins can be produced instead in the liver). Conversely, the CRP, a positive acute phase protein, is increased, confirming an inflammatory process.
- There is mildly increased total bilirubin and decreased urea, both probably related to the recent vomiting and inappetence.

Synovial fluid analysis

Table 2.11.

Cytology report
Aspirates from both carpi and one tarsal joint: 4 unstained slides submitted from each joint Fluid was not submitted for measurement of the protein concentration or nucleated cell count **Report:** There is a greatly increased cellularity in samples from all three joints, with >90% of nucleated cells in all three joints being mature, non-degenerate neutrophils. Larger, mononuclear cells are also observed. There is moderate blood contamination of slides from the right carpus. No micro-organisms or LE cells are observed. **Comment:** This appearance is consistent with immune-mediated disease of multiple joints. Bacterial culture is pending; available in 48 hours.

Imaging and infectious disease screening

- thoracic radiographs: unremarkable
- abdominal ultrasonography: unremarkable apart from mild thickening of the gastric wall
- radiographs of both carpi: no erosive lesions seen
- serology for *E.* spp.: negative
- serology for *Anaplasma* spp.: negative.

What is your refined problem list?

Jasper has inflammatory arthritis of multiple joints. Bacterial culture is pending, but the pattern of joint involvement is more suggestive of immune-mediated polyarthritis.

Consistent with this, there is an inflammatory leukogram, increased CRP and pyrexia, indicating a systemic acute phase response.

There is no apparent underlying cause for the IMPA after imaging of the thorax and abdomen and testing for infectious agents.

How would you like to proceed with this clinical case?

Even though IMPA was considered more likely here, it would be a high risk to start prednisolone at an immunosuppressive dose now in case these lesions are associated with a bacterial infection.

Sensible immediate treatment could therefore include:

- Analgesic: buprenorphine at 0.02 mg/kg IV q6–8h or methadone 0.1–0.2 mg/kg IV q4h.
- Antipyretic: paracetamol at 10 mg/kg IV q12h (note that paracetamol can be safely administered alongside corticosteroids). Paracetamol also has analgesic properties.
- Anti-inflammatory: dexamethasone at 0.05–0.1 mg/kg IV q24h. Note that this is an anti-inflammatory dose of this drug, not an immunosuppressive dose.
- Anti-emetic/anti-nausea: maropitant 1 mg/kg SC or IV q24h.

After 24 hours, interim bacterial culture is negative.

How would you modify the treatment plan?

Definitive treatment

This information should be sufficient to make a final diagnosis of primary, non-erosive IMPA. Consequently, immunosuppressive treatment may be started:

- dexamethasone 0.2–0.4 mg/kg IV q24h if Jasper is still inappetant, OR
- prednisolone 2 mg/kg PO per day if now eating.

As before, the glucocorticoid may be combined with another immunosuppressive agent to limit the dose of prednisolone. In this case, ciclosporin was added at 5 mg/kg PO q12h.

Jasper responded well to this treatment and was discharged with prednisolone and azathioprine 2 days later.

The dose of prednisolone was gradually decreased every 3 weeks, and he returned for re-examination 3 months later.

Re-examination

History

Jasper's owners report that he was making good progress but, since the previous dose reduction 3 weeks ago, he has seemed more lethargic and less willing to go for walks.

Clinical examination

- Jasper seems quiet but alert and responsive in the consultation.
- There are no palpable joint effusions, but Jasper seemed reluctant to flex the joints of his pelvic limbs and seems stiff when walking.
- Jasper has gained weight, increasing from 12 kg at diagnosis to 16.2 kg now.
- Jasper has mild bilateral alopecia of his flanks, and a mild pot belly.

Current medications:

- prednisolone 12.5 mg PO SID
- ciclosporin 60 mg PO BID.

What is your problem list for this visit, and how could you account for this?

Re-examination: problems

- Jasper now has some signs related to administration of glucocorticoids, including pot belly and non-pruritic, bilaterally symmetrical alopecia.
- Jasper has unexplained stiffness of some joints and is more lethargic. There are several possible reasons for this, including:
  - continued active arthritis
  - side effects related to glucocorticoids.

How could you establish whether Jasper is receiving appropriate treatment now?

Monitoring tests

We submitted a sample for measurement of CRP when Jasper was diagnosed with IMPA, so this can be repeated now to determine whether there is still active inflammation.

Table 2.12.

Parameter	Result	Reference interval
C reactive protein	18 mg/l	<20

This shows that Jasper probably does not have active inflammation. The stiffness in the pelvic limbs is more likely to be related to pseudo-myotonia, a rare complication of glucocorticoids that results in continuous muscle contraction.

Table 2.13

Parameter	Result
Ciclosporin pharmacodynamic monitoring (based on suppression of IL-2 expression in blood)	Moderate/high suppression

We could submit a blood sample for pharmacodynamic monitoring of ciclosporin, to help us decide how quickly to decrease the dose of prednisolone.

The results of this assay show that the ciclosporin dose is appropriate.

Note that this test requires submission of a fresh, chilled, 3 ml heparinized blood sample to the testing centre in the USA, so needs to be sent via courier. The sample should be obtained 2–3 hours after the last dose of ciclosporin, and the dog should have been receiving the current dose for at least 1 week.

How would you modify Jasper's treatment based on these results?

Revised treatment plan

Jasper's inflammation and original clinical signs appear to be well-controlled but he has side effects related to his immunosuppressive medications.

It would therefore be sensible to reduce the dose of BOTH medications now, and consider more rapid reduction or shorter intervals between reductions in future:

- Prednisolone: decrease to 12.5 mg PO every other day. The change to every other day dosing may help to limit side effects by giving a day for recovery of the endogenous adrenocortical axis.
- Ciclosporin: decrease to 50 mg PO BID.
- Arrange re-examination in 3 weeks.

Diagnostic imaging techniques

3

Amalia Agut Giménez

Chapter summary

In the past few decades the routine diagnostic procedures used in veterinary practice have changed. Whereas in the 20th century radiography ruled, in the 21st century ultrasound has come into its own. But both imaging modalities still very much have a part to play as diagnostic media.

Understanding the strengths and weaknesses of radiology versus ultrasound helps the veterinarian choose the most beneficial imaging modality. Take as an example the young vomiting dog. Previously, the diagnostic approach involved taking plain radiographs, followed by a time consuming (and messy) barium series. However, the modern first opinion practice is now equipped with ultrasound. In the hands of a skilled operator, a scan provides more information more quickly than a radiographic contrast study. However, if that same dog is regurgitating rather than vomiting, then radiography is still the modality of choice to check for the presence of megaoesophagus.

Interpretation of radiographs can be tricky. Detecting subtle differences between normal and diseased tissue may depend on obtaining the best possible radiograph. Achieving this depends on combining the correct exposure with great positioning and choosing the correct moment to take the radiograph. From patient preparation to selecting exposure factors, this chapter reviews how to take radiographs you can be proud to share with a specialist.

Key learning points

- How patient preparation and positioning aid optimal imaging.
- The use of Sante's rule to calculate the optimum kV for your patient, and how to select radiographic factors such as mAs.
- The legislation around radiographic safety, labelling of restricted areas, and good health and safety working practices around radiation.
- The principles of interpreting radiographs by understanding the five basic radiographic opacities.
- The principles of ultrasound use, selecting an appropriate transducer, appropriate equipment setting selection, and image orientation.

Radiographic technique

When taking radiographs, most unsatisfactory images arise from poor radiographic technique, such as poor patient preparation and incorrect positioning. Simply adopting a standardized technique can greatly improve the quality of the radiographs obtained. This section explains how to optimize radiographic technique in the small animal clinic.

Patient preparation

Obtaining good quality radiographs depends on **adequate preparation** of the area of the patient to be X-rayed and on the **technique** required. For example, when taking contrast studies, a preparatory enema may be needed. Also, to facilitate optimum exposure and prevent movement blur it is often necessary to **sedate** or even anaesthetise the patient.

Basic preparation includes **removing any objects**, such as collars, straps, or dirt on the hair, which may produce shadows on the radiograph.

How many projections are necessary?

Physical structures are three-dimensional, while radiographs produce a two-dimensional image. Therefore, at least **two orthogonal projections** (views at a 90-degree angle to each other) are necessary (Figure 3.1).

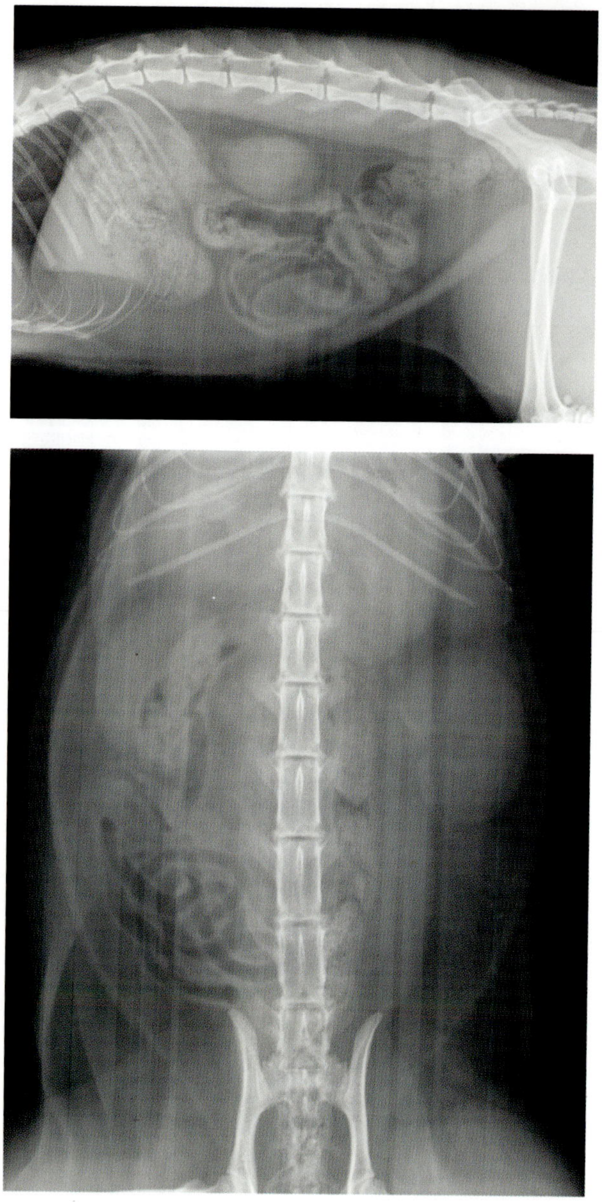

Figure 3.1. Two orthogonal projections. (a) Right lateral projection and (b) ventrodorsal projection of the abdominal cavity in a radiologically mature cat.

Typically these are:

- **lateral projection** (right or left)
- **ventrodorsal** (VD) or **dorsoventral** (DV) projection.

However, more than two projections are often needed, especially when using contrast techniques. For example, to fully assess gastrointestinal transit through the stomach and beyond, four views are needed.

Positioning of the patient

In order to prevent distortion, the area of the body to be radiographed must be positioned **parallel** to the cassette and as **close as possible** to it to avoid magnification.

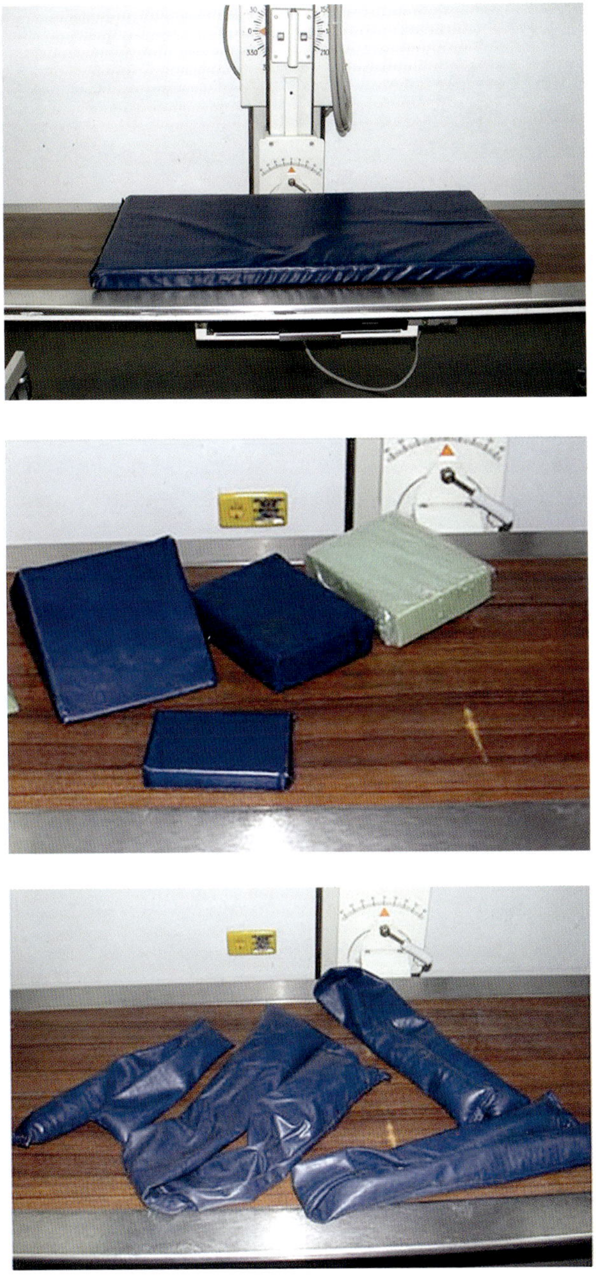

Figure 3.2 (a–c). Items to help with positioning of the patient while performing a radiograph.

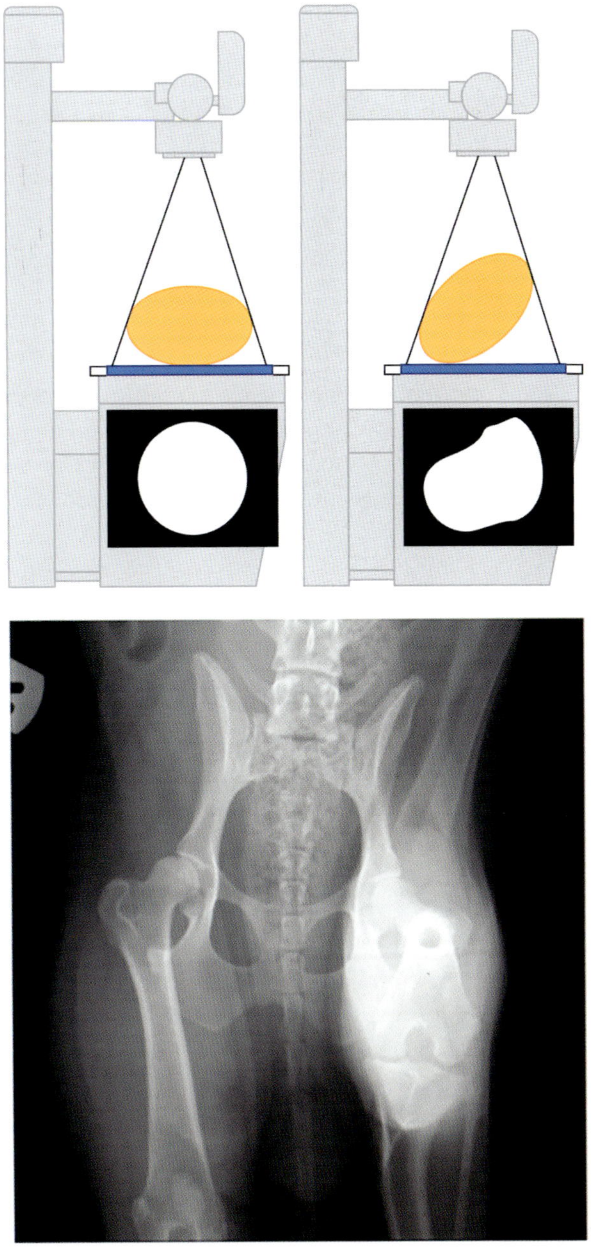

Figure 3.3. (a) The area which is to be radiographed should be parallel to the cassette so there is no distortion. (b) VD projection of the hips: the left hindlimb appears distorted as it is not parallel to the cassette.

To help with positioning of the animal, a good selection of supportive objects is essential. These may include the following items (Figure 3.2).

- A thin translucent foam mattress so the animal lies comfortably on the cold, hard X-ray table.
- Sandbags and pieces of foam rubber of varying sizes and shapes to help with positioning and to avoid rotation.

Central beam

The area to be radiographed should be placed in the **centre of the primary beam,** which is the area of **minimum distortion**. The beam diverges as it moves away from the central area, producing oblique projections of anatomy not aligned with the central beam (Figure 3.3).

Collimation

The **entire area of interest** should be included in the radiograph. Thus, when a lesion is suspected in a long bone, the whole bone with proximal and distal joints should be included.

Good collimation reduces scattered radiation and improves the quality of the radiograph, as contrast is increased.

Exposure factors

The X-ray tube has two electrodes:

- the cathode (negative electrode)
- the anode (positive electrode).

X-rays are formed when the electrons move at high speed from the cathode and collide with the focal point of the anode, causing a large amount of energy to be released as heat and some to be transformed into electromagnetic photons.

With reference to the X-rays produced, there are two fundamental factors to radiographic technique.

- The **number of rays**. This is determined by the **amount of electricity** and **time** given to the cathode, i.e., the **mAs.**
- The **quality of the rays**. The energy is the potential difference between the cathode and the anode and corresponds to the **penetration** of the X-rays, i.e., the **kVp**.

Santes' rule

This allows the optimal kVp to be calculated.

The formula involves doubling the thickness of the target area (in cm) and adding a conversion factor.

For example:

2 × thickness (cm) **+ 30 for the abdomen**
+ 40 for bony structures
+ 50 for the thorax

Example:

For a 10 cm thick thorax you would need:
(2 × 10) + 50 = 70 kVp.

An increase in kVp (>70) produces a lot of scattered radiation, which means a reduction in contrast and, consequently, background blur. To avoid scattered radiation, **a grid** is placed between the patient and the radiographic film.

Grids, which can be fixed or mobile (Potter–Bucky), are used when the thickness of the area to be X-rayed is greater than:

- **10 cm in abdomen**, head and extremities
- **15 cm in the thoracic** cavity.

Calculating mAs

The mAs determines the amount of radiation (number of X-ray photons) during the exposure. When the **mAs is increased** the **image becomes darker**, but does not directly affect the contrast.

These two parameters, mAs and kVp, can be used to control the darkness of the radiograph and therefore the contrast.When **low mAs/high kVp** are used, a **wide greyscale** is produced and a low contrast radiograph is obtained, which is useful for the thorax and abdomen.

When **high mAs/low kVp** are used, a **narrow greyscale** is produced, with whites and blacks, and a high contrast radiograph is obtained, which is useful for radiographs of bones and joints (head, spine and extremities).

Distance

The distance from the X-ray tube to the cassette is called the **film-focus distance (FFD)**. As the distance increases, the intensity of the X-rays decreases. Thus, when changing the FFD, the total amount of X-rays must be increased or decreased so that the exposure parameters adapt to the new distance.

Calculation of the change of mAs with FFD

$$\text{Previous mAs} \times \frac{(\text{New FFD})^2}{(\text{Old FFD})^2} = \text{New mAs}$$

FFD is an important exposure factor, so it should be **kept constant**. The distance commonly used in veterinary medicine is **100 cm**, except for the thoracic cavity where a distance of 120–150 cm can be used.

The object–film distance affects the detail of the radiograph and means that the patient should be as close as possible to the film.

Analogue radiology (conventional)

Cassette

The cassette is a rigid case which houses the **intensifying screen** and **protects** the film, with both in contact with each other. It has two sides, one of which is coloured to indicate the location of the screen.

There are different sizes of cassette, each with corresponding screen and film sizes.

Intensifying or reinforcement screens

X-ray films are much more sensitive to visible light photons than to X-ray photons, which is why reinforcement screens are used.

Intensifying screens are composed of layers of **phosphorescent crystals** that emit light when X-rays strike them. Their thickness and the size of the crystals can vary: the greater the thickness and the size of the crystal, the less radiation is necessary; more radiation causes a reduction in radiographic detail.

The crystals may be:

- **calcium wolframate or calcium tungstate**, which emit light within the blue spectrum (universal screens)
- **rare earth phosphor**, which emits light within the green spectrum (rare earth or orthochromatic screens).

The conversion of X-ray photons to visible light photons is four times greater in rare earth phosphor crystals than in calcium tungstate crystals.

Films

Radiographic film consists of a polyester base impregnated on both sides with an emulsion containing silver crystals. When the photons interact with the silver crystals, a latent image is created, which when developed becomes visible as an X-ray image.

There are two types of film.

- **With screen.** In these, the silver crystals have to be sensitive to the visible light photons that the screen will emit.
- **Without screen.** Films can be of varying speeds, according to the size of the crystals. There are also a wide range of densities or "film latitudes".

Taking all of the above into consideration, the film–screen combination should always be referred to when describing a technique.

Film processing

Development is the process by which the latent image becomes visible.

The stages of film processing are:

- exposure
- stop bath for fixation
- rinsing
- drying.

The process can be manual or automatic.

Digital radiology

In digital format the images are obtained directly, without passing through a radiographic film plate.

The advantages of this technique are that digital radiology:

- enables manipulation of the image
- facilitates storage of images
- enables viewing anywhere, which facilitates seeking an expert second opinion
- eliminates chemicals from the development process
- has rapid processing times.

However, good technique is still central to achieving quality radiographs.

Digital radiology systems

There are currently two types of digital radiology system: **computerized radiology (CR)** and **direct digital radiology (DR)**.

Computerized radiology

In this system the film, reinforcement screen and cassette are replaced with a photostimulable phosphor screen and CR cassette (Figure 3.4), and the development process with a digital image reader.

As soon as the CR cassette with the **phosphor screen is irradiated**, information is stored, and this is read by special equipment to become a digital image. Once the cassette is inside the reading device, the machine extracts the phosphor screen, places it in a **roller drag system** and sweeps each horizontal line of the plate with a **laser beam in the red wavelength.** Red laser light creates the **appropriate excitation for phosphor to emit the energy** accumulated during the irradiation with X-rays in the form of visible light photons in the blue to green wavelength range. A **fibre optic light guide** picks up much of the light emitted by the phosphor screen and takes it to a photomultiplier tube, which converts the light into an electrical signal, and thus forms the digital image (Figure 3.4).

The processor needs 60–90 seconds to produce the image from each cassette, before they can be reused.

The screens deteriorate with time, and last for approximately 10,000 exposures.

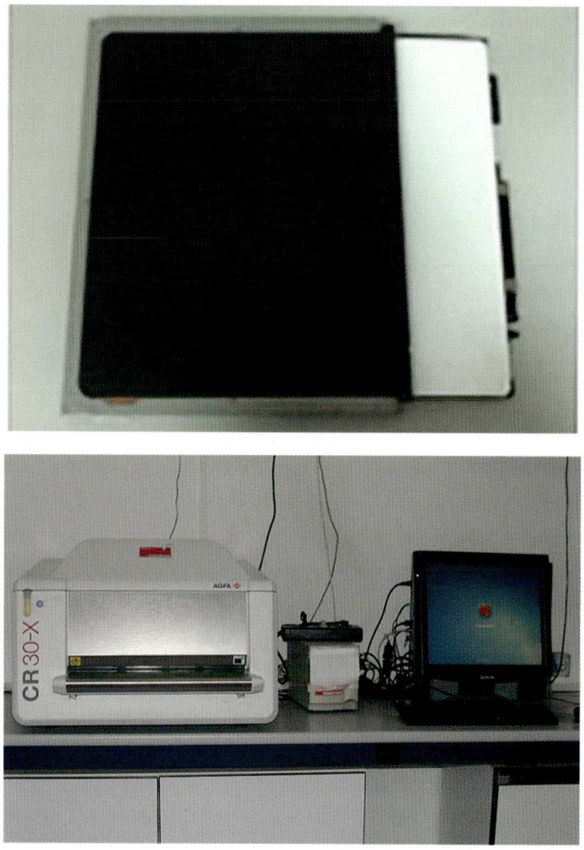

Figure 3.4. (a) Cassette with photostimulable screen used in computerized digital radiology (CR). (b) Digitizer and CR work station.

Direct digital radiology

DR produces a digital image instantaneously (within 4–10 seconds). With this system the film, the reinforcement screen and the cassette are replaced by direct capture equipment, in which the X-ray image is captured on a panel sensitive to electromagnetic photons that produces an image immediately, without the intermediate step of reading the panel.

Flat panel detectors

Systems based on **flat panel detectors (FPD)** collect information from the photons collect information from the X-ray photons through an active matrix through an active matrix and digitize it; the computer then stores the data file received from the detector, producing a digital image.

There are two types of FPDs.

- **Selenium detectors** (called direct conversion) directly convert the X-ray photons into electrical charge.
- **Silicon detectors** (called indirect conversion) convert the X-ray photons into visible light photons and these, in turn, into electrical charge.

In both systems, the reading of the charge stored in each pixel of the active matrix during an X-ray shot is initiated immediately after the equipment cuts the X-ray beam off.

They can be used in the X-ray equipment tray or on top of the table.

Charge coupled devices

There are also systems based on the incorporation of **charge coupled devices** into certain X-ray machines. However, their use in veterinary medicine is limited compared to CR and FPD.

Equipment

Monitors

Digital images are displayed on a computer monitor. To review them together with the owners in the consultation room, a low-resolution monitor is sufficient. But for diagnostic purposes, a high-resolution monitor is required, with at least 2 megapixels.

DICOM

DICOM (Digital Imaging and Communication in Medicine) is the format that standardizes medical digital images from all modalities and ensures the interoperability of the different teams that produce them.

Storage of digital images

As is the case with physical radiographs, digital images need to be stored as an integral part of the patient's clinical history.

There are several advantages presented by digital files compared to physical images.

- Less space is required for storage.
- They can be recovered and viewed quickly.
- The images do not degrade over time.

There are several storage options, from a network (PACS system, file system and communication) to removable recording media (CD, DVD, flash drives).

Radiation protection

Introduction

Radiation protection is a scientific and technical discipline whose purpose is the **protection of people and the environment** from the risks arising from the use of radioactive sources, both natural and artificial, in medical, industrial, research or agricultural activities.

General principles of radiation protection

Each country has their own legislation regarding ionizing radiation and safety. For example, in Spain, all functions of surveillance and establishment of standards are centralized within the National Security Council, following the regulations established by the International Commission on Radiological Protection (ICRP). Every clinic should be familiar with the relevant regulations and conform to them at all times.

The protection system recommended by the ICRP is based on three fundamental principles.

1. Justification.
2. Optimization.
3. Dose limitation.

Justification

The activity that involves radiation exposure must be **justified by the advantages** the system provides, which must outweigh the potential harmful effects.

Optimization

The **ALARA** criterion (**as low as reasonably achievable**) is followed, according to which all exposures to ionizing radiation should be kept as low as reasonably possible, taking into account certain economic and social factors. Individual doses, the number of people exposed and the likelihood of potential exposures occurring should be kept as low as reasonably achievable.

Dose limitation

In any case, the radiation dose that any individual can receive **must not exceed the values established as legal limits**, which guarantees the protection of the general public and in particular the professionals exposed to it.

Dosimetry

Limiting the effects of ionizing radiation is achieved by avoiding unjustified exposures and keeping the justified ones as low as possible.

Area dosimetry

When working with radioactive material, it is important to **frequently check the work area** and the environment are not contaminated. The dose rate should be measured in the environment, either with monitors or fixed dosimeters, to ensure it is as low as possible.

Personal dosimetry

When working with X-rays, personal dosimeters should be worn, which are based on photographic films or thermoluminescent crystals.

Legislation

Dose limits

The system of radiological protection currently established in Spain is included in the **Royal Decree 783/2001** which approves the Regulation on Health Protection against Ionizing Radiation. This Regulation **sets the dose limits** for professionally exposed personnel and trainees, students and the general public.

For workers who are exposed professionally, the effective dose limit is 100 mSv over a period of five calendar years (from January to December), subject also to a maximum effective dose of 50 mSv in any one calendar year. In addition, specific limitations are imposed to protect different parts of the body.

- **The eye**. Equivalent dose limit of 150 mSv per calendar year.
- **The skin**. Equivalent dose limit of 500 mSv per calendar year. This limit shall be applied to the average dose over any area of 1 cm^2, regardless of the area exposed.
- **The hands, forearms, feet and ankles**. 500 mSv per calendar year.

Classification and signage of work areas

The **owner of the business** must classify the workspaces, considering the risk of exposure and the probability and magnitude of potential exposures. This classification involves the following areas.

Controlled area

This is the area in which there is the possibility of receiving effective doses above 6 mSv/calendar year or an equivalent dose greater than 3/10 of the equivalent dose limits for the eye, skin and extremities. This also applies to areas in which it is necessary to follow work procedures, either to restrict exposure, to avoid the dispersion of radioactive contamination or to prevent or limit the probability and magnitude of radiological accidents and their consequences. It is signposted with a green trefoil on a white background (Figure 3.5).

Controlled areas can also be subdivided as follows.

Area of limited permanence. An area where there is a risk of receiving a dose which exceeds annual limits. It is signposted with a yellow trefoil on a white background.

Area of regulated permanence. An area where there is a risk of receiving a dose in excess of limits in a short period of time. It is signposted with an orange trefoil on a white background.

Prohibited access area. An area where there is a risk of receiving doses above annual limits in a single

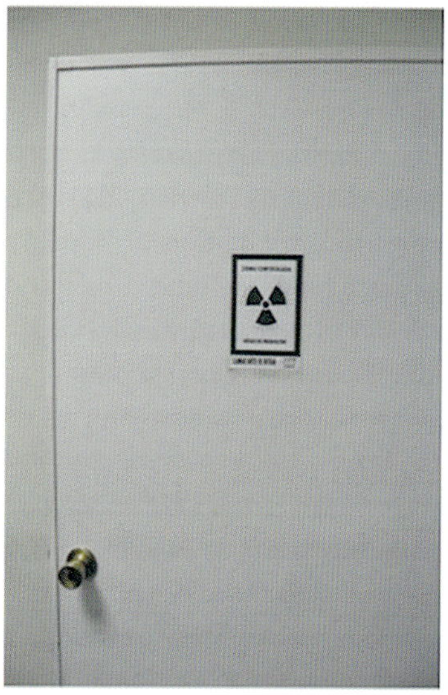

Figure 3.5. Signposting of controlled area.

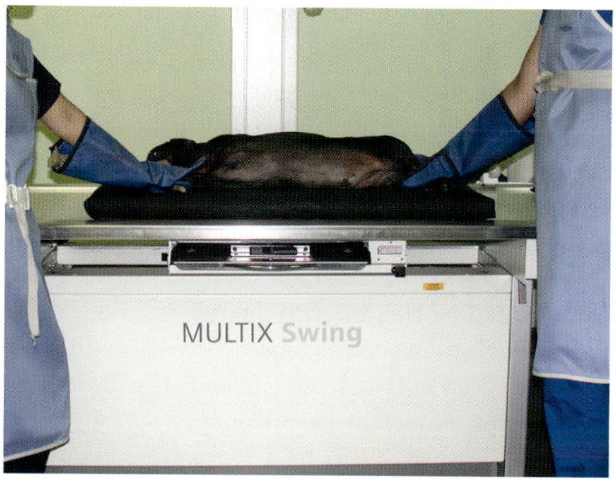

Figure 3.6. People involved in the immobilization of an animal should use lead-lined protective equipment (gloves, aprons, thyroid protectors) and position themselves outside the central X-ray beam.

exposure. It is signposted with a red trefoil on a white background.

Surveillance area. An area in which, although it is not a controlled area, there is a risk of receiving doses higher than 1 mSv/year or equivalent to 1/10 of the dose limits for eyes, skin and extremities. It is signposted with a grey/blue trefoil on a white background.

To specify the danger in more detail:

- the trefoil is bordered with **pointed tips** if there is a risk of **external irradiation**
- the trefoil is bordered by a **dotted field** if there is a risk of **radioactive contamination**
- the trefoil is bordered with **pointed tips on a dotted background** if the **two risks coexist**.

Radiation protection in diagnostic imaging services

In the clinic, quality diagnostic radiographs must be obtained while reducing the radiation dose to the minimum necessary. For this reason, the following general measures should be taken into account.

- Regarding the **X-ray machine**. **Quality control measures** for radiological equipment, image receivers, data recording, processing and visualization systems for the image according to the provisions of the Royal Decree 1976/1999, of 23 December, which establishes quality criteria in radio diagnosis.
- Regarding **radiological technique**. Justification and optimization in radiological examinations.
- Regarding **reduction of exposure**:
  - immobilization of the patient (sedation).
- Regarding **the personnel** involved in the immobilization, it is essential that:
  - personnel are kept to a minimum
  - they wear leaded protective equipment (gloves, aprons, thyroid protectors) (Figure 3.6)
  - they are positioned as far as possible from the X-ray tube and outside the line of the main X-ray beam
  - exposure time is reduced
  - structural shields are used.
- Surveillance measures:
  - **radiological surveillance** in work areas
  - **dosimetric and health surveillance** of exposed workers.

Principles of radiographic interpretation

Introduction

A radiograph is a **two-dimensional image** of a three-dimensional object, in black and white, that is visualized through a **greyscale** of shadows. Radiological interpretation is based on the visualization and analysis of these shadows and opacities, which are formed because:

- X-ray photons have the ability to penetrate tissues.
  - Some photons pass through tissue without changing.
  - Some photons are attenuated by the tissue, absorbed or scattered.

Absorption depends on the tissue's atomic number (Z), density and thickness (Figure 3.7).

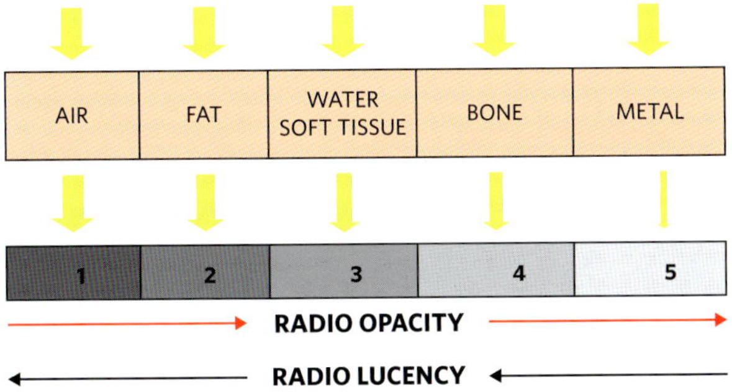

Figure 3.7. Differential absorption depending on density and atomic number of tissues.

- Tissues with a high Z value absorb more photons than those with a low Z value.
- Thicker tissues absorb more photons than thin tissues with the same Z value.

A radiograph shows **a range of opacities** from white to black through a greyscale, as a result of which an image is formed that is recognizable and can be interpreted.

Although air has a greater Z value than fat, it is much less dense and therefore less radiopaque (more radiolucent) than fat (Table 3.1).

By increasing the thickness of the same tissue, it appears more radiopaque (for example, the area where the two kidneys overlap).

Table 3.1. Density and atomic number of different substances.

Tissue	Z	Density (g/cm^3)
Air	7.8	0.001
Fat	6.5	0.92
Water	7.5	1.00
Muscle	7.6	1.04
Bone	12.3	1.65
Lead	82	8.7

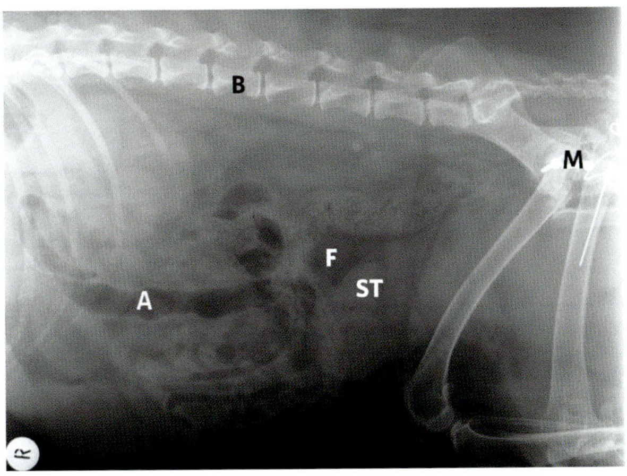

Figure 3.8. Basic radiographic opacities. A, air; F, fat; ST, soft tissue; B, bone/mineral; M, metal.

There are five basic radiographic opacities (Figure 3.8).

- **Gas** is the most radiolucent material visible on an X-ray. The transparency of gas provides contrast, allowing visualization of the thorax.
- **Fat** is more radiolucent than bone or soft tissue, but more radiopaque than gas. Fat's relative radio transparency serves as a contrast to visualize soft tissues that are surrounded by fat, especially in the abdomen.
- **Soft tissue/liquid**. Liquid and soft tissue have the same opacity. Thus, organs filled with fluid (for example, the bladder) and parenchymatous organs (for example, the liver) have the same opacity. Variations in the thickness and density of soft tissue lead to variations of opacities in radiography.
- **Bone** is the whitest physiological opacity seen on an X-ray. There are normal variations in the radiopacity of different types of bone (spongy, trabecular, cortical and medullary).
- **Metal** is the most opaque and appears white on a radiograph. This corresponds to contrast media and metallic foreign bodies.

An X-ray is an image comprised of these five opacities. However, within each there are **variations according to the thickness and density** of each structure. Also, these variations can be relative and depend on the opacity of the background (for example, a bladder stone) (Figure 3.9).

As previously defined, an X-ray is a two-dimensional image of a three-dimensional object. Therefore, the perception of depth is lost, and geometric factors can alter the image. It is therefore advisable to routinely use the same projections and become familiar with recognizing the different structures. The standard recommendation is as follows.

- Use two **orthogonal projections** (i.e., at an angle of 90°; Figure 3.1).
  - Place the area to be radiographed as **close as possible to the film**, to minimize magnification.
  - Place the area to be radiographed **parallel to the cassette** and perpendicular to the X-ray beam, to minimize geometric distortion (Figure 3.3).

Terminology

Listed below are some common radiographic terms.

- **Projections** are named according to the direction of the primary beam, first naming where it enters and then where it leaves and using the correct anatomical terminology.

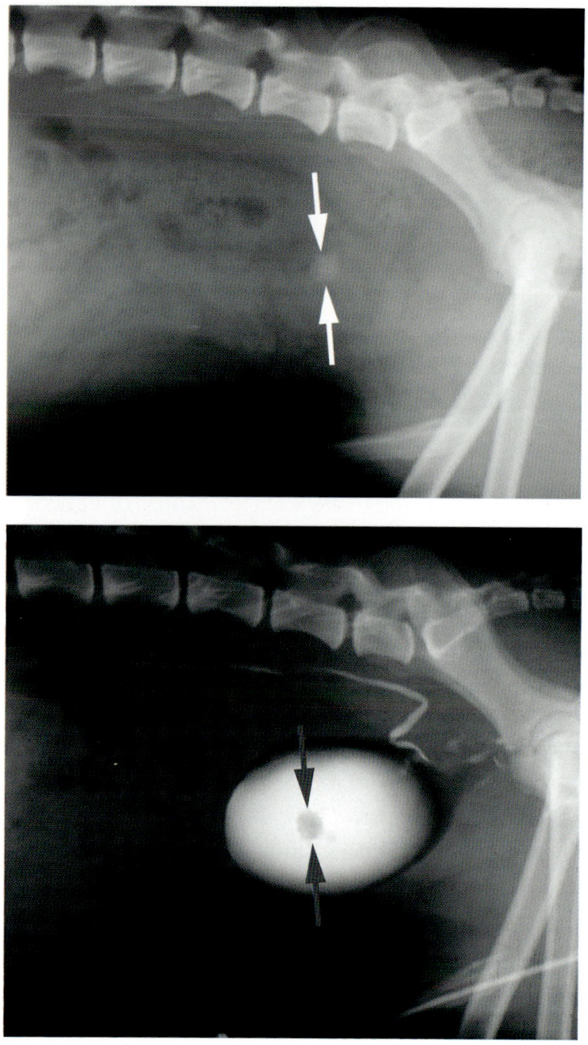

Figure 3.9. (a) Bladder stone with mineral opacity (arrows). (b) With a radiopaque background the stone is radiolucent.

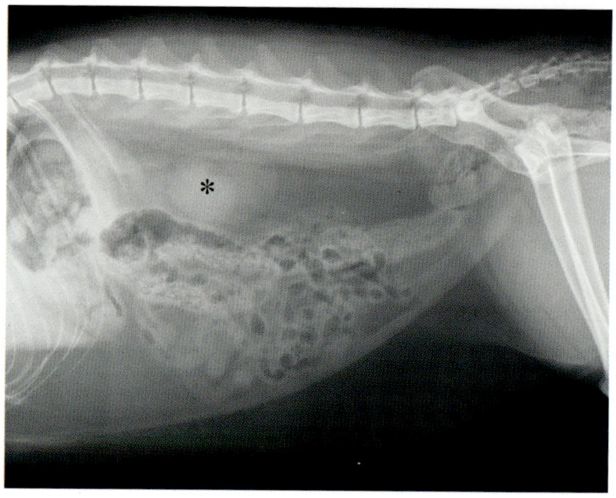

Figure 3.10. Summation sign. The two kidneys are superimposed (*), which gives the appearance of an area of increased opacity.

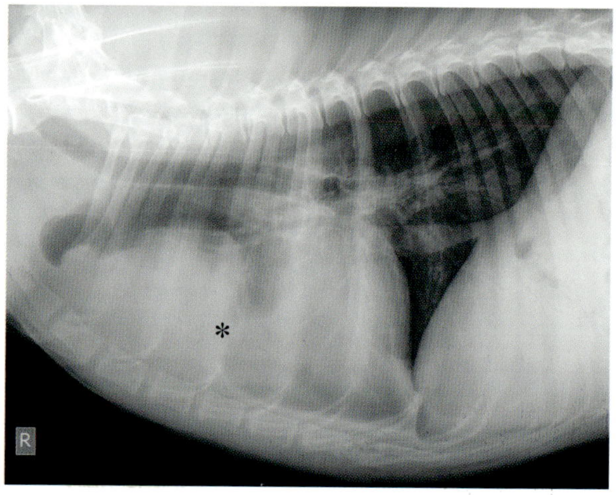

Figure 3.11. Silhouette sign. A mediastinal mass is in contact with the cardiac silhouette (*), whose border cannot be seen.

- **Radiopacity** refers to radio density or density, when the shadows as they appear on an X-ray are described.
- **Radiolucent or radio transparent** refers to structures that allow little absorption of electromagnetic photons; therefore more photons reach the film and the shadow is darker or black.
- **Radiopaque** is a term used for structures that absorb a lot of electromagnetic photons, so fewer of the photos reach the film and the shadow is paler or white.
- **Contrast** is the difference in tone between two radiopacities.
- **Summation sign.** This occurs when parts of a patient or objects located in different planes overlap. The result is a cumulative image representing the degree of absorption of X-rays of all superimposed objects (Figure 3.10). The summation sign may be radiolucent or radiopaque.
- **Silhouette sign** or border effacement (loss of visualization of the edges). When two structures with the same radiopacity are in contact, their margins cannot be seen (Figure 3.11). On the other hand, if two structures with the same radiopacity are not in contact and are separated by different radiopacities, their edges can be seen.

Radiological interpretation

Examination of radiographs should be done **systematically,** for which a negatoscope (for traditional radiographs) with two areas, or digital monitors with 2 megapixels, is necessary.

Radiographs should be placed on the monitor or negatoscope as follows.

- **Lateral projection**: place the head to the left and the dorsal area at the top of the image.
- **VD/DV projection**: place the left area of the animal to the right of the examiner and the cranial part at the top (Figure 3.1).

Basis for a radiological report

A report for any imaging technique must be structured and concise, and cover the points listed below.

Radiographic examination technique

This involves evaluation of the **technical quality** of the radiograph, including positioning, collimation, how it is centred, exposure factors and the absence of artefacts.

A thorough interpretation then has two further phases, the **analytical or recognition stage** and the **deductive stage**.

Analytical or recognition stage

It is very important to analyse the entire radiograph in a systematic way, either starting from the periphery and moving inwards, or **by organs** or systems. The five radiographic signs should be evaluated in either case.

1. Size.
2. Location.
3. Opacity.
4. Shape/contour.
5. Number.

To determine whether abnormalities are present it is important to be familiar with normal radiographic appearance and therefore it is useful to have an atlas of radiographic anatomy to hand.

At this stage all observations should be described using the correct vocabulary.

Deductive stage

A list of all **changes observed** (radiographic signs) and causes that could lead to these signs (differential diagnoses), ordering them from most to least likely, should be compiled. Together with the history and clinical signs other appropriate techniques should be employed to arrive at a diagnosis.

Therefore, the report for any imaging technique must have four sections.

1. Description.
2. Radiological diagnosis (summary of findings).
3. Differential diagnoses (the causes that could lead to these findings) in order of probability.
4. Other tests or techniques (ultrasound, FNA, etc.) to be performed.

Most common errors and artefacts on interpretation

The most common mistakes and artefacts on interpretation are as follows.

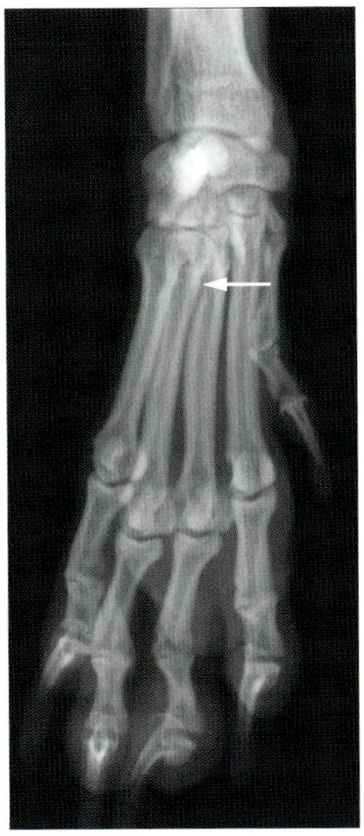

Figure 3.12. Mach bands. Dorsopalmar projection of the carpometacarpus of a dog. Radiolucent lines can be seen where the cortical abaxial and axial third and fourth metacarpus overlap, as if they were fissures (arrow).

- **Loss of visualization of the abdominal serosa** of a very thin animal. This can be confused with peritoneal effusion.
- **Normal anatomical variations** in the appearance of the organs **depending on the breed**.
- Superposition of the pulmonary vessels and ribs, which may appear as nodules.
- The thoracic nipples may look like masses.
- **Mach phenomenon.** Mach bands are optical illusions which are seen as radiopaque or radiotransparent lines with sharp edges between structures with a significant difference in opacity. They can appear between the bones, resembling fissures (Figure 3.12), or skin folds in a ventrodorsal projection, simulating a pneumothorax.
- Another optical illusion is the effect of the background contrast: structures superimposed on a more radiolucent background may appear more opaque than when on a radiopaque background.

Radiological contrast media

Introduction

Many structures or organs have a similar soft tissue opacity, which limits the information obtained from certain studies involving plain radiographs. To overcome this, contrast media are used. These agents either absorb more X-ray photons than soft tissue, making them appear white, or transmit more X-ray photons than soft tissue so they appear black.

The information obtained through the use of contrast relates to the anatomy of the organs (such as size, shape, position and margins) and, directly or indirectly, to their function. Indeed, contrast studies remain useful for certain conditions despite the availability of ultrasound or sectional imaging techniques such as computed tomography (CT) or magnetic resonance imaging (MRI).

Types of contrast media

There are two types of contrast: positive (radiopaque) and negative (radiolucent). When both types of contrast are used, this is termed double contrast.

Negative contrasts

These are **gases with a low physical density** (air, O_2, CO_2 and NO_2). They can be used to fill hollow organs or cavities and do not attenuate X-rays, so they produce **radiolucent** areas. They do not produce good mucosal detail (Figure 3.13).

Positive contrasts

These are elements with a **high atomic number**. They absorb a large number of X-rays and appear as more **opaque** areas than the surrounding structures (Figure 3.14).

Barium

Barium is used exclusively for imaging the **gastrointestinal tract** (GIT). It is an insoluble, inert contrast and is not absorbed through the GIT.

It can produce **granulomatous reactions** and adhesions if it enters the peritoneal or mediastinal cavity,

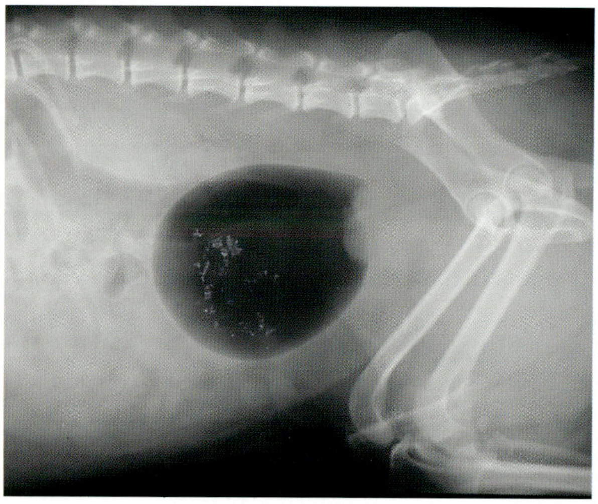

Figure 3.13. Negative cystography.

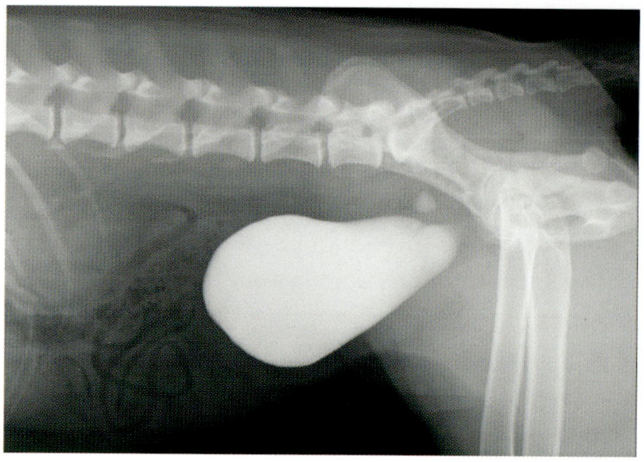

Figure 3.14. Positive cystography.

and if inhaled (for example, by animals with dysphagia or laryngeal paralysis) it can cause **aspiration pneumonia**.

When barium is used, endoscopy cannot be performed until 24 hours later.

Barium sulphate is available as:

- a colloidal suspension
- paste, in cases of ulcers
- powder
- barium impregnated polyethylene spheres (BIPS).

Hydrosoluble iodines

These are used for:

- **vascular** studies (upper urinary tract, cardiovascular and portal angiography)
- lower urinary tract
- digestive system
- arthrography
- sialography
- lacrimal sac
- fistulae
- lymphangiography
- **myelography**.

All iodinated contrasts are tri-iodinated benzoic acid derivatives which are soluble in water and are excreted by the kidneys. They can be ionic or non-ionic.

Ionic (hyperosmolar) iodinated contrasts

These are monomers derived from diatrizoate, metrizoic acid or sodium iothalamate combined with meglumine (Urografin, Gastrografin). They are ionic salts which dissociate in solution and are hyperosmolar.

They are viscous and should be heated before use.

They are contraindicated in patients with:

- hypotension
- dehydration
- kidney failure.

Non-ionic (low osmolarity) iodinated contrasts

These do not dissociate in solution and are considered iso-osmolar with respect to blood plasma. As they do not dissociate, they have no charge and can be used in myelograms.

They produce few side effects. Examples include iopamidol, iohexol and iopramide.

They are relatively innocuous, although they can produce some side effects such as:

- vomiting
- anaphylactic reactions
- idiosyncratic reactions.

Side effects generally occur with ionic contrasts, due to their high osmolarity (5–8 times normal), their ionic charge and their chemical toxicity. Reactions include:

- nephrotoxicity induced by contrast
- cardiovascular effects such as:
  - bradycardia
  - hypotension
  - hypertension.

Urinary tract studies

The most common **techniques** for evaluation of the urinary tract are:

- excretory urography (kidneys and ureters)
- cystography, positive or negative (bladder)
- retrograde vaginourethrography in the female
- retrograde urethrography in the male (urethra).

Patient preparation involves:

- fasting for 24 hours
- an enema 2–3 hours before
- deep sedation or general anaesthesia (for excretory urography)
- simple radiographs.

Excretory or intravenous urography (EU)

There are two ways of performing this technique.

Bolus method (low volume)

- **Dosage.** Rapid injection of contrast (dose 600–800 mg iodine/kg).
- **Shooting times.** Immediately and after 5, 10, 15 and 20 minutes.
- **Radiographic projections.** VD and, at 15 and 20 minutes, VD, lateral and lateral oblique to study the openings of the ureters into the bladder.

Infusion method (high volume)

- **Total dose.** 1200 mg iodine/kg, which is diluted with physiological saline and given at a dose of 5–10 ml/kg.
- **Administration.** Intravenously over 10–15 minutes.
- **Radiographic projections.** VD, lateral and lateral oblique at 5, 10 and 15 minutes after starting the infusion.

When the aim is to evaluate the outlets of the ureters, this technique is combined with negative cystography.

Interpretation

- **Vascular/arterial phase**. In the first few seconds after the rapid injection.
- **Nephrogram**. Between 30 seconds and 5 minutes after the injection. The kidneys appear more uniform with an increased opacity (Figure 3.15).
- **Pyelogram.** 2–5 minutes after injection, the contrast begins to appear in the diverticula, the renal pelvis and the ureters.
- **Ureters.** At 5–10 minutes, the ureters are observed as narrow lines of varying thickness, due to normal peristalsis, running caudally towards the bladder, ending in the vesical trigone and adopting a hook shape (Figure 3.15).

Normally, the outlets of the ureters are best visualized in oblique projections (Figure 3.16).

Cystography

Before performing contrast studies of the bladder, it should be catheterized and completely emptied of urine.

The projections used to evaluate the bladder are:

- lateral, immediately after administering the contrast
- ventrodorsal, when necessary.

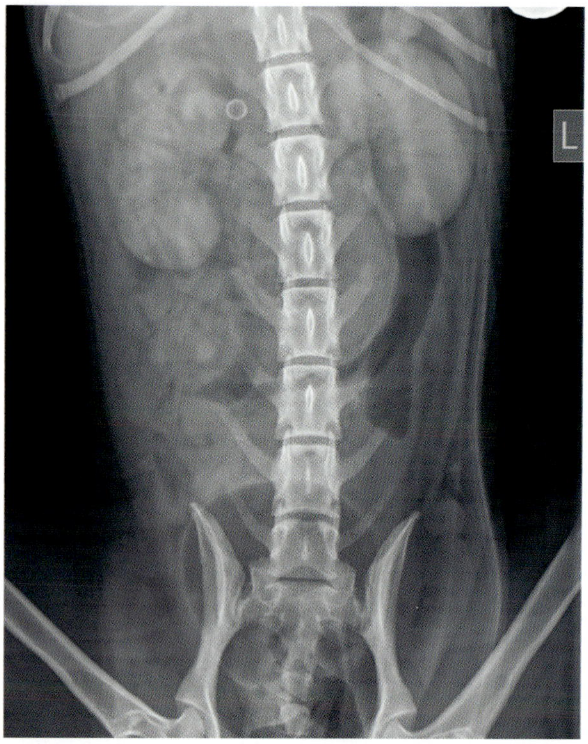

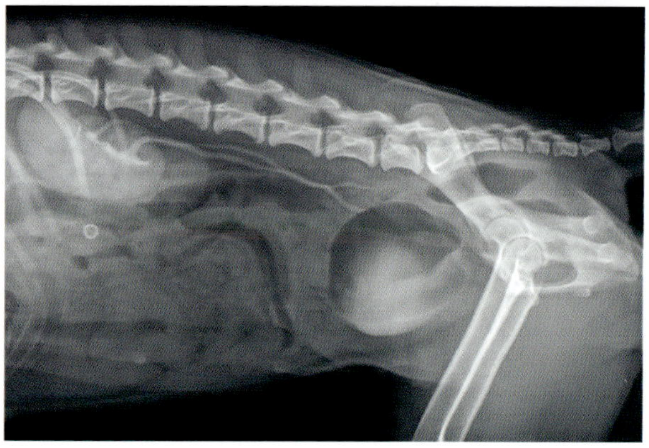

Figure 3.15. Intravenous urography. (a) Nephrogram phase. (b) Pyelogram phase.

Positive cystography

Contrast diluted to 5–10% in a volume of 50–300 ml depending on the size of the animal, is introduced into the bladder through a catheter (Figure 3.14). This provides good mucosal detail, although small lesions may be masked. It is indicated in cases of fistulas or wall breaks.

Negative cystography (pneumocystography)

Air is introduced into the bladder through a catheter, which is connected to a three-way tap to prevent leaks. The dose used is **6–10 ml air/kg** (Figure 3.13).

Pneumocystography is used to identify the location of the bladder. It does not produce good mucosal detail unless a large mass is present.

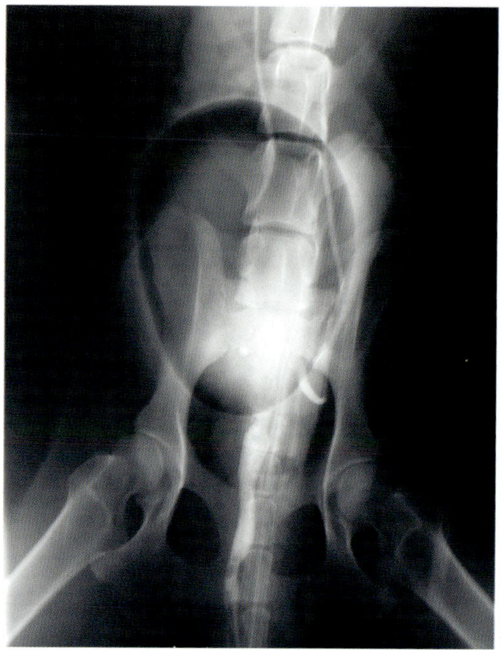

Figure 3.16. Oblique view to better visualize the outlet of the ureter.

Double contrast cystography

Contrast diluted to 20% in a volume of 5–10 ml is introduced into the bladder, which is then inflated with air (as in negative cystography).

This technique offers **good mucosal detail**, so that small lesions on the bladder wall and radiolucent stones can be seen.

Interpretation

The bladder should be uniformly distended, in the shape of a tear drop, with the wall intact, thin and of uniform thickness, without filling defects in the wall or lumen.

Retrograde urethrography (male)

Indications

- persistent haematuria
- dysuria
- urinary incontinence
- urinary obstruction
- prostatic disease
- urethritis/neoplasms.

Technique

1. Perform a negative cystography.
2. Inject 5–10 ml of diluted contrast (150–200 mg iodine/ml) through a catheter located in the penile urethra while the urethra is occluded.

3. Immediately perform lateral projections, pulling on the hindlimbs:
   a) cranially, to locate the ischiatic urethra
   b) caudally, to locate the penile urethra.
4. Perform a VD projection to identify:
   a) compression injuries
   b) displacement of the intrapelvic urethra
   c) prostatic lesions.

Retrograde vaginourethrography (female)

Indications

This technique is usually recommended to locate:

- abnormal communications of ureters with the urethra or vagina (ectopic ureters) (Figure 3.17)
- vaginal masses
- fistulae.

Technique

1. Fill the catheter lumen with the contrast to prevent the formation of bubbles.
2. Obtain a **negative cystography** and place a **Foley catheter** with the balloon filled with air in the vaginal vestibule. An intestinal clamp or uterine forceps can be placed on the lips of the vulva, to avoid the contrast refluxing.
3. Introduce diluted contrast at **150–200 mg iodine/ml (1 ml/kg)**.
4. Take a **lateral projection** immediately after introducing the contrast.

Interpretation

In males, the urethra should be visualized in its entirety, with smooth, uniform walls and no filling defects.

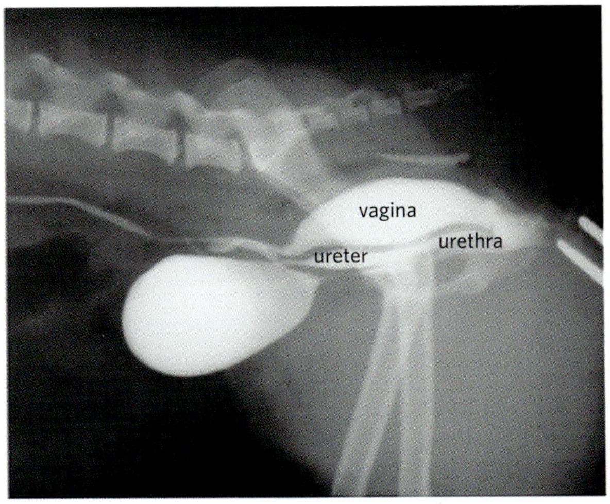

Figure 3.17. Lateral projection of a vaginourethrography. An ectopic ureter can be seen.

In females, both the urethra and the vagina should have smooth, uniform walls and no filling defects.

Studies of the gastrointestinal system

Currently, ultrasound and endoscopy are the techniques of choice to evaluate the GIT, having largely replaced radiographic techniques using contrast. However, radiographic or fluoroscopic studies (dynamic studies) that use **positive contrast media** such as barium are still important in the diagnosis of pathologies of the oropharynx, oesophagus and stomach. In fact, **fluoroscopy** is the technique of choice to evaluate **swallowing disorders** when functional changes are suspected.

Nowadays it is unusual to perform a gastrointestinal transit study using barium or an iodinated contrast, because this is expensive, time consuming, and the information gained is minimal compared to other techniques.

GIT studies (except for those of the colon) are performed with the patient conscious, since sedation interferes with motility and swallowing reflexes, with the risk of regurgitation and inhalation of contrast. If sedation is necessary, acepromazine (0.1 mg/kg) and pethidine (2 mg/kg) can be used.

The contrast media used are:

- barium sulphate
- barium impregnated polyethylene spheres (BIPS)
- sodium diatrizoate and meglumine (Gastrografin).

In cases of suspected gastrointestinal perforation, barium should not be administered, as it produces granulomatous peritonitis. Instead, a hydrosoluble iodinated contrast agent can be used, such as sodium diatrizoate and meglumine, which, in case of extravasation, is rapidly absorbed from the peritoneum. The drawback is that it has poor contrast and is diluted by the contents of the stomach and intestine.

Study of the oesophagus

Indications

- regurgitation
- gagging
- dysphagia
- vomiting undigested food after eating.

Technique

No preparation of the patient is needed. The recommended contrast is 100% barium sulphate mixed with food (without forgetting its contraindications).

The best projection to evaluate the oesophagus is a left lateral view of the cervical and thoracic areas.

In cases of dysphagia, an image amplifier should be used to visualize motility, and care must be taken so that aspiration of contrast does not occur, as this can lead to aspiration pneumonia.

On plain radiographs, two orthogonal projections should be performed to detect possible aspiration pneumonia.

To observe the transit of the bolus, the best technique is fluoroscopy.

Interpretation

The contrast bolus passes quickly from the base of the tongue to the pharynx, oesophagus and stomach. Contrast is observed in the oesophagus 30 seconds after swallowing.

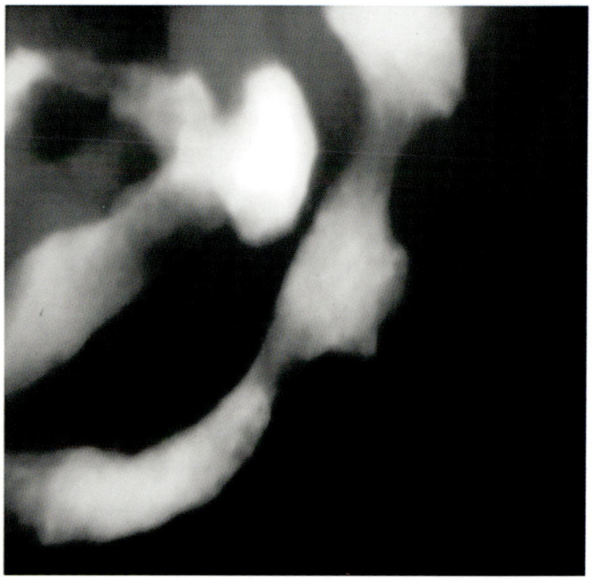

Figure 3.18. Peyer's patches (pseudo-ulcers).

Study of the stomach and intestine

Indications

- persistent vomiting
- haematemesis
- GIT displacement
- dilation of the small intestine.

Technique

The patient should be **fasted for 24 hours**, and if possible should not be sedated.

1. Perform plain radiographs (right lateral, left lateral, VD and DV).
2. Administer **5–10 ml/kg of barium sulphate suspension**.
3. Perform right lateral, left lateral, VD and DV radiographs (the appearance of the stomach will vary due to the displacement of gas and liquid to the dependent and non-dependent sides).
4. Lateral and VD projections should be repeated at 5, 10 and 15 minutes, and then every 15 minutes until the contrast reaches the colon.

During interpretation the following should be evaluated.

- **Gastric emptying.** If barium is used, this begins after 15 minutes but can be delayed for up to 30–45 minutes in nervous animals. The stomach takes 1–2 hours to empty partially and empties completely after 4 hours.
- **Gastrointestinal transit time.** This is the time that it takes contrast to reach the large intestine: 4 hours, if barium is used. In the case of water-soluble iodinated contrast, times are considerably reduced. In cats, transit times are shorter than in dogs.
- **Mucosal appearance.** The contrast column can be observed in the interior of the intestine, with regular borders, and **slits may be seen** in the antimesenteric border of the duodenum due to the **Peyer's patches** (Figure 3.18).

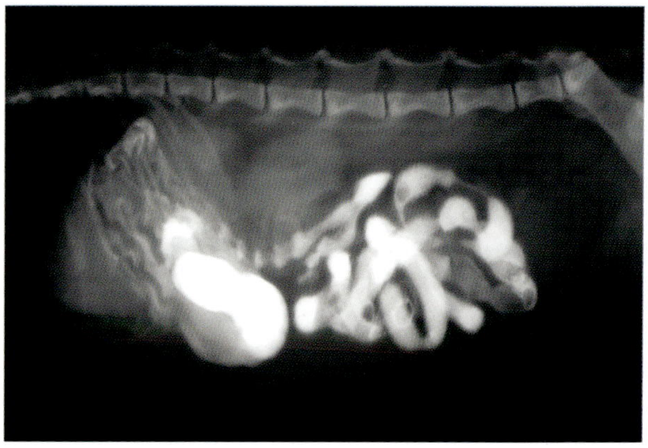

Figure 3.19. Gastrointestinal transit in a cat. The pearl necklace appearance can be seen in the duodenum.

In the cat, the **descending duodenum** may present a **segmented appearance** (pearl necklace) due to peristalsis (Figure 3.19).

Study of the large intestine

Endoscopy is the technique of choice for evaluation of the colon, so much so that it is currently unusual for positive or negative contrast to be used to obtain information about its condition.

Indications

- tenesmus
- melena
- chronic diarrhoea
- intrapelvic masses.

Technique

1. Administer a non-irritant enema 2–3 hours before.
2. Use strong sedation or general anaesthesia.
3. Create a pneumocolon. Inflate with **air (5–10 ml/kg)** through a Foley catheter.
4. Administer a barium enema. **Barium diluted with warm water (10 ml/kg)** is introduced slowly through a Foley catheter until the colon is fully distended.
5. Perform lateral and VD projections.

Interpretation

The pneumocolon is used to evaluate the size of the colon and differentiate it from the small intestine.

The colonic enema causes the edges of the colon to become clear and regular.

Other techniques

There are other contrast techniques available, such as myelography, arthrography, portography, angiocardiography, bronchography and cholecystography. However, these are now little used, either because specialized equipment is required or because they have been replaced by more modern imaging techniques such as ultrasound, CT or MRI.

Thoracic radiology

General considerations

To avoid and minimize the effects of cardiac and respiratory movements, which make it difficult to obtain a diagnostic chest X-ray, **exposure times of 1/60–1/120 s** are recommended. On the other hand, although the thorax is a region with high natural contrast due to the air contained in the lungs, to observe the structures with a soft tissue opacity contained within the lungs (vessels, interstitium, bronchi and possible small nodules) low contrast radiography is necessary (greyscale), so **high kV** (> **70**) and **low mAs** (high mAs, short exposure time) are used.

Projections

In a standard study, **at least two projections** are required: orthogonal (VD or DV) and lateral (left or right).

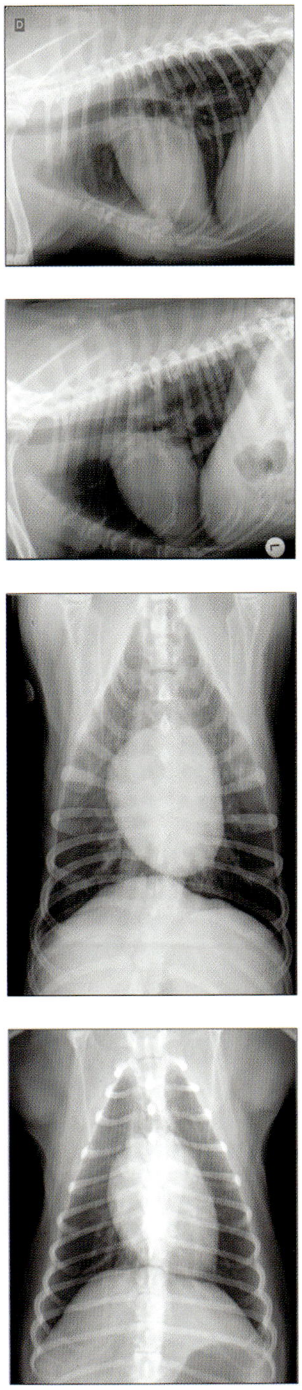

Figure 3.20. Thorax of a radiologically mature dog. (a) Right lateral projection. (b) Left lateral projection. (c) Ventrodorsal projection. (d) Dorsoventral projection.

However, the study is more complete with three projections (both lateral and one orthogonal), bearing the following points in mind (Figure 3.20).

- The **left lateral** projection is best for evaluating lesions in the **right lobes**, since these are better aerated, which increases the detail of the lung and soft tissue. However, it should be taken into account that in this projection the heart is visualized as more balloon-like and rounded.

- In the **right lateral** projection, the **left lobes** are better visualized.
- The **DV** projection is best for visualizing small amounts of **pleural fluid** and evaluating the size and **shape of the heart**.
- The **VD** projection is ideal for assessing **the lungs** and vascularization of the caudal lobes.

Thus, depending on the pathology in question, one or more of these projections should be used, as follows.

- **Cardiac changes**: right lateral and DV.
- **Pulmonary pathologies**: right lateral and VD.
- **Pulmonary metastases**: right lateral, left lateral and VD.

Positioning

Positioning is very important to avoid rotation, which can make interpretation difficult.

For **lateral projections**, the forelimbs should be placed cranially, and the neck extended. On certain occasions, in order to avoid axial rotation, the sternum should be raised slightly so that it is at the same height as the spine. If positioning is correct, the dorsal parts of the left and right ribs should be at the same height.

In **DV** or **VD projections**, the sternum and spine should be superimposed on the image.

The image should be collimated so that the thorax and the diaphragm appear intact. The **central beam** should be positioned on the **caudal edge of the scapula**.

Radiographs should be **taken at the end of the inspiration,** and this state should be evaluated in the lateral projection by the position of the lumbo-diaphragmatic recess (it must be at the level of T12 or caudal to it), the cardiac silhouette–diaphragm distance and the position of the diaphragmatic dome in the DV projection (which should be located at level T8 or caudal to it).

Interpretation

The following aspects of radiographic technique should be considered:

- exposure factors (the X-ray must have grey shades)
- whether the radiograph has been taken on inspiration
- whether there is any rotation.

The many factors which affect the normal appearance of the thorax should be taken into account, particularly in the canine species, including:

- breed
- age
- body condition
- respiratory phase
- cardiac cycle
- positioning.

The radiograph must be evaluated systematically, assessing all of the following:

- extra thoracic structures:
  - skin and subcutaneous tissue
  - spine
  - ribs and the costal cartilages
  - sternum
  - diaphragm
  - cranial abdomen
- intrathoracic structures:
  - mediastinum (cranial, middle [heart and great vessels], caudal)
  - lungs
  - pleural space.

For each structure, the five radiographic signs (number, position [location], size, shape [margins] and opacity) must be assessed individually and as a whole.

In addition, the relationship of possible differential diagnoses should be established, taking the patient's history and clinical signs into account.

Extrathoracic structures

Diaphragm

The diaphragm is a structure with soft tissue opacity, of which only the cranial surface can be visualized as this is in contact with the lungs, which are full of air. The caudal surface is in contact with the liver, which has the same opacity and therefore cannot be differentiated.

The diaphragmatic silhouette may be observed with varying appearances depending on the position of the animal, breed, age, obesity, the respiratory phase at exposure and where the X-ray beam is centred.

During normal breathing the diaphragm inserts dorsally between T9 and L1, depending on the depth of inspiration.

Intrathoracic structures

Mediastinum

The mediastinum is divided into three zones:

- cranial (cranial to the cardiac silhouette)
- middle (area of the cardiac silhouette)
- caudal (caudal to the cardiac silhouette).

Each of these zones is divided into two areas:

- dorsal
- ventral.

The oesophagus extends through the entire dorsal mediastinum, from the neck to the stomach, and is not usually visualized on X-rays unless it contains a small amount of air.

Cranial mediastinum

In VD or DV projections, the cranial mediastinum is superimposed on the spine, and the ratio of the widths of these structures (mediastinum:spine) is:

- in dogs: <2:1
- in cats: 1:1.

In obese animals, the cranial mediastinum can be wider due to the accumulation of fat, and its radiopacity can be confused with mediastinal masses.

Cranioventral mediastinal recess

This is identified on the lateral projection, cranial to the heart, just cranial to the right cranial lobe (Figure 3.21a).

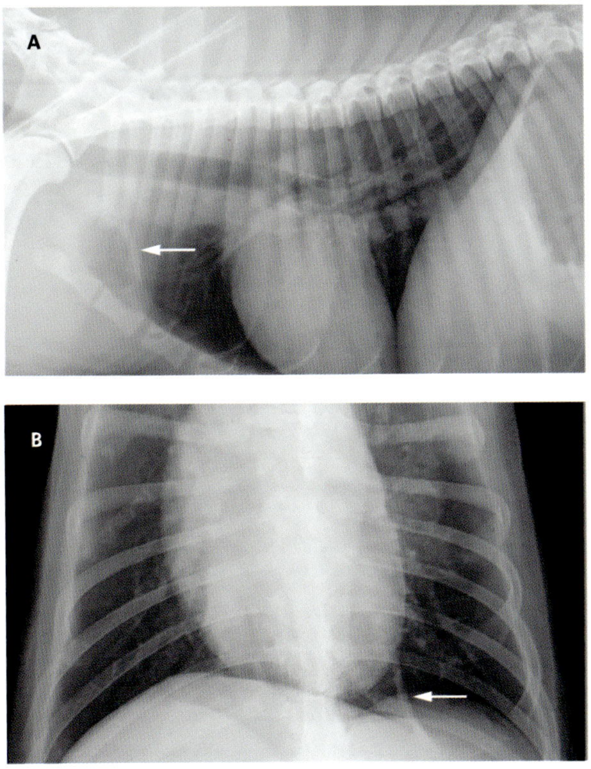

Figure 3.21. Thorax of a dog. (a) Right lateral projection. The cranioventral mediastinal recess can be seen as a radiopaque line cranial to the cardiac silhouette between the second and third sternebrae (arrow). (b) Ventrodorsal projection. The caudoventral mediastinal recess is seen as a straight radiopaque line in the left caudal hemithorax, extending from the area of the cardiac apex in a caudolateral direction towards the gastric fundus (arrow).

In the VD projection it appears as a curved radiopaque line with the concave part to the left of the animal, from T1 or T2 to the region of the main pulmonary artery.

Trachea

In the cranial mediastinum all structures, except for the trachea (air opacity), are of soft tissue opacity and cannot be seen due to the silhouette sign.

The diameter of the trachea is measured in lateral projections and should not be less than 20% of the distance between T1 and the manubrium (Figure 3.22), except in the Bulldog, where it can be 14%. Regarding the position of the trachea (lateral projection), in most dog and cat breeds it is slightly separated from the spine. Displacement towards the right side (in the VD projection) is normal in brachycephalic breeds.

Thymus

This can be seen in young animals (younger than 4–6 months) in VD projections, with a triangular or candle shape on the left side, in the space occupied by the cranioventral mediastinal recess (Figure 3.23). In the lateral projection, the thymus is not visualized because it overlaps the cardiac silhouette (silhouette sign).

Middle mediastinum

Cardiac silhouette

This is a conically shaped structure with soft tissue opacity. It is located obliquely (craniodorsal–caudoventral orientation) and is in contact with the sternum.

The **size of the cardiac silhouette** can be assessed in a lateral projection by either of two methods.

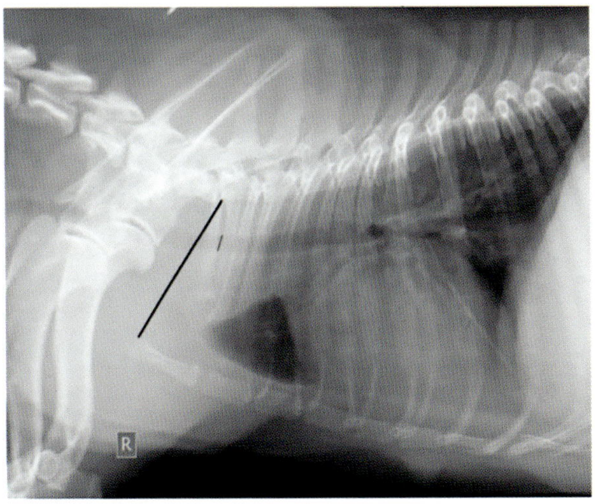

Figure 3.22. Evaluation of tracheal size (it should not be less than 20% of the distance between T1 and the manubrium).

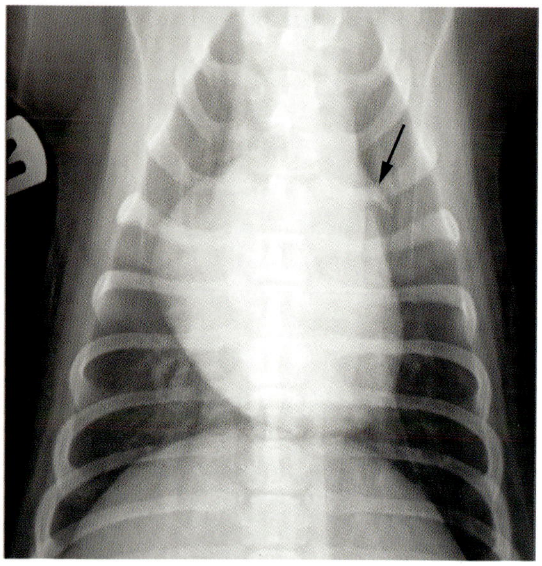

Figure 3.23. Ventrodorsal projection of a puppy's thorax. The thymus is visualized as a triangular or sail shape on the left side (arrow), in the space occupied by the cranioventral mediastinal recess.

In the **traditional method**, its **width** (or short axis, ventral to the caudal vena cava [CVC]) is:

- 2.5 to 3.5 intercostal spaces in dogs
- 2 to 2.5 intercostal spaces in cats.

Its **height** (or cardiac long axis, from the carina to the cardiac apex) must **not exceed two-thirds** of the total height of the thoracic cavity.

In an alternative method **using the vertebral bodies**, the short and long axes of the cardiac silhouette are transferred to the thoracic spine starting from the fourth thoracic vertebra, and the number of vertebrae that each of these two lines would encompass is assessed (Figure 3.24). The total of the two measurements should be as follows.

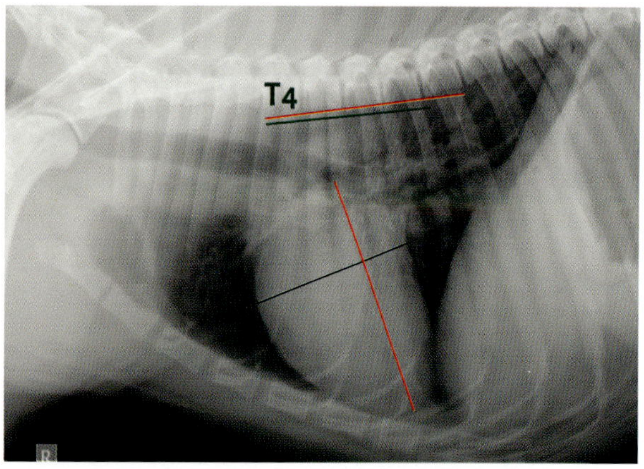

Figure 3.24. Lateral projection of the thorax in a dog. Using the vertebral body system to evaluate the size of the cardiac silhouette.

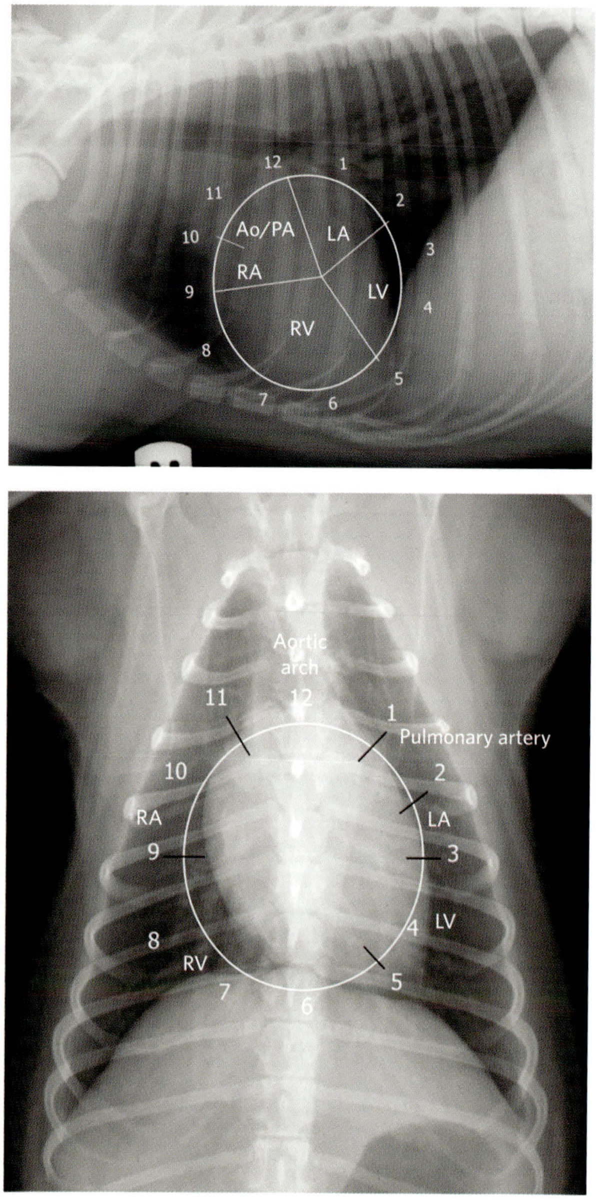

Figure 3.25. Thorax of a dog. (a) Lateral projection. (b) Ventrodorsal projection. The lines correspond to the different cardiac chambers. The cardiac silhouette resembles a clock. LA, left atrium; LV, left ventricle; RA, right atrium; RV, right ventricle. Ao: Aorta, PA: pulmonary artery

- **Dogs 9.7 ± 0.5**. However, in some breeds such as the Labrador Retriever, Boxer and Bulldog this may add up to 12 vertebral bodies.
- **Cats 7.5 ± 0.3**.

To evaluate which part of the cardiac contour corresponds to the different chambers of the cardiac silhouette, a comparison to a clock face is used (Figure 3.25).

Caudal mediastinum

Caudoventral mediastinal recess

This is visualized as a straight radiopaque line in the caudal left hemithorax, from the cardiac apex, in a caudolateral direction, to the gastric fundus (Figure 3.21b).

Pulmonary parenchyma

Generally, the space between pulmonary lobes is not seen on X-ray, unless the X-ray falls perpendicular to the pleura or there is fluid in the pleural space. Dogs and cats have two lungs, which are not symmetrical in terms of size and location (Figure 3.26).

The left lobe is formed of two lobes:

- left cranial lobe, divided into two segments:
  - cranial
  - caudal.
- left caudal lobe.

The right lobe is formed of four lobes:

- right cranial lobe
- right middle lobe
- right caudal lobe
- accessory lobe.

The lungs are composed mainly of **air**. The remaining structures are the pulmonary vessels, the bronchi, the bronchioles, the alveoli, the interstitial tissue, the lymph nodes and the pleura. The main **pulmonary vessels and bronchi** are usually seen in **the central area** near the hilus. In the middle area, usually only vessels that decrease in size towards the periphery are seen. The rest of the structures provide a general background opacity.

On a **lateral radiograph**:

- the pulmonary **artery is dorsal** to the bronchus
- the pulmonary **vein is ventral** to the bronchus.

The cranial lobar artery and vein should be approximately the **same size**, and their diameter at the level of the fourth intercostal space should not exceed the smaller diameter of the proximal portion of the fourth rib (Figure 3.27a).

On the **DV/VD projection**:

- the **vessels** are visualized better in the **DV** projection; the arteries and the caudal lobular veins can be identified, on the right and left
- the **arteries run lateral** to the veins and should be the **same size**, without exceeding the diameter of the ninth rib at the point where they intersect (Figure 3.27b).

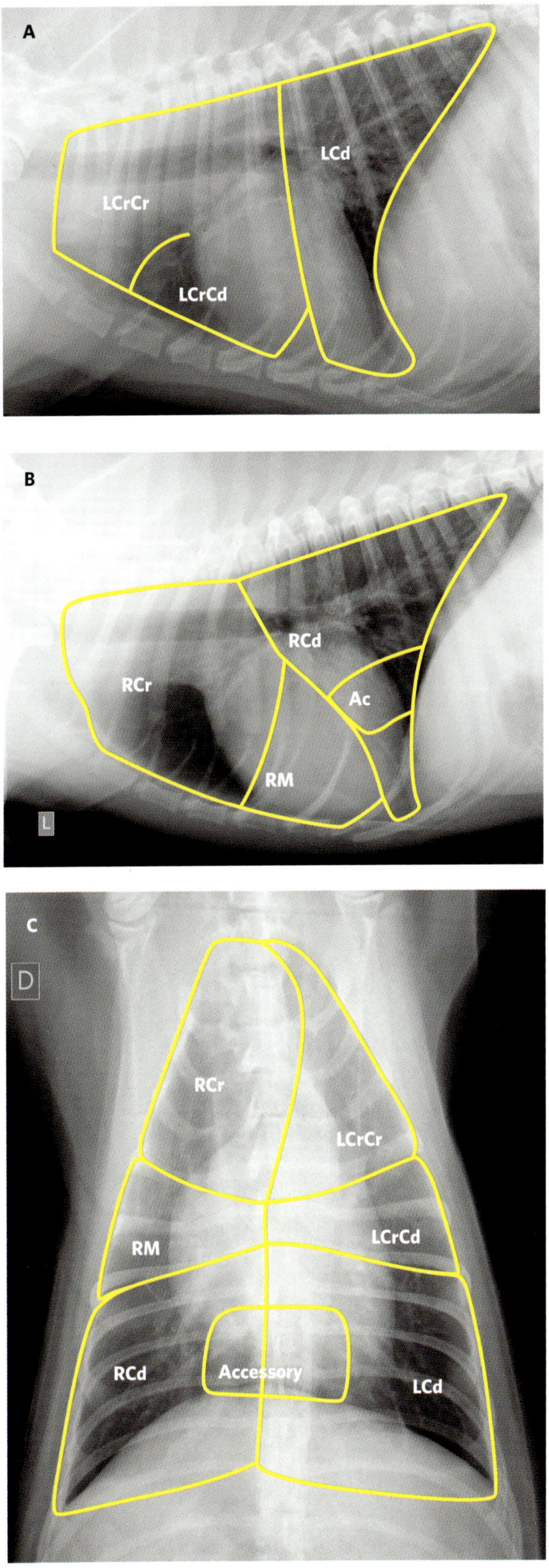

Figure 3.26. (a) Right lateral projection, (b) left lateral projection and (c) ventrodorsal projection of the thorax in a cat. Localization of the pulmonary lobes and fissures. LCrCr, cranial segment of the left cranial lobe; LCrCd, caudal segment of the left cranial lobe; LCd, left caudal lobe; RCr, right cranial lobe; RCd, right caudal lobe; RM, right middle lobe; Accessory, accessory lobe.

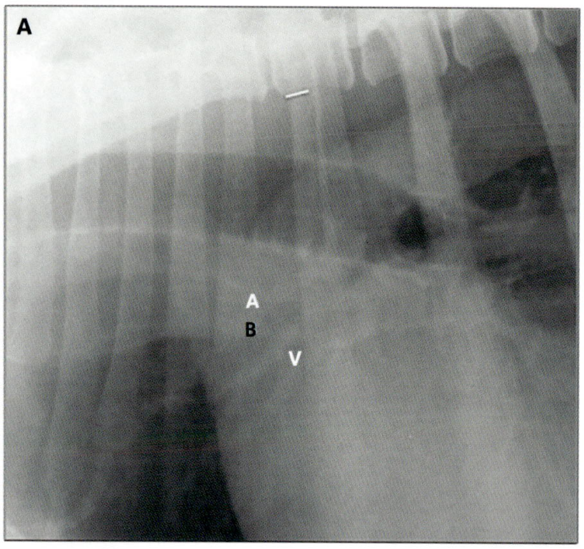

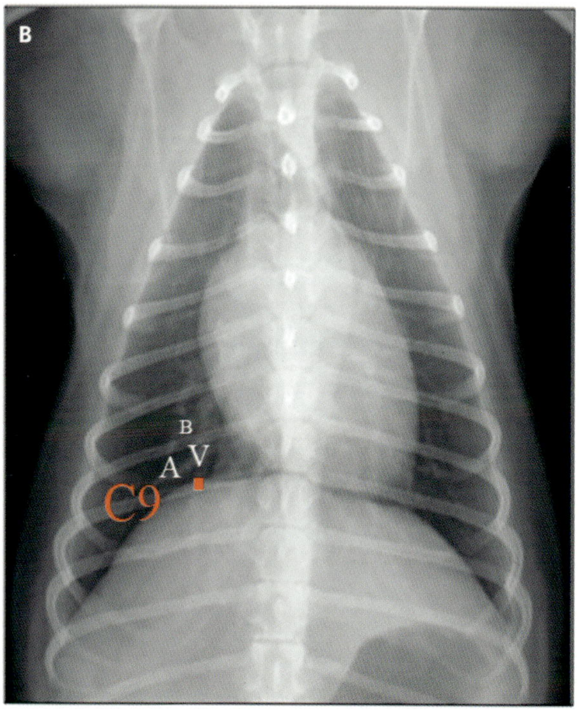

Figure 3.27. Thorax of a dog. (a) Lateral projection. (b) Dorsoventral projection. The size of the pulmonary vessels can be appreciated on the lateral projection by comparing them to the fourth rib (white line); and on the DV projection the vascularization of the caudal lobes is compared to the ninth rib (C9). A, artery; B, bronchus; V, vein.

Pleural space

The **pleura is too thin to be seen** on an X-ray in both the cat and the dog. However, there are circumstances in which the normal pleura can be **visualized as fine pleural lines**, in larger animals where there is **thickening or calcification**, or when the X-ray beam falls completely tangential to them. In obese animals there may be an accumulation of **fat between the fissures**; this is seen most frequently between the cranial and right middle lobes, and usually visualized in VD/DV projections. **Pleural fissures are not normally visible**; liquid or air must be present in the pleural space to observe them. However, it is important to know their location and direction (Figure 3.26).

Abdominal radiology

Technique

The organs and liquid contents of the abdomen have the same opacity and therefore little radiographic contrast. This makes good technique essential to obtain Preparation and inmobili maximum contrast.

Projections

At least **two projections** should be obtained: right or left lateral and ventrodorsal (Figure 3.1).

The dorsoventral projection is not recommended because it leads to superposition of organs and, consequently, poor visualization of the structures.

The **entire abdomen should be included** on the X-ray. For large/giant breeds, two X-rays (cranial abdomen and caudal abdomen) are necessary.

When pathologies affect the rectum, urethra and pelvic canal, the radiograph should focus on the pelvis. In males with urethral pathologies, the pelvic extremities must be retracted cranially to reduce the overlap of the urethra with the femurs.

Image acquisition

All abdominal radiographs should be taken on **maximum expiration**, which allows the abdominal wall to be relaxed, the diaphragm is displaced cranially, and there is a longer pause, thus reducing the possibility of artefacts due to respiratory movements.

Exposure times

To differentiate the attenuation between soft tissues and fat, a **moderate kV** (lower than that used for the thorax of same animal) should be used. In order to avoid respiratory movements, **exposure times must be short** (**mAs can be increased** to reduce them).

Preparation and immobilization of the patient

- Preparation
  - Clean, dry hair.
  - Fasted for 12 hours (contrast studies).

- Enemas 2 hours prior to the study (contrast studies).
- Immobilization
  - Sedation or anaesthesia as necessary.
  - Use translucent instruments (spoons, plastic skimmers) or compression bands (to facilitate definition of organs / masses and reduce necessary kV).
- To differentiate soft tissue from fluid, contrast studies can be used but ultrasound and endoscopy may be more appropriate.

Radiological anatomy of the abdomen

The following structures **can be visualized** in the abdomen:

- diaphragm
- stomach
- small intestine
- caecum
- colon
- liver
- spleen
- kidneys
- urinary bladder
- prostate
- os penis
- prepuce
- scrotum
- vulva
- ventral abdominal wall
- sublumbar fat (vessels, lymph nodes)
- sublumbar musculature
- thoracolumbar and lumbar vertebrae
- ribs
- pelvis.

The following abdominal structures **cannot be visualized**:

- adrenal glands
- mesentery
- mesenteric lymph nodes
- omentum
- pancreas
- aorta
- caudal vena cava
- gallbladder (ventral edge visible in some cats)
- ovaries
- uterus.

Of the structures named above, part or all may be more or less visible, as a function of their physiological or pathological status, depending on:

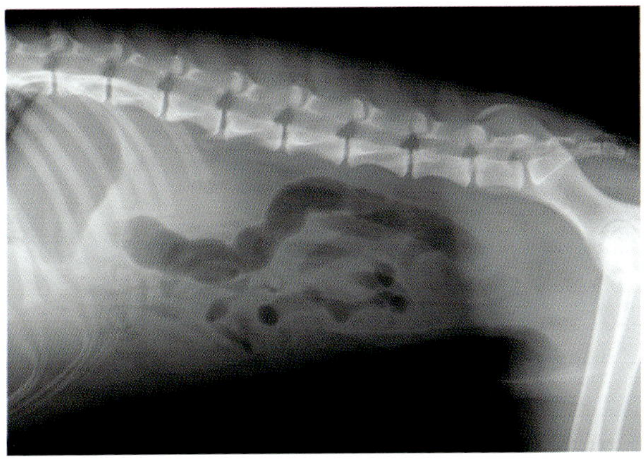

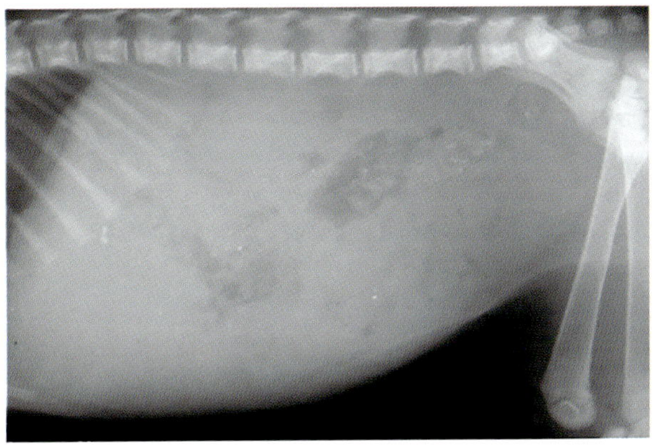

Figure 3.28. (a) Lateral projection of the abdomen in a thin dog. (b) Lateral projection of the abdominal cavity in a puppy. Both cases show poor visualization of the organs due to the small amounts of fat present.

- differences in opacity
- the amount of fatty tissue in the abdomen (Figure 3.28)
- intestinal contents
- the shape of the patient (deep chest, barrel chest, etc.).

Interpretation algorithm for the abdominal cavity

The following structures should be studied systematically on all radiographs of the abdominal cavity:

- extra-abdominal structures:
  - external limits of the cavity (ribs, vertebrae, pelvis, etc.)
  - diaphragm
- caudal thorax
- intra-abdominal structures:
  - liver
  - spleen
  - urinary system: kidneys, ureters, urinary bladder, urethra
  - reproductive system:
    - testicles, scrotum, prostate, os penis
    - uterus, vagina, mammary glands / nipples

- gastrointestinal system: stomach, small intestine, caecum, colon and rectum
- others: retroperitoneal space and cavity.

For each of the structures, the **five radiographic signs** (number, position [location], size, shape [margins] and opacity) should be assessed.

Extra-abdominal structures

The **edges of the cavity** should be examined, including the diaphragm, ventral abdominal wall, spine, pelvis and subcutaneous tissue.

Intra-abdominal structures

Liver

The **size of the liver** is measured by observing its **ventral edge**, which should be smooth and pointed and remain within the costal arch, and the position of the **longitudinal axis of the stomach**, which should be parallel to the ribs in the lateral projection (Figure 3.29a).

There are variations in the radiographic appearance of the liver between different breeds of dog.

- In **small breeds**, with a barrel-shaped thorax, the ventral hepatic lobe surpasses the costal arch.
- In **larger animals**, with a deep thorax, the liver almost slots into the costal arch.

On the VD projection (Figure 3.29b) the hepatic silhouette is not well visualized; its borders are marked by:

- the gastric fundus, on the left side
- the lesser curvature, in the central part
- the pylorus and the duodenal cranial flexure, on the right side.

In **cats**, if the stomach is empty, it is **often curved**.

The **liver has a** homogenous **soft tissue opacity.**

Spleen

On a **VD projection**, the head of the spleen is observed as a **triangular structure** of soft tissue opacity along the **left side** of the abdomen, caudal and lateral to the fundus of the stomach and cranial to the left kidney. The body and tail of the spleen can be orientated parallel to the longitudinal axis of the body, adjacent to the left side.

On a **lateral projection**, in the cat, the head of the spleen is seen as a **triangular structure** of soft tissue opacity in the **dorsal abdomen** between the fundus and the kidneys (Figure 3.30). As the spleen is shorter in the cat than in the dog, its tail and body are generally

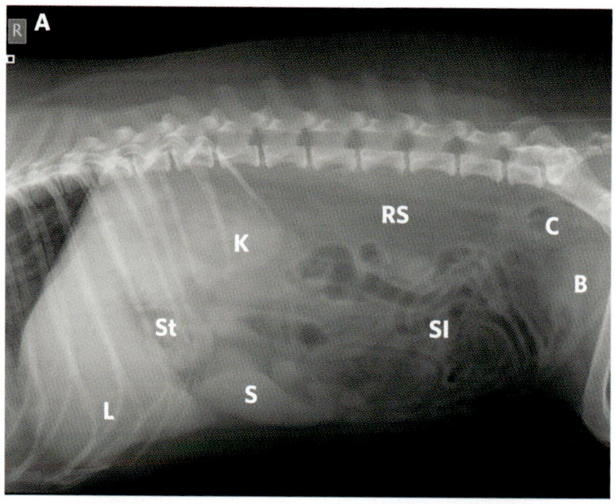

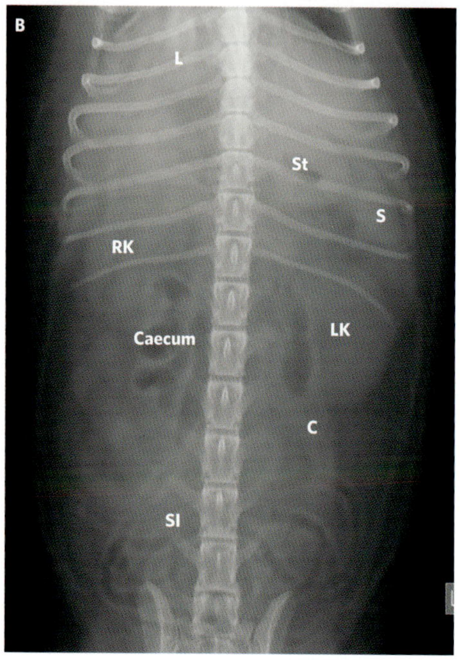

Figure 3.29. Abdomen of a dog. (a) Lateral projection. (b) Ventrodorsal projection. Localization of abdominal organs. B, bladder; C, colon; K, kidney; L, liver; LK, left kidney; RK, right kidney; RP, retroperitoneal space; S, spleen; SI, small intestine; St, stomach.

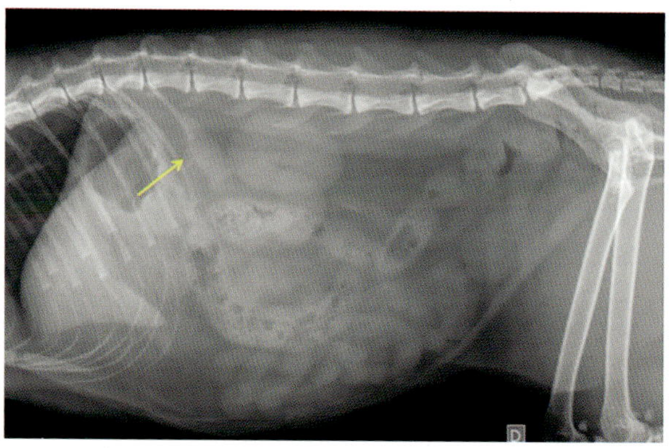

Figure 3.30. Lateral projection of a cat's abdomen. The head of the spleen (arrow) can be seen as a triangular structure with soft tissue opacity in the dorsal abdomen between the fundus and the kidneys.

less visible in the lateral projection when compared to the dog.

In the dog, the body and tail appear as a triangular structure located between the caudal ventral margin of the liver and the cranial border of the urinary bladder. This image is seen more frequently on right lateral projections than on left ones.

There are no references to determine the normal size of the spleen; it is more important to evaluate its morphology. Young and generally athletic dogs have larger spleens than geriatric and sedentary dogs. The German Shepherd has a larger spleen than other breeds of a similar size.

Urinary system: kidneys

The kidneys are located in the **retroperitoneal space** and their visualization on a plain radiograph of the abdominal cavity **depends on the amount of fat** that exists around them. Thus, in very thin animals or when there is fluid in the peritoneal or retroperitoneal space, no information can be obtained about the kidneys on plain radiographs. When they cannot be identified on a plain radiograph and more information is needed, an ultrasound examination can be performed.

If the kidneys can be identified, the following should be evaluated:

- number
- size
- shape
- margins
- opacity.

Size is evaluated by comparing it with the **length of L2** in the VD projection. The kidney should be:

- between 2.5 and 3.5 times larger in the dog
- 1.9–2.6 times larger in the castrated cat
- 2.1–3.2 times larger in the uncastrated cat.

It has also been described that in cats older than 10 years of age the renal size can be less than two times L2, with no evidence in laboratory tests of renal failure.

The **shape of the kidneys** is elongated, similar to a bean, and more rounded in cats. They have a soft tissue opacity, and sometimes a fatty opacity can be appreciated in the renal sinus area.

The **right kidney is more cranial** than the left, is in contact with the square lobe of the liver, and is located at the height of T13–L1. It can be difficult to visualize in:

- thin animals
- deep-chested animals
- animals with contents in the gastrointestinal tract.

The **left kidney is more caudal**, approximately half the length of the right kidney, and more ventral.

In cats, the right kidney is separated from the liver by fat and both kidneys are more easily identified.

Urinary system: ureters

These cannot be seen on a plain radiograph.

Urinary system: urinary bladder

Normally, the distended bladder can be localized within the abdominal cavity, with the neck over the edge of the pubis. In the bitch, a bladder located more caudally, with an intrapelvic neck, is often associated with sphincter mechanism incompetence and urinary incontinence, while in the male it appears this is not significant.

Urinary system: urethra

This cannot be seen on a plain radiograph.

Male reproductive system: prostate

In the young dog the prostate is located within the pelvic cavity, while in the old dog the increased size means it is located in the caudal abdomen, which can move the neck of the bladder to a more cranial position. Prostatomegaly is defined as when the cranial–caudal axis of the prostate exceeds 70% of the distance between the sacral protuberance and the pelvic floor. The prostate is rounded in shape with smooth edges and a soft tissue opacity.

Female reproductive system: ovaries

The ovaries are not usually radiographically visible.

Female reproductive system: uterus

Under **normal** conditions the **uterus cannot be seen**, although occasionally it can be seen in obese bitches with a lot of fat between the descending colon and the bladder.

During pregnancy, the following can be observed.

- Between the **third and fourth weeks of gestation**, small rounded masses with soft tissue opacity.
- Towards **5–6 weeks**, a tubular structure folded in the middle and caudal abdomen.
- At **6 weeks**, mineralization of the foetal skeletons.
- Towards the **end of gestation**, it is possible to visualize the presentation, size and number of foetuses.

Gastrointestinal tract: stomach

The stomach is located in the **cranial abdomen**, caudal to the liver. Its longitudinal axis is usually **parallel to the last rib**.

If it contains gas, sometimes the folds of the mucosa can be seen. In right lateral recumbency, the **pylorus** is usually filled with fluid and appears as a rounded or **oval structure** in the cranioventral area of the abdomen.

Gastrointestinal tract: small intestine

The small intestine occupies the entire central area of the abdomen. In the dog it usually contains liquid and gas; gas is rarely seen in the cat.

The diameter of an intestinal loop should not exceed the height of the central body of a lumbar vertebra.

Gastrointestinal tract: large intestine

The large intestine generally contains faecal matter and is easy to identify. The three sections can be seen:

- ascending (right side)
- transverse (caudal to the stomach)
- descending (left side).

Caecum

This is seen as a structure filled with gas in the medial and dorsal abdomen, on the lateral projection, and a structure in the right part of the middle abdomen in the ventrodorsal projection.

The diameter should not exceed the length of the body of L7.

Adrenal glands

These are not normally visible in the dog. They are only visible in the cat when calcified and this finding has no significance.

Pancreas

The pancreas cannot normally be seen on radiographs. It is located in the cranioventral abdomen, between the stomach, the transverse colon, and the descending duodenum to the right.

Peritoneal cavity

The peritoneum is a **serosal membrane** that lines the walls of the abdominal cavity and **forms folds** (the mesenteries, omenta and ligaments) that partially or totally surround a large part of the viscera located there, serving as a support for them. It is in contact, on one side, with the internal surface of the abdominal cavity and, on the other, with the external surface of the organs.

On a plain radiograph of the abdomen of an adult dog with good body condition, **fat acts as a contrast, enhancing the serosal surfaces** of the soft tissues in the abdomen. Generally, the adult cat has large deposits of fat in the peritoneum, particularly in the falciform ligament and the retroperitoneal space; the mesentery does not usually accumulate as much fat as in the dog.

In **emaciated animals**, the absence of fat results in a **reduction in the contrast** between the abdominal viscera, which decreases the ease with which structures can be differentiated. It may seem like there is free fluid, and that the abdomen is pendulous.

Until approximately 6 months, **neonatal and juvenile animals** have minimal amounts of fat, and the fat that is present has a large component of water, so **detail of the abdomen is poor.** This can be confused with free fluid. To differentiate it, the fascial planes in the retroperitoneal space and the pelvic canal should be observed.

Retroperitoneal space

The retroperitoneal space is the region of the abdomen **ventral to the spine** and **dorsal to the intestines.** The kidneys and the prostate protrude into the peritoneal cavity from the retroperitoneal space. Sometimes retroperitoneal fat delimits the kidneys and the ventral muscles of the spine. The aorta, the caudal vena cava and the ureters can sometimes be visualized in obese animals. The opacity of the retroperitoneal space is similar to that of the abdominal cavity.

Principles of ultrasound imaging

Introduction

Ultrasound is a non-invasive imaging technique that complements information obtained through the history, physical examination and other diagnostic tests. It has many uses in veterinary medicine.

- Examination of the abdominal cavity is perhaps the most common.
- Echocardiography is the second most important.
- Evaluation of pleural disease.
- Evaluation of mediastinal masses.
- Evaluation of peripheral pulmonary lesions.
- Diagnosis of musculoskeletal diseases.
- Ultrasound of the neck, particularly for evaluation of the thyroid lobes.
- Evaluation of the fundus in the eye in patients with mature cataracts.
- Fine-needle aspiration or ultrasound-guided biopsy.

Ultrasound examination

Since **ultrasound is a non-specific** technique, the visible changes may be similar in different pathologies. Thus, nodules or masses in the parenchyma can indicate a benign or malignant process, and cellular evaluation is needed for a definitive diagnosis. Ultrasound is a good technique to safely and accurately guide a needle into a nodule or mass, and in this way obtain a sample that allows a diagnosis to be reached.

Selection of a transducer

A fundamental part of the ultrasound device are **the transducers**, which are formed from **crystals with a piezoelectric effect**.

Currently, ultrasound devices can have **linear** array, **curvilinear** array (microconvex) and **phased array** transducers. The first two are used for abdominal and musculoskeletal ultrasound, and the third for echocardiography.

In addition to the arrangement of the crystals, the probes also come with **different frequencies**, which range from **2 to 18 MHz**. Nowadays, transducers can emit several frequencies, multi-frequencies; the choice of frequency depends on the depth of the structure to be examined.

- For **superficial structures, high frequency** transducers are used.
- For **deep structures, lower frequency** is used.

Generally, ultrasound examination is started using a frequency of:

- 3 MHz in large breeds of dog
- 5 MHz in medium-sized dogs
- 7.5 MHz for small breeds and cats.

Using a higher frequency gives higher resolution but less depth (Figure 3.31).

Equipment settings

The type of controls may vary from one device to another, but all devices have the following.

- **Power.** Regulates the intensity of the ultrasound output from the transducer. It should be adjusted **as low as possible** in order to obtain the best resolution and avoid artefacts.
- **Time gain compensation.** Amplifies the echoes differently depending on the depth of return.
- **General gain.** Amplifies all return echoes regardless of the depth at which they originated.
- **Focal area.** Area in which the beam has the best lateral resolution. This zone is indicated on the screen.

Examination technique

For an abdominal ultrasound examination, the **entire ventral area** of the patient's abdomen should be clipped. Most abdominal ultrasounds are performed with the animal in the supine position, although they can also be performed in right or left lateral recumbency and even with the animal standing.

This test requires a **systematic approach**. One method is to evaluate the abdomen working clockwise: start with the liver, followed by the spleen, the left kidney, the left adrenal gland (if present), the left ovary, the bladder, the uterus or the prostate, and then continue on the right side, examining the gastrointestinal tract, the pancreas and lastly the jejunal lymph nodes.

To examine the thoracic cavity using ultrasound, two different approaches can be used.

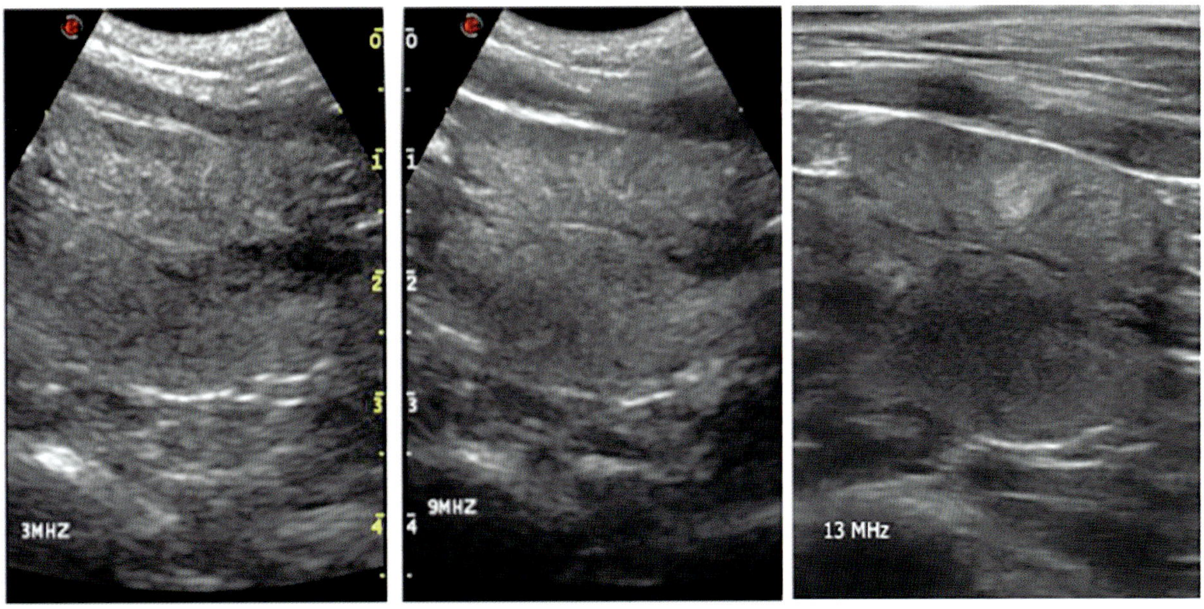

Figure 3.31. Ultrasound image of the prostate. As the frequency of the transducer increases a better resolution can be seen.

- **Intercostal.** Any intercostal space where the lesion is observed can be useful. Radiography helps to identify the location for the approach.
- **Subcostal.** The liver serves as an acoustic window. Useful for evaluation of a possible diaphragmatic hernia, or of lung masses in the caudal or accessory pulmonary lobes.

Pulmonary or mediastinal masses can present different sonographic appearances, it is normally useful to perform an aspiration of the mass to obtain a diagnosis.

Image orientation

The planes that are used are sections through the body (sagittal, transverse and dorsal).

In the **sagittal plane** with a ventral approach, the **cranial area** of the ultrasound image is located on the **left of the screen**, the ventral area at the top of the screen and the dorsal area at the bottom.

In a **transverse plane** from a ventral approach, the animal's right is on the left side, the ventral part at the top and the dorsal part at the bottom (Figure 3.32).

Terminology

- **Anechoic.** Without echoes (black, liquid) (Figure 3.33).
- **Hypoechogenic.** Less echogenicity than the surrounding tissue (grey, soft tissue).
- **Isoechogenic.** Same echogenicity as the surrounding tissue.
- **Hyperechogenic.** More echogenicity than the surrounding tissue (white, connective tissue, fat, air).
- **Mixed or complex.** A combination of various degrees of echogenicity.

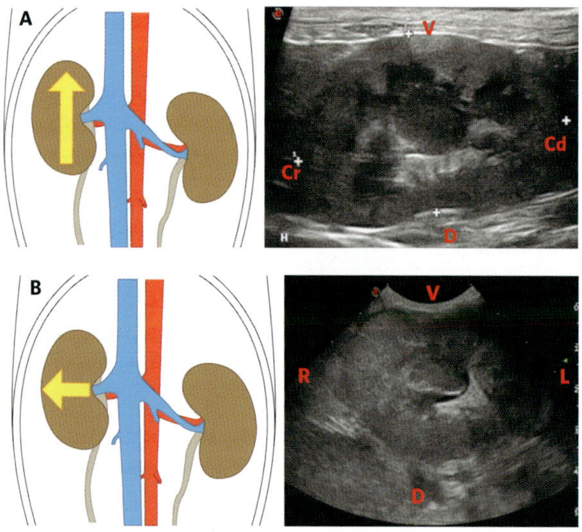

Figure 3.32. Image orientation. (a) Longitudinal section from a ventral approach. (b) Transverse section from a ventral approach. Cr, cranial; Cd, caudal; V, ventral; D, dorsal; R, right; L, left.

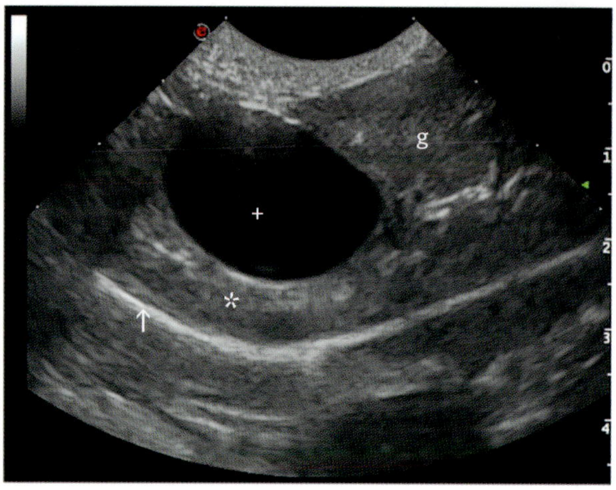

Figure 3.33. Terminology. An ultrasound image with anechoic (+), hypoechogenic (g) and hyperechogenic (arrow) areas, and a posterior enhancement artefact (*).

Artefacts

The most common artefacts are described below.

Reverberation. This is manifested by a succession of parallel hyperechogenic lines. It originates from multiple reflections between two highly reflective interfaces (for example, air) (Figure 3.34).

Mirror image. This artefact consists of the appearance of two symmetrical images separated by a hyperechoic line. It is observed mainly during the examination of the liver in the diaphragmatic region. The lung–liver interface completely reflects the ultrasound waves that hit it perpendicular to the diaphragm (Figure 3.35).

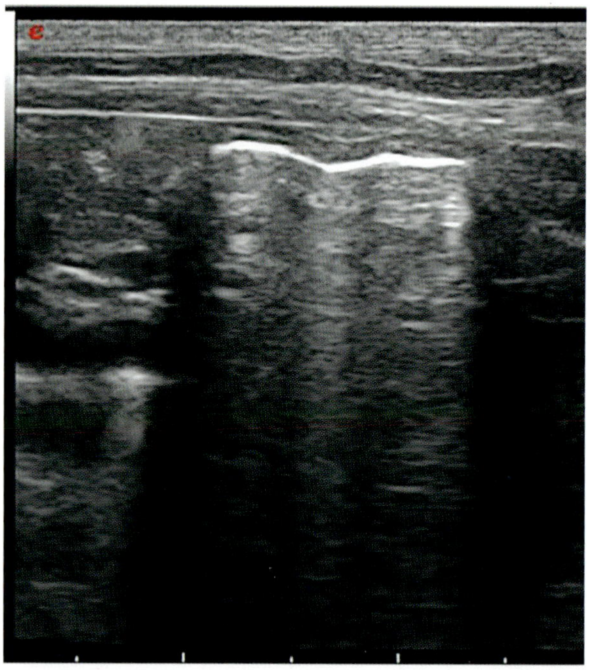

Figure 3.34. Reverberation artefact: a series of parallel hyperechogenic lines.

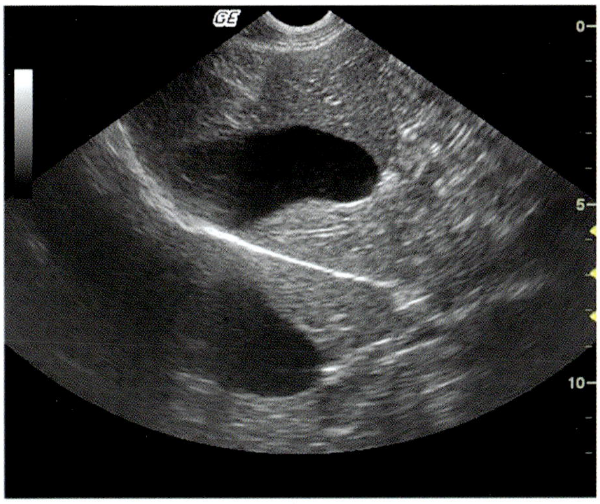

Figure 3.35. Mirror image artefact.

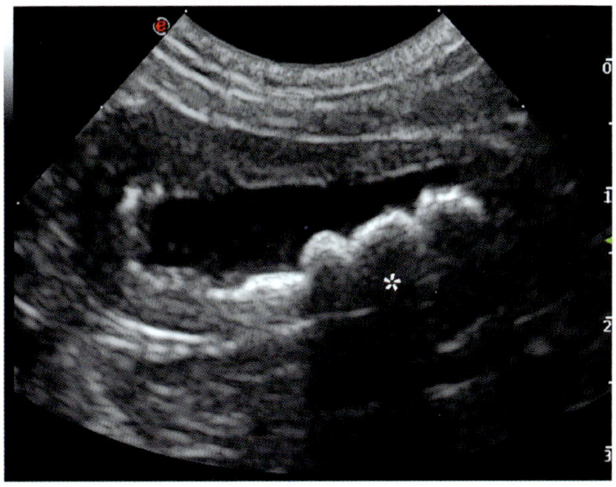

Figure 3.36. Acoustic shadow artefact (*).

Posterior enhancement. This appears as a more echogenic image, distally to a structure that does not attenuate ultrasound, such as the urinary bladder or gallbladder (Figure 3.33).

Acoustic shadow. This is observed as a dark cone, the result of the absence of ultrasound due to the total reflection of the ultrasound wave from a surface such as bone or stone (Figure 3.36).

Bibliography

Agut, A. (2014) *Diagnóstico por Imagen en Pequeños Animales*. Editorial Multimédica, Barcelona, Spain.

Barr, F. (2007) Getting the best results from ultrasonography. *In Practice* 29, 520–525.

Barr, F. and Gaschen, L., eds. (2011) *BSAVA Manual of Canine and Feline Ultrasonography*. BSAVA, Gloucester, UK.

Brinkman, E.L., Biller, D. and Armbrust, L. (2006) The clinical usefulness of the ventrodorsal versus dorsoventral thoracic radiograph in dogs. *Journal of the American Animal Hospital Association* 42, 440–449.

Caine, A. (2010) Digital image interpretation. A practical approach. *Irish Veterinary Journal* 61, 678–682.

Ewers, R. (2007) Getting the best results from radiography. *In Practice* 29, 464–469.

Holloway, A. and McConnell, F., eds. (2013) *BSAVA Manual of Canine and Feline Radiography and Radiology*. BSAVA, Gloucester, UK.

Scrivani, P.V. (2009) Nontraditional interpretation of lung patterns. *The Veterinary Clinics of North America. Small Animal Practice* 39, 719–732.

Strelec, S.D. and Lee, W.R. (2014) Why three is better than two: An overview of three vs. two view thoracic radiographic studies. Available at: http://veterinarymedicine.dvm360.com/why-three-better-two-overview-three-vs-two-view-thoracic-radiographic-studies-1 (accessed 28 June, 2019).

Warren-Smith, C. and Lamb, C. (2012) Abdominal radiography in small animals. *In Practice* 34, 454–461.

Test

1. **Regarding radiographic technique for the thorax, how can you tell if the radiograph was performed on inspiration or expiration?**
   A) According to the shape of the diaphragm.
   B) According to the shape of the heart.
   C) By the distance between the heart and the diaphragm.
   D) By the distance between the heart and the sternum.
2. **In a ventrodorsal view, in a 3-month-old dog, where is the thymus located?**
   A) On the right, cranial side.
   B) On the left, cranial side.
   C) On the right, caudal side.
   D) On the left, caudal side.

3. What is the radiographic opacity of urine?

A) Air.

B) Fat.

C) Soft tissue.

D) Bone.

4. If a ruptured bladder is suspected, what contrast technique should be used?

A) Positive cystography with iodinated contrast.

B) Negative cystography.

C) Excretory urography.

D) Positive cystography with barium sulphate.

5. What is a grid used for?

A) To eliminate the leakage of radiation.

B) To eliminate primary radiation.

C) To eliminate scattered radiation.

D) To eliminate radiation from the tube.

6. Under normal conditions, which of the following structures can be identified on a plain radiograph?

A) Liver.

B) Gallbladder.

C) Pancreas.

D) Ureter.

7. What is taken as a reference point to determine the size of the cranial mediastinum in the dog?

A) The width of a thoracic vertebral body.

B) The width of two thoracic vertebral bodies.

C) The length of two thoracic vertebral bodies.

D) The length of a thoracic vertebral body.

8. Which organ is used as reference to assess the size of the liver?

A) Left kidney.

B) Right kidney.

C) Stomach.

D) Intestinal loop.

9. If there is peritoneal effusion, what will be seen on a radiograph?

A) Generalized decrease in the opacity of the abdominal cavity.

B) Loss of visualization of the serosa of abdominal organs.

C) Enhancement of the serosa of abdominal organs.

D) Parts of abdominal organs that are not normally visible.

10. What is the radiographic sign of a mass in the cranial mediastinum with respect to the cardiac silhouette?

A) Silhouette.

B) Filling defect.

C) Summation.

D) Compartmentalization.

11. Which of the following statements is true?

A) Ultrasound is the preferred diagnostic imaging technique to study the lungs.

B) If the frequency of the sound wave increases, the resolution increases.

C) The gallbladder forms an artefact called an acoustic shadow.

D) If organ A is brighter than organ B, B is hypoechogenic with respect to A.

12. Which of the following structures is visualized on the left side in a ventrodorsal abdominal projection?

A) Caecum.

B) Head of the spleen.

C) Body of the stomach.

D) Pyloric antrum.

13. **What type of device does computerized radiology use to perform radiographs?**
    A) Flat panel detectors.
    B) Charged coupled devices.
    C) Photostimulable phosphor plate.
    D) Silicon detectors.
14. **The artefact produced by a kidney stone is called:**
    A) Posterior enhancement.
    B) Acoustic shadow.
    C) Lateral shadow.
    D) Reverberation.
15. **What contrast should not be used if oesophageal rupture is suspected?**
    A) Barium.
    B) Gastrografin.
    C) Iopamidol.
    D) Iohexol.
16. **With respect to the trachea in Bulldogs, up to what size is considered normal?**
    A) 16% of the ratio of the distance from T1–manubrium/trachea.
    B) 16% of the larynx/trachea ratio.
    C) 14% of the ratio of the distance from T1–manubrium/trachea.
    D) 14% of the larynx/trachea ratio.

Answers on page 117

Clinical case 1

A 6-year-old male castrated Yorkshire Terrier presents with pain on defaecation over the last 2 months. In addition, blood has been present in the urine for the last 5 weeks.

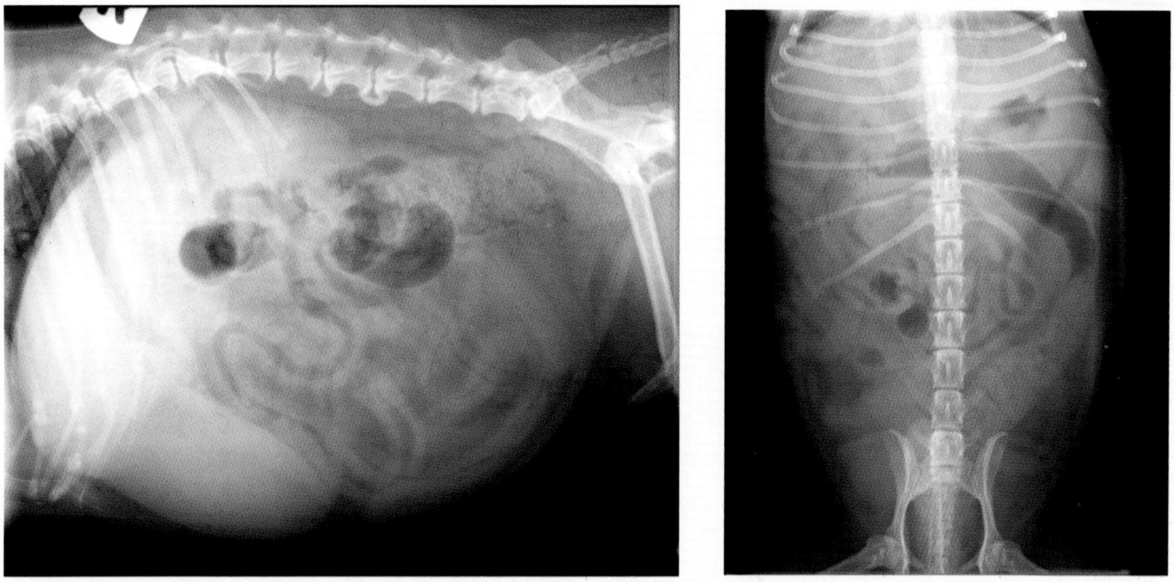

Figure case 1.1. Radiographs of the abdominal cavity. (a) Lateral projection. (b) Ventrodorsal projection.

1. **Describe the radiological findings.**
2. **What is the radiological diagnosis?**
3. **Establish a list of differential diagnoses.**
4. **What are your comments/recommendations?**

Answers on page 117

Clinical case 2

5. **Describe the radiological findings.**

A decrease in the T13–L1, L3–L4 and L4–L5 intervertebral spaces with sclerosis of the articular facets, associated ventral spondylosis and a transitional vertebra at L1 level (thoracolization) is seen. A pendulum abdomen is also seen. The rest of the limits of the cavity appear normal.

The liver is enlarged: it is seen caudal the last costal arch. It has rounded edges. There is a mild caudal displacement of the gastric axis. The neck of the urinary bladder presents with an abnormal morphology and inside it there is a small rounded structure with a mineral opacity. The prostate is enlarged (for a neutered dog), with regular borders and small areas of mineral opacity. In the region of the penile urethra, a linear structure with a mineral opacity compatible with a calculus is observed.

6. **What is the radiological diagnosis?**

- Spondylosis and thoracolization.
- Diffuse hepatomegaly.
- Abnormal morphology of the bladder neck.
- Structure with a mineral opacity inside the bladder and penile urethra.
- Prostatomegaly with areas of mineral opacity.

7. **Establish a list of differential diagnoses.**

- Disc disease, spondylosis and thoracolization.
- Steroid liver disease (due to hyperadrenocorticism), congestion, diabetes and neoplasia.
- Bladder stones or dystrophic mineralization. Calculi in the penile urethra.
- Prostatic neoplasia. The most likely, since it is a castrated male, and presents with mineralization.

8. **What are your comments/recommendations?**

Recommendation: perform an abdominal ultrasound.

Abdominal ultrasonography shows generalized enlargement of the liver, a diffuse increase in echogenicity, heterogeneous echotexture and rounded edges (Figure case 1.2). The gallbladder presents with mobile content which is echogenic and compatible with biliary sludge. Both adrenal glands are slightly enlarged (7 mm thick) with normal morphology and echogenicity. In the cranial region of the urinary bladder, a homogeneous overgrowth of the mucosa with well-defined borders can be seen. The neck of the bladder appears thickened with hyperechoic areas with acoustic shadows. The prostate presents a heterogeneous echogenicity with a multitude of hyperechoic foci with acoustic shadows and a small cyst which is 0.5 cm in diameter (Figure case 1.3).

The medial iliac lymph nodes are enlarged (short/long axis ratio 0.5) with normal morphology and echogenicity.

The ultrasonographical findings are compatible with:

- steroid liver disease
- biliary sludge
- hyperplasia of the adrenal glands

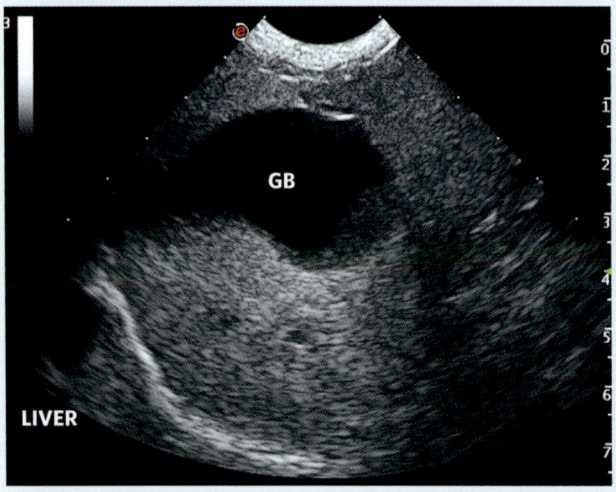

Figure case 1.2. Ultrasound image of a transverse plane of the liver. GB, gallbladder.

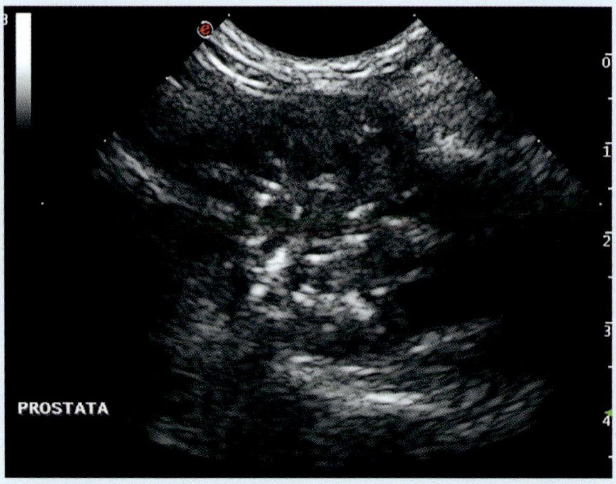

Figure case 1.3. Ultrasound image of a transverse plane of the prostate.

- gallbladder polyp
- prostatic neoplasia with probable invasion of the bladder neck.

Recommendations:

- fine-needle aspirate (FNA) of the prostate
- ACTH stimulation test or low dose dexamethasone suppression test.

On ultrasound-guided FNA of the prostate, a cell population compatible with an epithelial neoplasm was observed, possibly adenocarcinoma.

Correct answers

Test

1. C	7. B	13. C
2. B	8. C	14. B
3. C	9. B	15. A
4. A	10. A	16. C
5. C	11. B	
6. A	12. B	

4

Respiratory system disorders

Germán Santamarina Pernas

Chapter summary

From the sneezing kitten to the reverse-sneezing dog, patients with respiratory disease are a common presentation in small animal practice. However, for some conditions the symptoms are not always this obvious. This means that many patients with respiratory compromise are often not presented until the disease is well advanced. For example, the cat with a pleural effusion may go unnoticed until it stops eating and adopts an air-hunger position. By this stage, additional stress places the cat in danger of sudden decompensation and collapse, which means that the clinician must proceed with great caution.

This poses something of a dilemma. On the one hand the vet needs to diagnosis and treat the underlying condition but, on the other, doing so may push the patient into respiratory arrest. These issues are addressed in this chapter, with advice on emergency stabilization of the dyspnoeic patient and the prioritization of diagnostic tests.

The text takes a systematic approach to determine the anatomical origin of the condition, stabilize the patient and decide which diagnostic tests are most valuable. In addition, diseases of the upper and lower respiratory tract, and pleural diseases, are described, along with their treatment, all of which equips the vet in practice to handle with confidence the inevitable Friday evening case of a dyspnoeic dog.

Key learning points

- emergency stabilization and treatment of patients in respiratory distress
- localizing the anatomical region of the respiratory distress
- the presentation, clinical signs, diagnosis and treatment of upper respiratory tract, lower respiratory tract and pleural disorders.

General considerations

Patients with **respiratory symptoms are common** in small animal practice. Many of these cases are straightforward and respond well to conservative treatment. However, others are more complex and fail to respond so favourably, which makes obtaining a definitive diagnosis desirable.

However, there are difficulties associated with evaluating feline or canine respiratory disease since most of the **airway is encased by bony structures**, making palpation and visual evaluation difficult. Indeed, in some cases, the only way to reach a diagnosis is by observing the **response to treatment**.

Another consideration is that the respiratory system has a large ventilatory capacity and some regenerative capacity, which often means that clinical respiratory problems become evident only **once the disease is advanced**. In addition, **numerous pathologies affecting other organs** can lead to respiratory distress as a symptom, even though there is no respiratory system pathology.

As part of the diagnostic work-up, it is helpful to establish the **anatomical origin of the symptoms or disease**. For example:

- nasal cavity
- upper airways
- lower airways
- pulmonary parenchyma
- pleural space.

Table 4.1. Clinical signs providing clues to the presence of a respiratory disease.

Clinical signs
Nasal discharge
Cough
Respiratory sounds
Tachypnoea
Dyspnoea
Exercise intolerance

Clinical history

The clinical signs most frequently associated with respiratory problems are:

- exercise intolerance
- coughing
- syncope
- changes in respiratory pattern
- fever
- abdominal enlargement
- inappetence
- depression
- nasal discharge
- weight loss
- poor growth.

It is important to identify the **severity, duration and progression** of all symptoms. Subtle signs such as changes in bark or meow may indicate laryngeal dysfunction.

It is also desirable to know the vaccination status and deworming history, as well as the animal's normal habits. For example, the hunting activities of some cats predispose them to contracting pulmonary parasites (*Aleurostrongylus abstrusus* in hunting cats).

Breed predispositions can often indicate the origin of the problem. For example:

- chronic bronchitis in the Siamese cat
- laryngeal paralysis in the Labrador
- pulmonary fibrosis in the West Highland white terrier.

The presence of **concurrent diseases in other pets** in the household and the existence of environmental factors (such as an owner who smokes) provide important additional information.

Physical examination

Overall condition

Observe the body condition and mental state of the animal.

Mucous membranes

- **Pale mucous membranes** suggest peripheral vasoconstriction, decreased cardiac output or anaemia.
- **Cyanotic mucous membranes** indicate the presence of reduced oxyhaemoglobin in the peripheral circulation, which may be indicative of a severe pulmonary pathology or a cardiac defect with a right-to-left shunt.

- **Red, congested or injected** mucous membranes suggest toxaemia or septicaemia.
- **Oedematous, congested** mucous membranes are sometimes seen in cases of severe right-sided heart failure.

Capillary refill time

The capillary refill time is assessed using the buccal or gingival mucous membranes. A **normal refill time is less than two seconds**, and an increase suggests hypotension and shock.

Examination of the oral cavity

It is important to examine the oral cavity to check for issues such as nasopharyngeal polyps, masses or foreign bodies. Examination of the nasopharyngeal area may be difficult in the conscious animal.

Respiratory rate

A normal resting respiratory rate is **12–24 breaths per minute.** The rate is influenced by excitement, anxiety and exercise immediately prior to the consultation.

Respiratory pattern

Evaluate the **respiratory pattern** to determine whether there is hyperpnoea, tachypnoea, abdominal breathing and/or dyspnoea (inspiratory or expiratory). **Orthopnoea**, where the animal presents with an open-elbow (abduction) posture with neck extended trying to capture air (Figure 4.1), indicates severe pulmonary pathology.

Cough

In **dogs** a cough can be indicative of a **heart problem or primary respiratory** disease. In **cats**, however, a cough usually indicates a **respiratory cause** since they rarely cough with heart disease.

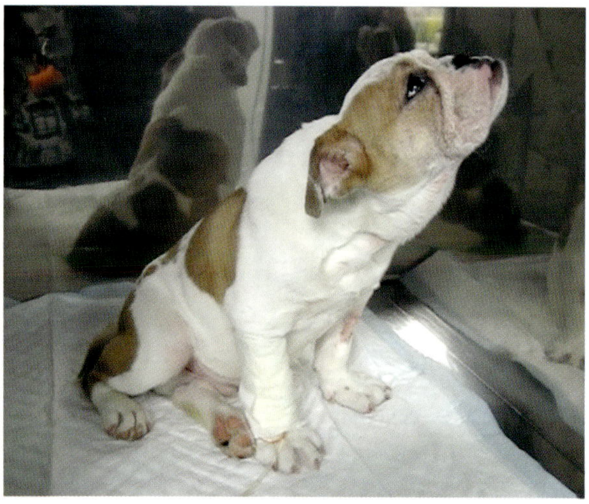

Figure 4.1. Orthopnoeic position.

Palpation

Cervical larynx

Gentle pressure on the side of the larynx may exacerbate the signs of laryngeal paralysis, and allows detection of physical asymmetries.

Cervical trachea

Palpate the cervical trachea for signs of collapse. Also, if tracheal inflammation is present, this palpation readily induces a cough.

Femoral pulse

The quality of the femoral pulse is a good indicator of cardiac output. The rhythm, regularity and pulse quality should be assessed.

Thoracic auscultation

This allows detection of cardiac murmurs, gallop rhythms or arrhythmias.

Respiratory sounds should be categorized as follows:

Discontinuous sounds. Perceived only during inspiration

- **Fine crepitations** (high frequency, low intensity and short duration). Occur when the **small airways re-open** upon inspiration.
- **Coarse crepitations** (low frequency, high intensity and short duration). Heard when diameter airways are opened and **obstructed by secretions**.

Continuous sounds. These are heard during inspiration and expiration.

- **Wheezing, rales and pulmonary** rubbing are associated with narrowing of the airways.
- Low-intensity **grunting sounds** are caused by rapid movements of air in the main airways (normal when associated with exercise).
- **Gurgling** is associated with the mixture of fluid and air in the airways–for example, in bronchopneumonia.

Thoracic percussion

Should be performed in a dorsoventral (along a rib) and cranial–caudal (from one rib to another) direction, to locate muted or non-resonant areas of the chest.

- **Pleural effusion** generally causes a **symmetrical dull sound** on percussion of the ventral chest.
- **Neoplasms** and **consolidated pulmonary lobes** can show **localized areas of low** or no resonance.

Increased resonance is present with a pneumothorax.

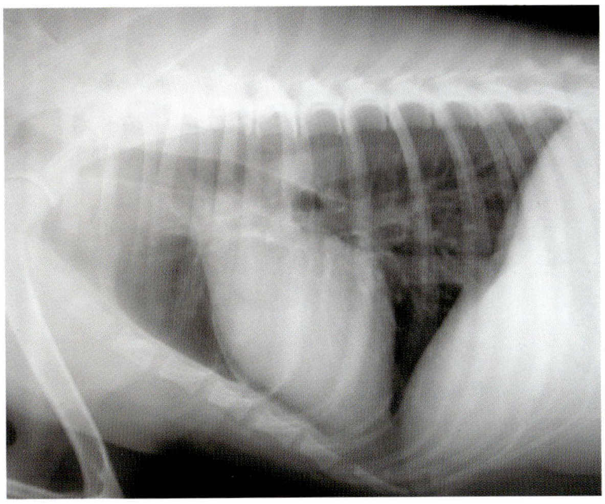

Figure 4.2. Bronchial pattern in a dog (chronic bronchitis).

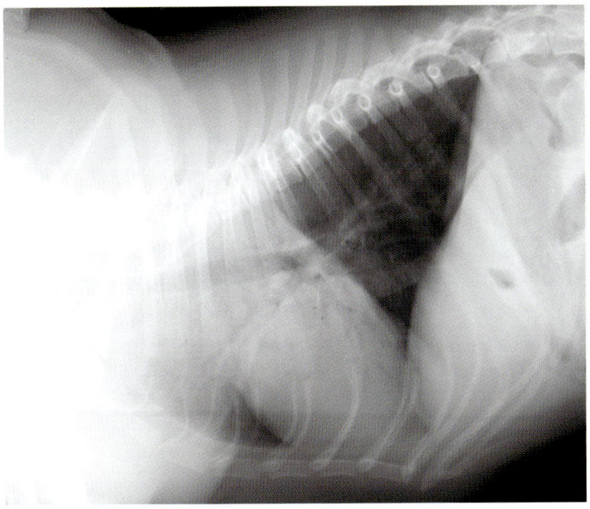

Figure 4.3. Alveolar pattern in a dog, cranial lobes (pneumonia).

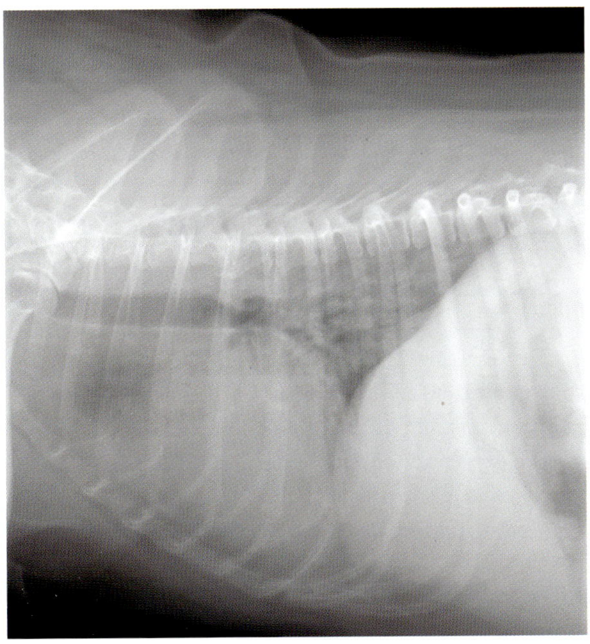

Figure 4.4. Interstitial pattern in a dog (pulmonary fibrosis).

Chest compression

In **young cats** with respiratory signs, the **compressibility of the cranioventral thorax** should be assessed. A reduction in compressibility may be due to a cranial mediastinal mass such as a thymoma.

Laboratory techniques

Blood tests

Routine complete blood count, serum biochemistry and electrolytes tests are required.

Complete blood count findings may not be specific (for example, an inflammatory leucogram), but may suggest certain conditions. For example, although not diagnostic, high levels of **circulating eosinophils** may suggest **parasitism or an allergic** respiratory disease (feline asthma). Serum biochemistry helps rule out systemic processes.

Faecal analysis

When **pulmonary parasitism** is suspected, stool samples should be subjected to **faecal flotation tests**. Significant examples are the larvae of *Angiostrongylus vasorum* and *Oslerus osleri* in the dog, and *Aleurostrongylus abstrusus* in the cat.

Thoracic radiography

Thoracic radiography is essential for the assessment of numerous respiratory conditions. Obtaining good-quality radiographs is crucial for the interpretation of fine pulmonary details. To facilitate this, it may be necessary to sedate the animal. The decision to sedate or not, and the type of sedation used, depends on the degree and severity of the cardiopulmonary compromise. **Acepromazine and butorphanol** usually produce adequate sedation for thoracic radiographs. A combination of **ketamine and midazolam** can also be used in cats.

The following projections are required:

- **right and left lateral views**, to effectively assess all pulmonary fields
- **ventrodorsal**, in respiratory cases
- dorsoventral, useful to assess the cardiac silhouette.

High exposure speeds are necessary to avoid kinetic blur (high kilovoltage and low milliamperage).

Ideally radiographs should be taken on the **inspiratory peak** to obtain the **maximum contrast** between air and soft tissue, and to make a more accurate assessment of lung fields. **Expiratory radiographs** can **simulate pulmonary pathologies** and lead to diagnostic errors.

On the other hand, the signs of **intrathoracic tracheal collapse** can **only be identified on expiratory X-rays.** However, to assess dynamic changes such as tracheal collapse, **fluoroscopy** is more accurate.

Lung patterns

Vascular pattern

Arteries and veins can be evaluated at the following points when they cross:

- The **fourth rib**, in the lateral view. The vessels should not be thicker than the base of this rib.
- The **ninth rib**, in the dorsoventral view. The vessels should be of a similar thickness to the ribs.

The pulmonary arteries and veins are usually of **equal thickness**.

- **Veins wider** than the arteries usually suggest **left-sided congestive heart** failure.
- **Arteries wider** than the veins are seen in **pulmonary hypertension**, pulmonary thromboembolism or filariasis.
- Lung **vasculature wider** than normal is present in cases of **pulmonary over-circulation**, such as persistent ductus arteriosus and ventricular septal defects.
- **Pulmonary vasculature narrower than normal** is observed in haemorrhages and severe dehydration (hypovolaemia), pulmonary stenosis and tetralogy of Fallot.

Bronchial pattern

The **bronchi are not usually visible**, but are **delineated by the adjacent artery and vein**. Diseases that affect the walls of the bronchi render them visible. In such cases, the bronchial walls are visualized as **train tracks when viewed longitudinally** and as **doughnuts when sectioned transversely**. Bronchitis, bronchiectasis, calcification and inflammatory or neoplastic infiltrates can lead to a bronchial pattern.

Alveolar pattern

This is seen when the **alveolar space is filled with fluid** or exudate, which causes a loss of visualization of the pulmonary vasculature and increased visualization of the air that fills the bronchi (air bronchogram).

Interstitial pattern

The pulmonary interstitium gives the lung parenchyma a diffuse, grey appearance. Diseases that affect the interstitium cause an **increase in the opacity** of this tissue and a patchy loss of pulmonary detail, obscuring the vasculature and the airways in a similar way.

Mixed pattern

Mixed patterns can be seen in different situations; the most common is probably the mixed alveolar–interstitial pattern associated with pulmonary oedema. This pattern can have a perihilar distribution but it can also be diffusely distributed, especially in the cat.

Echocardiography and thoracic ultrasound

Echocardiography can rule out congestive heart failure as the underlying cause of respiratory signs.

When differentiating respiratory disease from a cardiac one, it is important to assess the size of the cardiac chambers, paying special attention to **dilatation of the left atrium** and **enlargement of the right side of the heart**.

Dilation of the left atrium suggests an underlying cause of **congestive heart failure**. The degree of dilatation of the left atrium should be **considered in the context** of the severity of the congestive signs. For example, in a dog with severe respiratory compromise, pulmonary oedema and/or pleural effusion, mild dilation of the left atrium is unlikely to account solely for these signs.

Echocardiography can also confirm **pulmonary hypertension**, without the need for cardiac catheterization or measurement of pulmonary capillary pressure. Indications of pulmonary hypertension include **dilatation of the pulmonary arteries**, before and after the bifurcation. There may also be evidence of **atrial and right ventricular dilation** and, if the hypertension is long-standing, **right ventricular hypertrophy** is observed. **Tricuspid insufficiency** is often present, and the regurgitation jet shows a high velocity (> 2.8 m/s).

Pulmonary hypertension can develop as a consequence of:

- **Pulmonary over-perfusion** in the presence of ventricular septal defects or large persistent ductus arteriosus. In these situations, damage can occur in the arterioles and alveolar capillaries, their muscle layer hypertrophy increasing vascular resistance and the development of pulmonary hypertension, in what is known as Eisenmenger syndrome.
- **Increased resistance to blood flow through the lungs** for other reasons, such as chronic or recurrent bronchopneumonia, eosinophilic pulmonary infiltrates or interstitial pulmonary fibrosis (in the West Highland white terrier).

Non-cardiac thoracic ultrasound is useful to clarify changes observed on radiography, such as the presence of **pleural effusion, lung or mediastinal masses**. Thoracic ultrasound also allows **guided aspiration** of pleural fluid and aspiration or biopsy of masses close to the chest wall.

Rhinoscopy

Rhinoscopy (Figure 4.5) is an important technique when there are clear signs of **upper airway obstruction**.

The nasal chambers can be visualized very effectively using a **narrow, rigid endoscope (2.7 mm)** to identify the numerous conditions that affect the nasal cavity and nasopharynx. It is always performed under **general anaesthesia**. A flexible endoscope can be used for the retrograde examination of the caudal area of the nasal cavities.

Bronchoscopy

Rigid endoscopes offer better image quality and, in small animals, these smaller-diameter endoscopes allow examination without compromising the tracheal lumen. They are **limited by their length** (maximum 35 cm), which impedes their use in large animals, and are less easily controlled than flexible endoscopes.

Flexible endoscopes usually have a working channel that allows introduction of different **tools for sampling** areas of interest. Thus, using this technique, biopsies can be obtained and cytological sweeps or bronchoalveolar lavages can be performed.

Bronchoscopy requires **general anaesthesia**, so its use is limited to animals that do not have a severe respiratory distress. Animals that must undergo anaesthesia for bronchoscopy should be **maintained with 100% oxygen**, since the endoscope occludes the airway. Animals should be placed in lateral or sternal recumbency.

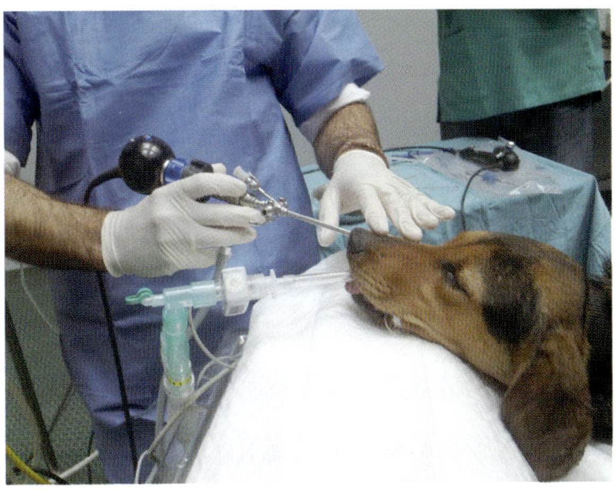

Figure 4.5. Rhinoscopy.

In most patients, if a bronchoscope of adequate dimensions is used, visualization of the **trachea to the carina** is possible. The visualization of the main bronchi is possible in large dogs using a small-diameter bronchoscope.

In the dog, **normal airways** have mucosa with a **pale pinkish mucosa** appearance and the vessels of the submucosa are clearly visible. In the cat, the tracheal mucosa is also pale but the blood vessels are less apparent.

The airways should be **inspected systematically**, starting with **laryngeal function** and evaluating the movements of the arytenoid cartilages and vocal cords. Dogs with laryngeal paralysis will show a loss of lateral movement during inspiration in one or both arytenoid cartilages; the left is the most frequently affected. In dogs with brachiocephalic respiratory syndrome, special attention should be paid during examination of laryngeal and **tracheal dimensions**, and whether the **laryngeal saccules** are everted.

Any excessive **exudate, mucous production** or purulent material in the trachea should be assessed. The colour and **texture of the mucosa** should be observed, looking for signs of redness, inflammation, roughness or diverticula. The **width and any signs of collapse** (ventral bulge during inspiration) should be assessed on the ligament and dorsal tracheal muscle. In addition, the presence of nodules associated with *O. osleri* infection should be ruled out.

The main bronchi should be examined as far as possible, which is dependent on the diameter of the bronchoscope, the size of the dog and operator skill.

If an area of suspected pathology is located, it should not be touched before taking samples.

Bronchoalveolar lavage

Bronchoalveolar lavage (BAL) is a diagnostic technique for taking **cytological samples** from the alveoli and lower airways, and is useful in the evaluation of specific diseases affecting the lung parenchyma. For example, the definitive diagnosis of an eosinophilic pulmonary infiltrate is achieved only through bronchoalveolar lavage.

This lavage is performed by using a bronchoscope, which is advanced into the lower airways to occlude the secondary bronchus of the lobe from which the samples are to be obtained. **25 ml of physiological saline** are introduced through the endoscopic channel, which is immediately re-suctioned using the same syringe. Two boluses are used to wash each of the lobes examined. In **small dogs and cats, 10 ml boluses** are used in each lobe and the procedure is **repeated up to four or five times**. At the end of the process, more than 50% of the fluid introduced is recovered and the remaining fluid is quickly reabsorbed through alveolar tissue. Patients should be carefully monitored for signs of hypoxia during the recovery period after bronchoalveolar lavage.

To perform bronchoalveolar lavage without a bronchoscope, probes of appropriate length and size are used, introduced via the endotracheal tube.

Transtracheal and endotracheal lavage

In some animals, transtracheal samples can be obtained without general anaesthesia.

For **transtracheal lavage** (Figure 4.6), an area of hair is clipped around the proximal area of the trachea and cleaned with antiseptic. The skin is infiltrated with **local anaesthetic** over the cricothyroid ligament, the head of the dog is placed vertically and a **12–14 G needle** or catheter inserted through the cricothyroid ligament, **directing the tip ventrally** towards the trachea.

A **urinary or nasogastric** tube is then advanced through the catheter into the trachea. The end of the probe must not go further than the bifurcation of the carina, so the saline is distributed between the two sides of the lungs. Therefore the tube's length should be measured from outside the dog and go no further than the fifth costal space.

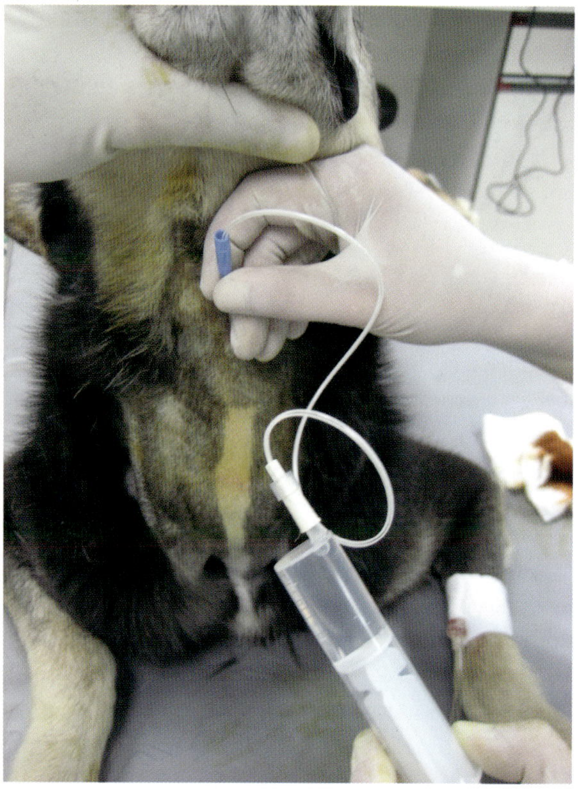

Figure 4.6. Transtracheal lavage.

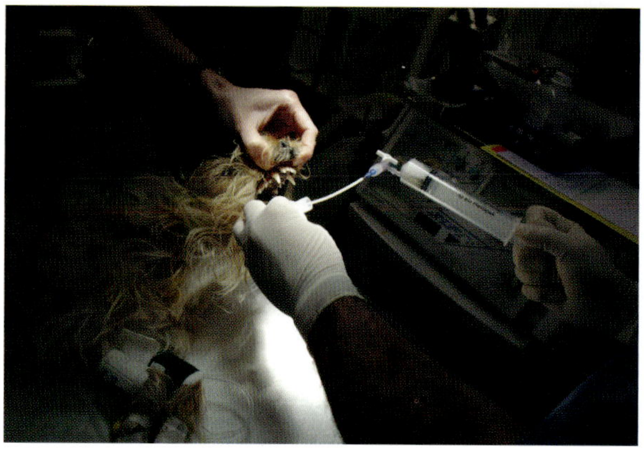

Figure 4.7. Endotracheal lavage.

The needle/catheter is removed, leaving the urinary catheter in the lumen of the trachea. Through this, sterile physiological saline should be injected and recovered in the same way as in bronchoalveolar lavage. The volume used in each aliquot is **4–5 ml in small dogs and cats**, and **10–20 ml in large dogs**. The process is **repeated three or four times**, until an adequate sample is obtained.

Tracheal lavage can also be performed using the endotracheal technique (Figure 4.7) by inserting a nasogastric catheter or urinary catheter directly through a sterile endotracheal tube.

Processing the samples

Samples obtained by BAL and transtracheal lavage should be transported in two separate containers:

- **One for cytology**. This sample can be left without additives if it is going to be examined in less than 24 hours; otherwise, it should be stored in EDTA tubes.
- **Another for bacteriology**. The sample for culture should not contain any additives.

Thoracoscopy

Thoracoscopy is an invaluable aid in deep exploration of the pleural cavity or pulmonary parenchymal disease.

It involves **general anaesthesia** and requires **intermittent positive-pressure ventilation** (IPPV).

It can be performed to obtain biopsies if a lung tumour is suspected, and is less invasive than a complete thoracotomy. Once negative pressure is removed from the pleural space (the pleural vacuum), the lung collapses and, due to the rigidity of the rib cage, inflation with air is not necessary for exploration of the pleural cavity.

Parasternal access from the xiphoid allows access to **both pleural spaces** with the animal in dorsal decubitus. Intercostal access can also be used, which allows a more localized visualization of that one side, with the animal in lateral recumbency. A **5 mm x 35 cm endoscope tube** allows for complete examination of the pleural cavity, even in large dogs.

Thoracotomy

Thoracotomy can be performed using the intercostal or sternal approach. Indications include:

- Without previous thoracoscopy, when thoracotomy is the only way to obtain a definitive diagnosis in conditions affecting a specific area of the lung or pleural cavity.
- Post-thoracoscopy, in which a lesion is diagnosed that affects a pulmonary lobe and can be removed only by thoracotomy.

Even when using opiates for pain relief, both thoracoscopy and thoracotomy cause a certain degree of **postoperative discomfort** and should be performed only when there is a minimum certainty that the benefit will outweigh the disadvantages.

Lung biopsy

Currently, lung biopsy is not used routinely in veterinary practice. Among other reasons, there is a **significant risk of pneumothorax**, especially in biopsies with forceps in ventilated lung parenchyma.

In areas of pulmonary lobe consolidation or neoplastic infiltration, biopsies can be readily obtained by thoracoscopy since consolidation prevents the area of the biopsy from subsequent ventilation. Biopsy of a complete lung lobe can be performed by thoracotomy.

Thoracoscopy techniques are improving, and the thoracoscopic ligation of a pulmonary lobe and its removal is now quite routine in human medicine, either for the removal of an isolated tumour or for biopsy. Biopsy of the lung lobe allows histological classification of the changes present in the lung parenchyma and can help to differentiate among infectious, inflammatory and allergic diseases of the respiratory tract.

Respiratory distress

Introduction

Patients in respiratory distress are a common presentation in emergency veterinary medicine, and one that can pose a diagnostic and therapeutic challenge to the clinician.

Patients with respiratory distress are very unstable, so stress induced by diagnostic processes must be minimized to avoid decompensation that evolves into cardiorespiratory arrest. Oxygen supplementation can aid short-term stabilization.

The clinician should quickly determine the cause of respiratory distress based on clinical history, examination and non-invasive diagnostic tests.

Dyspnoeic patients should be rapidly categorized into groups defined by the probable anatomical location of their disease:

- upper airways
- pulmonary parenchyma
- pleural space
- thoracic wall.

Initial management of a patient presenting in severe respiratory insufficiency

1. **Minimize stress and anxiety**. Avoid handling the patient, and even postpone the diagnostic tests until stabilized. On many occasions it is necessary to resort to sedation to relieve anxiety and facilitate treatment.
2. **Ensure the airways are patent.** Explore the nasal and oral cavities, pharynx, larynx and trachea to ensure air passage.
3. **Urgently administer oxygen** (oxygen therapy) using the most appropriate method for the circumstance and the patient.
4. **Place an intravenous catheter**, for the administration of fluids or drugs.
5. **Assess for intubation and mechanical ventilation**, when the above procedures are not sufficient to guarantee adequate gas exchange.

Depending on the cause, to relieve respiratory distress, different emergency techniques may be necessary, such as:

- oxygen supplementation
- pharmacological intervention
- thoracentesis
- placement of thoracotomy tube
- tracheostomy
- positive-pressure ventilation.

Clinical picture

The **clinical signs of severe respiratory distress** include:

- tachypnoea and breathlessness
- open-mouth breathing (especially in the cat)
- nasal flare during breathing (in the cat)
- anxiety, and inability to remain recumbent at rest
- fixed, anguished gaze
- head in an orthopnoeic posture with the neck extended (Figure 4.8)
- Abdominal breathing and paradoxical breathing (abdominal movements are opposite to those of the thorax).

Cats show more subtle clinical signs of respiratory distress than dogs.

Types of dyspnoea

Identifying on physical examination the type of dyspnoea present helps determine its origin, and therefore minimizes the use of diagnostic tests.

Inspiratory dyspnoea

There are often easily audible respiratory sounds without the need for a stethoscope (stridor and snoring). The duration of inspiration is longer than that of expiration, and **inspiratory effort is greater than the expiratory** effort (Table 4.2). In severe cases, during inspiration, when an extreme negative intrathoracic pressure is created, the **abdomen expands while the thorax collapses** due to retraction of the intercostal muscles. This type of dyspnoea may be due to **upper respiratory tract conditions** (pharynx, larynx and trachea).

Table 4.2. Pathologies that present with inspiratory dyspnoea.

Pathologies
Brachycephalic syndrome
Masses or foreign bodies
Laryngeal oedema
Laryngeal paralysis
Trauma
Cervical tracheal collapse
Nasopharyngeal polyps (in the cat)

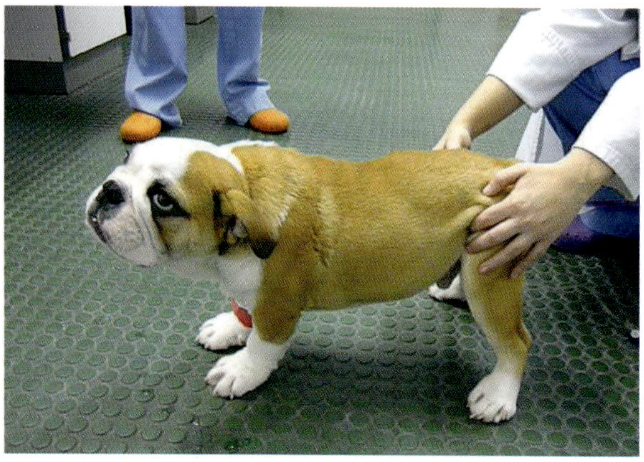

Figure 4.8. Signs of respiratory distress: head in an orthopnoeic position and neck extended.

Expiratory dyspnoea

Respiratory sounds are easily audible, and distress is more evident on expiration. The duration of **expiration is longer than that of inspiration** and is usually accompanied by respiratory **wheezing** on auscultation. This type of dyspnoea is caused by changes that cause **obstruction of the lower airways**, and there is often a previous history of coughing (Table 4.3).

Mixed dyspnoea

Respiratory difficulty during **inspiration and expiration**. The animal often breathes with its mouth open and manifests paradoxical breathing, anxiety and orthopnoea, but sometimes it is coughing and gagging. It is usually accompanied by crackles on auscultation. This type of dyspnoea is caused by **conditions affecting the lung parenchyma**, and the clinical manifestations vary depending on the cause (Table 4.4).

Fast, shallow breathing

Short, shallow breaths are observed with intermittent attempts at deep breathing.

Cardiorespiratory sounds are attenuated on auscultation and changes are also perceived on thoracic percussion, with **dull sounds** (in the case of **effusions, masses and diaphragmatic hernias**) and tympanic sounds (in the case of pneumothorax) (Table 4.5).

Modification of the respiratory rhythm

There is hypoventilation/**bradypnoea**, a decrease in range of thoracic movements and abdominal

Table 4.3. Pathologies that present with expiratory dyspnoea.

Pathologies
Intrathoracic tracheal collapse
Bronchial constriction
Feline asthma
Chronic canine bronchitis
Foreign bodies
Neoplasms

Table 4.4. Pathologies that present with mixed dyspnoea.

Pathologies
Pulmonary oedema (cardiogenic and non-cardiogenic)
Pneumonia
Pulmonary haemorrhage
Pulmonary contusion
Acute respiratory distress syndrome
Pulmonary thromboembolism

Table 4.5. Pathologies that present with rapid and superficial breathing.

Pathologies
Pleural effusion
Pneumothorax
Intrathoracic masses
Diaphragmatic hernia

Table 4.6. Pathologies that occur with modification of respiratory rhythm.

Pathologies
Intracranial (trauma, neoplasia, etc.)
Extracranial (hepatic encephalopathy, hypoglycaemia, medications, etc.)
Of the spinal cord (trauma, herniated discs, polyradiculitis, etc.)
Neuromuscular (myasthenia, polyneuropathy, etc.)

effort. These are abnormal respiratory movements associated **with neurological or neuromuscular disorders**. Other neurological signs related to the underlying disorder are almost always present (Table 4.6).

Emergency treatment

Oxygen supplementation

Oxygen supplementation should be administered to any animal showing signs of respiratory distress. More precisely, oxygen supplementation should be considered in patients with arterial oxygen pressure (PaO_2 >70 mmHg) or **arterial haemoglobin saturation (SaO2) <93%**.

The objective is to increase the inspired fraction of oxygen (FiO_2) to try to raise arterial oxygen partial pressure and haemoglobin saturation, in order to increase arterial oxygen and, consequently, its distribution to tissues. In most cases a FiO_2 of 30–40% provides the patient with an adequate amount of oxygen with a wide safety margin.

When oxygen is supplemented, prolonged exposure of more than 24 hours with FiO_2 >60% or more than 12 hours with FiO_2 >100% should be avoided. **Oxygen poisoning** can cause irreversible pulmonary fibrosis due to the production of cytotoxic free radicals. Inspired concentrations <50% are considered safe.

It is advisable to **humidify the oxygen**, since the administration of dry oxygen produces mucosal dehydration, increased viscosity of secretions, degeneration of the respiratory epithelium, alteration of the mucociliary apparatus and an increased risk of respiratory infections. Humidification is particularly necessary when oxygenation methods that bypass the nasal or oral cavities are used, preventing natural humidification of the gas (for example, nasal or tracheal catheter).

The choice of method for administering oxygen (Table 4.7) depends on the target FiO_2 to be achieved, estimated duration of treatment and patient temperament.

Nasal catheterization

For nasal catheterization, a catheter or probe of 1–3 mm in diameter with multiple fenestrations at the end is used so as not to damage the nasal mucosa with the jet of oxygen. It is introduced through the nasal fossa after having applied a local anaesthetic (lidocaine 2%), advancing the tip through the alar in a ventromedial

Table 4.7. Techniques for oxygen administration.

Technique	Advantages	Disadvantages	Observations
Face mask	Simple Cheap Always available FiO2 40–50%	Requires high oxygen flow (2–5 l/min) In large breeds this can reach 10 l/min In brachycephalic dogs and cats it can be difficult to fit the mask The patient must be constantly monitored so that the mask remains in place	Useful for initial oxygen supply
Continuous flow (flow-by)	Simple Cheap Always available Not stressful for the animal	Requires high oxygen flow (2–5 l/min) FiO_2 25–40% lower The patient must be constantly monitored to keep the tube near the face, 2–4 cm from the nose or mouth	Useful to supplement oxygen in emergencies Alternative for animals that cannot tolerate the face mask

Table 4.7. Continued.

Technique	Advantages	Disadvantages	Observations
Buster collar	Simple and economical	The initial oxygen flow must be kept high for 2 min to fill the oxygen chamber, and then it can be reduced to 1–5 l/min, thus reaching an FiO_2 of 30–40% (although this cannot be measured exactly) Causes hyperthermia, high humidity and CO_2 retention Some patients cannot tolerate it, some dyspnoeic dogs can become more stressed	The front part of the Elizabethan collar is covered with cellophane, creating a chamber in which the oxygen source can be introduced. A hole is made in the upper part to let out the moisture, heat and the CO_2 produced
Nasal catheter	More freedom of movement for the patient Lower oxygen flow (<2 l/min)	Cannot measure the exact level of FiO_2 that is reached (about 44%) An excessive flow of oxygen can cause gastric dilation	Practical and effective way to raise tracheal O_2 concentration Very useful for tolerant patients who require oxygen therapy over several days
Oxygen cage	Non-invasive Less stressful for the patient Allows precise control of FiO_2, humidity and temperature	Requires a high oxygen flow (>10 l/min) to maintain an adequate FiO_2 (40–50%) Opening of the cage leads to a decrease in FiO_2 Expensive	
Intratracheal (catheter or tube)	A catheter can be placed in an emergency and then the placement of an endotracheal tube can be commenced FiO_2 40–80% depending on whether a catheter or tube is used	Endotracheal tube placement requires sedation or anaesthesia of the patient Requires continuous monitoring	

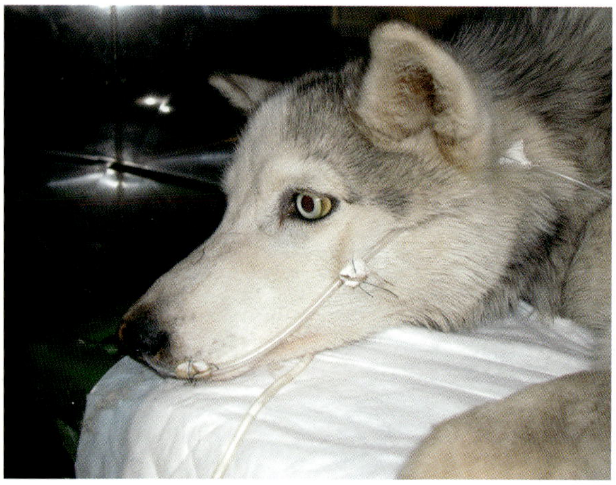

Figure 4.9. Oxygenation using a nasal catheter.

direction to the level of the medial canthus of the eye (previously measured from outside) (Figure 4.9).

The outside of the catheter is attached with a suture or glue to the dorsal area of the snout and head and connected to the oxygen source. In patients with reduced mobility or under sedation, the nasal tubes used in humans (which are placed in both nostrils) can be useful. The flow of O_2 must **not exceed 50–100 ml/kg/min**, to avoid damage to the nasal mucosa or gastric dilatation. In this way, with flows generally lower than 2 l/min, a FiO_2 of 40–50% can be achieved.

Transtracheal catheterization

The placement of a transtracheal catheter is performed by inserting a **14–16 G needle** or trocar through the cricothyroid ligament or between two tracheal rings, after desensitization of the area (1–2 ml of 2% lidocaine SC). A long, flexible catheter with a fenestrated distal edge is inserted through the needle, and the needle is subsequently removed. The end of the catheter should not reach the carina, approximately at the height of the **5th intercostal space** (it must be measured before inserting it). With this system, the highest levels of FiO_2 (40–60%) are achieved using very low oxygen flow rates (**10–50 ml/kg/min**), which should always be humidified.

Oxygen administration in a cage

See Figure 4.10.

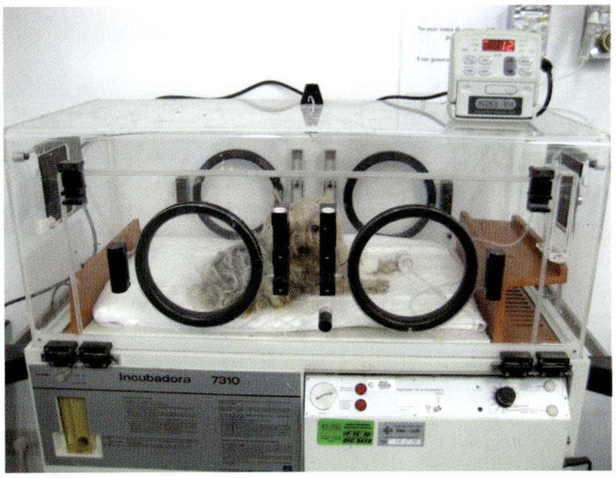

Figure 4.10. Oxygenation in a cage.

Positive-pressure ventilation

Patients who will need high FiO_2 for long periods are candidates for the application of positive-pressure ventilation.

Intubation almost always requires **sedation** with benzodiazepines or opiates, alone or in combination:

- in the dog, diazepam 0.4 mg/kg IV + fentanyl 2–5 mg/kg IV
- in the cat, butorphanol 0.005–0.4 mg/kg IM/IV.

If this is not enough, induction with propofol (2–7 mg/kg IV), with a high dose of opiates or with halogenated agents (sevoflurane or isoflurane) administered with a mask, can be resorted to.

Emergency tracheostomy

Emergency tracheostomy is used when it is not possible to clear the upper respiratory tract by less invasive methods.

If the animal is cyanotic and requires oxygenation, while everything is made available for the tracheostomy it can be oxygenated by placing a 14 or 16 G catheter through the cricothyroid ligament and connecting the oxygen source to a humidifier.As soon as mucous membranes return to a good colour, sedation or anaesthesia should be administered to perform the tracheostomy.

Table 4.8. Candidates for the application of ventilation with positive pressure.

Candidates
Animals with fatigue
Animals in respiratory arrest
Animals in a coma
Animals with increased intracranial pressure
Animals that do not respond to oxygen supplementation

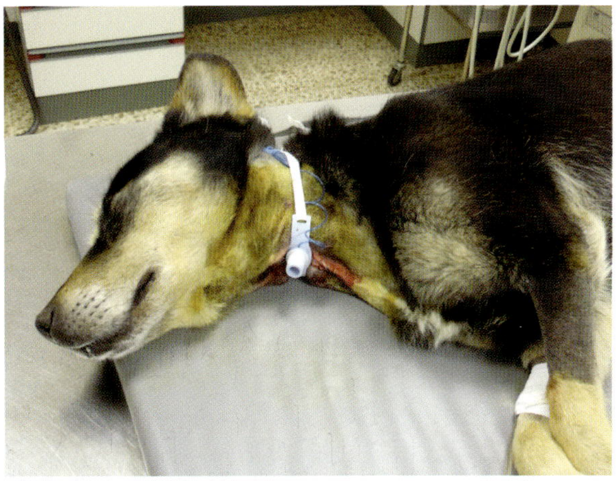

Figure 4.11. Emergency tracheostomy.

- The patient should be placed in **dorsal recumbency** with a towel or cushion under the neck to optimize exposure of the incision site.
- Clip the area and instil **local anaesthesia with 2% lidocaine**.
- Make a skin incision between the **4th and 6th tracheal rings** and exteriorize the trachea.
- Make an incision through the annular ligament between two rings, cutting **40–60% of the tracheal circumference**.
- **Two sutures** should be placed holding the proximal and distal rings and pulling them so that the incision is opened.
- **Introduce the tracheostomy cannula**. These cannulae usually have a balloon that does not need to be inflated unless mechanical ventilation is necessary (and should never be inflated with great pressure as this risks causing necrosis of the tracheal mucosa).
- The **skin suture** around the cannula does not need to completely seal the orifice, to allow the escape of air that is lost between the incision of the trachea and the tube, and thus prevent it from leaking through the subcutaneous tissue to the mediastinum and causing a pneumo-mediastinum.
- The tube should be **irrigated every 2–4 hours** with sterile physiological saline (2 ml in cats and 5–10 ml in dogs) and secretions aspirated. The tube should always be connected to an oxygen source with humidification.

Thoracentesis

Thoracentesis is indicated when the presence of air or fluid in the pleural space causes respiratory distress.

The only contraindication, due to the risk of haemorrhage, is when the effusion is the result of a coagulation problem.

To perform thoracentesis, the puncture site must be clipped and disinfected. Use an **18–21 G needle** or a butterfly connected to an extension with a three-way tap, which in turn is connected to **20–60 ml syringe** to perform the aspiration. The needle is usually inserted into the **7th or 8th intercostal space**, but can sometimes be guided by ultrasound to help choose the best area for aspiration.

The needle should be placed more dorsally for a pneumothorax and more ventral for an effusion. Introduce the needle close to the **cranial edge of the rib** to avoid damage to the vessels and nerves that run along the caudal edge. The surface of the bevel of the needle should preferably be orientated towards the dorsal part, in order to reduce the risk of laceration of the lung and, once introduced, must be manoeuvred to try to place it parallel to the costal wall. If the patient tolerates the procedure well, as much fluid or air as possible should be aspirated. Occasionally, it may be necessary to aspirate multiple areas of the thorax to ensure maximum fluid or air withdrawal.

Thoracic drainage placement

A drainage tube should be placed when continuous withdrawal is required of fluid or air from the pleural space.

Drainage tubes can be placed under local anaesthesia, but it is always better if it is done under **general anaesthesia**. Clip and disinfect the area. The location of introduction should be the **dorsal third of the 7th or 8th intercostal space**, but the skin incision will be a few centimetres more caudal. The chest tube should be measured and marked (from the point of introduction to the end of the sternum). To make the incision, an assistant should pull the skin cranially by sliding it over the ribs. An incision is made and the trocar inserted with the tube (blunt dissection of the intercostal muscles can facilitate this).

Once in the pleural space, the fenestrated tip of the tube is advanced cranially, **clamping the outer end** to prevent the entry of air. Once introduced, tension on the skin is released so that a cutaneous tunnel forms, the point of entry of the tube into the skin being further caudal than the entry point into the thoracic cavity. The tube should be sutured to the skin using a **Chinese finger trap**, and for further security anchored to the periosteum of the rib. It is fixed by creating a butterfly with some tape and suturing it to the skin. The tube is then connected to the suction/drainage device and suction performed. Finally, a sterile compress with antiseptic cream should be placed on the tube and the thorax covered with an elastic bandage, avoiding excessive tension.

A thoracic radiograph must always be performed to verify correct placement of the tube, and repeated later to check the viability of the drain.

Content can be aspirated continuously or intermittently. Continuous drainage is achieved with drainage systems based on three bottles or spaces placed in series: the first space acts to retain the fluid drained from the thorax; the second, as a water seal that allows only unidirectional escape of air; and the third, as a negative pressure regulator. It is in the last chamber where suction should be applied: water is added to the bottle and the depth of the water column determines the amount of negative pressure applied.

Pharmacology in respiratory emergencies

Sedation

In many patients with respiratory distress, sedation is necessary to relieve anxiety in order to facilitate treatment. A low dose should be used initially and increased according to effect. If the cardiovascular system is stable, acepromazine (0.0–0.05 mg/kg IV, up to 0.1–0.4 mg/kg IM or SC), with or without butorphanol (0.1–0.4 mg/kg IV or IM) and diazepam or midazolam (0.2–0.5 mg/kg IV or IM) can safely be administered.

Bronchodilators

In the management of lower airway obstruction that requires emergency treatment (such as feline asthma), induction of bronchodilation is required. Protocols differ depending on the severity of the case.

The selective β2-adrenergic agonists (terbutaline, salbutamol) are most widely used, since usually these do not have undesirable side effects. However, their use should be avoided in patients with heart disease.

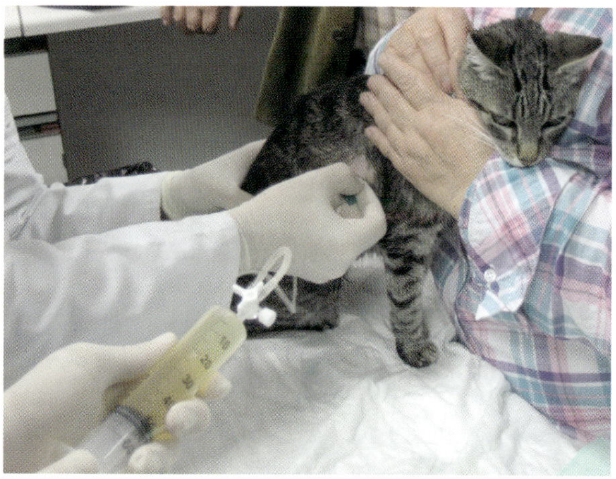

Figure 4.12. Thoracentesis in a cat using a butterfly needle.

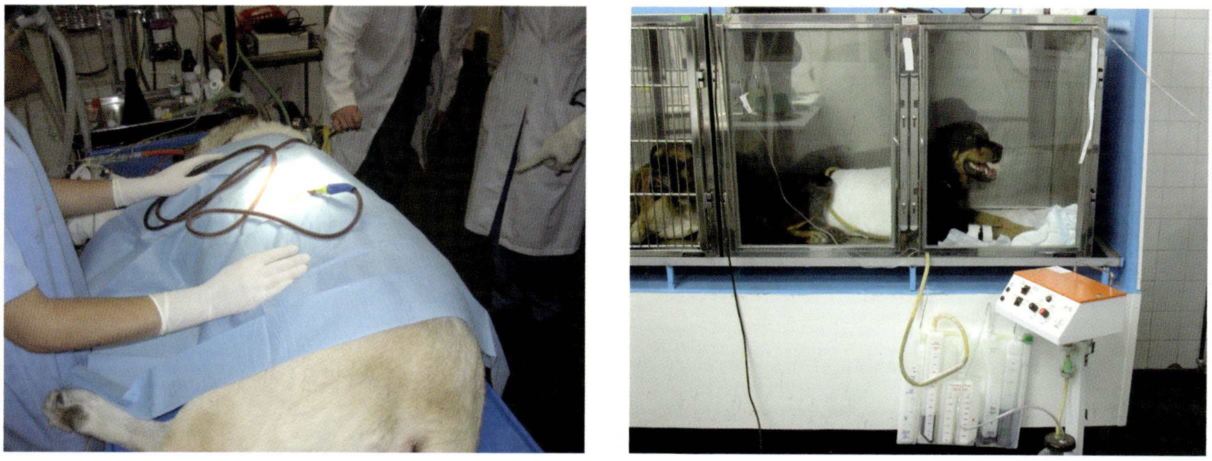

Figure 4.13. (a) horacic drainage tube; (b) thoracic drainage system.

In emergency situations, among the bronchodilators of choice is terbutaline (0.01–0.05 mg/g/4–12 h IV, IM, SC).

Salbutamol is frequently used as an aerosol for the management of **feline asthma** and **chronic canine bronchitis**. The dose for the management of asthma attacks is one inhalation every 30 min up to a maximum of eight. The bronchodilatory effect, if tolerated, is usually immediate.

In mild cases, methylxanthines can be used. The one used in cases of emergency is aminophylline (5 mg/kg IV). Intravenous administration should be slow, because this can cause hypotension.

Anti-inflammatory agents

If bronchoconstriction of **allergic aetiology** or another immune-mediated inflammatory process is suspected as the cause of respiratory distress, administration of a fast-acting corticosteroid is indicated: dexamethasone 0.25–1 mg/kg IV or methylprednisolone succinate 2–4 mg/kg IV.

Diuretics

Diuretics are indicated when the symptoms, history and clinical examination are highly suggestive of congestive heart failure.

In general, severe **pulmonary oedema** responds well to repeated doses of furosemide. Ideally, furosemide should be administered **intravenously** to achieve a more rapid effect, and to take advantage of the vasodilator properties it has when it is given via this route. However, if this is not possible without stressing the patient, the subcutaneous or intramuscular routes are appropriate. In severely dyspnoeic patients, doses of furosemide 2–4 mg/kg/1–2 h IV may be administered until the desired effect is obtained. Cats are especially sensitive to furosemide and should receive no more than up to three doses of 4 mg/kg every two hours. During treatment, the state of hydration and diuresis should be closely monitored.

In canine patients with severe heart failure, a more effective alternative is a continuous infusion of furosemide. After an initial bolus of 0.5–1 mg/kg, the estimated dose for 24 hours should be administered in a constant rate infusion of approximately 1 mg/kg per hour.

Venodilators

Nitro-glycerine is a potent venodilator administered as an ointment that is absorbed through the skin (gloves must be used when applied), and can be used when fulminant pulmonary oedema is suspected. Generally, in dogs it is used in 2% nitrogylcerin cream, rubbing it on the skin inside the pinna or on the inside of the thigh, depending on the size of the dog, at a rate of 1–4 cm every 6 hours. Care should be taken if the animal is hypotensive.

Like nitroglycerin, sodium nitroprusside can be administered together with furosemide to control fulminating pulmonary oedema. It is administered as a continuous infusion of sodium nitroprusside (0.5–2.5 µg/kg/min), always monitoring blood pressure to avoid excessive hypotension. In any case, the period of administration should not exceed 48 hours.

Anticoagulant and fibrinolytic treatments

Any problem that causes endothelial damage, venous stasis or hypercoagulability can cause the appearance of **thromboembolic** alterations (for example, pulmonary thromboembolism).

The management of pulmonary thromboembolism includes the general management of respiratory distress and administration of anticoagulatory treatment. Initially IV heparin (200 IU/kg) followed by

100–200 IU/kg/6 h SC can be administered. The goal is to keep the activated partial thromboplastin time (APTT) 1.5–2 times longer. Heparin does not dissolve the existing thrombus, but may prevent the formation of additional thrombi. The recommended doses for the use of low-molecular weight heparins are: 1 mg/kg/12 h SC for enoxaparin and 100 IU/kg/12 h SC for dalteparin.

Although rarely used due to their price and possible complications (haemorrhage), some authors recommend the use of fibrinolytics in an attempt to destroy the thrombus:

- streptokinase: loading dose 3400 IU/kg IV in 30 minutes, followed by 1500 IU/kg/h over 6–24 hours
- tissue plasminogen activator (r-TPA): loading dose 4400 IU/kg IV in 10 minutes, followed by 4400 IU/kg/h over 6–24 hours.

Evaluation of respiratory function

Whenever possible, the patient's respiratory function should be assessed. The most reliable technique is arterial blood gas, which provides information on ventilation, oxygenation and the state of the acid–base balance.

Pulse oximetry

Through **pulse oximetry**, the **oxygen saturation of arterial haemoglobin** can be measured non-invasively and an indirect estimate of arterial oxygen pressure made. It also allows for heart rate measurement. The most common sites of application of the probe are the tongue, the lips, the pinna, the axillary fold and the inguinal fold. A rectal probe can also be used.

A haemoglobin saturation of 90% corresponds approximately to an arterial blood pressure (PaO_2) of 60 mmHg. If the reading on the pulse oximeter is **<90%, treatment should be started to improve oxygenation**.

Capnography

Capnography monitors analyse the concentration of **CO_2 in exhaled air**. The exhaled CO_2 (end-tidal) measuring plate reflects alveolar CO_2 that, given the high diffusion of this gas, will be only about 2–5 mmHg lower than the value of the arterial pressure of CO_2 ($PaCO_2$).

CO_2 measurement is usually performed with the patient intubated, pairing the probe with the endotracheal tube. The value of exhaled CO_2 can be useful to identify hypoventilatory states. For example, if the monitor reflects a **high $PaCO_2$** it means that the patient is **hypoventilating**.

Upper respiratory tract disorders

Rhinitis

Definition

Rhinitis is a **generic term** that describes all conditions where there is an inflammatory reaction in the nasal cavity with sneezing, discharge and nasal discomfort. It is not a diagnostic term – **it is a symptom** of possible condition affecting the nasal cavity (it is also present in cases of frontal sinus and extra-nasal diseases).

Clinically, most of the processes that cause inflammation of the nasal cavity (and/or sinusitis) are addressed as '**patients with nasal discharge**'. Nasal discharge is a relatively frequent problem that requires a systematic evaluation to correctly determine the underlying problem. The complementary tests are standardized in a **phased study** (Table 4.9).

Not all patients require the entire range of tests (Table 4.9); sometimes the signalment and physical examination are sufficient to determine the aetiology of the condition. However, in other cases, diverse and expensive complementary studies are necessary. These studies should be prioritized according to the main suspicions that emanate from each animal's clinical history. Regardless of whether or not the technology or skills are available to carry them out, it is important to be aware of when to use the different tests to reach a correct diagnosis and establish an appropriate treatment.

Aetiology

Two causes should be considered:

1. Primary conditions **outside the nasal cavity** such as, for example, infectious processes involving other areas of the respiratory system, coagulopathies, dermatopathies of the nasal plane, or hypertension.
2. Primary conditions **inside the nasal cavity** (Table 4.10). These are addressed in the text.

Despite a wide knowledge of the causes of clinical sneezing and nasal discharge, there are many occasions when both diagnosis and treatment strategies fail. The reasons are multiple and the following highlighted:

- The treatment options available to the patient depend on the motivation and economic resources of their owners.
- The difficulty of the approach and adequate visualization of anatomical structures due to the small size of the cavity.

Table 4.9. General diagnostic approach to the dog and cat with chronic nasal discharge.

Stage I: non-invasive tests			
All patients	Dogs	Cats	Dogs and cats with nasal haemorrhage
History		Evaluation of nasal cytology from a swab (cryptococcosis)	Complete blood count Platelet count
Physical examination Examination of the fundus of the eye Thoracic radiographs	*Aspergillus* titre	*Cryptococcus* titre and antigen Viral tests: FeLV FIV ± herpesvirus ± calicivirus	Coagulation times Buccal mucosal bleeding time Test for vector-transmitted disease (dogs) Arterial pressure Von Willebrand factor test (dogs)
Stage II: all patients (requires general anaesthesia)			
Nasal radiography or CT Oral examination Rhinoscopy: nasal cavity and nasopharynx Nasal biopsy/histological examination Deep nasal culture: – Fungi – Bacteria (the significance of their growth is unclear)			
Stage III: all patients (usually need to be referred)			
CT (if not done before) or MRI Exploration of the frontal sinus, if it has been affected, using CT, NMR or RX			
Stage IV: all patients (consider referral)			
Repeat stage II using CT or MRI Exploratory rhinotomy with turbinectomy			

- Identification of pathogens that are not the cause of structural changes.
- The indeterminate nature of some conditions.
- The lack of adequate treatment for some conditions.

Clinical picture

History and physical examination allow a list of probable diagnoses to be made, and establish the urgency of the complementary tests and/or whether a symptomatic treatment approach is appropriate. Bear in mind that **sedation is often necessary** to achieve a thorough examination.

Diagnosis

The tests detailed below should be performed **based on suspected diagnoses** arising from the patient's information – that is, not all patients require the whole range of diagnostic tests.

For example:

- An unvaccinated, stray, 3-month-old cat with nasal and ocular discharge is very likely to suffer from herpesvirus and, unless the symptoms do not improve with the usual treatment, no further tests are necessary. A nasal swab for PCR of respiratory pathogens could be taken, but this test may be more useful if the condition becomes chronic (Figure 4.14).
- An 8-year-old dog with epistaxis and nasal discharge for the last 4 months is very likely to have a neoplasm or a fungal condition, and therefore requires additional evidence to help confirm or rule out these suspicions (Figure 4.15).

Table 4.10. Primary conditions within the nasal cavity.

Non-infectious contagious causes	Infectious contagious causes
Congenital Cleft palate Ciliary dyskinesia Nasopharyngeal stenosis Atresia of nares	**Viral** In the cat, rhinotracheitis and calicivirus (very common) In the dog, adenovirus, herpesvirus, distemper
Inflammatory Lymphoplasmacytic rhinitis (diagnosis requires histopathological study) Allergic rhinitis (diagnosis by exclusion of other causes) Chronic rhinitis (diagnosis by exclusion of other causes)	**Bacterial** Not very frequent as a primary aetiology Usually present as secondary and sometimes make the symptoms of rhinitis due to another aetiology becoming more evident and/or perpetuate it (especially in the cat)
Nasopharyngeal polyps	Multiple species may be involved, among the most prominent being *Staphylococcus* spp. and *Streptococcus* spp.
Polypoid rhinitis Nasopharyngeal stenosis secondary to chronic conditions	*Bordetella bronchiseptica* and *Pasteurella multocida* Pathogenic potential *per se*
Neoplasms Adenocarcinomata Squamous cells carcinomata In the cat, lymphosarcomata	**Fungal** On many occasions, associated with systemic disease In the cat: *Cryptococcus neoformans* and *gattii* (there are still a few cases described in Spain) In the dog: *Aspergillus fumigatus* (worldwide distribution)
Dental conditions Tooth root abscess Oronasal fistulae	**Parasitic** In the cat: *Pneumonyssus caninum* (nasal mite)
Foreign bodies Especially of plant origin, such as grass seeds	
Trauma	
Vascular malformations	

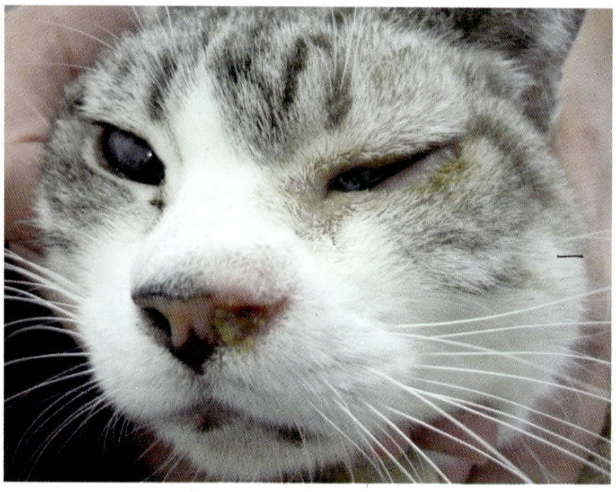

Figure 4.14. Nasal and ocular secretions in a cat.

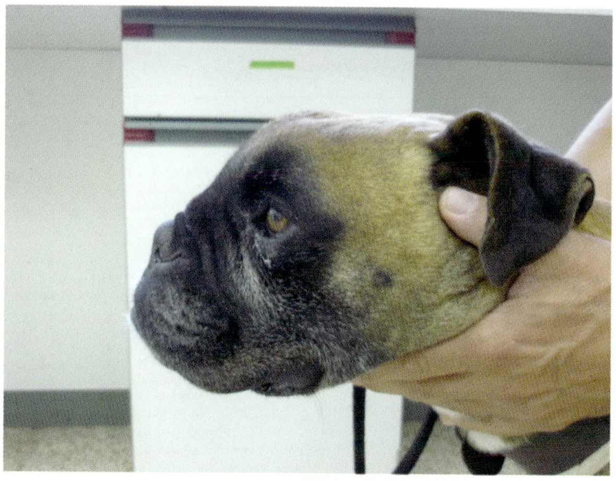

Figure 4.15. Deformation of the nasal plane in a dog.

Complete blood count

A complete blood count is indicated if there are systemic signs or as a pre-anaesthetic assessment. It is usually inconclusive and rarely reveals the specific cause of rhinitis. In haemorrhagic cases a coagulation test should be included.

Specific serology and molecular genetics

This includes testing for **infectious disease** in an area of high prevalence (e.g. Ehrlichia, Leishmaniosis).

In cats: **FeLV and FIV** may contribute to disease but are not primary causes.

Table 4.11. Differential diagnoses, diagnostic suspicion.

	Finding	Diagnostic suspicion
Patient's age	Young	Infectious diseases, congenital (dyskinesia, stenosis, palatal lesions)
	Adults	All are possible
	Senior and geriatric	Neoplasia
Morphology	Dolichocephalic dogs	Inflammatory, neoplastic and fungal pathologies
Duration of signs	Acute	Frequent in viral conditions and with foreign bodies; empirical treatment is justified
	Chronic	Need for multiple tests; empirical treatments usually only partially control the signs
Systemic involvement (apathy, anorexia, fever, etc.)	Rare for only the nasal cavity to be affected	Usually indicates a pneumonic process or systemic disease
Type of secretion	Serous	Viral, foreign bodies, parasitic, initial phases of multiple conditions prior to infection
	Mucosal	Possible bacterial contamination
	Mixed with blood	Destruction or intense inflammation
	Epistaxis	Destructive processes or extra-nasal causes
Unilateral or bilateral secretion	Unilateral start	Suggests local disease such as neoplasia, foreign bodies, fungal infections or dental lesions
	Bilateral involvement	Indicates diffuse infectious or inflammatory causes
Presence of signs that indicate space-occupying lesions (masses or proliferative lesions) lack of soft palate depression		Airflow patency, ocular retropulsion
Other signs	Facial asymmetry	
	Pain	
	Lymph node enlargement	Periosteal involvement and/or local invasion
	Nasal depigmentation	40% of dogs with aspergillosis

PCR for FHV and FCV. This can be done using nasal or nasopharyngeal swabs. Negative results do not exclude a possible initiating role. In certain chronic feline rhinitis, these viruses may initiate the process and cause a lesion which, after the disappearance of the initiating virus, becomes chronic.

Where suspicion arises:

- Measurement of **Ag due to *Cryptococcus*** (sensitivity 90–100% and specificity 97–100%, but gives false negatives in case of localized nasal disease).
- Determination of **Ac due to *Aspergillus*** (sensitivity 90% and specificity 100%).

See Table 4.11 for differential diagnoses.

Cytology of secretions

This is **rarely diagnostic**, and the most common cytological finding is non-specific rhinitis with a predominance of neutrophils. Ideally cytology should be performed on deep samples taken by nasal lavage or samples obtained by endoscopy. The results from spontaneous secretion are difficult to interpret and should be rejected.

Bacterial and fungal cultures

Generally culture **does not provide any useful information**, and interpretation is dubious due to the presence of saprophytic bacteria in the nasal cavity. The most useful cultures are those performed on deep samples taken under endoscopic guidance. These can be of help in:

- some fungal conditions – for example, *Aspergillus*
- dogs, in which a significant isolation can be made of bacteria including *Bordetella bronchiseptica* and *Pasteurella multocida*.

Examination of the oral cavity and ears

Under anaesthesia and prior to imaging tests, a detailed examination of the oral cavity and ears should be performed. This provides information on possible nasopharyngeal masses, palatal changes, dental alterations and nasopharyngeal polyps.

Radiography

Although not conclusive for diagnosis (except for certain dental conditions), radiographs can show changes in the density and symmetry of the nasal cavity. At least two views are required – lateral and ventrodorsal with an open mouth.

In the case of neoplasms (and severe fungal conditions), destruction of the nasal turbinates may be observed. These signs (rather than being a diagnosis) should **be considered indicative of the duration of the condition**, the degree of involvement and the invasive potential of the underlying disease.

Computed tomography and magnetic resonance imaging

These techniques offer a more detailed picture of the condition, and are indicated when **nasal neoplasia** is suspected. They allow the extent of the tumour invasion to be evaluated and detection of small-size neoplasia, as well as ensuring that approaches by rhinoscopy are safe since they locate the injury or the suspicious finding (Figure 4.16).

Rhinoscopy and biopsy

Although rhinoscopy is useful, it should be **performed after less invasive imaging studies**, such as CT and MRI so that neither inflammation nor bleeding can interfere with the imaging studies.

It requires special equipment (flexible small-bore endoscopes) which, on certain occasions and in small-sized animals, is considered a limitation.

Rhinoscopy facilitates evaluation of changes in the nasal mucosa and collection of biopsies, which yield a definitive diagnosis in approximately 85% of cases. It is much more sensitive for diagnosis than blind biopsy or aspiration biopsy (introduction of a biopsy tool through the nasal passage and extraction of a sample without visual assessment of the area being biopsied).

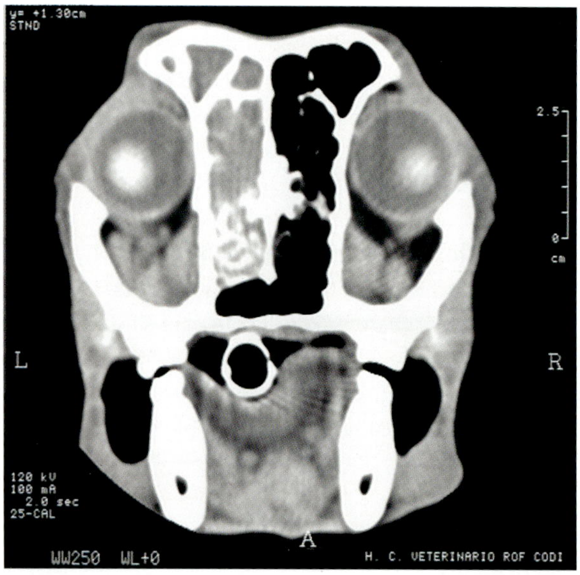

Figure 4.16. CT showing a nasal tumour.

Treatment

Symptomatic

- Cleaning and **moistening of secretions**.
- **Supportive care**, such as maintaining hydration status.
- **Decongestants**: Their effectiveness has not been proven, but they are sometimes utilized. When used, the most complicated aspect is usually their local administration, because few patients tolerate them (oral administration is also possible). The most commonly used are phenylephrine, pseudo-ephedrine/diphenhydramine and chlorpheniramine (agents that exert their effect through an antihistaminic and vasoconstrictive mechanism).
- If secretions are mucopurulent, the **prophylactic use of antibiotics** is recommended, which will solve the problem if there is primary infection and will provide a transient improvement in the case of secondary infection.

Specific

- **Foreign bodies**: extraction of the foreign body.
- **Tooth root abscesses, dental fistulae or others**: surgical treatment and dental prophylaxis.
- **Fungal infections**: the use of **oral antifungals** is recommended, but these therapies, generally prolonged and expensive, are not 100% successful. In the case of aspergillosis, treatment with topical fungicidal agents (such as enilconazole or clotrimazole) has been seen to have a high success rate. Local administration requires the patient to be anaesthetized, with introduction and maintenance of the treatment for a certain amount of time, which can be minimized with the use of depot fungicide solutions.
- **Acute viral infections**: symptomatic treatment and administration of antibiotics for the management of secondary infections in patients with marked clinical manifestations. These tend to become chronic and are a frequent problem in the cat.
- **Chronic rhinitis in the cat**: Secondary bacterial rhinitis (cultures of deep nasal specimens) is ideally **treated for 6–8 weeks** and at least two weeks after the symptoms subside, especially if there are signs of osteomyelitis. **Saline nebulization** or administration of two drops in each nostril (2–4/d) are both useful. Periodical nasal flushing, to reduce the intensity of symptoms, requires general anaesthesia. It is advisable to avoid corticosteroids but, if the biopsy shows lymphoplasmacytic infiltrates, their administration can be considered topically; systemically these can exacerbate the infection.

- **Parasitic infections:** specific treatment: For example, in the case of nasal mites (*Pneumonyssoides caninum*) the use of subcutaneous ivermectin is recommended.
- **Neoplasms**: Benign tumours can be treated by **surgical ablation**. With malignant tumours, excision of the tumour and affected tissues is considered a palliative treatment because in most cases the tumour recurs. Improvement in survival rate usually requires combined protocols of surgery, radiotherapy and/or chemotherapy.
- **Allergic rhinitis**: use of **corticosteroids** until control of the condition is achieved via the minimum effective dose. Identify the allergen and avoid contact where possible.
- **Lymphoplasmacytic rhinitis**: **Glucocorticoids** are administered systemically until control of the condition at the minimum effective dose. It been shown recently that glucocorticoids are not effective in all animals with lymphoplasmacytic rhinitis. In these refractory patients there may be a certain hypersensitivity to sustained inhalation of fungal spores and, although glucocorticoids can partially control, recurrence is common when treatment is stopped. The lack of knowledge of its true aetiology means that the literature proposes therapeutic alternatives as disparate as the use of itraconazole (5 mg/kg/12 h VO for 3–6 months) or the long-term combined use of antibiotics with immunomodulatory effects and non-steroidal anti-inflammatory drugs. The recommended doses are: piroxicam (0.3 mg/kg/24 h) together with doxycycline (3–5 mg/kg/12 h) or azithromycin (5 mg/kg/24 h). If improvement is seen after 4–8 weeks, piroxicam is maintained but the frequency of doxycycline is reduced to 24 hours or azithromycin to twice per week. This treatment may be necessary for a **minimum of 6 months**, and sometimes indefinitely.

Sinusitis

Definition

The paranasal sinuses are invaginations of the bony cavities of the skull which are covered in mucosa. Therefore, the sinuses have the same risks of developing disease as any other organ in the upper respiratory tract, and fundamentally the **same as the nasal cavity**. The term sinusitis refers to the **inflammation of the paranasal sinuses**.

Aetiology

In small animals, the nasal cavity and paranasal sinuses are usually affected simultaneously. In these cases, the most commonly affected sinus is the **frontal sinus**.

When the condition arises as a result of an injury or **dental condition** there is usually involvement of the **maxillary sinus**.

Clinical picture

The initial presentation is often unilateral **nasal discharge** (bilateral if there is involvement of the nasal cavity), which varies between serous and mucopurulent. In cases where extensive tissue necrosis exists, secretions often acquire a foul odour.

Other clinical signs include:

- dullness on percussion of the affected sinus
- nasal deformation
- sometimes an ocular discharge
- mandibular lymphadenopathy
- sometimes pyrexia and signs of systemic involvement (due to infection in a confined space).

Diagnosis

Radiography (in small animals the ideal is a **CT scan**) is the method of choice. It shows changes in density and a line of fluid inside the sinuses.

In many cases centesis (or trepanation) of the sinus is required to take a **cytology and culture** in order to determine the underlying cause.

Treatment

The **underlying pathology should be treated** (for example, dental problems must be rectified for the symptomatic treatment for sinusitis to be successful) and secondary infection controlled (with drainage of the cavity and daily lavage using trepanation of the sinus and placement of a catheter).

The use of **local antibiotics** is recommended, chosen according to bacterial susceptibility. Polymicrobial infections are frequent, and therefore it is important to submit samples for culture and sensitivity.

If there is **general involvement**, administration of **parenteral antibiotics** may be necessary. Treatment should be performed based on sensitivity studies (pending the results of the antibiogram, penicillin). In some patients, the use of **anti-inflammatory drugs** has also been recommended. Generally, in uncomplicated cases, local treatment over 10–14 days is usually sufficient. Response is assessed by a reduction of secretions.

Chronic cases and those in which it is not possible to perform specific treatment may require **long-term treatment** and even permanent trepanation of the sinuses. These tend to be very **refractory to treatment** and only partial or incomplete resolution of the symptomatology is achieved.

Laryngeal paralysis

Definition

Laryngeal paralysis is the absence of movement of the arytenoids during the respiratory cycle. This is characterized by a **lack of abduction of the vocal folds and arytenoid cartilages** during inspiration and is caused by a **loss of innervation** to the intrinsic musculature of the larynx, whose motor innervation comes from the recurrent laryngeal nerves. In small animals the condition is more frequent in the dog than the cat, although it can occur in the latter.

Types

- **unilateral**: rarely causes a clinically manifest disease
- **bilateral**: presents with **intense inspiratory dyspnoea**, which is clinically evident.

Aetiology

Laryngeal paralysis is **congenital in certain breeds** – Bouvier des Flandres, Irish setter and Siberian husky. These animals usually present with the disease between 4 and 8 months and before 2 years of age.

The **idiopathic form** is the most frequent and mostly affects medium- to large-sized breeds such as the Irish Setters, Afghan hound, Pointers and Labrador retriever. Males have an incidence rate two to three times higher than females, and the average age of onset is >10 years of age.

Other less frequent causes

- **Neoplasmia**: malignant tumours of the thyroid gland, lymphomas and thymomas
- **Trauma or surgery**: iatrogenic causes that damage the recurrent laryngeal nerve
- **Immune-mediated, endocrine**: hypothyroidism and hypo-adrenocorticism
- **Systemic polyneuropathies**: hypocalcaemia and certain toxins
- Certain **neuromyopathies** such as myasthenia gravis
- In older animals it can occur as a result of the **ankylosis of the cricoarytenoid joint**.

Clinical picture

Clinical signs develop acutely or may be more chronic, and are closely linked to the degree of deterioration of respiratory function.

- **Inspiratory stridor**: the main and most constant finding
- **Exercise intolerance** or, at least, exacerbation of symptoms during exercise
- Changes in **vocalization**, such as a hoarse bark
- **A cough** associated with the ingestion of food or water, due to aspiration resulting from incomplete closure of the larynx or uncoordinated swallowing
- **Heat intolerance** or exacerbation of signs with heat
- **Collapse** and loss of consciousness are possible
- There may be **pulmonary oedema** and/or **aspiration pneumonia**.

Diagnosis

Diagnosis is made by **direct observation of the larynx** under light sedation so as not to interfere with normal movement (doxapram 2.2 mg/kg IV).

The larynx must be inspected over several respiratory cycles. Usually the arytenoid cartilages and vocal folds separate in a coordinated way at the beginning of each inspiration. However, when laryngeal paralysis is present these structures do not come together or separate completely, but rather **remain in a neutral position**. The **absence of abduction (lateralization)** of the arytenoids during the **inspiratory phase** is the basis for the diagnosis of laryngeal paralysis.

If the dog is calm, movement of the arytenoid cartilages can be inspected without sedation using ultrasonography of the larynx.

Radiography is of no use for the diagnosis of laryngeal paralysis. It can be used to:

- eliminate other differential diagnoses (cervical or intralaryngeal masses)
- eliminate possible causes of laryngeal paralysis
- eliminate the possibility of aspiration pneumonia
- identify respiratory anomalies caused by laryngeal paralysis.

Emergency treatment

- oxygen supplementation
- corticosteroids (dexamethasone or prednisone)
- sedation (acepromazine)
- cooling.

Surgical treatment

The main objective of surgery is to **increase the fixed diameter of the larynx**, allowing a flow of air compatible with the normal physical activity of the animal. This is indicated in the following cases:

- if exercise intolerance is not acceptable
- if collapse occurs due to respiratory failure
- if there is an inability to cope with heat or stress.

A good candidate for surgery is an animal with exercise intolerance, cyanosis and syncope, without underlying disease.

A poor candidate for surgery is:

- suffering from one or more of the following symptoms: cough, nausea/regurgitation or dysphagia
- one that presents with a significant involvement of the function of the hind legs due to a polyneuropathy
- one with another age-related comorbidity, such as a thoracic mass or renal failure.

Brachycephalic syndrome

- In brachycephalic dogs several anatomical anomalies are common:
- The cartilaginous skeleton of the external part of the nostrils is usually shorter and thicker, displaced medially and secondarily obstructs the nostrils. This leads to **stenotic nares**.
- The size, shape and position of the nasal turbinates are modified, which causes **intranasal stenosis**.
- The soft palate, which under normal conditions reaches the epiglottis, extends 1–2 cm beyond. In many cases the **palate is not only longer but thicker** than normal.
- **Hyperplasia of the tongue and tonsils** is also frequent.
- **Protrusion of the laryngeal ventricles** towards the laryngeal lumen.
- The trachea of certain breeds (especially the British Bulldog) is **hypoplastic**, which further reduces the entry of air.

See Figures 4.17–4.19 and Table 4.12.

These anatomical anomalies generate a **multifocal obstruction** in the upper respiratory tract, which in turn causes secondary functional alterations. Due to stenosis of the nostrils and nasal passages, animals must produce a greater negative pressure to breathe adequately. After this inspiratory effort, the cuneiform and corniculate cartilages are dragged into the entrance of the glottis, which causes **laryngeal collapse**, inspiratory stridor and even suffocation. In these animals, the laryngeal saccules are usually everted towards the laryngeal lumen.

Clinical picture

Typical clinical signs include rales, stridor, snoring, coughing, exercise intolerance, increased respiratory effort, hyperthermia, cyanosis and even, in the most severe cases, episodes of syncope.

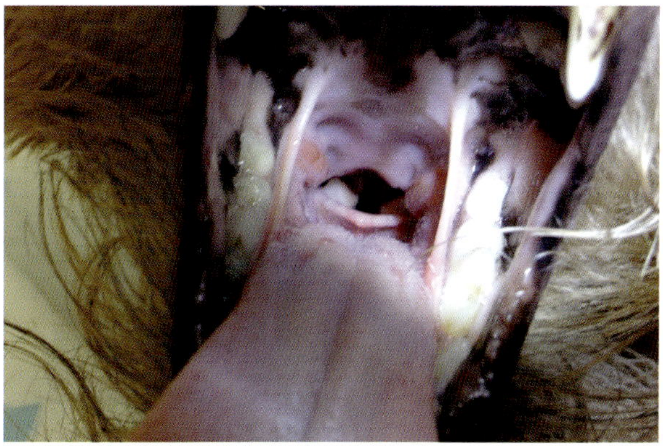

Figure 4.17. Direct observation of the larynx.

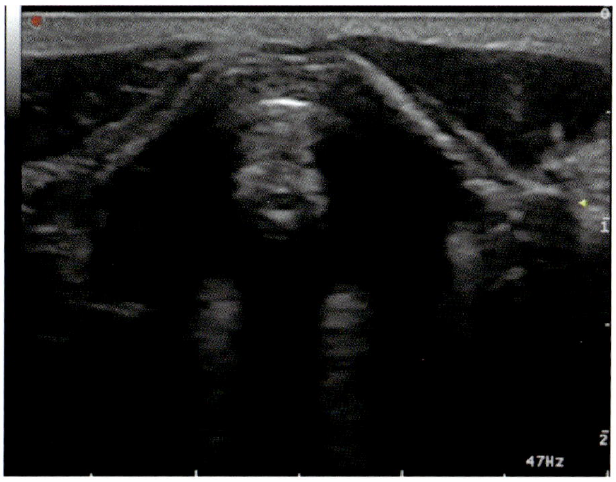

Figure 4.18. Laryngeal ultrasound.

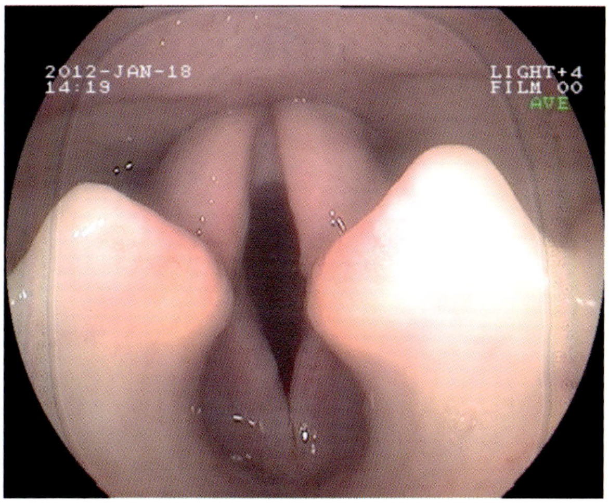

Figure 4.19. Laryngeal endoscopy.

These problems are often **aggravated by stress, exercise and heat**. It is interesting to note that some of these can occur during sleep (which cause great alarm to the owner) as a consequence of laryngeal relaxation, a form of **sleep apnoea**.

Being a progressive disease, clinical signs may vary from a minimum increase in respiratory effort to a severe respiratory crisis due to closure of the airways

Table 4.12. Primary and secondary structural defects (result of inflammation associated with increased flow and pressure) due to brachiocephalic syndrome (source: https://www.acvs.org/small-animal/brachycephalic-syndrome).

Anatomical structure	Defect	Observations
Nasal opening	Stenotic nares Stenosis of the nasal vestibule caused by the inner part of the nasal ala	Resect nostrils when they are narrow, especially if they present paradoxical movement during inspiration
Nasal cavity	Obstruction of the respiratory tract due to hyperplastic and dysplastic turbinates Obstruction due to rostral aberrant turbinates (RAT)	
Nasopharyngeal meatus and turbinates	Obstruction due to an aberrant growth of the turbinates in a caudal direction (CAT)	
Nasopharynx	Elongated soft palate (87% of cases) Severe increase in thickness of soft palate	One of the most common problems It should be corrected as soon as possible to avoid the appearance of secondary signs (increase in thickness)
Tonsils	Increase in the size of tonsils	This is not a structural change, but in all those animals that show a visible increase in tonsillar size, and is contributing to airway obstruction, the tonsils should be eliminated
Larynx	Collapse as a consequence of laryngomalacia Eversion of laryngeal saccules Laryngeal collapse Laryngeal oedema	In the Pug, laryngeal collapse appears in a primary form; in other breeds, it appears in the final stages caused by a failure in the cartilage, secondary to the inflammation and due to the increase in inspiratory effort The appearance of laryngeal oedema necessitates treatment with steroidal anti-inflammatory drugs in some cases

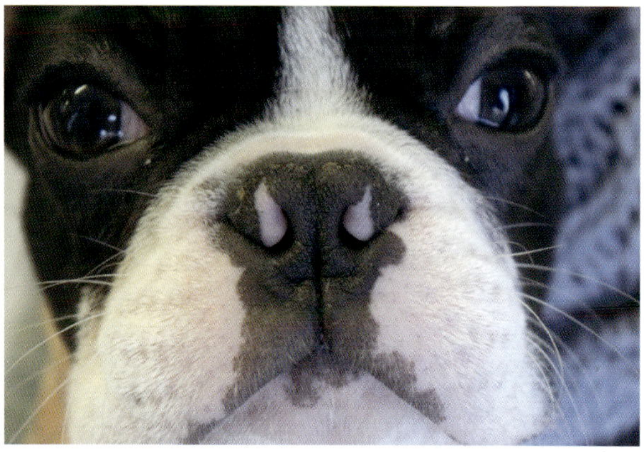

Figure 4.20. Brachycephalic breed: stenosis of the nasal orifices.

and laryngeal collapse that requires urgent medical intervention.

Concomitantly, they usually suffer from **gastrointestinal disorders**: frequent vomiting, regurgitation, salivation, hiatal hernias and/or pyloric stenosis. In a study of 73 brachycephalic dogs, 97.3% presented with one of these abnormalities: distal oesophagitis (37%), diffuse gastric inflammation (89%) and diffuse duodenal inflammation (53%).

Diagnosis

Examination of the upper airway using a **light anaesthetic** (ideally with the use of a bronchoscope for deeper visualization) can be performed to evaluate the soft palate, laryngeal function, the tonsils and the saccules. In some breeds, antegrade and retrograde rhinoscopy is recommended to establish whether the turbinates are normal. During the same procedure, if digestive signs are observed an **anterior gastrointestinal endoscopy** is usually recommended.

A **CT scan** may be performed to evaluate the length and thickness of the soft palate, as well as other mucosal hyperplasias or nasal abnormalities, and **thoracic radiographs** are recommended to diagnose tracheal hypoplasia or possible aspiration pneumonia.

Because sedation and anaesthesia can cause episodes of acute respiratory distress, before proceeding preparations should be made to handle a possible emergency.

Treatment

Medical

Weight control is the basis of medical treatment. In addition, avoid activities that increase respiratory effort.

Emergency

- **Cooling**.
- **Oxygenation** with mask or cage. In severe cases, rapid induction of anaesthesia with endotracheal intubation should be performed.
- Often, during an acute respiratory crisis, **sedation** with acepromazine (0.005–0.02 mg/kg IV or SC), butorphanol (0.2–0.4 mg/kg IV, IM or SC) or diazepam (0.2 mg/kg IV) is necessary.
- **Short-acting anti-inflammatories**: Dexamethasone sodium phosphate (0.1–0.2 mg/kg IV) or prednisone (0.5–1 mg/kg IV) may be useful for reducing inflammation during the crisis.

Surgical

This is preferably preventive, before the proliferative and inflammatory changes cause more damage:

- **rhinoplasty** or correction of stenotic nares, as young as 3–4 months (Figure 4.21)
- Resection of the soft palate or **palatoplasty**, at the time of neutering or castration.

Reverse sneezing

Definition

The reverse sneeze involves a strong **paroxysmal inspiratory effort against a closed glottis** to remove irritants from the nasopharynx. This is a reflex similar reflex to sneezing (involving the nose) or coughing (trachea).

Aetiology

Reverse sneezing may be due to:

- inflammation of the posterior part of the choana due to an **allergic response** to environmental stimuli
- anything that causes momentary or permanent **irritation of the throat** (including repeated vomiting, perfumes, etc.)
- In brachycephalics, **suction of the soft palate**
- **Foreign bodies**
- **Nasal mites**.

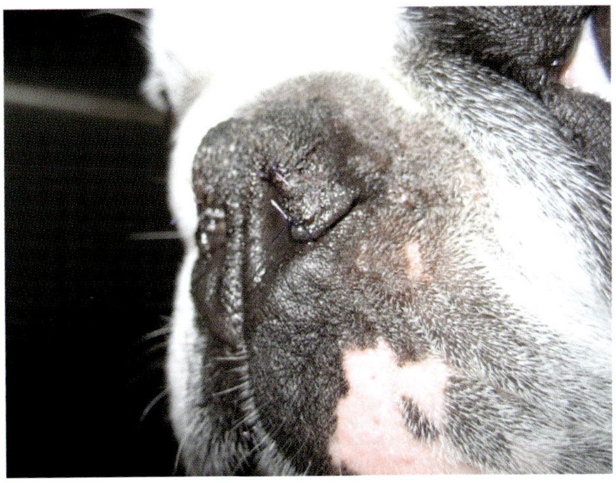

Figure 4.21. Rhinoplasty: widening of the nasal orifices.

Diagnosis

Generally, the history and normality between episodes point towards the diagnosis.

Additional examination is indicated if the appearance of the reverse sneeze is accompanied by syncope, exercise intolerance or other signs of respiratory disease, or if the reverse sneeze is pronounced, progressive or has become a chronic problem. In those cases, the following tests should be performed:

- Direct and/or **endoscopic visualization** (to rule out masses, nasal or pharyngeal foreign bodies, etc.).
- Biopsy: This is often inconclusive, with histopathology suggestive of an allergic process.

Treatment

Some dogs have these episodes throughout their lives, while others develop them as they get older. In the majority, it is a temporary problem that disappears on its own. Effective measures to alleviate signs have been demonstrated such as:

- **massaging the throat**, covering the nose, stimulating swallowing, etc.
- administering **antihistamines**: some animals require corticosteroids to control inflammation
- giving an empirical **treatment for nasal mites** (selamectin, one application every two weeks (three treatments)).

Lower respiratory tract disorders

Canine infectious tracheobronchitis

Definition

Canine **infectious tracheobronchitis (ITB)** is an **acute** disease, which occurs in the airways and is **highly contagious**, caused by one or several infectious agents, including canine adenovirus type 2, parainfluenza virus and *B. bronchiseptica*, with other microorganisms as secondary pathogens.

Clinical picture

An intense **dry cough** develops shortly after contact with an affected animal. The cough can be easily

provoked by tracheal palpation, with exercise or when the neck is compressed with a collar. Sometimes there may also be gagging and/or nasal discharge. Uncomplicated cases do not show signs of systemic disease.

Secondary respiratory complications rarely occur:

- When it affects newborn animals or those with immune problems, it can evolve into a pneumonic condition.
- Dogs with chronic diseases of the airways or with tracheal collapse can experience acute and severe exacerbations of their condition.

Diagnosis

The diagnosis of ITB is usually based on clinical signs, its acute onset and the history of recent contact with infection.

When signs suggest a more serious disease or when they do not improve with empirical treatment, a complete blood count, thoracic radiographs and tracheal lavage are indicated.

In uncomplicated cases, the thoracic radiograph and complete blood count are not helpful since these rarely show significant change, and a tracheal wash sample usually indicates the presence of acute inflammation. The **bacterial culture** of the sample can be useful to identify any bacteria involved, and culture useful when choosing antibiotics, especially in patients that do not respond to initial treatment.

Treatment

Uncomplicated canine ITB is **self-limiting**. Rest is recommended for at least 7 days, avoiding exercise and excitement to minimize episodes of excessive coughing. Antitussives are useful, but should not be used if the cough is productive or if the presence of lung secretions are suspected through radiographs or auscultation. In some patients affected by *Bordetella* spp. the **cough may persist for up to 30 days**. Glucocorticoids should not be used.

In the cases with symptoms of **systemic involvement**, the use of **antibiotics** is indicated. The ideal is to choose these based on culture results of respiratory secretions but, in the absence of these data, amoxicillin, enhanced sulphonamides, doxycycline and enrofloxacin can be good choices.

Prevention

ITB can be prevented by minimizing exposure to microorganisms (isolation of patients) and by **vaccination**. Injectable and intranasal vaccines are available against the major pathogens: canine adenovirus type 2, parainfluenza virus and *B. bronchiseptica*.

The ability of a dog to respond to infection without developing severe symptoms is maximized with proper nutrition, regular deworming and avoidance of stressful situations.

Tracheal collapse

Definition

Tracheal collapse is the dynamic reduction of the luminal diameter of the trachea as a consequence of the weakening of its cartilaginous support.

Anatomical components involved in tracheal collapse include **flattening of the tracheal rings**, which normally occurs in a dorsoventral direction. The latter results in **stretching of the dorsal tracheal membrane** which, when prolapsed towards the lumen, contributes another component of tracheal collapse.

Epidemiology

Tracheal collapse mainly affects **small-breed dogs** (Poodle, Yorkshire Terrier, Pomeranian, Maltese, Pug and Chihuahua), and rarely medium/large breeds. Although dogs of all ages can suffer from this disease, it is more frequent in middle-aged animals. The condition is rare in felines.

Aetiopathogenesis

The aetiology is unknown, but a **primary anomaly of the tracheal cartilage** is assumed, leading to weakness (hypocellularity and alterations in composition). Possible triggers for this weakness include **congenital factors**, nutritional deficiencies and metabolic factors.

There are also certain **secondary factors** that can trigger the process and cause a patient suffering from asymptomatic cartilaginous weakness to become symptomatic. These changes include diseases causing obstruction of the upper airways, chronic respiratory pathologies of the lower airways, obesity and concurrent cardiac alterations that present with cardiomegaly.

Localization of tracheal collapse

Changes can be located either in the **cervical or thoracic trachea**, in both locations simultaneously and even, in severely affected patients, in the bronchial tracts.

The condition is defined as **dynamic** because (depending on the area affected) the symptoms are observed in one phase or another of the respiratory cycle:

- Patients affected in the **neck area** may collapse or show symptomatology during **inspiration**.
- Patients affected in the **intrathoracic region** may collapse and/or manifest symptoms during **expiration** as a consequence of increased intrapleural pressure.

Clinical signs

Affected dogs usually have a long history of chronic cough, which is rough, dry, unproductive and often described as a '**goose honking**'.

Initially the cough is occasional, but over time it becomes paroxysmal or even continuous. Often these coughing attacks appear associated with moments of **excitement**, pressure on the collar, the ingestion of food or water or environmental changes such as extreme cold.

There may be some **exercise intolerance**, although this depends on the patient's activity level. Severely affected dogs show varying degrees of **tachypnoea and dyspnoea** and, in the case of severe airway compromise, **cyanosis and syncope**.

Physical examination

The animal may appear normal at rest, but **agitation induces a honking cough** and causes dyspnoea. Marked **tracheal sensitivity** is typical, such that gentle palpation precipitates a crisis.

Cervical tracheal collapse results in **inspiratory difficulty**, and auscultation may reveal wheezing or wheezing inspiratory sounds. **Intrathoracic collapse** is associated with **expiratory dyspnoea**. When it affects a wide segment, it is possible to auscultate a clicking noise. Affected dogs often have hepatomegaly for reasons that are still unclear.

Diagnosis

Tracheal collapse can be suspected based on the clinical picture, the animal's signalment and physical examination. Diagnostic confirmation and assessment of the degree of involvement require radiography and bronchoscopy.

Radiography

Radiographs facilitate a diagnosis of tracheal collapse in the majority of cases, but CT may also be helpful (Figures 4.22 and 4.23).

Lateral radiographs should be taken on inspiration and expiration to identify cervical or intrathoracic collapse, respectively, or radioscopy or fluoroscopy can be used.

An advantage of radiography is that it allows the pulmonary field and the cardiac image to be assessed at the same time to identify possible concurrent pulmonary disease or heart failure.

Bronchoscopy

Bronchoscopy is the ideal technique to confirm tracheal collapse, but is not considered essential and, in reality in most practices a diagnosis is made using radiography. However, the identification of bronchial involvement usually requires bronchoscopy.

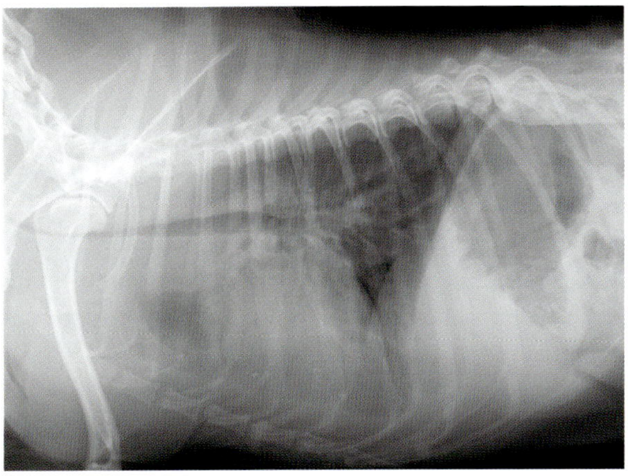

Figure 4.22. Radiography: cervical tracheal collapse.

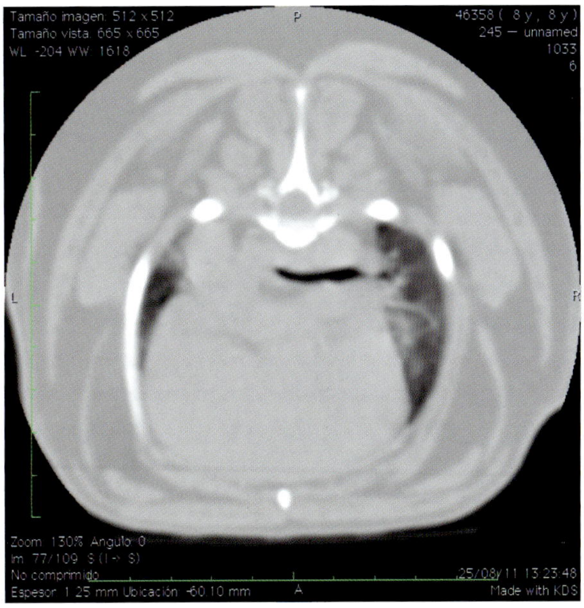

Figure 4.23. CT: intrathoracic tracheal collapse.

Among the advantages of this technique over radiography is that it allows determination of the degree, extent and severity of the collapse.

Graduation of the severity of collapse (this does not necessarily correspond to clinical signs):

- **grade 1**: almost normal, slightly pendulous dorsal tracheal muscle
- **grade 2**: 50% reduction in size of the tracheal lumen
- **grade 3**: 75% reduction in size of the tracheal lumen, with the dorsal tracheal muscle contacting the ventral surface
- **grade 4**: flattened tracheal cartilages, leaving less than 10% of the lumen visible; when the tracheal muscle is in contact with the ventral surface of the trachea, a double lumen is observed.

Bronchoscopy can be used to assess status and **functionality of other respiratory structures** (larynx, laryngeal saccules), and to take samples from the respiratory tract for bacterial culture and cytology and thus identify a possible infection or underlying lung inflammation.

Treatment

There is no universal or permanent treatment, so periodic check-ups are required. With frequent monitoring and modifications depending on the symptoms of the patient and the management of concurrent conditions, success rates of up to 70% have been achieved.

Medical

Hygienic/dietetic measures to manage obesity with diet and exercise. Avoid situations that could aggravate the condition such as collars, excess humidity, heat and excitement.

Treatment of co-existing problems that may aggravate the condition is essential, including laryngeal paralysis, laryngeal saccule eversion, bronchitis, heart failure and other lower respiratory tract diseases.

The use of bronchodilators is controversial, since there are few patients where bronchoconstriction has been documented.

Corticosteroids reduce tracheal inflammation, but cause weight gain which is counterproductive. They are **not indicated in long-term** treatment, but are indicated in cases of clinical exacerbation of the condition when oedema and inflammation of the tracheal mucosa occurs as a consequence of mechanical trauma caused by the long coughing episodes. The most commonly used glucocorticoid is prednisone at anti-inflammatory doses (1 mg/kg divided into two doses) for a short period of time (5–7 days), which is then reduced gradually (23 weeks).

Antitussives are recommended in long-term treatments to reduce mechanical irritation of the epithelium.

The use of antibiotics is justified when an infection has been confirmed using culture or cytology, but in other cases they do not provide any benefit.

Surgical alternative

In animals that do not respond to treatment, surgical or endoscopic insertion of **tracheal/bronchial prostheses** (tracheal stents or extraluminal rings) can be used as a last resort.

Prognosis

A complete cure is not possible; the animal will have a variable symptomatology throughout its lifetime, sometimes even uncontrollable, potentially causing a serious threat to its life.

Chronic bronchitis

Definition

Chronic bronchitis is defined as a **chronic, progressive inflammatory disorder** (with bronchial remodelling), which occurs with a recurrent or **persistent cough** accompanied by excessive production of mucus, which occurs consecutively (most days) for a period of at least **two months** in the year preceding diagnosis. It is one of the most frequent chronic respiratory problems in the dog.

Aetiology

The specific aetiology or the inciting cause is rarely determined. The following have been suggested as possible aetiologies or triggers:

- **air pollutants** such as tobacco smoke or pollution
- **allergic** response to certain antigens (type I hypersensitivity)
- **chronic infections** that decrease the response threshold of the bronchial receptors, resulting in hyper-reactivity to irritants such as cold, dust or environmental pollution (non-specific hyper-reactivity).

Epidemiology

Most commonly affects small to medium-sized breeds, with clinical signs from middle age (>6–8 years) onwards.

Clinical signs

The typifying sign is **a chronic dry cough** of several months' duration. This cough is the result of attempts to eliminate mucus from the airways. It is typical for **tracheal palpation to cause coughing**, and the end of each coughing episode may be accompanied by gagging. Auscultation of the respiratory tract may reveal **wheezing**, increased bronchovesicular sounds and, occasionally, **crackles** due to the presence of secretions.

Generally, a **prolonged expiration phase** is observed, sometimes accompanied by an abdominal effort. Exercise intolerance, dyspnoea on exertion, cyanosis and even syncope can be noted.

Signs of systemic involvement are rare, unless the process is complicated by a pneumonic process. Obesity exacerbates the symptoms.

Diagnosis

A diagnosis of chronic bronchitis is made based on the clinical history and performance of complementary tests to rule out other conditions with similar symptoms.

Radiography

Thickening of the bronchial walls (peribronchial cuffs) is often observed. However, there is not always a correspondence between evident lesions affecting the bronchial mucosa seen on bronchoscopy and thoracic radiographs (which appear normal).

Bronchoscopy and bronchial cytology

This helps rule out the presence of foreign bodies and helps in the assessment of obvious changes, such as mucosal oedema, hyperaemia, the presence of mucus and reduction in bronchial lumen. **Tracheobronchial cytology** usually reveals an **inflammatory (non-septic)** response with a predominance of neutrophils (Figure 4.24).

Treatment

Anti-inflammatories, specifically **glucocorticoids**, are the basis of treatment. Given that treatment is long-term, short-half-life glucocorticoids (prednisolone or prednisone) are recommended, with PO administration, preferably in the **mornings**.

It is advisable to start with prednisone or prednisolone at a dose of 0.5 mg/kg, or even double, every 12 hours for 5–7 days. If remission of clinical signs is induced with this dose, is can be **reduced by half every 10–15 days** until the minimum dose capable of controlling the condition is reached. Most patients require a minimum treatment of 2–3 months, and some need it on a continuous or intermittent basis throughout their lives.

If an improvement is not achieved solely with glucocorticoid administration, a therapeutic trial of at least two weeks with a combination of **prednisone and a bronchodilator**, either sustained-action theophylline or salbutamol, can be performed. The bronchodilators should be discontinued if no improvement is perceived after two weeks of treatment, but they should be administered in the long term if an improvement is observed.

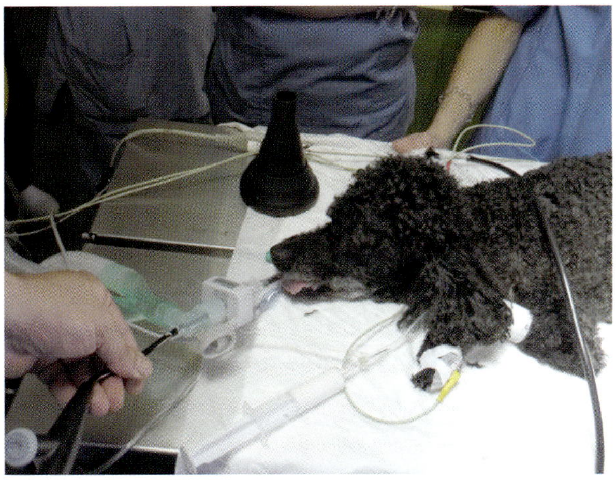

Figure 4.24. Bronchoscopy in a patient with chronic bronchitis.

Antibiotics are indicated only if culture suggests the existence of an additional infection or the patient suffers an exacerbation of symptoms.

Antitussives are indicated only when coughing does not allow the animal or its owners to rest, or when it is so severe it causes syncope.

Feline asthma

Introduction

Bronchitis, or feline asthma, is an **inflammatory disease of the lower airways** characterized by bronchial hyper-reactivity to different stimuli. Bronchitis and feline asthma are the **most frequent causes of cough in this species**.

Feline asthma and chronic bronchitis are slightly different:

- **Feline asthma** is a spontaneous and **reversible bronchoconstriction** (type I hypersensitivity) usually caused by **hypersensitivity**.
- **Chronic bronchitis** is a **chronic inflammatory** process that involves **irreversible changes**.

On a practical level, differentiating between these can be complex because functional tests not routinely available are required. In addition, both conditions present a large clinical and lesional overlap, and may in fact be the same condition but in different stages or phenotypes:

- **Bronchoconstriction** (type I hypersensitivity) is a spontaneous and **reversible** bronchial hyper-reactivity that causes contraction of the smooth muscle, with a consequent decrease in the diameter of the bronchial lumen.
- **Chronic** condition with bronchial remodelling:
  - hypertrophy/-plasia of goblet cells and mucous glands, causing **excessive accumulation of mucus** and changes in its viscosity
  - hypertrophy of the smooth muscle of the bronchial wall and parietal oedema that involves **thickening of the wall**
  - **fibrosis** of the lamina propria, in very advanced stages.

Clinical signs

These vary depending on the severity of the condition, but the classic signs include **coughing**, wheezing, distress, orthopnoea, tachypnoea and dyspnoea with pronounced **expiratory effort**.

They can be constant or intermittent; mild, moderate or severe. In mild cases, they may be limited to brief and occasional coughs. These signs are often chronic and progress slowly. Some cats may even remain asymptomatic between occasional episodes of acute airway obstruction.

In severe cases, cats may present with a daily, persistent cough accompanied by frequent acute dyspnoeic crises with respiratory distress. Clinical signs may be induced or exacerbated by exposure to potential allergens or irritants such as a new bed, cigarette or chimney smoke, cleaning products or scented air fresheners, dust or seasonal pollens, and they usually become worse with stress or exercise.

During a dyspnoeic crisis, cats usually adopt a characteristic position: pressed close to the floor in sternal recumbency with the head and neck extended, wheezing with the mouth open. If the bronchoconstriction lasts a long time, the animal may **become cyanotic** and the **thorax can become barrel-shaped** due to entrapped air. The intensity of dyspnoea is assessed by the degree of **lateral retraction of the nose** and labial commissures.

Physical examination

Many cats with asthma appear to be normal on physical examination at rest. In severely affected cases, there is marked expiratory distress accompanied by adventitious noises such as crackles. Wheezing is usually noticed when the disease is advanced, or during episodes of acute aggravation. Trapped air distal to the obstructed airways decreases chest compressibility, causing the chest to have a barrel-like appearance.

Diagnosis

Radiography

The classic radiographic pattern in a cat with asthma usually shows **bronchial wall thickening** (generally described as doughnuts and railway tracks); there may also be increased radiolucency, flattening and caudal displacement of the diaphragm. It is important to emphasize that cats with asthma can present with normal chest radiography, so the diagnosis should not be ruled out based solely on the absence of radiographic signs (Figure 4.25).

Computed tomography

See Figure 4.26.

Bronchoscopy and bronchial cytology

Bronchoscopy reveals **erythema and oedema of the mucosa**, reduction of the luminal diameter of the airways and, sometimes, excessive mucus and **mucous plugs**. The cytological findings are not pathognomonic – evidence of airway inflammation with an increased number of eosinophils is generally obtained.

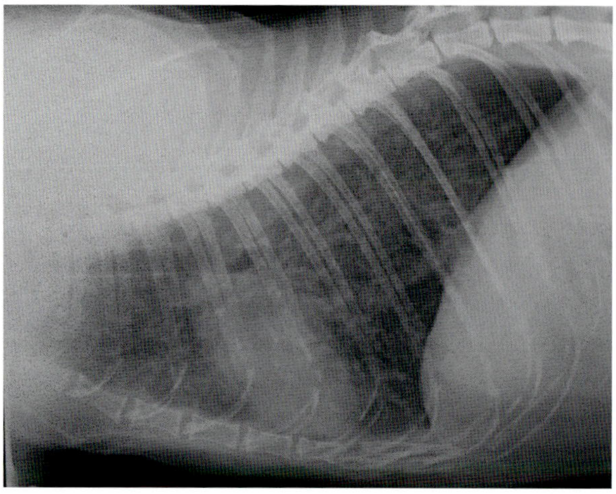

Figure 4.25. Radiography: feline asthma.

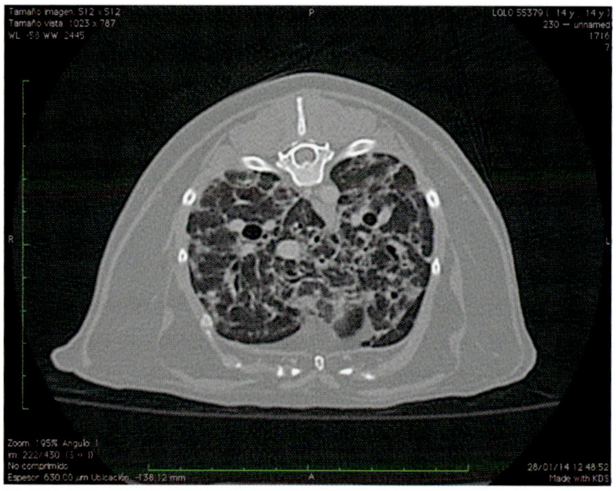

Figure 4.26. CT: chronic feline asthma.

Cultures can be taken from aseptic samples of the wash, taking into consideration that organisms considered pathogenic, such as *Klebsiella* s *Pseudomona* spp., can grow in samples obtained from healthy cats. In fact, it is most likely that bacteria that are isolated from the airways of the asthmatic cat reflect **colonization rather than infection**. A finding of *Mycoplasma* is an important dilemma even today: initially it was believed that it was isolated only in patients with bronchial disease, but recent studies seem to contradict this.

Treatment

Not all asthmatic cats are affected in the same way by the disease and, therefore, management varies according to the severity of the condition.

Therapeutic strategies for the treatment of asthma are focused on the **suppression of inflammation** and the **reversal of bronchoconstriction**.

For mild symptoms

When the symptoms occur **less than once per week**, it is considered that there is no active chronic inflammation of the airways and bronchodilators can be used safely for treatment on demand: inhaled salbutamol (100 µg). If the frequency of use is greater than twice per week, treatment should be reconsidered.

For persistent, moderate symptoms

Oral glucocorticoids are the basis of chronic treatment of feline asthma and are recommended even in asymptomatic cats, since inflammation of the airway is a very important component of this pathology. It is advisable to start with prednisone or prednisolone at a daily dose, divided into two doses, of 1–2 mg/kg (and even 3 mg/kg if the patient does not respond) for 7–10 days and then to carry out a gradual reduction until the minimum effective dose is reached, which is generally estimated around 2.5 mg every two days. In animals which are difficult to handle, **depot solutions** (methylprednisolone acetate 10–20 mg IM, one dose every 4–8 weeks) can be used.

Bronchodilators (terbutaline 0.625 mg/12 h or sustained-action theophylline 25 mg/kg, night-time intake) can be added to treatment when glucocorticoids alone fail to control clinical signs or when prednisolone doses >10 mg every two days are required to control them. Bronchodilators appear to be more effective for acute episodes rather than long-term management.

Bacterial infections are rarely associated with bronchial disease in cats, and therefore the use of antibiotics is indicated only if cultures of tracheobronchial secretions show significant growth or grow *Mycoplasma* spp.

Some patients can **tolerate inhaled glucocorticoids** administered through inhalation chambers via a mask; the most commonly used aerosolized glucocorticoids are fluticasone and budesonide. Theoretically these drugs have no systemic effects, which would allow indefinite maintenance of corticotherapy (certain studies have revealed that the benefits associated with steroid therapy on airway remodelling are lost when it is discontinued).

In a crisis

- **careful handling**: avoid stress and postpone diagnosis
- **oxygen** therapy
- **bronchodilators** to combat acute bronchoconstriction:
- fast-acting β2-adrenergic agonists such as **salbuterol** (terbutaline if available); can be administered inhaled (Figure 4.27)
  - positive response is expected between 15 and 30 minutes – that is, a decrease in frequency and respiratory effort of 50% or more
  - can be used **every 30–60 minutes** for up to 4–6 hours without causing serious adverse effects
- administration of a **short-acting corticosteroid** such as dexamethasone at a dose of 1 mg/kg IV or IM (documented dose 0.25–2.5 mg/kg).

Pulmonary parenchymal disorders

Pneumonia

Introduction

The term pneumonia includes all conditions that produce **inflammation of the lung parenchyma**, whether attributable to infectious or non-infectious causes.

Non-infectious causes include:

- inhalation of toxins or irritants
- inflammatory and immune-mediated processes.

These should be considered as possible causes in patients with a history suggestive of exposure to toxins or irritants, and in those in which identification of an aetiological agent fails.

Infectious agents include:

- bacteria
- viruses
- fungi
- parasites.

Bacterial aetiology is the most prevalent in the small animal clinic (Table 4.13).

From an anatomical point of view, the term **pneumonia is restricted to inflammation of the lung parenchyma**. When the process also **involves the airways (terminal bronchioles) and peribronchial tissues, the term bronchopneumonia** is used. In clinical practice, the distinction between pneumonia and bronchopneumonia is difficult. It is not easy to specify to what extent

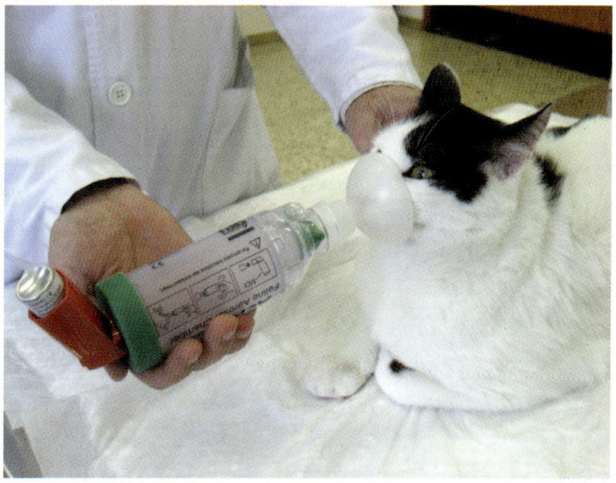

Figure 4.27. Inhalation therapy in a cat with asthma.

Table 4.13. Organisms commonly isolated in feline and canine patients with respiratory tract infections.

	Species	Samples (*n*)	Percentage (%)	Gram stain characteristics
Dogs	Enteric	53	46	Gram-negative bacilli
	Escherichia coli	36	31	
	Klebsiella	8	7	
	Others	15	13	
	Pasteurella spp.	26	22	Gram-negative bacilli
	β-Haemolytic Streptococcus	14	12	Gram-positive cocci
	Streptococcus/Enterococcus	14	12	Gram-positive cocci
	Obligate anaerobes	25	22	Gram-positive or -negative cocci
	Bordetella bronchiseptica	14	12	Gram-negative coccobacilli
	Staphylococcus coagulase^{+}	11	10	Gram-positive cocci
	Pseudomonas	9	8	Gram-negative bacilli
	Mycoplasma	6	5	Absence of wall
	Others	18	16	
Cats	*B. bronchiseptica*	12	30	Gram-negative coccobacilli
	Pasteurella spp.	9	22	Gram-negative bacilli
	Mycoplasma	6	15	Absence of wall
	Escherichia coli	5	12	Gram-negative bacilli
	Streptococcus	6	15	Gram-positive cocci
	Others	2	5	
	Obligate anaerobes	1	1?	

the bronchioles are affected, which is why the most commonly used term is bronchopneumonia.

Aetiopathogenesis of bronchopneumonia

Bronchopneumonia is almost always related to **bacterial invasion** of the lung parenchyma. However, we must bear in mind that there are other possible aetiologies such as viruses, parasites, fungi and, more rarely, hypersensitivity reactions (eosinophilic and allergic pneumonia).

It is rare for a primary infection to occur in a patient with effective defence mechanisms. These allow the establishment of factors such as the existence of viral infections, aspiration of foreign bodies, chronic bronchial diseases or any other respiratory disease.

Colonization of the lower respiratory tract may occur due to:

- Airborne infection or by **inhalation**. Therefore, it is most common for many of the bacteria isolated in patients with pneumonia to be part of the normal flora of the trachea and bronchi.
- **Haematogenous** spread. This usually occurs in hospitalized animals, mainly in cases of bacteraemia associated with the use of an intravenous catheter.
- Direct **extension of an infection** from neighbouring structures. Occurs after the penetration of foreign bodies into the chest, penetrating oesophageal lesions or the use of contaminated endotracheal tubes.

Viral pneumonias, with the exception of distemper virus, canine influenza virus and feline calicivirus, are **usually self-limiting**. Unless complicated by secondary bacterial contamination, they rarely cause systemic signs or severe symptoms.

Fungal pneumonias (blastomycosis, histoplasmosis, cryptococcosis and coccidiomycosis) show a distribution that is highly dependent on **geography** and a more extensive tropism than just the simple respiratory parenchyma. There is often **multi-systemic involvement** (gastrointestinal, ocular, musculoskeletal, etc.).

The main **parasitic pneumonias** (pulmonary nematodiasis) are caused by:

- *Oslerus osleri* and *Angiostrongylus vasorum* in the dog
- *Aelostrongylus abstrusus* in the cat.

Aetiopathogenesis of aspiration pneumonia

Occurs after **aspiration of food, fluid, gastric** contents or any other foreign substance from the oropharynx.

This condition differs from a bronchopneumonia of infectious origin in two ways:

1. The **underlying pathologies**. In aspiration pneumonia there is frequently an underlying pathology. The latter predisposes to the repeated or large-scale aspiration of foreign material, which overflows the normal depurative mechanisms of the respiratory tract. Examples of these predisposing factors include, among others:

- Certain oesophageal diseases:
  - megaoesophagus
  - oesophagitis due to reflex
  - oesophageal obstructions
  - pharyngeal dysfunction
- Diseases or conditions that occur with repeated vomiting (especially in weakened, recumbent or sedated animals)
- Iatrogenic causes such as:
  - poor placement of feeding tubes
  - incorrect administration of substances orally

2. The **physio-pathogenic mechanisms**. In aspiration pneumonia, lung damage is caused by a combination of irritative damage (gastric acid causes a chemical-type lesion as a consequence of its low pH), airway obstruction (by inhaled particles or material) and/or infection (usually bacteria from the oropharynx or that are present in the aspirated material).

History
Pneumonia does not usually occur in previously healthy patients, especially if they are adult animals. Usually there is a predisposing cause, whether known or unknown.

Risk factors
These include:

- age – higher morbidity in young animals
- immune status
- congenital disorders, such as megaoesophagus or ciliary dyskinesia
- environmental factors, especially the quality of accommodation, ventilation and hygiene
- exposure to crowded environments at a breeder, shelter or pet shop
- certain infections (e.g. calicivirus, distemper, adenovirus and parasitosis).

Some animals, especially puppies, have a history of exposure to groups with upper respiratory tract conditions. They may show signs such as exercise intolerance, tracheal reflex and cough but are systemically stable. The condition very often progresses to involve the lung parenchyma and cause rapid deterioration.

Clinical signs
Clinical signs vary from **mild to severe** depending on the severity and extent of lung involvement. If the patient suffers from a predisposing disease, the symptoms of this can dominate while those attributable to pneumonia go unnoticed. This occurs until either there is an exacerbation of the condition or pneumonia is identified with the help of complementary tests.

Non-specific signs such as lethargy, anorexia and weakness are present in most patients, and are sometimes the only characteristics of the disease, since not all affected animals show signs attributable to the respiratory system.

Respiratory signs resulting from pneumonia:

- respiratory difficulty
- tachypnoea
- productive cough
- nasal discharge (there may be swallowing of secretions, so the discharge may not be obvious)
- exercise intolerance
- fever (50% of cases).

In extreme situations:

- cyanosis
- orthopnoeic positions
- a state of shock.

In the **cat**, unlike the dog, most **pneumonias are asymptomatic** to the point where 40% of cats with histologically confirmed pneumonia may not present symptoms related to the respiratory system, and the presence of symptoms can be considered an indicator of an advanced, severe respiratory condition.

Auscultation
Reveals an increase in normal **bronchovesicular sounds, crepitations and wheezing**. Occasionally, areas of consolidation are detected by the absence of respiratory sounds or by a marked auscultatory asymmetry between each hemithorax.

Diagnosis
Symptoms, along with a **complete blood count** and **radiography**, may be sufficient to make a presumptive diagnosis of bacterial pneumonia.

Thoracic radiography
Radiography is essential in the diagnosis and monitoring of patients with pneumonia. In the early stages of the disease, an interstitial pattern appears that usually progresses to an alveolar pattern. The majority of the animals show **alveolar consolidation** with a **cranioventral distribution** in which, in addition, **air bronchograms** may be present (Figure 4.28).

Laboratory tests
A complete blood count may show **leucocytosis with a left shift** (in approximately 50% of cases). A certain degree of dehydration that results in a slight increase in total proteins and haematocrit may also be observed.

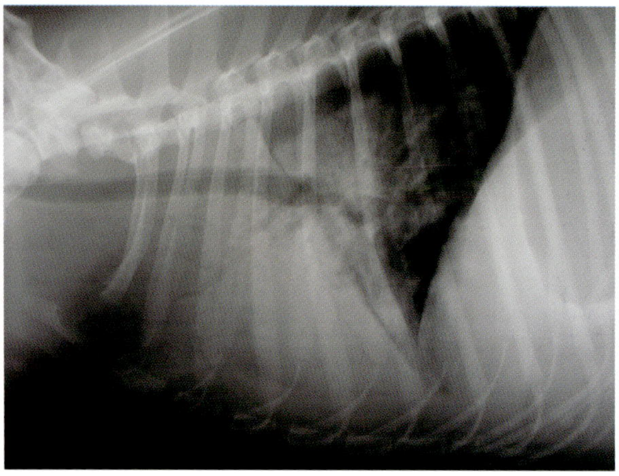

Figure 4.28. Radiography: Pneumonia with a cranioventral alveolar pattern.

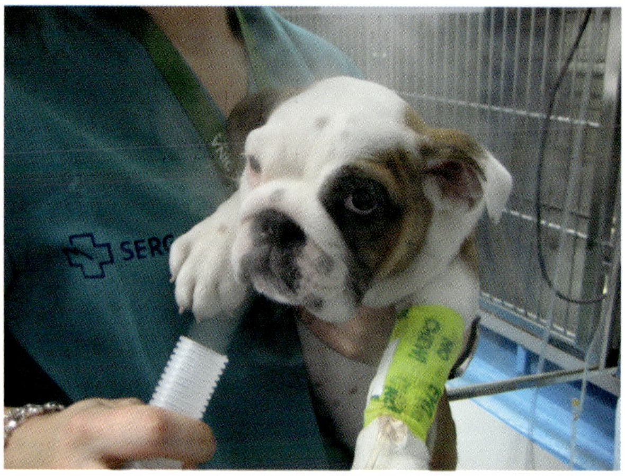

Figure 4.29. Nebulization in a puppy with pneumonia.

The biochemistry profile hardly changes (except for a slight hypo-albuminaemia in severe cases); if present, changes are related to the underlying disease.

Cytology and culture of secretions

Diagnostic confirmation of bacterial pneumonia is based on the cytological study and **culture of the secretions** obtained by procedures such as tracheal lavage (transtracheal or endotracheal) or bronchoalveolar lavage using bronchoscopy.

Cytology and the culture of tracheal or bronchoalveolar samples, although fundamental to the choice of a specific antibiotic treatment, **may not be indicated in unstable patients**. In the latter the risks associated with sampling may exceed the initial benefits. In animals in which there is no specific diagnosis of the causative agent, empirical treatment is a starting point according to the immediate needs of the patient, which may vary throughout the course of the disease forcing a diagnostic rethink, which includes the taking of samples.

Treatment

Supportive treatment

Recovery from pneumonia depends on eliminating retained secretions, by utilizing the cough reflex and mucociliary escalator.

There are numerous treatments that can facilitate this clearance:

Administration of parenteral fluids. It is considered very useful to maintain an optimal degree of hydration and avoid drying and thickening of secretions.

Nebulization of the respiratory tract. This can be used to **hydrate respiratory secretions** and facilitate their elimination. This is very beneficial in patients suffering from diseases that cause excessive production of mucus or for it to become trapped in the airways (Figure 4.29).

Moderate exercise

To achieve lung expansion and **therapeutic thoracic percussion**. It can also stimulate the cough reflex and mobilize retained secretions.

Administration of mucolytics, such as N-acetylcysteine

These help to expel secretions and viscous mucus and any purulent material from the lower respiratory tract, by breaking the sulphur bonds. Many authors recommend its use by **inhalation via nebulization**, but special care must be taken because some patients experience episodes of bronchospasm. In these cases, it is recommended to pre-treat with bronchodilators or even reconsider its usefulness. The exact dose for oral use has not been established, but an **empirical dose of 30–60 mg/kg** (not exceeding 600 mg/kg per patient) is prescribed two or three times per day.

Bronchodilators. Their efficacy has not been fully demonstrated, but they help to reverse irritative bronchoconstriction and decrease the level of fatigue in respiratory muscles in the dyspnoeic animal.

Whenever possible, **the use of antitussives should be avoided**, as these suppress the beneficial effect of coughing.

Antibiotic treatment

Ideally antibiotic selection should be based on the results of culture and sensitivity tests. However, despite the importance of specific antibiotic treatment, tracheal lavage may not have been performed, either because of economic limitations or because it is not 100% indicated in highly unstable patients. In any case, whilst waiting for the results to arrive, the choice of an antibiotic is based on the patient's general condition.

Empirical antibiotic treatment is almost never optimal but sometimes it is necessary and, in many cases, it saves lives.

Not all patients with pneumonia have life-threatening infections, and it is not always necessary to resort to hospitalization and parenteral therapy. Oral administration and ambulatory follow-up in the first 48–72 hours are adequate for stable patients that are active and alert, without evidence of hypoxaemia, with a good appetite and able to maintain an adequate hydration status. However, those with **severe clinical signs** or in a state of sepsis must be hospitalized and administered **intravenous antibiotics during the first 3–7 days**. Once the results of the antibiogram have been obtained and/or the patient is stable, administration can be switched to the oral route and, therefore, home management.

Antibiotics should be administered for a minimum of **three weeks**. However, the duration of treatment depends on the resolution of the clinical and radiographic changes, and it is optimal to continue treatment for at least two weeks after these have disappeared. And, since symptomatic improvement occurs before radiological improvement, a radiographic follow-up to determine the adequate duration of the therapy is necessary. **Thoracic radiographs should be evaluated every 1–2 weeks** for the duration of treatment, and 7–10 days after it is stopped, in case there is a persistent focus of infection that would suggest the presence of a foreign body or abscess, which would require more aggressive treatment (Figure 4.30).

Antibiotic selection is tabulated in Tables 4.14 and 4.15.

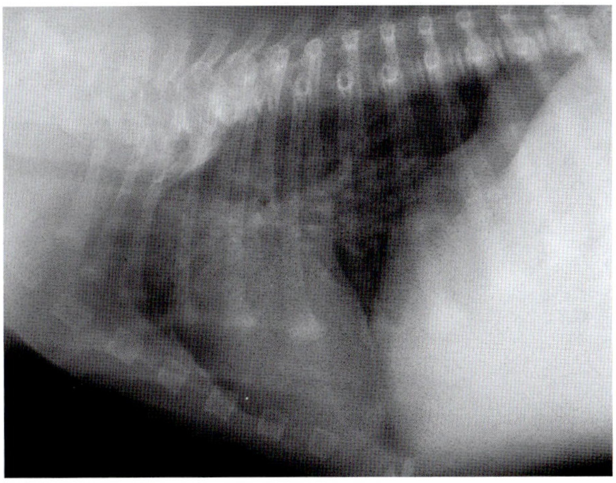

Figure 4.30. Pneumonia. Radiographical monitoring: initial radiograph.

Causes of treatment failure

The most frequent causes of treatment failure are the following:

1. **Incorrect choice of antibiotic, dose or frequency**. In this sense, if 48–72 hours after the introduction of an empirical treatment the animal's condition has deteriorated or remains unstable, a change of antibiotic treatment is justified. The efficacy of this measure will be questionable in the absence of previous collection of tracheal samples for the identification of the causative agent and the performance of a specific antibiogram.
2. **Failure of the elimination of secretions**. In some patients, despite an adequate choice of antibiotic, the lack of additional measures directed at clearing or eliminating secretions may delay improvement.
3. **Insufficient duration of treatment as a consequence of failure to follow up**. That is, when the decision to suspend treatment is based on the

Table 4.14. Recommendations for the selection of antibiotics based on clinical parameters (Ford, 2009).

			Treatment	
		Clinical picture	**First choice**	**Alternative**
Canine	**Stable patient**	Cough, lethargy, some exercise intolerance, possible fever, reduced appetite	Trimethoprim-sulphonamide 15–30 mg/kg/12 h VO or SC	Cephalexin 20–40 mg/kg/8 h VO Amoxicillin-clavulanic acid 22 mg/kg/8 h VO
	Unstable patient	Respiratory failure, fever, leucocytosis and immature neutrophilia	Cefazolin 15–25 mg/kg/6–8 h IV	Ampicillin 20–40 mg/kg/6–8 h IV or SC with enrofloxacin 2.5 mg/kg/12 h SC If there is suspicion of an anaerobic microorganism, ampicillin should be replaced with clindamycin 10–20 mg/kg/12 h IV or SC
Feline	**Stable patient**	Cough, decreased activity, increased respiratory effort and radiological changes	Amoxicillin-clavulanic acid 10–20 mg/kg/8 h VO	Trimethoprim-sulphonamide 15–30 mg/kg/12 h VO or SC Cephalexin 22–44 mg/kg/8 h VO
	Unstable patient	Respiratory failure (tachypnoea or dyspnoea at rest), radiographic changes	Cefazolin 33 mg/kg/8–12 h IV	Ampicillin 20–40 mg/kg/8 h IV or SC with enrofloxacin 2.5 mg/kg/12 h SC

Table 4.15. Choice of empirical antibiotics in patients with pneumonia (Veterinary Clinics of North America Small Animal Practice (2014) 44, 143–159).

Clinical picture	Treatment
Stable patients, mild clinical signs	**Monotherapy:** Trimethoprim sulphate 30 mg/kg/12 h VO Amoxicillin-clavulanic acid Dog: 13.75 mg/kg/12 h VO Cat: 62.5 mg/12 h VO
Moderate clinical signs	**Monotherapy:** Trimethoprim sulphate 30 mg/kg/12 h VO Amoxicillin-clavulanic acid Dog: 13.75 mg/kg/12 h VO Cat: 62.5 mg/12 h VO **Combination therapy:** Amoxicillin-clavulanic acid Dog: 13.75 mg/kg/12 h VO Cat: 62.5 mg/12 h VO **and** Enrofloxacin 10 m/kg/24 h VO/IV **or** Amikacin 15 mg/kg/24 h SC
Critical patients, severe clinical signs	**Monotherapy:** Ticarcillin-clavulanic acid 50 mg/kg/6 h IV Meropenem 24 mg/kg/24 h IV Imipenem 10 mg/kg/8 h IV **Combination therapy:** Amoxicillin-clavulanic acid Dog: 13.75 mg/kg/12 h VO Cat: 62.5 mg/12 h VO **and** Enrofloxacin 10 m/kg/24 h VO/IV **or** Amikacin 15 mg/kg/24 h SC

absence of clinical signs and follow-up radiographs are not carried out.

4. **Impossibility of management of the underlying disease** that causes constant aspiration of material from the oropharynx.
5. **Necrosis or abscess in a pulmonary lobe**. This is usually associated with the presence of a foreign body or pulmonary consolidation that acts as a focus favouring recurrent infection.
6. **Incorrect diagnosis**. Presence of a neoplasm, pulmonary lobe torsion or bronchopneumonia of different aetiology to that suspected (viral, fungal, parasitic, non-infectious aetiology).

Interstitial pneumonia

Introduction

Interstitial pneumonias encompass a **heterogeneous group of pulmonary diseases** with **similar clinical, radiological and functional manifestations** that affect the alveolar-interstitial structures of the lung and, in many cases, its surrounding tissue (small airways and pulmonary vasculature). They are **characterized by the presence of different degrees of inflammation**, which probably starts with restorative purposes but, in many cases, through complex immune system responses ends up causing important structural changes, including the deposition of collagen with **fibrosis of the lung parenchyma**.

The causes most frequently identified in veterinary practice are **infectious pneumonias** and **lung tumours**, but there are other conditions (neither neoplastic nor infectious) that can cause changes to the distal lung parenchyma with involvement of the interstitial region. For correct diagnosis, **histological studies are generally required** and, in the usual clinical setting, this requirement for lung tissue samples often prevents the clinician reaching a conclusive diagnosis.

Eosinophilic pneumonia

Definition

Eosinophilic pneumonia is also called **eosinophilic bronchopneumonia** or pulmonary infiltrates with eosinophilia syndrome. This encompasses a group of lung diseases characterized by the presence of **numerous eosinophils in the terminal bronchioles, alveoli and the bloodstream**.

Aetiopathogenesis

In human medicine, the condition is **classified according to the aetiology** and the role of eosinophils in its pathogenesis:

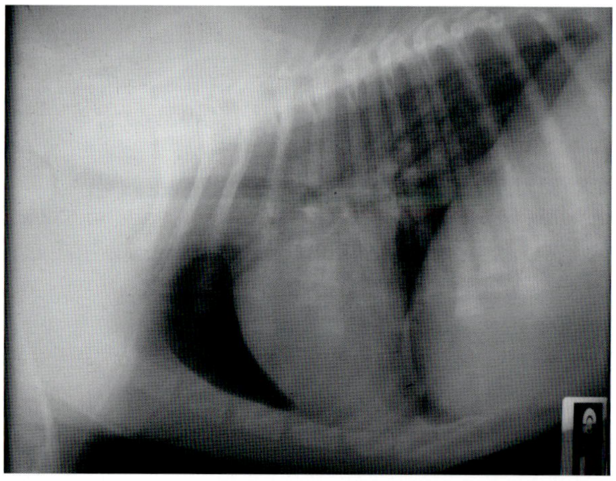

Figure 4.31. Pneumonia. Radiographic monitoring – resolved.

- Eosinophilic pulmonary diseases. Among the known causes of eosinophilic pneumonia are certain drugs, chemical vapours and fungal and parasitic infections.
- Lung diseases associated with eosinophilia.

In veterinary medicine it is suspected that **inhaled allergens** are involved in the aetiopathogenesis, but why eosinophils accumulate in the lungs has not been determined. The most frequent type of inhalation allergy in veterinary medicine is atopic dermatitis, but very few of these animals simultaneously show respiratory symptoms.

However, despite this lack of correlation between respiratory and dermatological symptoms, it is likely that the allergens are the same. It may be a **hyper-reactivity process**, although it differs substantially from asthma in that reversible obstruction of the airway is not identified. On the other hand, it is considered that **dirofilariasis and parasitism contribute** to eosinophilic pulmonary diseases and hence the inclusion of anti-parasitic medications in treatment protocols for eosinophilic pneumonia.

Epidemiology

Affected patients are usually **middle-aged dogs** (4–6 years). In studies, **females** presented with a higher incidence.

A certain breed predisposition (Siberian husky) is described, but it has also been identified in numerous breeds of varying size (Labrador retriever, German shepherd, Alaskan malamute, Jack Russell, Fox terrier, Belgian shepherd).

Clinical picture

The **course of eosinophilic pneumonia is very variable**, with some patients being diagnosed three weeks after the onset of symptoms and others suffering subtle symptoms for years.

The most common sign is **a cough, which is usually dry and persistent** and often accompanied by final gagging (in some texts it is defined as a smoker's cough). Certain patients also have exercise intolerance and some degree of respiratory distress. Half of those affected may show **nasal discharge**, but signs of systemic involvement are rarely found.

The presentation of these symptoms can be either **acute**, even with dyspnoea that endangers the life of the patient, or feature **chronic** episodes of occasional cough.

Auscultation may be normal, or **crackles and wheezing** can be present.

Diagnosis

Eosinophilic pulmonary syndromes can be suspected for four reasons:

1. presence of radiological infiltrates and eosinophilia in peripheral blood
2. presence of abundant eosinophils in bronchoalveolar lavage (BAL)
3. histopathological findings of lung tissue obtained by biopsy
4. rapid response of the condition to corticosteroids.

An eosinophilia in peripheral blood is suggestive of the disease, but its absence does not exclude the process since it occurs in only 50–60% of cases.

If eosinophilic pneumonia is suspected, **parasite studies** are very useful. In areas where filariasis is endemic, testing is obligatory. In addition, as in any patient with chronic cough, a flotation test and a Baermann test should be requested to try to identify any pulmonary parasites. However, be aware that the ability to detect parasites by these methods, when a single sample is used, is only 30–70%.

As a hypersensitivity process is speculated, numerous studies with intradermal reaction tests have been performed in patients but the results are difficult to interpret and have little clinical utility.

Radiography

Thoracic radiography usually shows a diffuse type **broncho-interstitial pattern**, which is more marked than in chronic bronchitis. The peribronchial cuffs appear 20% of the time, as does marked thickening of the bronchial walls. The presence of bronchiectasis suggests a certain chronicity. Occasionally, some alveolar pattern may be present. In general, the severity of radiological abnormalities usually correlates with the severity of clinical signs, however, none of the changes described above are pathognomonic for this process.

Bronchoscopy and bronchial cytology

Bronchoscopy cannot diagnose the condition but is useful for harvesting cytology samples. Bronchoscopy

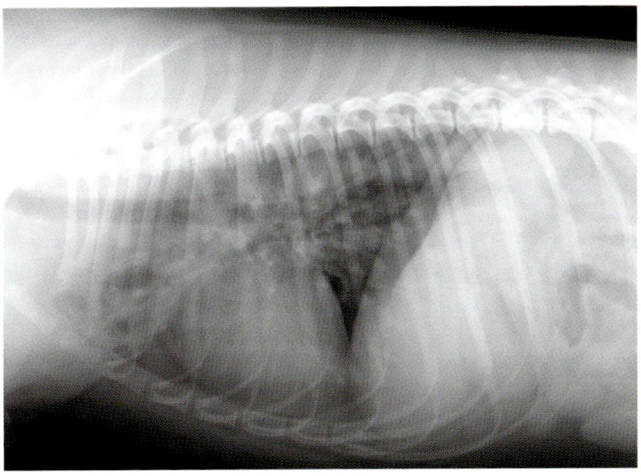

Figure 4.32. Eosinophilic pneumonia. Thoracic radiograph.

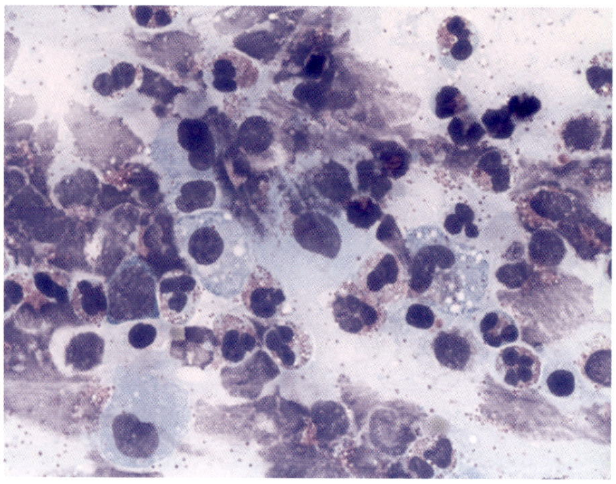

Figure 4.33. Eosinophilic pneumonia. Cytology of a bronchioalveolar lavage.

usually shows yellowish-green mucous secretions, thickening of the mucosa with a polypoid appearance and marked hyperaemia.

Cytological washes are essential and often diagnostic, with the presence of a marked increase in **eosinophils (50–90%) and the presence of neutrophils** at a lower proportion. The total eosinophil count in healthy patients is usually not higher than 5% and the predominant cells are usually macrophages. However, eosinophils may also be a major population in neoplasms, fungal processes and pulmonary parasitism.

Treatment

The fundamental goal of treatment is to reduce inflammation and thereby decrease the intensity of the clinical signs. A complete cure may not be achieved, and the owner must be informed of this.

Management requires the long-term use of corticosteroids (initial dose 1 mg/kg/12 h), over an expected average duration (including induction and then gradual reduction) of 4–6 months. Since treatment is expected to be long-term, **inhaled corticosteroids** can be useful in reducing the dose of oral steroids and adverse side effects. A decrease in peripheral eosinophilia and radiographic improvement accompany the clinical improvement of the patient and can serve as a criterion for the gradual reduction of steroid dosage. The response to treatment is usually satisfactory after a few months and, in some cases, it can be completely withdrawn.

Once treatment is stopped, patients may suffer relapses, especially those in which the treatment is interrupted abruptly or are managed irregularly with depot formulations. However, some dogs have shown complete resolution.

Given the relatively low sensitivity of methods used for the detection of parasites and the intermittent nature of egg elimination in faeces, the empirical use of anthelmintic therapy is recommended: a 14-day cycle of fenbendazole at a dose of 50 mg/kg.

Idiopathic pulmonary fibrosis

Definition

Idiopathic pulmonary fibrosis (IPF), also known as cryptogenic fibrosing alveolitis, is a specific form of interstitial pneumonia associated with the histological appearance of usual interstitial pneumonia on lung biopsy. It is a **chronic, progressive disease** of the pulmonary interstitium caused by **replacement of the functional tissue of the lung by fibrous tissue**, which progressively converts the lungs into extensive scar tissue leading to the loss of ability for gas exchange.

Aetiopathogenesis

Idiopathic pulmonary fibrosis is a condition described in humans, dogs and cats. Its **aetiology remains unknown** and its pathophysiology is the subject of much debate. In veterinary medicine it is considered a relatively modern entity, since the first publications of case series date from only 1999.

The process of fibrosis and deposition of collagen is of great importance for tissue repair, and plays a key pathophysiological role in pulmonary fibrosis: **IPF is characterized by the abnormal accumulation of collagen in the pulmonary interstitium.**

The fibrotic lung represents a process **of aberrant remodelling as a response to injury**. The most widely accepted pathophysiological theory for IPF states that the process begins with inflammation of the pulmonary alveoli in response to lesions produced by various agents. The objective of this stereotyped inflammatory response would be to neutralize or destroy the causal agent and restore tissue normality. However, when the lesion is too extensive or affects tissues with no regenerative capacity, repair occurs by replacing normal tissue with connective tissue (fibrosis and scarring). In pulmonary fibrosis, this process does not stop and there is a progressive fibrosis of the connective tissue that supports the alveolar walls and, occasionally, the small airways and pulmonary vasculature.

The progressive substitution of the alveoli by fibrous tissue leads to:

- hypoxaemia
- respiratory insufficiency
- pulmonary hypertension
- right-sided heart failure.

Although the theory of an inflammatory component is widely accepted, questions are raised given that anti-inflammatory and immunosuppressive drugs are not effective in the treatment of the disease. It is believed the main factor in the development of IPF may be **cellular injury to the alveolar epithelium** stimulating the development of fibrosis, meaning that the classical theory of **inflammation plays a secondary role**. Although its aetiology is unknown, it is likely to be a consequence of the action of external agents in individuals with a genetic predisposition.

In both dogs and cats, lesions are characterized by **collagen deposition in the alveolar septum** but, unlike in humans, no foci of fibroblasts are usually detected.

It is speculated that in the West Highland white terrier it is the result of an aberrant regulation of collagen, while the forms described in cats are more similar to human IPF caused by a defect in type II pneumocytes.

Epidemiology

The incidence of pulmonary fibrosis in small animals is unknown. It appears **more prevalent in the terrier breeds**, particularly the West Highland white terrier, while other breeds, such as the Staffordshire bull terrier, Jack Russell and Cairn terrier are also affected.

In a study conducted on 29 West Highland white terriers, approximately 60% of individuals with pulmonary fibrosis were male and 30% female, but in order to confirm this sex predilection, analysis of a greater number of cases would be necessary.

Clinical signs

This is a disease of slow progression, which shows symptoms only late on. Dogs usually manifest with chronic and progressive lung signs such as dyspnoea and exercise intolerance. In cats the clinical evolution is more rapid, sometimes showing signs within a period of 2 days to 2 weeks.

The clinical signs are:

- Exercise intolerance
- Dyspnoea, in about 30% of cases
- Laboured breathing. The owner may notice these symptoms, but often attributes them to the animal's advanced age rather than to a lung disease.
- Coughing is not a predominant sign and usually appears later, but it may be the only reason why the owner visits the vet.
- Possible additional clinical findings:
- intermittent cyanosis
- syncope.

Most affected dogs are over 9 years of age and have other, concomitant health problems that can complicate the condition, such as:

- skeletal, muscular or endocrine disorders (hypothyroidism, Cushing's)
- obesity
- tracheal collapse
- chronic bronchitis.

However, dogs with this disease usually behave normally, are alert, have a good appetite and seem to enjoy an optimum quality of life.

Diagnosis

Auscultation

- Dry 'Velcro-like' crepitations. This is one of the signs most frequently observed in these patients. However, crepitations are not heard in some patients due either to an early diagnosis or to difficulties of auscultation in severely affected animals with rapid, superficial breathing.
- Wheezing is noted in around half of patients.
- Tachypnoea with uncomplicated expiration, unlike that in bronchitis.

Radiography

A **diffuse interstitial lung pattern** is observed with different degrees of bronchial involvement, usually without involvement of the pleura or adenopathies.

Cats may show a patchy or diffuse pattern, predominantly interstitial, alveolar or bronchial.

In dogs, about 50% of the cases studied present radiographic evidence of cor pulmonale, but the relationship of this finding with survival has not been evaluated.

Serial radiographs are considered very useful for monitoring the disease. Radiographic findings, together with the patient's clinical signs, can be used in classifying the severity of the process (Figure 4.34).

CT

Shows fairly conclusive images that correlate well with the severity of the disease (Figure 4.35).

Early stages

- frosted-glass images.

Advanced stages

- irregular septal thickening
- traction bronchiectasis
- honeycomb images.

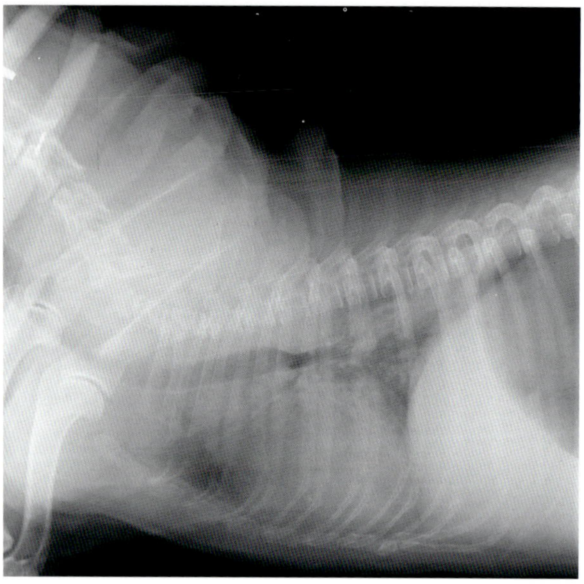

Figure 4.34. Pulmonary fibrosis. Thoracic radiograph.

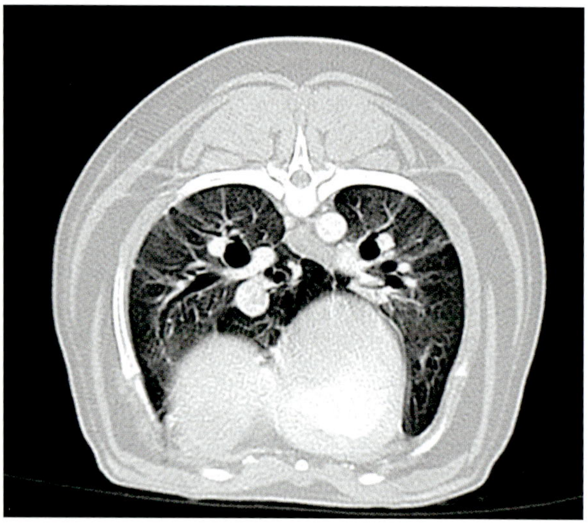

Figure 4.35. Pulmonary fibrosis. CT scan.

Bronchoscopy and bronchial cytology

These are not diagnostic per se, but are a fundamental for differentiation from other pulmonary pathologies.

In dogs with pulmonary fibrosis, BAL is normal or shows a slight presence of inflammatory cells. The most frequent findings are usually mucosal irregularity and some degree of tracheobronchomalacia. To what extent IPF produces bronchial changes or is an independent phenomenon remains unanswered. Cytological findings on BAL normally correspond with increase in neutrophils, macrophages and mastocytes. And, as occurs in human medicine, lymphocytosis is an infrequent finding; in fact, the lymphocyte count is usually lower than that obtained in patients not affected by respiratory conditions. It has not been demonstrated that the serial practice of BAL is of use in the prognosis or response to treatment.

Lung biopsy

Biopsy is generally necessary to confirm the diagnosis and should be considered whilst the patient is stable, rather than left until the damage is terminal.

Transbronchial biopsy, performed by fibroendoscopy, may allow the diagnosis of some interstitial pneumonias but it is not effective for pulmonary fibrosis.

Trans-parietal needle biopsy should not be used, due to the small size of the samples obtained and the high incidence of secondary pneumothorax.

Since lesions are distributed heterogeneously, **biopsy must be taken by thoracotomy**. It is established that while one area of lung tissue shows fibrosis, others may have only an active inflammatory process. **Areas in the final stages should not be biopsied**, since this does not provide relevant information for diagnosis. In short, open-lung biopsy guided by CT findings is preferred.

The changes most consistent with IPF are:

- interstitial fibrosis
- hyperplasia of type II pneumocytes
- presence of prominent intra-alveolar macrophages
- architectural distortion
- emphysematous changes.

These findings correspond in part with those observed in humans, although foci of fibroblast proliferation (a histopathological criterion for diagnosis in human medicine) are not frequently observed. The honeycomb image is very interesting – in humans it is considered that the effects of corticosteroids in these patients will be minimal – while if the histopathology reveals an active cellular process (neutrophils and macrophages), benefits will be greater.

Despite the usefulness of biopsy, in the usual clinical setting it is rarely carried out due to the potential **risks of morbidity and mortality**, and also in part due to the lack of technical means (thoracoscopy) and experience. However, it is considered that all patients where there are strong suspicions of interstitial involvement would benefit from **referral to a specialist centre**.

Measurement of blood gases

This is not commonly used, but it is important to be aware that affected individuals have **hypoxia with normo- or hypocapnia**, and alveolar arterial oxygenation gradients show a ventilation and perfusion (V/Q) disorder as a consequence of alteration in the diffusion barrier.

6-minute walk test

The objective is to **assess exercise tolerance** by provoking physiological stress in the cardiorespiratory and muscular systems in conditions where there is an aerobic demand. In humans it is considered a valuable tool in evaluation of the physiological impact of the deterioration of lung function on the ability to perform exercise in patients with chronic respiratory diseases. Recently the first references to it have been published in the veterinary literature.

This easy-to-carry-out test consists of measuring the maximum distance walked on flat terrain over a 6-minute period, following a standard protocol. Although reference values are scarce, it can be an excellent monitoring tool, comparing the results obtained at a given time with those previously obtained by the same patient.

Biological markers

Their usefulness has been investigated to differentiate between chronic bronchitis and IPF. Measurement of the **pro-collagen precursor** is a direct expression of the process of fibrosis – that is, of the balance between the production and deposition of collagen. In this sense, although pro-collagen III levels are elevated in patients with IPF, they do not seem to be of any use in the identification of different respiratory diseases.

Treatment

The main treatment is the administration of **corticosteroids and bronchodilators**. Experience in humans shows that the addition of **azathioprine or cyclophosphamide** may be useful in some cases. Older patients who develop pulmonary hypertension benefit from its management. When the cough is intense, pharmacological suppression can improve the quality of life of both dog and owner.

Colchicine, a drug with antifibrotic properties, is an alternative in patients with a low tolerance to glucocorticoids or other immunosuppressants.

Studies carried out in humans show that **N-acetylcysteine** administration helps to enhance reduced concentrations of glutathione in the pulmonary epithelial fluid of patients with IPF. There is evidence that an important part of the pathogenesis of IPF is an imbalance between oxidants and antioxidants. Considering that excessive oxidative stress in the respiratory tract can play an important role, low glutathione may play a decisive role as a major component of the antioxidant defence system of the human lung. Given that N-acetylcysteine has a high safety margin and is well tolerated, plus the theoretical advantages, it would not be unwise to include this drug in the treatment of IPF. At the present time, and from a theoretical point of view, there are no studies that demonstrate its true usefulness.

In principle, the most appropriate treatment for IPF should include:

- an antifibrotic drug
- an immunosuppressant
- an antioxidant.

Prognosis

Due to the few studies carried out, it is difficult to give a prognosis. However, the latter is usually unfavourable due to the advanced degree of the disease at the time of diagnosis, because the subtlety of the initial clinical symptoms contributes to diagnostic delay.

The **average survival of dogs is 18 months** from the onset of clinical signs, with survival of up to >3 years.

In the cat practically 50% die or are euthanized within a few weeks of their diagnosis, and only 30% survive more than 1 year.

Pleural disorders

Effusions and pleural effusions

Introduction

The pleura is a serous membrane of mesodermal origin that covers the pulmonary parenchyma, the mediastinum, the diaphragm and the internal surface of the thoracic wall. Anatomically it is subdivided into:

- **visceral pleura** covering the pulmonary surface
- **parietal pleura** covering the inner surface of the chest wall, lateral aspect of the mediastinum, and diaphragmatic wall.

The two pleural layers consist of a layer of mesothelial cells that rest on a thin basement membrane, beneath which is a layer of connective tissue that contains abundant collagen and elastin and where the blood and lymphatic vessels and nerve branches are located.

Between the two sheets is a closed virtual space called the **pleural space cavity**, whose interior contains a **small amount of fluid (0.1–0.3 ml/kg body weight)** and whose function is to facilitate the smooth sliding of the lungs during respiratory movements within the chest and to maintain the independence of the pleural membranes. The amount of fluid present in the pleural space remains constant, due to the continuous equilibrium between its production and absorption.

Pleural fluid is a plasma filtrate that arises from the capillaries of the parietal pleura (systemic circulation) that deliver blood constantly into the pleural space. It is mainly reabsorbed by the lymphatics of the parietal pleura (whose mesothelial cells possess stomata which are in contact with the lymphatic vessels of the pleura) and capillaries of the visceral pleura (pulmonary circulation) that drain into the left side of the heart. In this way, the volume and composition of the pleural fluid depend primarily on lymphatic drainage, oncotic and hydrostatic pressure gradients through the mesothelium and capillaries, and the permeability of both pleural membranes. Any problem (local or systemic) that alters this delicate balance will result in an abnormal accumulation of fluid that, depending on the aetiology of the underlying process, can be of a diverse nature (transudate, exudate, blood or lymphatic fluid) and that at a clinical level is referred to as a pleural effusion or effusion.

Aetiology

Pleural fluid can accumulate pathologically as a result of increased formation or decreased resorption. This may occur due to increased hydrostatic pressure or permeability, decreased oncotic pressure or impaired lymphatic drainage. These causes are common to numerous conditions, meaning that a **pleural effusion is not a disease in itself but a sign of an underlying disease**.

Clinical picture

The accumulation of fluid in the pleural cavity causes a decrease in lung volume, so the capacity for lung expansion is reduced by varying degrees depending on the compression exerted by the leaked fluid. Although many pleural effusions may be asymptomatic or simply occur with non-specific signs common to many diseases, the main symptoms arise as a consequence of the interference in lung expansion, and include **dyspnoea and exercise intolerance**. Although this dyspnoea may present acutely, adequate questioning frequently identifies the presence of subtle signs of discomfort in the preceding weeks.

The volume of the effusion may influence the degree of dyspnoea, but this is not always a direct relationship. It is possible that pain, an underlying pulmonary or cardiac pathology, or the speed of fluid accumulation, explains this dissociation. It is considered that **30 ml/kg of fluid may be sufficient to cause some symptoms**, and that 60 ml/kg could cause obvious signs of respiratory distress. Dyspnoea is characterized by a **prolonged inspiratory phase and a short, effortless expiration**. Inspiration is accompanied by a marked abdominal component. In some patients, obvious signs of respiratory compromise are observed, such as orthopneic positions, open-mouth breathing and cyanosis.

Many patients also suffer from a **dry, unproductive cough** that can occur as a result of pleural irritation, an existing lung disease or a mediastinal mass causing tracheal compression. Coughing may be the first clinical sign of chronic pleural effusion, and often precedes the development of respiratory failure a week or two later, which is the main reason for consults in patients with severe effusions.

The accompanying signs vary depending on the type of pleural pathology and its degree of involvement:

- Common **non-specific signs** such as anorexia, depression, dehydration and weight loss may be present and be a consequence of the underlying condition.
- Fever is more common in pyothorax.
- **Pale mucous membranes** may accompany haemorrhagic-type effusions.
- Auscultable **murmurs and arrhythmias** often accompany cardiogenic effusions.
- The presence of **Horner's syndrome** (enophthalmos, palpebral ptosis, protrusion of the third eyelid and miosis) may indicate the existence of a mass in the anterior mediastinum.

In felines the **presence of hypersalivation** is not infrequent and is associated with a **poor prognosis**. The mechanism by which it occurs is not fully understood, but it is possible the accumulation of fluid in the pleural cavity causes a type of dysphagia, the patient is in pain or there is an underlying secondary liver failure.

On physical examination, common findings include the elimination of vesicular breath sounds in the ventral region, increased bronchovesicular noises in the dorsal area and the **dampening of cardiac sounds**.

Percussion of the thoracic region can show the **presence of a liquid line** delineated by the existence of deeper noises in the ventral region.

Diagnosis

The signalment and findings from a physical examination suggest the presence of the pleural effusion, and thoracic radiography allows its presence to be confirmed.

The primary objective of diagnostic tests is to **determine the cause of the effusion**; therefore, these patients should be studied systematically.

Occasionally, information from the clinical history or physical examination may suggest the cause of the pleural effusion, such as cardiomegaly and signs of heart failure or a recent history of rodenticide consumption. However, most frequently different tests are needed to reach a definitive diagnosis. Additional diagnostic tests have to be assessed according to each clinical case and

Table 4.16. Pathophysiological mechanisms associated with the various causes of pleural effusion.

Physiopathological mechanism	Fluid type	Differential diagnosis
Decreased oncotic pressure, in the presence of hypalbuminaemia (<1.5 g/dl)	Transudate	Protein-losing nephropathy Protein-losing enteropathy Liver disease
Increase in systemic hydrostatic venous pressure	Transudate/modified transudate	Congestive heart failure Pericardial effusion Pulmonary thromboembolism Pulmonary lobe torsion Vena cava syndrome Diaphragmatic hernia Neoplasia
Increase in vascular permeability (occurs mainly when the pleura itself is involved in the pathological process)	Exudate	Systemic inflammation Local infection or abscess (pneumonia or pyothorax) Systemic infection (vasculitis, FIP) Pancreatitis Anaphylactic reaction Neoplasia Repeated centesis
Increased lymphatic pressure or rupture of the thoracic duct	Modified transudate/ chylothorax	Cardiac disease Vascular or lymphatic abnormalities Lymphatic obstruction (lymphosarcoma, mesothelioma, pulmonary or metastatic carcinoma, chronic effusions) Lymphangiectasia Trauma Idiopathic disease
Haemorrhage	Serohaemorrhagic/ haemorrhagic	Platelet disorders Secondary haemostatic disorders (rodenticide poisoning) Coagulopathies due to ingestion Thoracic trauma Neoplasms

the availability of appropriate equipment at each practice (Table 4.16).

Radiography

Diagnostic imaging is the most effective means to confirm the presence of a pleural effusion, whether it is unilateral or bilateral participation, and to evaluate the possible presence of pulmonary or mediastinal masses (Figure 4.36). **Dogs and cats have a fenestrated mediastinum** that allows **free communication between both hemithoraxes**, so effusions are usually bilateral; however, many pathological conditions (producing fibrin) can occlude these fenestrations.

Special attention should be paid to the severity of the animal's dyspnoea. In some cases, drainage of the pleural fluid to **stabilize the patient is recommended before carrying out a radiographic study**. The extraction of even small amounts of liquid significantly improves the ventilatory capacity of the animal and allows it to be handled with less risk. If this is not the case, when there is severe respiratory distress, dorsoventral or lateral projections using the **horizontal beam** are recommended, which are less stressful.

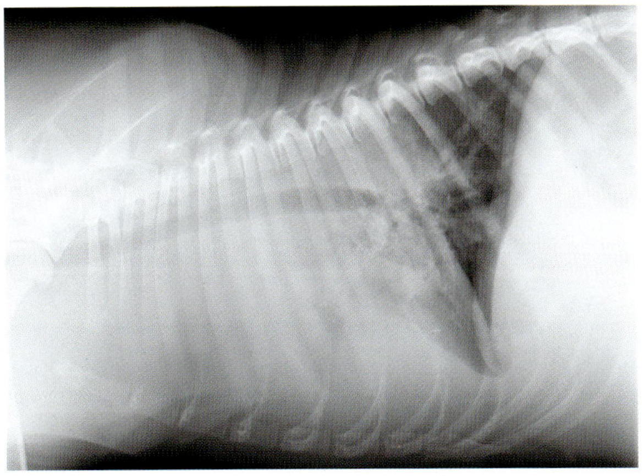

Figure 4.36. Pleural effusion. Thoracic radiograph.

The radiographic signs of pleural effusion in the **lateral view** are:

- increase in soft tissue density dorsal to the sternum
- loss of visualization of the cardiac silhouette and the diaphragmatic dome

- presence of marked, rounded interlobar fissures
- retraction of the pulmonary lobes and separation from the costal wall.

Fluid tends to accumulate in the lower areas, which means that the dorsoventral projection usually shows less definition of the cardiac silhouette and a wider mediastinal space than the ventrodorsal view, in which pleural fissures are better defined.

Although it is not common, special attention should be paid to potential **pleural thickening** (fibrosing pleuritis) that appears in chronic effusions, since pleural fissures can be marked and easily confused with a pleural effusion. This can occur with exudative effusions, in which morphological and functional changes take place in the mesothelial cells that give rise to greater fibrin formation (or a lower capacity for fibrinolysis) and an increase in collagen that induces the growth of fibroblasts within the thick exudate covering the visceral and parietal pleural surfaces. This causes the formation of a membrane lacking elasticity, called the **pleural cortex**.

The presence of pleural fluid makes it difficult to visualize intrathoracic masses, especially when there is an accumulation of large amounts of fluid with the consequent dorsal displacement of the trachea and severe pulmonary collapse. If this is the case, the use of other imaging techniques such as ultrasound or computed tomography is necessary to reach a diagnosis.

Ultrasound

Thoracic ultrasound is a non-invasive procedure that is easy to perform in the presence of fluids, since these provide a good acoustic window. It may be indicated to help identify the primary cause (pulmonary or mediastinal masses, abscesses, pulmonary neoplastic nodules or cardiac alterations) or, in the case of encapsulated effusion, to locate the most appropriate place to perform thoracentesis (Figure 4.37).

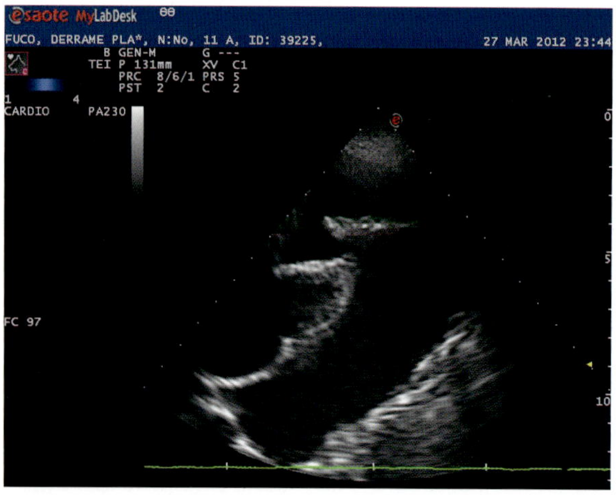

Figure 4.37. Pleural effusion. Thoracic ultrasound.

Pleural effusion has a variable appearance, depending on the amount and type of fluid, and is recognized as **anechoic or echogenic material** within the pleural space:

- **Anechoic** pleural effusion usually corresponds to a **transudate or chyle**.
- **Exudates and haemorrhage** are more **echogenic**.

The presence of free bands floating within an anechoic pleural effusion, with simple linear septa and complex septations, usually corresponds to an exudate.

Small amounts of fluid, which are seen as slight separations of the parietal and visceral pleurae, can be difficult to detect. This can be seen through intercostal windows with separation of the pulmonary surface of the thoracic wall or small spaces between the lung and diaphragm.

Moderate or large effusions are immediately recognized from virtually any window to the thorax.

Ultrasound can also be used to make decisions about the suitability of one treatment over another. The presence of **fibrin or adhesions** between both pleural layers may be an indication of the suitability of surgical debridement versus the placement of a drainage tube.

CT

This is not often used in veterinary practice for this condition. Its general reasons for use are to:

- differentiate pleural from pulmonary pathology
- determine the characteristics of the underlying pathology (pulmonary and/or mediastinal)
- determine whether the effusion is free or encapsulated
- serve as a guide for treatment
- detect the complications of effusions and residual changes secondary to these (Figure 4.38).

Free pleural fluid is easily recognizable on CT scans, with **attenuation values very close to those of water (0 Hounsfield units)**, and therefore they are easily distinguishable from pleural thickening and pleural masses. Evaluation of pleural fluid attenuation is of limited value in differentiating between exudates, transudates and chylothorax, but **haemorrhagic effusions can be identified by their greater density** (**>50 Hounsfield units**). Pleural thickening and reinforcement after contrast are more frequently observed in pyothorax and chronic conditions (Figure 4.38).

In transverse section, effusions can be of varying appearance depending on whether they are encapsulated:

- **Free effusion** has a rectilinear or discretely concave upper edge, probably due to pressure from the adjacent lung.

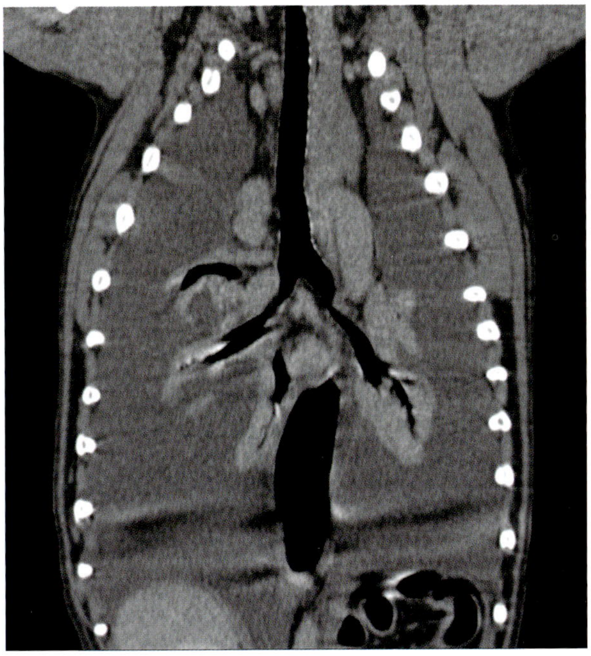

Figure 4.38. Pleural effusion. CT.

- An **encapsulated effusion** presents with a bi-convex lens shape with respect to the lung, or is located in the anatomical lung fissures and lacking continuity with the remainder of the effusion.

Thoracentesis

All pleural effusions should be sampled via thoracentesis, except if they are of very small volume or it is known they are secondary to congestive heart failure.

Thoracentesis can be carried out with the animal in lateral or sternal recumbency, although generally patients with dyspnoea **tolerate sternal recumbency better**. In addition, lateral recumbency is not helpful when obtaining samples of a small-volume effusion (Figure 4.39).

The necessary consumables are easily available and include a 50 ml syringe, an extension tube with a three-way tap and a butterfly or coated catheter:

- 20–22 gauge butterfly for cats and small dogs
- 14–18 gauge catheter with extension for large dogs.

Depending on the patient's temperament, this procedure can be performed either with the animal awake or lightly sedated. A simple nerve block of the intercostal nerve with local anaesthesia and/or a small incision where the catheter is to be inserted can usually be performed without sedation.

The site for thoracentesis is selected either empirically at the **7th–9th intercostal space** at the level of the costochondral junction, or guided by chest radiography, physical examination or ultrasound.

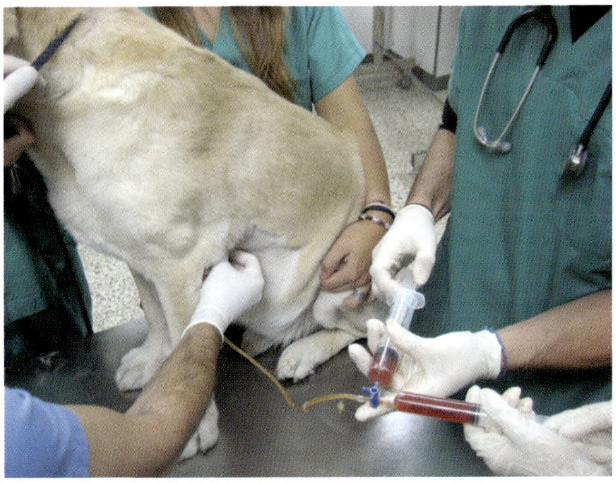

Figure 4.39. Thoracentesis for extraction of pleural fluid.

The skin should be disinfected. An injection of 2% lidocaine is used to anaesthetize the entire route from the skin to the parietal pleura. Subsequently, the needle or catheter is inserted perpendicular to the chest wall, following the **cranial edge of the rib** to avoid damaging the neurovascular bundle located in the costal groove of the caudal border. Once the chest wall is penetrated, gentle suction is applied until liquid is obtained.

If a butterfly is used, the needle should be angled until it is as parallel as possible to the pleural surface, in order not to damage the lung parenchyma, and extraction commences.

If a catheter is used, the catheter should be advanced a little and the cannula should be fully inserted into the pleural cavity. The needle is removed quickly to avoid the entry of air, and the catheter connected to the extension tube with the three-way tap to start the fluid aspiration.

For **diagnostic thoracentesis**, extract sufficient liquid to perform the laboratory tests. For **therapeutic thoracentesis**, to relieve the patient's dyspnoea the entire volume of fluid is removed.

Tubes without and with anticoagulant (EDTA) should be used together with a container large enough to collect significant amounts of liquid.

Cytology, biochemistry and culture (**aerobic and anaerobic**) of the liquid are of great help and are considered essential in the diagnostic process. If only small volumes are obtained, **cytology is the test that takes priority**:

- If cellularity is marked, cytological extension can be performed directly.
- If cellularity is moderate or scarce, cytology of the sediment should be performed after centrifugation.

Effusions and pleural effusions are classified according to the nature of the liquid contained in the cavity.

These characteristics are taken from its macroscopic aspect, cytological characteristics and protein content. The traditional differentiation between transudates, modified transudates and exudates is considered the initial step in the investigation of any pleural effusion. Although it does not determine the disease responsible, the number of options when making a list of differential diagnoses may be reduced. However, there may be an overlap of values between the different categories, which means that this classification is often not useful, especially when trying to differentiate a modified transudate from an exudate. Therefore, a classification that also includes chymal, neoplastic and haemorrhagic effusions, categorized according to their aetiology, may be more useful from the clinical point of view (Table 4.17).

The **measurement of glucose can be used to identify septic effusions**, although there may be some overlap with neoplastic effusions. The normal value in pleural fluid is similar to that of plasma, but this decreases when mesothelial cells have increased metabolic activity, which occurs frequently with pyothorax. In such cases, the glucose level can be close to zero.

In felines, the concentration of pleural lactate dehydrogenase and the ratio of pleural liquid to whole-blood protein are useful to establish a clear differentiation between exudates and transudates, with a sensitivity of 100 and 91%, respectively, and a specificity of 100%, according to a recent study.

Based on these parameters a diagnostic approach, applicable exclusively to the cat, includes the measurement of lactate dehydrogenase as a starting point:

- **≤200 IU/l lactate dehydrogenase** confirms the presence of a transudate and no further analysis is necessary, as most cases are caused almost exclusively by congestive heart failure, hypoproteinaemia and excess intravenous fluids.

Table 4.17. Classification of pleural fluid.

Type of effusion	Colour and turbidity	Total protein (g/dl)	Density	Total cells (n)	Differential	Observations
Transudate	Clear and transparent	<2.5	<1.017	<1500	Macrophages, lymphocytes and mesothelial cells	
Modified transudate	Serous and transparent or moderately cloudy	2.5–5	1.017–1.25	1000–7000	Macrophages, lymphocytes, non-degenerate neutrophils, mesothelial cells and red blood cells	
Non-septic exudate	Serosanguinous or straw-coloured and turbid	>3	>1.025	>5000	Non-degenerate neutrophils, macrophages, mesothelial cells and occasional red blood cells	In case of FIP, positive Rivalta test (PPV 86%, NPV 97%). Albumin/globulin ratio 0.5
Septic exudate	Purulent, creamy, serosanguinous and turbid and with floccules	>3	>1.025	>5000	Degenerate neutrophils, mesothelial cells and red blood cells Intracytoplasmic bacteria	Positive bacterial culture. A culture for aerobic and anaerobic bacteria and an antibiogram should be performed on all samples containing degenerate neutrophils, even though no bacteria are detected on cytology A cloudy, yellowish appearance with the presence of so-called sulphur granules is highly suggestive of the presence of *Nocardia* or *Actinomyces* spp.

Table 4.17. Continued.

Type of effusion	Colour and turbidity	Total protein (g/dl)	Density	Total cells (n)	Differential	Observations
Chyle	White, pinkish, milky and opaque	>2.5	>1.018	Variable	Lymphocytes, non-degenerated neutrophils and mesothelial cells	Compared with serum, it has a higher level of triglycerides and the cholesterol/triglyceride ratio is <1 The presence of high cholesterol levels in the pleural fluid is suggestive of pseudo-chylothorax Pseudo-chylothorax has a milky appearance due to the high lipid content, but is not caused by thoracic duct injury Tends to be due to chronic effusions in which cholesterol arises from the degradation of white and red blood cells within the pleural space
Haemorrhagic	Bloody and opaque	>3	>1.025	>1000	Similar to peripheral blood Presence of erythrophagocytosis	The presence of a small amount of blood (1–2 ml or 1–5%) can cause a bloody appearance in a pleural effusion, but a haemothorax is considered to be present when the haematocrit of the pleural fluid is ≥ that of the peripheral blood It does not coagulate, because continuous movement produces defibrination; this helps to differentiate the effusion from the accidental puncture of a vessel
Neoplasia	Serosanguinous and turbid	>2.5	Variable	Variable	Macrophages, lymphocytes, non-degenerate neutrophils, mesothelial cells and the presence of neoplastic cells	Special attention should be paid to erroneous interpretations of reactive mesothelial cells by inflammatory stimuli, which can be confused with neoplastic cells With the exception of lymphoma, most require tissue biopsy for a definitive diagnosis Most lymphoblastic lymphomas are easily identifiable by cytology (larger cells with prominent nucleoli, and evidence of mitosis)

- **200 IU/l lactate dehydrogenase** indicates that this is an exudate and additional measurements are necessary.
- **pH ≤6.9**: there is a high probability that it is a pyothorax.
  - In addition, these fluids usually have glucose levels <30 mg/dl.
  - Cytology shows the percentage of neutrophils >85%.
- **pH ≥7.4**: suggests an effusion associated with malignancy.
  - Glucose is usually 10–80 mg/dl.
  - The neutrophil count is <30%.
  - A high red blood cell count in the absence of trauma or coagulopathy is also highly suggestive of neoplasia.

Treatment

Treatment depends on the underlying aetiology. In the case of pure transudates, the only treatment is that specific to the initiating disease.

When the volume of effusion is significant and produces dyspnoea, initial treatment is aimed at stabilizing the animal through generic management of respiratory emergencies, delaying aetiological diagnostic studies.

Generalized pleural effusion

Regardless of its aetiology, **narrow or wide thoracic drainage** should be put in place depending on the nature of the fluid. This may enable the thorax to be adequately re-evaluated by means of radiography, and make possible identification of underlying causes that were hidden due to the fluid. In addition, it stabilizes the patient sufficiently to proceed with other diagnostic studies.

Recurrent pleural effusion

As with most cases of neoplasia or chylothorax, pleurodesis can be performed. In order to go ahead with the procedure, it is important that the dyspnoea is due mainly to the effusion and that the lung is able to re-expand once all the pleural fluid is evacuated. Several substances have been used for pleurodesis, the most common being talcum powder and chlortetracycline.

When life expectancy is short, as an alternative to repeated thoracentesis and to facilitate management at home, a permanent pleural catheter (pleural port device) may be implanted.

Pyothorax

Aetiology

The main cause of pyothorax is the **presence of an infectious agent in the pleural cavity** resulting in an inflammatory response and the accumulation of fluid in the pleural space. Practically speaking, 80–90% of patients with pyothorax have **bilateral involvement**.

In the majority of cases, neither the specific cause nor the route of infection is identified. There are reports of pyothorax caused by grass seeds, penetrating wounds, extension of lung abscesses, foreign bodies that perforate the oesophagus and even a distant infectious focus (haematogenous route).

In cats the most common causes identified include:

- pneumonia (parapneumonic pyothorax)
- upper airway infection
- perioperative aspiration
- parasitic migration
- Direct inoculation by a cat bite. This is suspected as the isolated flora is similar to the normal bacterial flora of the oropharynx, and affected patients frequently live alongside other cats.
- haematogenous spread
- extension from adjacent viscera.

Treatment

There are different options for controlling a pyothorax, but there is no single optimal or universal approach that is recommended for all patients. Recent studies have shown that surgical intervention is beneficial. In dogs, surgery was 5.4 times more successful than medical treatment, and cats managed surgically had a higher survival rate than those treated medically.

However, excellent prognoses have been described in dogs and cats with conservative treatment. Recently, one study described 15 dogs treated satisfactorily with a single drain and long-term antibiotic treatment (none of these presented with evidence of lung masses, abscesses or effusions of granular appearance that could have indicated the presence of *Actinomyces*).

The general recommendation is for **less invasive treatments to be used first** and, in the case of a poor response, more invasive options are resorted to. As a minimum, **systemic antibiotic treatment and supportive care** are required. In older patients, ideally the removal of pleural fluid should be attempted either through therapeutic thoracentesis or placement of thoracic drainage to facilitate the elimination of pleural fluid.

The criteria used to determine whether conservative treatment for pyothorax has failed have yet to be established. However, if these procedures are not effective after 48–72 hours, additional imaging tests and the possibility of surgical intervention should be considered to rule out the following possibilities:

- The **thoracic drain is obstructed** by liquid, fibrin or blood, or it is bent or incorrectly placed (it is important that the tube is seated on the sternum, in the ventral part of the thorax).
- **The effusion is septate** so it cannot be completely eliminated with a thoracic drain, and/or a fibrous layer has formed on the visceral pleura preventing expansion of the underlying lung. In these circumstances, thoracotomy is required to eliminate fluid and infected or necrotic tissue, debride the pleural surface, identify and eliminate any foreign material and wash the entire pleural cavity to decrease the number of bacteria and allow better penetration of antibiotics.

Thoracoscopy may also be an option, since this allows examination of the thoracic cavity, biopsies to be taken and adhesions debrided (provided they are not extensive), drainage of the pleural cavity and optimal placement of a drainage system.

Systemic antibiotic treatment

If the pathogen is unknown, an empirical approach should include antibiotics active against the bacteria that most frequently cause pyothorax. Once the results of stains and cultures are received, the antibiotic treatment initially prescribed should be adjusted and, at the same time, treatment against anaerobes continued, since these are difficult to isolate.

The agents that cause infection in the pleural cavity usually consist of a combination of **obligate anaerobes and facultative bacteria**. Few differences are observed between the feline and canine species with respect to the pathogens involved, except for the Gram-negative bacilli: in the case of the dog, *E. coli* predominates and, in the case of the cat, *Pastereulla* spp. Most samples, especially in cats, contain obligate anaerobes.

No single antibiotic is able to cover this spectrum and, therefore, an intravenous combination of drugs with activity against **obligate anaerobes** (ampicillin, amoxicillin-clavulanic acid, clindamycin or metronidazole) and **facultative bacteria** (amikacin, gentamicin or ceftizoxime) is, a priori, a good choice. Most of these drugs, with the exception of aminoglycosides, present good penetration of the pleural space and a wide dosage margin without causing adverse effects. Enrofloxacin could also be an appropriate option to cover **coliform bacteria**.

The duration of treatment is established based on the resolution of the changes detected in each patient, but the average time shown in some studies is **4–6 weeks**. The isolation of **filamentous bacteria from the genus *Actinomyces*** requires a special mention. These pathogens are almost **entirely transported by plant material (usually grass seeds)** and, therefore, once the results of the culture have been obtained, if their presence is detected the source should be identified and eliminated, which can sometimes be impossible. In these cases, the duration of the treatment must be prolonged. Relapses are frequent, as it is very difficult to sterilize plant material that remains within tissues.

Evacuation of pleural fluid

Repeated thoracentesis with a needle is not efficient for a complete thoracic drainage, since the fluid is usually thick, flocculated and reaccumulates rapidly.

Thoracic drains facilitate complete emptying of the pleural cavity while also allowing lavage. The choice of the side of the thorax for placement of the drainage tube is made based on radiographic findings, and on the volume and distribution of the fluid. Sometimes it is necessary to place drains in both hemithoraxes because, although the mediastinum is permeable, it may be septate.

For a long time it was recommended that the size of the drainage tube should approximate the diameter of the main bronchus of the animal, since this diameter greatly facilitates the drainage of viscous fluids such as those found in pyothorax. Relatively recently in veterinary medicine, however, the advantages of using small drains have been discussed:

- **advantage**: can be introduced by untrained personnel, and with light sedation
- **disadvantage**: a priori they are not indicated for very dense effusions and clog easily.

After tube placement and initial thoracic drainage, continuous suction is performed using commercial aspiration devices or intermittently by aspiration. In most practices, **intermittent suction is performed every 2–6 hours during the first 24–48 hours**. Lavage of the cavity provides benefits, such as modification of intra-cavitary pH and reduction in fluid viscosity and the number of purulent particles and bacteria. Frequently, a **warm sterile isotonic solution is administered at a volume of 10–20 ml/kg**. The benefits of adding heparin to the solution have also been demonstrated in some studies, and is a technique commonly used. The **fluid is left in place for 5–10 minutes** and the pleural cavity is then drained, with recovery of >75% of the introduced volume advisable. This procedure can be carried out **between two and four times per day**.

Every two days, an analysis of the fluid obtained should be carried out to check progress of the condition. Favourable criteria are considered to be:

- negative cultures
- absence of intracellular bacteria

- decrease in the number of inflammatory cells
- decrease in fluid production
- increase in the initial pH.

The tube is removed when drainage is <2–3 ml/kg/24 h of serous fluid and there is considerable improvement in thoracic radiographs.

Chylothorax

Definition

This is the accumulation of chyle in the pleural space.

Chyle has a milky aspect due to its high lipid content. It arises from absorption from the intestinal lymphatic vessels, which drain into the chyle cistern and from there to the thoracic duct, which ends in the caudal vena cava. The thoracic duct may be single or multiple, and drains lymph from almost the entire organism – with the exception of the right anterior limb and the right part of the head and neck.

Epidemiology

The incidence of chylothorax in small animals is not high and does not seem to present any sex or age predisposition, although there are some breeds in which there is a higher incidence:

- **Dogs**: Mastiffs and Afghan Hounds (the latter also frequently suffer from pulmonary lobe torsion; the relationship between the two conditions is not entirely clear).
- **Cats**: Abyssinian and Siamese.

Aetiology

Chylothorax is associated with:

- trauma to the thoracic duct
- generalized lymphangiectasia
- inflammation
- obstruction of lymphatic flow
- heart disease (especially feline cardiomyopathies and tricuspid dysplasia in the dog)
- neoplasia.

Often, despite diagnostic efforts, no underlying cause can be demonstrated and it is then considered idiopathic.

Treatment

Initial treatment depends on the severity of the effusion and the underlying disease. It is important to manage the underlying disease because in some cases this is sufficient, but in others drainage of the pleural space with a pleural drainage tube is necessary. The great dilemma with chylothorax is not only that it involves a respiratory problem, but also the loss of lymph can be associated with hypalbuminaemia, hypoproteinaemia and T lymphocytes, with immunological deficits.

Medical

The first choice of treatment is medical. The effusion may resolve spontaneously in a period of weeks to months. A **low-fat diet** may be helpful, although clinical studies have not confirmed that the volume of lymph flow through the thoracic duct is reduced. Some patients benefit from this measure and, although the flow may not decrease, lymph with lower lipid content can be reabsorbed more quickly. Possibly the reason for the lack of efficacy lies in the requirement for extreme lipid restrictions with an additional supply of medium-chain triglycerides as an energy source that can be absorbed through the portal circulation, and this is rarely done. Pharmacological treatment is based on the administration of a natural benzopyrone, sold in herbal medicine shops and indicated for lymphatic oedema, although its mechanism of action is not very clear.

Surgical

Indications for a surgical intervention are usually:

- Failure to reduce the flow of lymph after 5–10 days of medical management (need for thoracentesis more than once a week).
- Chyle losses greater than 20 ml/kg/d for more than 5 days.
- Constrictive pleuritis.
- Signs of protein-calorie malnutrition and hypoproteinaemia.

There are several surgical options which may be required in isolation or combination. Ligation of the thoracic duct with partial pericardiectomy is the most widely used technique and possibly has the highest success rate:

- **Advantage**: if successful, it completely resolves the effusion (which is not the case with palliative interventions such as pleuroperitoneal shunts or diaphragmatic omentalization).
- **Disadvantage:** the need to perform a lymphangiography to recognize at what point the thoracic duct appears as a single vessel, in order to ensure no branches are left permeable.

Pleural drainage may be considered as part of the treatment protocol (Figure 4.40).

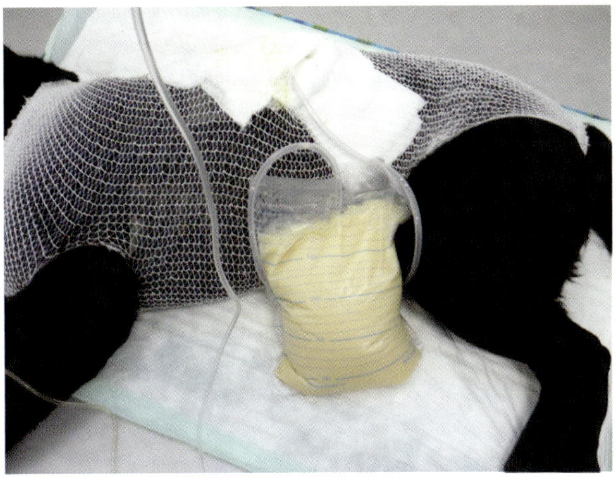

Figure 4.40. Pleural drainage in a dog with chylothorax.

Haemothorax

Aetiology

The accumulation of blood in the pleural space can occur as a consequence of:

- trauma
- systemic coagulopathy
- pulmonary lobe torsion
- neoplasia
- rodenticide poisoning – the most common cause.

Clinical picture

In some cases of rodenticide poisoning, the systemic **signs of shock** caused by acute blood loss predominate and the identification of pleural effusion is based on the **suspicion of rodenticide use** the previous week rather than on clinical signs. Not all patients present with bleeding in the pleural cavity, with pulmonary haemorrhage or haemorrhages in other parts of the body (abdomen, skin, eyes, spinal canal, etc.) also being common.

Other aetiologies cause more subtle and slow-onset signs.

Diagnosis

Radiography and ultrasound are useful to determine possible underlying causes, and in the case of coagulopathies there are usually marked abnormalities on coagulation tests.

Treatment

If a **coagulopathy is identified, chest drainage is not usually necessary** since dyspnoea is often due to parenchymal bleeding and/or blood loss itself (decreased oxygen transport capacity and increased sympathetic tone) rather than the direct effect of the effusion. When performing thoracentesis, it is advisable to extract only the volume necessary to relieve dyspnoea because, if the basic problem is corrected, practically 90% of red blood cells will be reabsorbed within 4 days.

In the case of rodenticide poisoning, the administration of vitamin K (phytomedione) should be started at a loading dose of 5 mg/kg, but its effects take a few hours to manifest. Therefore, to stop bleeding (especially if the animal is anaemic) fresh frozen plasma at a dose of 6–10 ml/kg or whole blood is required. Subsequently, vitamin K is maintained at a dose of 1.5–2.5 mg/kg twice daily orally, together with food (facilitates the absorption of vitamin K, which is fat-soluble) for as long as necessary, depending on the half-life of the ingested antagonist. The treatment is usually maintained for a 3-week period, and prothrombin time is measured 36 hours after it is stopped (extrinsic F VII pathway, half-life 6 hours):

- If the prothrombin time is extended, the treatment should be continued.
- If the prothrombin time is normalized, administration of more vitamin K is not necessary.
- In the case of trauma without active bleeding, conservative management may be sufficient; however, if bleeding is persistent, surgical intervention may be required.

Bibliography

Ancochea, J. (2010) Consenso para el diagnóstico de las neumonías intersticiales idiopáticas. *Archivos de Bronconeumolia* 46(5), 2–21.

Byers, C.G. and Dhupa, N. (2005) Feline bronchial asthma: pathophysiology and diagnosis. *Compendium of Continuing Education for Veterinarians* 27(6), 418–425.

Byers, C.G. and Dhupa, N. (2005) Feline bronchial asthma: treatment. *Compendium of Continuing Education for Veterinarians* 27(6), 426–431.

Clercx, C., Peeters, D., Snaps, F., Hansen, P., McEntee, K., Detilleux, J., Henroteaux, M. and Day, M.J. (2000) Eosinophilic bronchopneumopathy in dogs. *Journal of Veterinary Internal Medicine* 14(3), 282–291.

Clercx, C. and Peeters, D. (2007) Canine eosinophilic bronchopneumopathy. *Veterinary Clinics of North America Small Animal Practice* 37(5), 917–935.

Cohn, L.A. (2009) Inhalant therapy: finding its place in small-animal practice. *Veterinary Medicine* 104, 336–341.

Cohn, L.A., Norris, C.R., Hawkins, E.C., Dye, J.A., Johnson, C.A. and Williams, K.J. (2004) Identification and characterization of an idiopathic pulmonary fibrosis-like condition in cats. *Journal of Veterinary Internal Medicine* 18(5), 632–641.

Corcoran, B.M. Clinical approach to coughing. In: Fuentes, V.L., Johnson, L.R. and Dennis, S. (eds) *BSAVA Manual of Canine and Feline Cardiorespiratory Medicine*, 2nd edn. British Small Animal Veterinary Association, Gloucester, UK, pp. 11–14.

Corcoran, B.M., Cobb, M., Martin, M.W., Dukes-McEwan, J., French, A., Fuentes, V.L., Boswood, A. and Rhind, S. (1999) Chronic pulmonary disease in West Highland white terriers. *Veterinary Record* 144(22), 611–616.

Dempsey, S.M. and Ewing, P.J. (2011) A review of the pathophysiology, classification, and analysis of canine and feline cavitary effusions. *Journal of the American Animal Hospital Association* 47, 1–11.

Dethioux, F. and Goy-Thollot, I. (2008) *Manual del veterinario: Guía práctica de urgencias en perros y gatos*. Royal Canin, Paris, France, p. 47.

Ettinger, S.J. and Feldman, E.C. (eds) (2010) *Textbook of Veterinary Internal Medicine*, 7th edn. WB Saunders, Philadelphia, PA, USA.

Fasanella, F.J., Shivley, J., Wardlaw, J.L. and Givaruangsawat, S. (2010) Brachycephalic airway obstructive syndrome in dogs: 90 cases (1991–2008). *Journal of the American Veterinary Medical Association* 237, 1048–1051.

Ford, R. (2009) Bacterial Pneumonia. In: Bonagura, J.D. and Twedt, D.C. (eds) *Kirk's Current Veterinary Therapy XIV*. Saunders Elsevier, MO, USA, pp. 412–421.

Forrester, D. and Moon, M. (1997) Diseases of the Lower Airways and Lungs. In: Leib, M. and Monroe, W. (eds) *Practical Small Animal Internal Medicine*. WB Saunders Company, Philadelphia, PA, USA, pp. 1153–1185.

Foster, S.F., Martin, P., Braddock, J.A. and Malik, R. (2004) A retrospective analysis of feline bronchoalveolar lavage cytology and microbiology (1995–2000). *Journal of Feline Medicine and Surgery* 6(3), 189–198.

Hawkins, E. (2000) Enfermedades del parénquima pulmonar. In: Nelson, R. and Couto, G. (eds) *Medicina interna de animales pequeños*. Editorial Inter-Médica, Buenos Aires, Argentina, pp. 323–340.

Henninger, W. (2003) Use of computed tomography in the diseased feline thorax. *Journal of Small Animal Practice* 44, 56–64.

Johnson, L.R. (ed.) (2014) Canine and feline respiratory medicine. *Veterinary Clinics of North America Small Animal Practice* 44(1).

Johnson, L.R. and Drazenovich, T.L. (2007) Flexible bronchoscopy and bronchoalveolar lavage in 68 cats (2001–2006). *Journal of Veterinary Internal Medicine* 21(2), 219–225.

Johnson, L.R. (ed.) (2010) *Clinical Canine and Feline Respiratory Medicine*. Wiley-Blackwell, Ames, IA, USA.

Johnson, V.S., Corcoran, B.M., Wotton, P.R., Schwarz, T. and Sullivan, M. (2005) Thoracic high-resolution computed tomographic findings in dogs with canine idiopathic pulmonary fibrosis. *Journal of Small Animal Practice* 46(8), 381–388.

King, L.G. (ed.) (2004) *Textbook of Respiratory Disease in Dogs and Cats*. WB Saunders; Philadelphia, PA, USA.

Larson, M.M. (2009) Ultrasound of the thorax (noncardiac). *Veterinary Clinics of North America Small Animal Practice* 39, 733–745.

Lewis, D.H., Armitage-Chan, E., Chan, D.L. and Garden, O. (2009) Septic pneumonia and pyothorax in dogs. *Veterinary Record* 164(12), 378.

Llabrés-Díaz, F. (2007) Practical radiography in small animal practice II: coughing patients. *Irish Veterinary Journal* 60(8), 489–494.

Macdonald, E.S., Norris, C.R., Berghaus, R.B. and Griffey, S.M. (2003) Clinicopathological and radiographic features and etiologic agents in cats with histologically confirmed infectious pneumonia: 39 cases. *Journal of the American Veterinary Medical Association* 223(8), 1142–1150.

Martin, M. and Corcoran, B. (eds) (1999) *Enfermedades cardiorrespiratorias del perro y del gato*. Ediciones S, Barcelona, Spain, pp. 259–293.

McNeill, E. (ed.) (2010) Respiratory diseases. *Veterinary Focus* 20(2).

Murphy, K. and Papasouliotis, K. (2011) Pleural effusions in dogs and cats 1. Diagnostic investigation. *In Practice* 33, 462–469.

Murphy, K. and Papasouliotis, K. (2011) Pleural effusions in dogs and cats 2. Placement of tubes and treatment. *In Practice* 33, 526–530.

Norsworthy, G. et al. (2006) Lung Parasites. In: *The Feline Patient*, 3rd edn. Blackwell Publishing, Ames, IA, USA, p.175.

Padrid, P. (2000) Canine and feline pleural disease. *Veterinary Clinics of North America Small Animal Practice* 30, 1295–1307.

Padrid, P. (2006) Use of inhaled medications to treat respiratory diseases in dogs and cats. *Journal of the American Animal Hospital Association* 42(2), 165–169.

Padrid, P. (2010) Asthma. In: August, J.R. (ed.) *Consultations in Feline Internal Medicine*. WB Saunders, Philadelphia, PA, USA, pp. 447–458.

Plickert, H.D., Tichy, A. and Hirt, R.A. (2014) Characteristics of canine nasal discharge related to intranasal diseases: a retrospective study of 105 cases. *Journal of Small Animal Practice* 3(55), 145–152.

Quimby, J. and Lappin, M.R. (2009) Feline focus: Update on feline upper respiratory diseases: Introduction and diagnostics. *Compendium of Continuing Education for Veterinarians* 31(12), E1–E7.

Quimby, J. and Lappin, M.R. (2010) Update on feline upper respiratory diseases: Condition-specific recommendations. *Compendium of Continuing Education for Veterinarians* 32(1).

Rand, J. (2006) Cat with Lower Respiratory Tract or Cardiac Signs. In: *Problem-Based Feline Medicine*. Saunders Elsevier, Australia, p. 47.

Reed, N. and Gunn-Moore, D. (2012) Nasopharyngeal disease in cats: 1. Diagnostic investigation. *Journal of Feline Medicine and Surgery* 14, 306–315.

Reed, N. and Gunn-Moore, D. (2012) Nasopharyngeal disease in cats: 2. Specific conditions and their management. *Journal of Feline Medicine and Surgery* 14, 317–323.

Reinero, C.R. and Cohn L.A. (2007) Interstitial lung diseases. *Veterinary Clinics of North America Small Animal Practice* 37(5), 937–947.

Scott, J.A. and Macintire, D.K. (2003) Canine pyothorax: Pleural anatomy and pathophysiology. *Compendium of Continuing Education for Practising Veterinarians* 25, 172–179.

Secrest, S.A., Bailey, M.Q., Williams, K.J. and Smarick, S.D. (2008) Imaging diagnosis: feline idiopathic pulmonary fibrosis. *Veterinary Radiology and Ultrasound* 49(1), 47–50.

Sherding, R. (2009) Respiratory Parasites. In: Bonagura, J.D. and Twedt, D.C. (eds). *Kirk's Current Veterinary Therapy XIV*. Saunders Elselvier, MO, USA, pp. 666–670.

Venema, C.M. and Patterson, C.C. (2010) Diagnosing and managing canine eosinophilic bronchopneumopathy. *Veterinary Medicine* June, 272–282.

Test

1. **In relation to the problems in the nasal cavity we can affirm that:**
   A) In a 6-month-old cat, with sneezing and bilateral serous nasal discharge of acute onset, the presence of a neoplasm should be suspected.
   B) In a middle-aged dolichocephalic dog with sneezing, chronic haemorrhagic discharge and nasal deformation, the most likely diagnosis is fungal rhinitis or nasal neoplasia.
   C) Diagnostic imaging tests (RX, CT, MRI) provide little information; therefore, in the diagnostic study of any patient with a nasal condition, rhinoscopy with biopsies taken from the nasal cavity is always recommended as a first-line test.
   D) Bacterial aetiology is the most frequent primary cause of rhinitis in small animals; therefore, most animals respond satisfactorily to the use of antibiotics for 7–14 days.
2. **A 10-year-old Collie dog presents in a consultation suffering from a haemorrhagic nasal discharge and sneezing over the last month. The patient is alert, active, afebrile, has a unilateral ocular discharge and some degree of facial deformation and tenderness around the affected area. Based on this information, which of the following decisions do you consider most appropriate?**
   A) The aforementioned history suggests that it is most likely a dental problem. Therefore, anaesthetizing the patient to perform a detailed study of the oral cavity, including a radiographical study, is recommended.
   B) The history indicates that it is most likely a viral condition (calicivirus or herpesvirus), and the recommended treatment is symptomatic with administration of antibiotics to prevent secondary infections.
   C) The history suggests that it is most likely a foreign body, so a fibro-endoscopic study under general anaesthesia should be performed to confirm or rule out the diagnosis.
   D) The history indicates that it is very likely to be a tumour, so a detailed imaging study (CT) and a subsequent biopsy by means of fibro-endoscopy should be recommended.
3. **An 11-year-old Labrador retriever is brought in due to noisy breathing over the last four months. Clinical signs began associated with episodes of excitement, during exercise and with heat. The symptomatology has progressed and currently the patient shows clear signs of exercise intolerance. There are also changes in the tone of the bark and occasional coughing after the ingestion of food or water. During the physical examination the presence of inspiratory stridor is detected, which is more evident after exercise, showing a marked respiratory effort and signs of cyanosis after running. Based on this information, which of the following is the most likely diagnosis?**
   A) pulmonary oedema
   B) tracheal collapse
   C) laryngeal paralysis
   D) laryngeal oedema.
4. **Which of the following is not a component involved in brachycephalic syndrome?**
   A) stenotic nares
   B) presence of hyperplastic and dysplastic turbinates and rostral aberrant turbinates
   C) tracheal collapse
   D) laryngeal collapse.
5. **In tracheal collapse, which of the following is true?**
   A) It is a frequent pathology in the feline species that presents with a chronic cough and respiratory distress.
   B) It is a frequent pathology in dogs due to trauma, fundamentally bites, which involve the neck region.
   C) It mainly affects small-breed dogs and invariably occurs with tachypnoea, dyspnoea, cyanosis and syncope, with coughing being a very occasional sign.
   D) Radiography (preferably fluoroscopy) is usually sufficient for diagnosis, but bronchoscopy is considered more useful since it determines the extent and severity of the collapse.
6. **Which of the following statements is false regarding kennel cough and infectious canine tracheobronchitis?**
   A) It is an acute and very contagious disease of the upper airways that affects canines.
   B) The agents involved include canine adenovirus type 2, parainfluenza virus and *Bordetella bronchiseptica*, as well as other secondary pathogens.
   C) It always requires long-term antibiotic treatment (4–8 weeks) and antitussives.
   D) Uncomplicated cases usually present with a sudden, severe dry cough without signs of systemic disease.

7. In relation to feline asthma, which of the following is true?

A) It mainly affects older and obese cats.

B) Clinical manifestations include coughing, wheezing and reduced activity, with marked signs of systemic involvement such as fever, anorexia and vomiting.

C) Patients that are severely compromised show persistent daily coughing and frequent episodes of respiratory distress, with increased expiratory effort and wheezing.

D) The tracheobronchial cytology usually shows an inflammatory response with marked eosinophilia, because in all cases a parasitic cause lies behind it.

8. In which of the following cases is feline asthma one of the main differential diagnoses?

A) 2-year-old Siamese cat, coughing daily over the last week, with wheezing, peripheral eosinophilia and a bronchial pattern and signs of hyperinflation on radiography.

B) 5-month-old Common European cat (CE), with a cough and difficulty breathing and the presence of wheezing; on radiography there is a marked bronchial pattern and *Aelurostrongylus abstrusus* larvae in faecal matter.

C) 9-month-old Ragdoll cat, with sudden onset of respiratory distress, sporadic coughing starting a week ago, decreased lung sounds in both hemithoraxes, hyperglobulinaemia and uveitis.

D) 12-year-old CE cat, which recently underwent a mastectomy and is losing weight, as well as showing exercise intolerance, persistent dyspnoea and crepitations on pulmonary auscultation.

9. Indicate which statement is correct regarding the treatment of chronic canine bronchitis.

A) Most patients respond appropriately to antibiotic treatment administered for at least two weeks after the resolution of clinical signs.

B) Many patients are completely cured after prolonged therapy with bronchodilators, especially if these are administered by inhalation therapy.

C) Corticosteroids are the basis of treatment, and some animals can do without them temporarily while others will need maintenance doses for life.

D) In dogs with chronic bronchitis that present with a productive cough and abundant mucus, the use of antitussives such as codeine or butorphanol is considered highly effective.

10. An 11-year-old Cocker spaniel with intense respiratory distress, tachypnoea, crepitations, a pinkish foamy discharge and systolic grade V/VI murmur with a maximum intensity point on the left apex is brought in for a consultation. Based on this information, what would be the most appropriate clinical action?

A) Administer an ACEI (benazepril or enalapril) and oral furosemide and wait for it to stabilize. Normally, since it takes 24 hours for the effects of this medication to be seen, it is better to send the patient home.

B) Immediately perform radiography (right and left lateral) and echocardiography to determine the aetiology of the condition, and prescribe a specific treatment for possible cardiac involvement.

C) Rest the patient, oxygen therapy and administration of intravenous furosemide until stabilization is achieved, after which the relevant complementary tests can be performed.

D) Rest the patient, and administration of a fast-acting corticosteroid intravenously.

11. Which of the following statements is true regarding pulmonary oedema?

A) The most frequent causes of pulmonary oedema in small animals are those related to reduced oncotic pressure, since a slight decrease in plasma albumin is enough to cause pulmonary oedema.

B) From a clinical perspective, it can be said that most dogs and cats that develop pulmonary oedema do so as a result of heart disease.

C) In a patient with a heart murmur and severe signs of pulmonary oedema, immediate radiography and echocardiography are recommended to determine the aetiology of the condition and thus to establish a specific treatment.

D) The most appropriate diuretic for the management of acute pulmonary oedema is spironolactone.

12. Which of the following statements is true with regard to pneumonia?

A) There are many diseases that underlie the development of aspiration pneumonia, but the cause is very rarely oesophageal or gastric disease.

B) In addition to respiratory symptoms (respiratory distress, tachypnoea, productive cough, bilateral nasal discharge), patients with pneumonia usually show fever, lethargy, anorexia and weakness.

C) Radiography is very useful in diagnosis, since almost all patients usually present with a broncho-interstitial pattern with caudodorsal distribution.

D) Regardless of the symptoms presented by the animal (stable/unstable with severe respiratory distress), tracheal or bronchoalveolar lavage is mandatory to obtain samples for culture and antibiogram.

13. Which of the following statements is correct regarding the treatment of bronchopneumonia?

A) In patients with pneumonia, parenteral fluids are totally contraindicated since these pose a high risk of pooling of fluid in the lungs and increased respiratory distress.

B) The duration of treatment is established based on the total WBC count, so that it is maintained for at least a week after it has reduced to within normal parameters.

C) In bacterial pneumonia, administration of antibiotics for at least two weeks after the resolution of the clinical and radiographic changes is recommended.

D) The oral administration of antibiotics, bronchodilators and antitussives is the first choice of treatment for a patient with clear signs of respiratory distress, fever and leucocytosis, and chest radiography where pulmonary consolidation and air bronchograms are seen.

14. Which of the following measures is not indicated in the treatment of bacterial pneumonia?

A) Nebulization and humidification of the respiratory tract to facilitate the elimination of secretions by reducing their viscosity.

B) Oral administration of antibiotics in stable patients.

C) Administration of intravenous antibiotics during the first 3–7 days in unstable patients (respiratory insufficiency, fever, leucocytosis and immature neutrophilia), as well as management of complications.

D) Oral administration of antibiotics for 2 weeks or, at least, up to 3 days after the resolution of the clinical signs.

15. A 1-year-old Persian cat presents in consultation with signs of respiratory distress. A week previously, it had experienced decreased appetite and reduction in physical activity. Physical examination shows a patient in good body condition, afebrile and with a restrictive respiratory pattern. Auscultation shows the absence of sounds in all lung fields except for the dorsal ones, and heart sounds are barely audible. The pulse can be palpated and is normal and rhythmic. On biochemistry there is a marked elevation of serum globulins. Based on this information, which of the following statements is correct?

A) For the signs described, the most likely diagnosis is a pleural effusion. Therefore, rest in an oxygen cage and thoracentesis until stabilization allows additional diagnostic tests to be performed, should these be recommended.

B) For the signs described, the most likely diagnosis is asthma. Therefore, rest in an oxygen cage and administration of corticosteroids until stabilization allows additional diagnostic tests to be performed, should these be recommended.

C) For the signs described, the most probable diagnosis is cardiogenic pulmonary oedema. Therefore, rest in an oxygen cage and administration furosemide until stabilization allows additional diagnostic tests to be performed, should these be recommended.

D) For the signs described, the most likely diagnosis is bronchopneumonia. Therefore, thoracic radiographs and sedation for sampling by tracheal lavage should be recommended.

16. Indicate which statement is correct regarding pleural cavity pathologies.

A) Restrictive respiratory pattern, exercise intolerance, existence of muffled and inaudible heart and lung sounds in ventral areas, and the presence of respiratory sounds in dorsal areas suggest pleural effusion.

B) In the case of pleural effusion, thoracic radiographs are not considered to be of diagnostic utility, since other conditions such as bronchopneumonia or pneumothorax show the same radiographic changes.

C) Thoracentesis is so high-risk for the patient that it should be performed only after confirmation by radiography that there is a condition affecting the pleural cavity.

D) In dogs, the most frequent pneumothorax is the spontaneous and traumatic open type seen in frequency.

Answers on page 178

Clinical case 1

Patient's signalment: 2-year-old castrated male Common European cat, weighing 4 kg.
Reason for consultation: symptoms of respiratory distress that began 2 hours ago. The cat maintains a sternal position and there are moments when it seems like he is drowning. It has never previously been to the vet for this problem (Video 1. http://publication.improveinternational.com).

History: vaccinated and dewormed. There are no more animals in the household, and the owner is a frequent smoker. The cat has had occasional coughing episodes, which recur at least once per week. Apart from this, the veterinarian defines him as a healthy, playful cat (Video 2. http://publication.improveinternational.com).
Physical examination: with minimum handling of the patient, signs of high-risk dyspnoea become evident. With handling kept to a minimum, the following information is obtained:

- respiratory rate 70 bpm
- superficial respiration with an obvious abdominal component
- pulmonary sounds in all lung fields
- presence of wheezing
- heart rate 200 bpm
- no murmurs or galloping heart sounds are heard.

1. **Taking the information provided into account, what would you do immediately? Choose which of the following options you consider to be most appropriate, and justify your response.**
   A. placement of a catheter
   B. fluid therapy
   C. thoracic radiography
   D. endotracheal wash
   E. oxygen therapy and rest
   F. thoracentesis
   G. slight sedation/tranquillization
   H. administration of a corticoid
   I. administration of theophylline
   J. administration of salbutamol
   K. administration of doxycycline and/or enrofloxacin
   L. blood sample for complete blood count
   M. blood sample for biochemistry.
2. **What would you do immediately? Justify your answer. In regard to administration of any type of medication, the route that seems most convenient at the time should be used, taking the weight of the patient into account, to perform the appropriate calculations depending on the chosen drug.**
3. **Two hours after the procedure, the patient is more stable, respiratory rate is 40 bpm and handling is not as risky (Figure 4.41). Would you?**
   A. place a pink catheter
   B. place a blue catheter
   C. place a yellow catheter
   D. perform thoracic radiography
   E. take blood sample for complete blood count
   F. take blood sample for biochemistry
   G. perform endotracheal wash
   H. perform stool analysis.

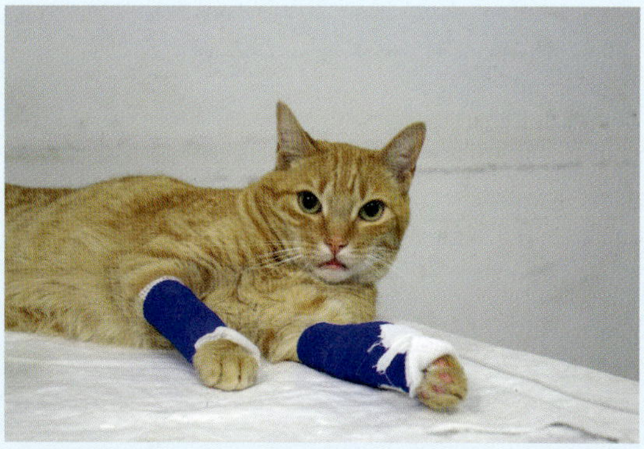

Figure 4.41.

4. **This is the patient's radiograph (Figure 4.42). Which findings are the most significant?**
   A. alveolar pattern
   B. interstitial pattern
   C. vascular pattern
   D. bronchial pattern
   E. cardiomegaly
   F. microcardia
   G. fractured rib
   H. flattened diaphragm
   I. hepatomegaly
   J. tracheal collapse
   K. pleural effusion
   L. pneumothorax
   M. hyperdistention
   N. right cranial lobe atelectasis
   O. It is poorly positioned and is not of diagnostic value.

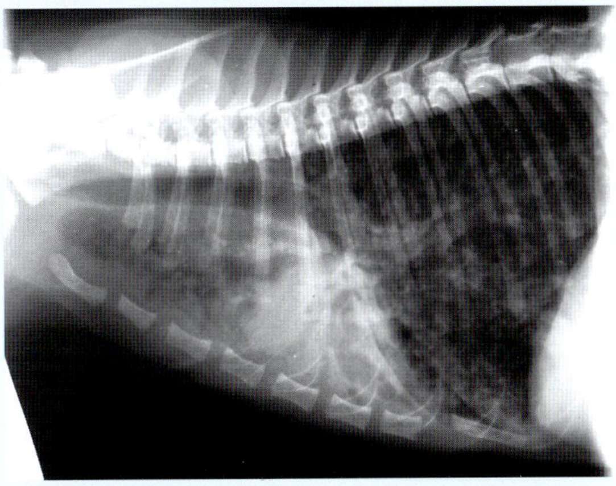

Figure 4.42.

5. **Based on history, examination and radiological findings, what is the most likely diagnosis?**
6. **What other differential diagnoses should be considered?**
7. **What complementary tests would you recommend and what would each of them contribute?**
8. **A sample has been extracted for a complete blood count; what would be the findings that were compatible with this condition?**
9. **24 hours go by and the animal is stable and goes home. What treatment and other recommendations would you give? Choose between the drugs available in the pharmacy (Case Study Table 1) and do not forget the dosage and long-term management until the next check-up, which will be in 15 days, so it is advisable to carefully write all instructions down for the owner.**
10. **The patient continues with treatment as recommended, and at the first check-up the owner mentions that he has not had more serious episodes like the previous one, but that occasionally he suffers from coughing fits (twice per week). The owner has been checking on the Internet and has seen that inhalers can be used. Give appropriate instructions regarding an inhaler and how to use it.**

Case Study Table 1 Pharmacy stock.

Pharmacy stock
Alsir 10 (enrofloxacin): each tablet contains 50 mg enrofloxacin
Cefa-cure 200 (cefadroxil): each tablet contains 200 mg cefadroxil
Calmo neosan (acepromazine): each millilitre contains 5 mg
Clavaseptin 50 mg (amoxicillin-clavulanic acid): each tablet contains 50 mg amoxicillin
Dacortin 5 (prednisone): each tablet contains 5 mg prednisone
Dormicum (midazolam): each millilitre contains 5 mg
Estilsona drops (prednisolone): each ml of suspension contains 13.30 mg prednisolone steaglate
IV euphyllin (theophylline): injectable solution, 200 mg/10 ml
Flixotide (fluticasone): suspension for inhalation, 250 mcg/application
Fortecortin (dexamethasone): 4 mg tablets and 4 mg/ml injectable solution
Panacur 250 (fenbendazole): each tablet contains 250 mg fenbendazole
Ronaxan 100 (doxycycline): each tablet contains 100 mg doxycycline
Terbasmin oral solution (terbutaline): each 5 ml contains 1.5 mg terbutaline sulphate
Theolair retard (theophylline): each tablet contains 175 mg theophylline
Urbason (methylprednisolone): several presentations – injectables 8, 20 and 40 mg per 2 ml
Valium (diazepam): each millilitre contains 5 mg
Ventolin (salbutamol): inhaler, 2 mg tablets and 0.5 mg/ml injectable solution

Answers on page 178

Clinical case 2

1. **Taking the information provided into account, what would you do immediately? Choose which of the following options you consider to be most appropriate and justify your response.**
   A. Placement of a catheter.
   It is an option, but it can further stress the patient and the drugs that we are going to use can be administered perfectly well using the intramuscular route.
   B. Fluid therapy.
   It is not an option.

C. Thoracic radiography.
   It is an option, but only when the cat is more stable; right now there are urgent procedures that should be performed.
D. Endotracheal wash.
   It is not an option.
E. Oxygen therapy and rest.
   It is one of the pillars of the management of patients with respiratory distress.
F. Thoracentesis.
   It is not an option; the physical examination does not suggest the presence of pleural fluid.
G. Slight sedation/tranquillization.
   It is an option, especially if handling of the patient produces stress. It is not essential immediately, but it should be evaluated soon after administration and effect of other drugs.
H. Administration of a corticoid.
   It is essential, because the history suggests an asthmatic crisis.
I. Administration of theophylline.
   It is not an option unless there is intravenous access.
J. Administration of salbutamol.
   It is an option, especially if inhalers and inhalation chambers are available. The oral route would be too slow, and its administration could induce greater stress in the patient. The dose for the parenteral route is not established.
K. Administration of doxycycline and/or enrofloxacin.
   It is not an option.
L. Blood sample for complete blood count.
   It is not an immediate option.
M. Blood sample for biochemistry.
   It is not an option.

2. Initial treatment for severe clinical signs

- oxygen therapy
- inhalation of albuterol (100 μg q30–60 min until respiratory distress is resolved) or terbutaline (0.01 mg/kg SC or IM until every 4 h).
- dexamethasone (1mg/kg IV or IM)
- consider the administration of magnesium.

After stabilization:

- prednisolone (1 mg/kg/12 h PO 5 days, then 1mg/kg/24 h PO 5 days, then 1mg /kg/48 h PO 5 days)
- fluticasone (250 μg every 12 h, and progressively decrease to the lowest dose possible)
- inhaled albuterol (100 μg as needed).

Oxygen therapy and careful management should be provided using the least stressful method possible (cage, Elizabethan collar, by-flow, etc.) and would increase the fraction inspired by oxygen.

Initially, bronchodilators should be administered to combat acute bronchoconstriction. Albuterol (Ventolin) can be administered via inhalation using a spacer chamber. One pulse is administered (100 mcg) and a positive response is expected after 15–30 minutes, which is manifested by a decrease in respiratory frequency and effort of 50% or more. If the cat does not respond favourably in that time, the dose should be repeated every 30 minutes for up to 4–6 h, without causing serious adverse effects.

Fast-acting corticosteroid such as dexamethasone at a dose of 1 mg/kg IM (total dose 1 ml of Fortecortin injection).

If the patient is very stressed despite the treatment administered, sedation can be carried out; for this, a low dose should always be used to start with and continued according to the effect. If the cardiovascular system is stable, acepromazine 0.02 mg/kg IM ± butorphanol 0.1 mg/kg IM ± midazolam 0.2 mg/kg IM can be used.

Stress caused by handling in the cat suffering an asthmatic crisis is very dangerous: in these cases administration of butorphanol (0.2–0.4 mg/kg IM) can be useful for its sedative and antitussive effects, and the cat can be left in an oxygen cage while the treatment is effective (sedative, bronchodilator and corticosteroid).

3. Two hours after the procedure, the patient is more stable, respiratory rate is 40 bpm and handling is not as risky. Would you?

B, D and E.

4. This is the patient's radiograph. Which findings are the most significant?
D, H, M and N.

5. Based on history, examination and radiological findings, what is the most likely diagnosis?
Feline asthma.

6. What other differential diagnoses should be considered?
Based on the clinical presentation and the findings on radiography:

- parasitic
- infectious bronchitis
- pulmonary parasites
- *Aelurostrongylus* spp.
- *Paragonimus* spp.
- *Capilaria* spp.
- infectious bronchitis
- *Bordetella*
- *Mycoplasma*
- Foreign body.

7. What complementary tests would you recommend, and what would each of these contribute?
Stool study. In endemic areas, lung parasites should be checked for by appropriate faecal tests that include flotation with or without centrifugation (to find *Paragonimus* and *Capillaria* eggs) and Baermann sedimentation (to detect *Aelurostrongylus larvae*).

Tracheal wash. The cytological findings obtained from endotracheal lavage and/or bronchoalveolar lavage are not pathognomonic of feline asthma. Generally, in cats with asthma, evidence of airway inflammation is obtained with an increase in the number of eosinophils recovered from bronchial secretions. However, numerous studies have made it clear that a prevalence of eosinophils (20–25% of the total cell count) recovered from tracheobronchial washings can be found in many normal cats. For this reason, eosinophilia in the lavage fluid of the airways should not be used for the definitive diagnosis of asthma in felines.

If aseptic samples are obtained from endotracheal or bronchoalveolar lavage, cultures and antimicrobial sensitivity tests can be performed for aerobic bacteria and *Mycoplasma* spp.

Endotracheal lavage and blind BAL

The collection of respiratory tract samples for cytological analysis and culture is a key component in the diagnostic evaluation of a cat suspected of having asthma. In general practice, BAL and endotracheal lavage can be performed blindly, without the use of a bronchoscope, to obtain adequate samples of the airway:

- 2 h before the induction of general anaesthesia, terbutaline should be administered 4 mg/kg SC to prevent bronchospasm, which can be induced by the procedure.
- After induction of general anaesthesia, the cat should be placed in left lateral decubitus recumbency and intubated with a sterile endotracheal tube.
- 0.9 % sterile saline solution is then infused into the respiratory tract by one of the following techniques.

Endotracheal lavage

A volume of 5 ml/kg warm sterile saline is infused directly into the lumen of the endotracheal tube using a 20 ml syringe, which is attached to a syringe adapter inserted at the end of said tube. Immediately afterwards, suction is applied using the same syringe to recover a part of the fluid. This procedure should be repeated twice.

Blind BAL

A volume of 5–10 ml of warm sterile saline is infused through a 6- or 8-calibre sterile French red rubber urinary catheter, which has been passed through the endotracheal tube into the distal airway (Figure 4.43). Immediately afterwards, suction is applied using the same syringe to recover a part of the fluid. The procedure should be repeated once.

The caudal half of the cat can be raised to aid in the recovery of the liquid. The recovery of 40–50% of the infused volume should be expected.

After the procedure, 100% oxygen is administered through the endotracheal tube for 5 minutes.

Immediately after collection, aliquots of the sample should be made and a small amount transferred to a sterile tube for general aerobic culture and mycoplasma culture.

The rest of the sample should be centrifuged immediately or placed on ice until it can be processed.

After centrifugation, a sample of the sediment cells should be taken and placed on a microscope slide, air dried and stained with Wright or Romanowsky stain (Diff-Quik).

At least 200 cells should be counted per field to determine the differential cell count.

Bronchoscopy. Involves a certain risk and will rarely be necessary to establish an accurate diagnosis of asthma in a feline patient. However, sometimes it can be useful to try to eliminate other pathological processes for differential diagnosis. Bronchoscopy in feline asthma reveals erythema and oedema of the mucosa, and a reduction of airway luminal diameter; excessive mucus and mucous plugs can sometimes be observed.

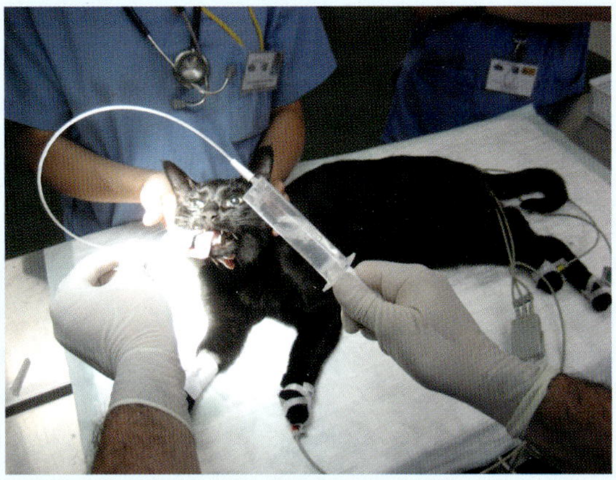

Figure 4.43. Blind bronchoalveolar lavage.

8. A sample has been extracted for a complete blood count. What would be the findings that are compatible with this condition?

In cats with asthma there may be a stress leucogram, but it is not specific. Similarly, 20% of cats with feline asthma have peripheral eosinophilia.

9. 24 hours go by and the animal is stable and goes home. What treatment and other recommendations would you give? Choose between the drugs available in the pharmacy, and do not forget the dosage and long-term management until the next check-up, which will be in 15 days; it is therefore advisable to carefully write all instructions down for the owner.

Long-term oral glucocorticoids with a periodical reduction in dose until the cat stabilizes: Estilsona drops 0.6 ml/12 h PO (1 ml of Estilsona contains 6.6 mg of prednisolone) for 5 days. Another possibility is Dacortin 5, 1 tablet/12 h PO (5 mg prednisone per tablet) for 5 days. After 5 days the corticoid should be administered every 24 hours and then every 48 hours. This dosage can be modified according to the patient's response.

Bronchodilators such as Terbasmin oral solution can be administered at a rate of 2 ml/24 h PO (0.625 mg of terbutaline); or Theolair retard, PO half a tablet at night (87.5 mg of theophylline).

10. The patient continues with treatment as recommended, and at the first check-up the owner mentions that he has not had more serious episodes like the previous one, but that occasionally he suffers from coughing fits (twice per week). The owner has been checking on the Internet and has seen that inhalers can be used. Give appropriate instructions for an inhaler and how to use it.

Inhalation chambers can be purchased through the website www.aerokat.com, and the instructions for administration using the inhalers are available on the website and in the instruction manual.

It can also be purchased through Henry Schein, and the cost from this company – which has a good distribution network to veterinary clinics – is approximately 110 euros (as of 2019).

This inhalation chamber can be used for the administration of inhaled glucocorticoids such as Flixodite (250 mcg fluticasone/application), applied twice per day for at least 10 days. Subsequently the dose can be reduced according to the patient's clinical response and periodic veterinary check-ups, with up to one application every 2 days.

It can also be used for the administration of bronchodilators such as Ventolin (salbutamol 100 mcg/application), but always depending on the patient's needs (asthma attacks).

How to administer inhaled medication to a patient:

A. Shake the inhaler several times and insert the metered dose inhaler into the spacer chamber connected to the mask.
B. Keep the unit on the face of the cat to avoid leaks.
C. Press the inhaler as far as it will go, to introduce the drug into the spacer chamber.
D. Keep it in place for 10–15 breaths.
E. If two inhalations are necessary, wait at least 1–2 minutes before repeating the procedure.
F. If the animal is frightened when pressing the inhaler, it can be pressed before placing the mask on the cat, but doing so means that a lower dose is available for intake and therefore a second application may be necessary to ensure the administration of sufficient levels of medication.
G. In the case of giving fluticasone and albuterol together, always start with the bronchodilator.

Inhalation therapy with glucocorticoids

Fluticasone propionate is an inhaled glucocorticoid administered by metered dose inhaler connected to a spacer chamber and mask, and can be used as an alternative to systemic steroid therapy. The doses used range between 100 and 250 µg every 12 or 24 hours, depending on the severity of the condition. Due to its low oral bioavailability, fluticasone is not associated with the same adverse effects seen with the long-term use of prednisolone.

During the first 10 days of inhalation therapy, prednisolone should be administered concomitantly, 14 mg/kg/1–2 h VO, to allow time for fluticasone to reach its maximum effect.

Material necessary for the administration of inhalation therapy in cats: metered dose inhaler that dispenses the product into the spacer chamber, and face mask to adapt to the patient's face.

To administer pharmaceutical products via inhalation in a cat, the mask must remain firmly placed on the face of the patient for 7–10 breaths.

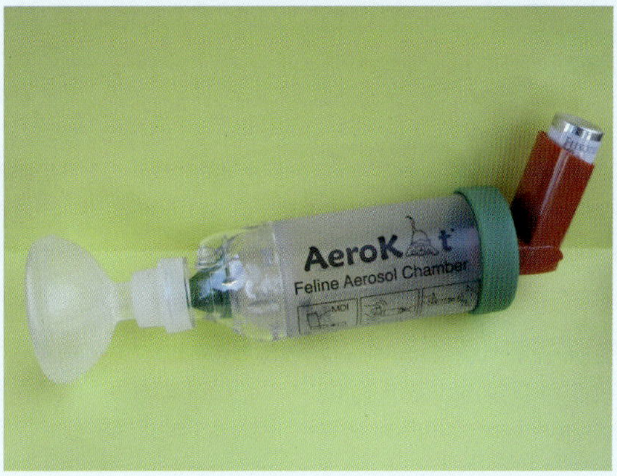

Figure 4.44. Metered dose inhaler and face mask.

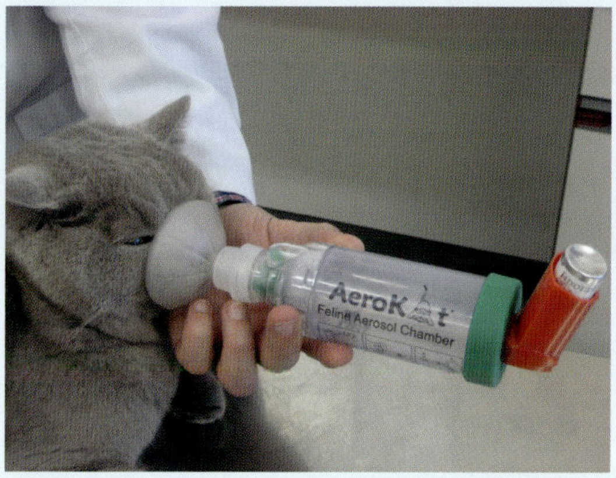

Figure 4.45. Administration of inhaled medications in a cat.

Correct answers:

Test

1. B	7. C	13. C
2. D	8. A	14. D
3. C	9. C	15. A
4. C	10. C	16. A
5. D	11. B	
6. C	12. B	

Cardiovascular system disorders

5

Ma Josefa Fernández del Palacio

Chapter summary

During the average working day in practice, most vets can expect to see several animals that have some form of heart disease. This may be the puppy presented for vaccination that has a murmur, or the elderly cat presented collapsed with a gallop rhythm. One of the challenges facing the clinician is to assess the significance of the clinical signs and decide what form of investigation is warranted or, indeed, whether the condition is life-threatening and requires urgent stabilisation.

To answer these questions the clinician has a number of tools, not least of which is a thorough clinical examination. Something as simple as standing back and watching the patient's demeanour, body condition and breathing pattern gives valuable information about whether the problem is acute or chronic.

Also invaluable is an understanding of the significance of different heart sounds and rhythms, along with clinical findings such as pulse quality and mucous membrane colour. This enables the clinician to make crucial decisions about whether emergency stabilisation is necessary or whether it is acceptable simply to monitor the patient at regular intervals.

Tests such as radiology, ultrasound and electrocardiographs are helpful in making this diagnosis. But this requires the clinician to feel confident about their use and interpreting the data obtained. The purpose of this chapter is to equip the veterinarian with the information necessary to fulfil all of the above. The chapter includes a comprehensive overview of common cardiac diseases, both congenital and acquired, in the dog and cat, to give the reader a sound grasp of the diagnosis, treatment and prognosis of those heart conditions likely to be encountered in practice.

Key learning points

- Understand the significance of different types of heart murmur.
- Acquire competence at performing echocardiography.
- Interpret electrocardiograms (ECGs).
- Understand the different types of heart disease.
- Know how to treat arrhythmias.
- Understand heart therapeutics and drug selection.

The prevalence of cardiovascular conditions

Heart disease is common. Of those animals presented at veterinary clinics, around 2–5% of dogs and 3–4% of cats have some form of cardiopathy (although the exact percentage varies depending on whether the centre is a first opinion practice or a referral centre).

Risk factors

There are numerous risk factors that predispose small animals to cardiovascular disease. The most significant factors are listed below.

- **Species**: There are important differences between congenital and acquired heart diseases in dogs and cats.
- **Age**:
  - Young animals are more likely to present with congenital disorders than acquired disease. This said, if the defects are minor they can lead a normal life for years, until detected by chance in adulthood.
  - Older animals are more likely to present with acquired conditions, such as degenerative mitral valve disease in dogs or restrictive cardiomyopathy in cats.
  - Certain conditions, such as dilated cardiomyopathy in dogs and hypertrophic cardiomyopathy in cats, can affect a wide range of ages. However, they mainly present in adult animals.

- **Breed**: In dogs, certain breeds are prone to congenital or acquired disease. In cats there is a breed predisposition to hypertrophic cardiomyopathy.
- **Sex**:
  - Dogs: Males are particularly susceptible to atrioventricular valve insufficiency (endocardiosis) and dilated cardiomyopathy. Patent ductus arteriosus mainly affects females.
  - Cats: Males appear more susceptible than females to hypertrophic cardiomyopathy.
- **Extracardiac disorders**: Some systemic disorders have the potential to affect the heart. For example, hypoadrenocorticism can cause arrhythmias, while chronic renal disease and hyperadrenocorticism can cause hypertension.
- **Geographical location**: Parasitic diseases such as dirofilariasis and leishmaniasis are prevalent in warmer regions. They can trigger heart disease as a result of cor pulmonale and also systemic hypertension (secondary to chronic renal insufficiency). Also, in dogs, certain bloodlines have a higher prevalence of heart disease, according to their distribution in different countries.

Despite all the different risk factors one statistic is clear, which is that acquired heart diseases are more common than congenital cardiac problems.

Prevalence of acquired heart disease in dogs

Chronic valvular disease

Representing **44% of all cardiopathies**, chronic valve disease is the most common heart disease in older, small-breed dogs.

The **breeds** which are commonly most affected include the Poodle, Maltese, Pekinese, Pomeranian, Miniature Schnauzer, Yorkshire Terrier, Dachshund, Chihuahua, Lhasa Apso and mongrels.

Cavalier King Charles Spaniels are an exception with regards to age, as they can present with the disease at any age from 1 year old onwards. Some medium and large dog breeds, such as the Cocker Spaniel, Boxer and German Shepherd, can also suffer from chronic valvular heart disease. Males are have a higher predisposition than females.

Dilated cardiomyopathy

Dilated cardiomyopathy constitutes **15% of all heart diseases** and affects middle-aged to old dogs of medium and large breeds: American Cocker Spaniel, Doberman, Boxer, Great Dane, Irish Wolfhound, German Shepherd, Spanish Mastiff and Neapolitan Mastiff.

Portuguese Water Dogs are an exception with respect to age, as they can present with a juvenile form of dilated cardiomyopathy. Males are usually more commonly affected than females (with a ratio of 2:1).

Pericardial effusions and cardiac neoplasms

Pericardial effusion and cardiac neoplasms constitute **10% of all heart diseases**.

Idiopathic pericarditis is the most common pericardial disorder. **Neoplasia** is the cause of effusion in 35–50% of cases. The most common primary neoplasms are right atrial haemangiosarcomas in German Shepherds and Golden Retrievers, and chemodectomas of the heart base in brachycephalic breeds.

The breeds which are most commonly affected are the Golden Retriever, German Shepherd, Labrador Retriever, German Pointer and Akita.

Primary arrhythmias

Primary arrhythmias constitute approximately **8% of all heart diseases**. They can be secondary to structural heart disease, but also primary disorders associated with certain breeds.

The most common primary arrhythmias are as follows.

- **Sick sinus syndrome**. This has a high incidence in Miniature Schnauzers, with a female to male ratio of 3:1. Breed predisposition has also been described in Pomeranians, Boxers, Cocker Spaniels and West Highland White Terriers.
- **Persistent atrial standstill**. In Springer Spaniels and Labradors and also in Siamese cats.

Other processes

Other less common processes, which represent 3–5% of all heart disease, include endocarditis, systemic hypertension and dirofilariasis.

Prevalence of congenital heart disease in dogs

Congenital heart diseases constitute **0.5% to 1.5%** of the canine clinical population and **18% of all heart diseases**.

The breeds worst affected by the most commonly diagnosed congenital heart diseases are listed below (from most to least commonly affected).

- **Patent ductus arteriosus**. Maltese, Poodle, Keeshond, Bichon Frise, Pomeranian, Yorkshire Terrier, English Springer Spaniel, Alsatian, Cocker Spaniel, Chihuahua, Miniature Schnauzer, German Shepherd, Collie, Golden Retriever and Labrador Retriever. This anomaly affects females more often than males, with a ratio of 3:1.

- **Pulmonary stenosis**. Bulldog, Scottish Terrier, Miniature Schnauzer, West Highland White Terrier, Chihuahua, Samoyed, Yorkshire Terrier, Cocker Spaniel, German Shepherd, Collie, Golden Retriever, Labrador Retriever and Beagle.
- **Aortic/subaortic stenosis**. Newfoundland, Boxer, Golden Retriever, Rottweiler and German Shepherd. Some authors have also mentioned the Samoyed, Great Dane and English Bulldog.
- **Ventricular septal defect**. West Highland White Terrier, English Springer Spaniel, Basset Hound, English Bulldog, Akita, Shih Tzu, Poodle, Husky, Chow Chow, Beagle and Labrador Retriever.
- **Tricuspid valve dysplasia.** Labrador and Golden Retrievers, German Shepherd and English Shepherd.
- **Mitral valve dysplasia.** Great Dane, German Shepherd, Bull Terrier and Newfoundland.
- **Tetralogy of Fallot**. Breeds which very commonly suffer from pulmonary stenosis and ventricular septal defects are at risk: West Highland White Terrier, Wire Fox Terrier and Keeshond, in particular.
- **Atrial septal defects**. Boxer and Newfoundland. Some authors have suggested a predisposition in the Doberman and Samoyed.

Prevalence of acquired heart disease in cats

Acquired heart diseases constitute **80% of all feline** heart diseases. The most common of these are listed below.

- **Cardiomyopathies**. Hypertrophic (the most common), restrictive, dilated, not classified and arrhythmogenic right ventricular cardiomyopathy. These constitute 70% of all heart diseases. Although hypertrophic cardiomyopathy can occur in any breed, the most commonly affected breeds include the Maine Coon, Persian, Norwegian Forest, Sphynx, American and British Shorthair and Ragdoll.
- **Other disorders**. Pericardial effusion, neoplasia, arrhythmias and systemic hypertension constitute 8% of feline heart disorders.

Prevalence of congenital heart disease in cats

These constitute approximately **12%** of all feline heart disease.

- **Septal defects** are the most common, followed by atrioventricular valve dysplasia, tetralogy of Fallot and, less often, pulmonary stenosis, aortic stenosis and patent ductus arteriosus.

Clinical history and physical examination of the cardiovascular system

Certain heart diseases can be **detected** at an **early stage** on a routine physical examination. This is a characteristic peculiar to the cardiovascular system, in contrast to other organs and systems.

Data obtained from medical records and the physical examination also provide valuable information to establish a diagnosis, monitor disease progression and determine initial interventions (such as oxygen therapy). The physical exam can also suggest additional procedures and techniques required to complete the examination, such as arterial pressure, radiology, electrocardiography, echocardiography and laboratory analysis.

Clinical history

The purpose of the clinical history is to **detect** heart disease, **differentiate** between cardiac, respiratory and systemic disorders, and monitor how a condition is progressing and/or the **response** to treatment.

Information about the animal's signalment is key, as certain heart diseases are more prevalent in a particular species, age group, breed or sex.

The consultation (anamnesis) with the animal's owner enables information about the patient's signalment (species, age, breed and sex) to be collected, and the medical history plus the reason for consultation (current clinical signs) ascertained.

Questions can be grouped into three sections as described below.

#1: General questions

Questions about signs relating to **general health** such asking about diet, parasite control, vaccination status, exposure to infectious disease and any current medication. This also includes asking about the reason for the consultation.

#2: Questions about signs frequently associated with cardiac disorders

General questions including **onset and duration** of clinical signs (acute or chronic), behaviour and level of exercise tolerance.

The client's awareness of clinical signs related to the cardiovascular system and progression of heart disease are significantly different in cats and dogs.

In dogs, heart disease tends to develop gradually.

Cat owners rarely observe early clinical signs related to heart disease. **Acute** and progressive onset (24–48 hours) is the most common presentation, with difficulty breathing and/or paralysis (aortic thromboembolism). Signs such as lethargy and reduced appetite may have appeared previously and be of variable duration, but not attributed to heart disease.

#3: Questions about signs related to other body systems or organs

This includes questions about appetite, water consumption, urinary habits, defaecation, vomiting or regurgitation, seizures, syncopal episodes, reproductive state, lameness (possible endocarditis) or paresis, previous illnesses or injuries, geographical location where the animal lives, or has been living (dirofilariasis).

Signs most frequently associated with heart disease

Exercise intolerance

This is usually due to the inability of the cardiovascular system to maintain cardiac output and tissue perfusion. Fatigue is caused by deviation of deoxygenated blood to the systemic circulation and, in disorders such as tetralogy of Fallot, secondary polycythaemia.

Respiratory signs

The clinician should try to discern whether the clinical signs are of **cardiac or respiratory** origin.

One of the most typical clinical signs is a **cough**. This reflex is stimulated by mechanical or chemical agents which mainly affect the pharynx, larynx, trachea and main bronchi.

- **In cats**, coughing is associated with **bronchial disease** and only rarely with heart disease.
- **In dogs**, coughing is caused by **tracheobronchial** conditions (tracheobronchitis, tracheal collapse, neoplasms) as well as by **heart diseases** which give rise to dilation of the left atrium, compressing the left main bronchus. This occurs in small-breed dogs with chronic degenerative mitral valve disease. In these cases, coughing can be the result of a combination of both conditions (cardiopathy and tracheobronchial disorders).

The nature of the cough and the time of day at which it occurs can help differentiate the condition responsible.

- Coughs with a **cardiac origin** are **worse at night**, except in late stages, when they also occur during the day.
- **Tracheal collapse** produces a characteristic **'goose honk'** cough, caused by nervousness, pressure from a collar or drinking water.

Syncope

Syncope can be defined as a sudden and **temporary loss of consciousness** and postural tone with spontaneous recovery.

It is caused by a sudden **cessation of blood flow** to the brain and it can be secondary to **heart** diseases (arrhythmias, heart failure) or **vasovagal** (neurocardiogenic), but the cause is impossible to determine in over 50% of patients, given the complexity of its aetiology.

Clinical signs do not always present in the same way; when blood flow is only partially reduced, symptoms are characterised by weakness, collapse or ataxia, without syncope.

When cerebral hypoxia is prolonged, **convulsions** may occur, particularly in severe bradyarrhythmias. In cats, syncope of cardiovascular origin can occasionally present with neurological signs, so it is important to differentiate between the two. In general, the prognosis for neurological syncope is better than for those associated with heart disease.

Other signs related to cardiovascular disorders

Different types of heart disease present different signs.

In dogs:

- Reduced growth (patent ductus arteriosus [PDA] in large dog breeds, tetralogy of Fallot).
- Weight loss (late-stage congestive heart failure).
- Vomiting and diarrhoea (right-sided heart failure).
- Oliguria (reduced renal perfusion due to left-sided heart failure).

In cats:

- Hindlimb paralysis (aortic thromboembolism secondary to heart disease).

Physical examination

Despite advances in technology, the **traditional methods** of examination (inspection/observation, palpation, percussion and auscultation) persist. They are very cost-effective and highly appropriate for patients in a critical state. Data obtained from physical examination can indicate whether clinical signs may be due to a cardiac disorder or are pathognomonic of one, and whether they should influence the **differential diagnoses**.

The physical examination should be carried out **systematically** to ensure nothing is overlooked. The examination should be extended to other organs and systems because non-cardiac disorders can be involved in the functioning of the cardiovascular system and certain clinical signs can be common to different systems.

Physical examination consists of **general observation** of the patient and examination of the:

- head (mucous membranes)
- neck (jugular veins)
- thorax (palpation of the precordium, auscultation)
- abdomen (presence of effusion, organomegaly)
- extremities (temperature, femoral pulse).

General observation of the patient

The first thing to consider is the animal's posture, and the pattern, frequency, duration and effort of respiration. This helps determine whether the condition can be managed or urgent intervention (oxygen therapy) is required. The patient's body condition and behaviour are also important.

Posture

Dogs refuse recumbency when suffering from pulmonary oedema or pleural effusion. Patients with pulmonary alveolar oedema adopt an **orthopneic position** (or 'air hunger' position) characterised by abducted elbows, extended neck and open mouth breathing.

Cats with breathing difficulties often position themselves in **sternal recumbency**.

Respiratory rate and rhythm

Tachypnoea and panting in dogs can be caused by excitement during examination, but can also be signs of respiratory insufficiency.

Respiratory pattern/dyspnoea

Dyspnoea consists of laboured and abnormal breathing, which in severe cases constitutes an emergency. The respiratory phase in which the dypsnoea occurs (inspiratory, expiratory, restrictive, paradoxical) should be determined, along with the degree of breathing difficulty.

The aetiology can often be determined from the form the dypsnoea takes.

- **Inspiratory dyspnoea** is characterised by a prolonged and **laboured inspiratory phase**. It is a sign of upper respiratory tract obstruction when accompanied by breathing sounds (brachycephalic syndrome and laryngeal disorders in dogs, and upper respiratory tract infection in cats) or difficulty expanding the lungs (pleural effusion, diaphragmatic dysfunction or profuse peritoneal effusions).
- **Expiratory dyspnoea** is characterised by **difficulty eliminating air** from the lungs due to reduced pulmonary elasticity (pulmonary oedema, pneumonia) or narrowing of the lower airways (feline bronchial disease).
- **Restrictive dyspnoea** is characterised by rapid, short, forced breaths, which are a sign of pleural effusion, pneumonia and pulmonary oedema.

A **paradoxical respiratory pattern** is characteristic of fractured ribs and diaphragm dysfunction.

Causes of **acute dyspnoea** include foreign bodies, laryngeal oedema, massive pulmonary embolism and pneumothorax.

In cats, acute forms of congestive heart failure with pulmonary oedema and pleural effusion can be detected by the owner.

Chronic dyspnoea tends to be due to bronchial conditions (feline asthma), interstitial lung disease and heart disease.

Body condition

Animals with congestive heart failure can appear weakened and **emaciated** (loss of muscle mass) due to insufficient tissue perfusion and the release of cytokines. Many dogs with chronic **pulmonary diseases** (bronchitis, fibrosis, tracheal collapse) are **obese**.

Examination of the head

This includes examination of the **mucous membranes** (pink, pale, dark red, cyanotic) and **capillary refill time**, as well as possible buccal conditions, as described below.

- **Pale mucous membranes** can be due to anaemia, insufficient cardiac output or increased sympathetic tone (stress during the consultation).
- **Dark red coloured** mucous membranes can be a sign of polycythaemia, sepsis or nervousness.
- **Cyanosis** (blue-coloured mucous membranes) can be a sign of **airway obstruction**, conditions affecting the pulmonary parenchyma and pleural space, **pulmonary oedema**, congenital heart defects which cause a left–right shunt, hypoventilation and **shock**. When cyanosis predominates in the caudal mucous membranes (differential cyanosis) this indicates shunt reversal (pulmonary artery towards the descending aorta) through a PDA (although no murmur is detected).
- **Increased capillary refill time** (**>2 s**) may suggest low cardiac output (subaortic and pulmonary stenosis), but also dehydration, increased sympathetic tone and vasoconstriction.

Cats with **heart disease** can present with **normal mucosal colour** and capillary refill times.

Examination of the neck

Examination of the **jugular veins** provides valuable data on central venous pressure (right-sided chambers). When

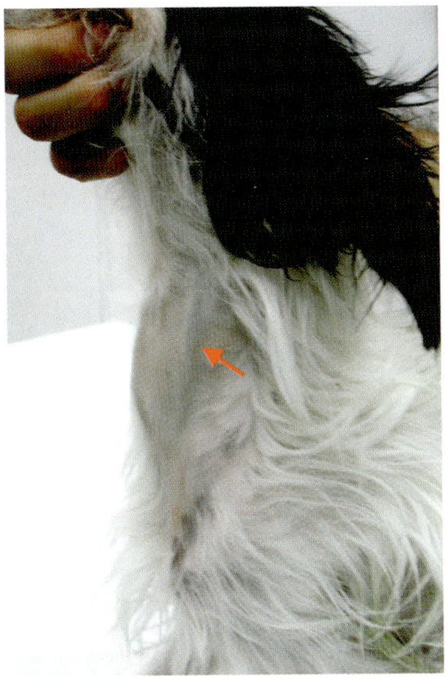

Figure 5.1. Image of the neck of a dog with significant tricuspid insufficiency, showing distension of the left jugular vein (arrow).

the animal is standing, with the head and neck in a normal position, the jugular veins should not be distended.

Distension occurs when right heart filling pressures increase (tricuspid stenosis, pericardial effusion/tamponade) or the superior vena cava is obstructed, making venous return difficult (Figure 5.1). In dogs with neoplasms in the mediastinum or heart base which constrict the superior vena cava, there may be variable degrees of swelling of the neck and thoracic inlet (superior vena cava syndrome).

Distension combined with pulsation (up to the level of the scapula) is observed during the course of various right-sided heart diseases, with reduced compliance (ventricular hypertrophy, severe tricuspid insufficiency) or atrioventricular (AV) dissociation (complete AV block). As a rule, **distension of the jugular veins** in a dog with **ascites** suggests **cardiac** aetiology. This distension can be accentuated by pressing the abdomen with both hands just behind the xiphoid process of the sternum (hepatojugular reflux).

Examination of the thorax

Evaluation of the thorax includes observing respiratory movements (as described above), palpation of the precordium, percussion and auscultation.

Palpation and percussion

The thorax should be palpated to detect anomalies such as pectus excavatum, and changes in heartbeat intensity or precordial fremitus. Palpable heartbeat intensity is a product of the pressure in the ventricular chamber and its diameter against the thoracic wall. An increased intensity can be interpreted as due to increased force of contraction or ventricular dilation. Heartbeat intensity is also high in animals which are very thin or hyperdynamic due to anaemia and fever.

The palpable heartbeat can be reduced or absent in obese animals, but this can also be indicative of fluid (pleural or pericardial effusion) or a mass interposed between the heart and the thoracic wall. Detection of precordial fremitus (a vibration transmitted to the chest wall) is indicative of a loud heart murmur (5/6 and 6/6).

Although currently less widely used, percussion of the thorax can be useful to determine the presence of pleural effusion or pneumothorax in animals with dyspnoea.

Auscultation

Despite technical advances in cardiac diagnostics, chest auscultation, which is safe for critically ill patients and accessible to all clinicians, continues to be considered a key part of cardiac semiology. It should be carried out systematically, auscultating the respiratory system and heart separately as it impossible to concentrate on both at the same time.

Auscultation of the respiratory system

Normal sounds are called bronchovesicular sounds, and are soft sounds produced by the passage of air through the airways. These are more audible in the trachea and its bifurcation, and intensity decreases in the distal areas of the lungs. They can be accentuated in cases of tachypnoea, nervousness or stress, and intensity diminishes with fluid or pneumothorax.

Pathological sounds audible on auscultation are listed below.

- **Crepitations**. These are sounds similar to those produced by opening velcro and there are two types.
  - **Soft and inspiratory**, generated by the movement of air through a fluid. These are associated with pulmonary oedema, pneumonia and pulmonary haemorrhage.
  - **Strong and discontinuous**, generated by sudden equalisation of pressure between open and closed airways. These are specific to fibrosis and chronic bronchitis.
- **Whistling**. Musical sounds, usually continuous, caused by the movement of air through narrow airways. These occur in primary bronchial diseases (bronchitis and feline asthma).

Auscultation of the heart

This includes evaluation of heart rate, rhythm and sounds. Some factors must be considered before starting auscultation, such as the stethoscope to be used and the main areas of auscultation for heart sounds.

The use of an appropriate stethoscope is essential for detailed auscultation. The use of a paediatric stethoscope is recommended in cats and small-breed dogs, to avoid exceeding the cardiac projection area. The diaphragm can be used to assess most high-frequency heart sounds (first and second heart sounds and systolic murmurs) and respiratory sounds and the bell transmits low-frequency sounds better (gallop heart sounds and some diastolic murmurs). Sufficient time (1–2 minutes) should be dedicated to auscultation, to enable detection of discrete murmurs and transient arrhythmias.

The clinician may sometimes need to hold their breath momentarily so that heart and respiratory sounds can be differentiated. Auscultation should therefore be considered a dynamic examination, encompassing the whole thorax, covering each valve area, the thoracic inlet and the carotid arteries (to detect normal sounds and their propagation). Simultaneous auscultation and palpation of the pulse is essential in a thorough cardiovascular examination.

The two main areas of auscultation include the heart apex and base in each hemithorax. The first heart sound is heard best at the apex, in the mitral area, and the second sound over the left heart base (pulmonary area).

Heart sounds can be accentuated in cases of cardiomegaly and in hyperdynamic states, and they can be muffled by most pericardial and pleural effusions. Displacement of heart sounds can indicate thoracic masses or peritoneal–pericardial diaphragmatic hernias.

Heart rate

Heart rate varies greatly according to species, age, breed and nervous state.

Normal values range from 70–140 bpm in dogs and 140–200 bpm in cats. Heart rate can be raised in patients with heart failure and also those in hyperdynamic states.

Heart rhythm

In **dogs**, regular sinus rhythm and **sinus arrhythmia** (a regularly irregular rhythm) are considered physiological.

Sinus arrhythmia is common in brachycephalic breeds and is associated with **increased vagal tone.** It usually coincides with the respiratory phase; the heart accelerates during inspiration and slows during expiration. In these cases, the intensity of normal heart sounds may be variable. Sinus arrhythmia disappears in patients with heart failure and can be accentuated in patients with severe pulmonary disease.

In cats, only **regular sinus rhythm** is considered normal.

A femoral pulse which does not coincide with the heartbeat is indicative of **premature beats** or **atrial fibrillation**; in the case of the latter, a pulse rate of 100 bpm and a heart rate of 180–220 bpm is typical. Other clinically significant arrhythmias, such as **ventricular tachycardia**, cause an abrupt change in heart rate and heart sound intensity. In the group of **bradyarrhythmias**, complete (third-degree) heart block causes bradycardia with a marked increase in pulse strength.

Heart sounds

Normal heart sounds heard using auscultation of the heart in healthy dogs and cats are as follows.

- **First heart sound (S1),** generated by vibrations and tension from closure of the atrioventricular valves.
- **Second heart sound (S2),** generated by closure of the aortic and pulmonary valves.

Abnormal sounds, usually associated with heart diseases, are called murmurs and are described below.

Murmurs

Gallop sounds include the combination of **S1 and S2**, together with **S3 or S4**. S3 is a low-frequency sound, generated by rapid ventricular filling and systolic dysfunction (dilated cardiomyopathy). S4 is caused by contraction of the atrium forcibly ejecting blood towards a ventricle with reduced compliance (hypertrophic or restrictive cardiomyopathy).

Murmurs are more prolonged than normal S1 and S2 sounds. They are produced by vibrations within the cardiovascular system, caused by **turbulent blood flow** in heart diseases. Typical causes include valvular insufficiencies, obstruction of the ventricular outflow tract (pulmonary and aortic stenosis), communication between chambers and great vessels (septal defects, patent ductus arteriosus) and reduced blood viscosity (anaemia).

However, some murmurs are not related to heart disease; these include physiological murmurs associated with hyperdynamic states and exercise, and innocent murmurs, typical of puppies, which tend to disappear after 16 weeks of age.

Classifying murmurs according to the phase of the cardiac cycle in which they are heard, intensity and pitch, and area of maximum intensity can assist with their interpretation. Both innocent and physiological murmurs occur during systole and are low intensity. They are auscultated better at the heart base, can change with heart rate from one day to the next, and also vary with body position.

Murmurs in the cardiac cycle are classified according to their timing and duration.

Systolic murmurs are the **most common** murmur in small animals. They appear during systole, from the onset of S1 to the onset of S2 and are divided into the following types.

- **Holosystolic**. Occupy the whole of systole but allow normal sounds to be heard.
- **Pansystolic**. Prevent normal sounds being heard.
- **Crescendo–decrescendo or ejection murmurs**. Characteristic of ventricular outflow tract obstruction (left, subaortic stenosis; right, pulmonary stenosis) and increased blood flow (anaemia, stress, fever, physiological).

Diastolic murmurs are uncommon in small animals. They occur during diastole, between the onset of S2 and the onset of S1. They can be classified as follows.

- **Protodiastolic**. Characteristic of aortic and pulmonary regurgitation.
- **Mid-diastolic**. Characteristic of mitral and tricuspid stenosis.
- **Continuous murmurs**. Start in systole and end in diastole, as the pressure gradient which permits blood to flow from an area of high pressure to one of low pressure is maintained throughout the entire cardiac cycle. Typical of patent ductus arteriosus, pulmonary arteriovenous fistula and aortopulmonary defects.
- **To-and-fro murmur**. When systolic and diastolic murmurs co-exist. Characteristic of dogs with aortic insufficiency associated with subaortic stenosis or ventricular septal defects (prolapse of one of the sigmoids through the defect).

Murmurs are graded according to intensity, as follows.

- **Grade I/VI murmur**. Very quiet and only detectable in a quiet room after auscultation for several seconds.
- **Grade II/VI murmur**. Also quiet, but easily auscultated.
- **Grade III/VI murmur**. Moderately loud.
- **Grade IV/VI murmur**. Loud, with no accompanying fremitus.
- **Grade V/VI murmur**. Very loud, accompanied by fremitus.
- **Grade VI/VI murmur**. Very loud murmur which is heard even when the stethoscope is raised just above the thoracic wall.

In dogs, there is positive correlation between murmur intensity and the severity of pulmonary and aortic stenosis, and the clinical stage of chronic degenerative mitral valve disease.

The area of maximum intensity corresponds to the area in which the murmurs are most intense and easily audible (Figure 5.2).

Mitral valve area. The area of maximum intensity for the murmurs caused by mitral valve diseases (mitral valve dysplasia, degenerative mitral valve disease and dilated cardiomyopathy). This is located over the left ventricular apex (5th intercostal space towards the sternum), although these murmurs sometimes radiate towards the heart base and right hemithorax.

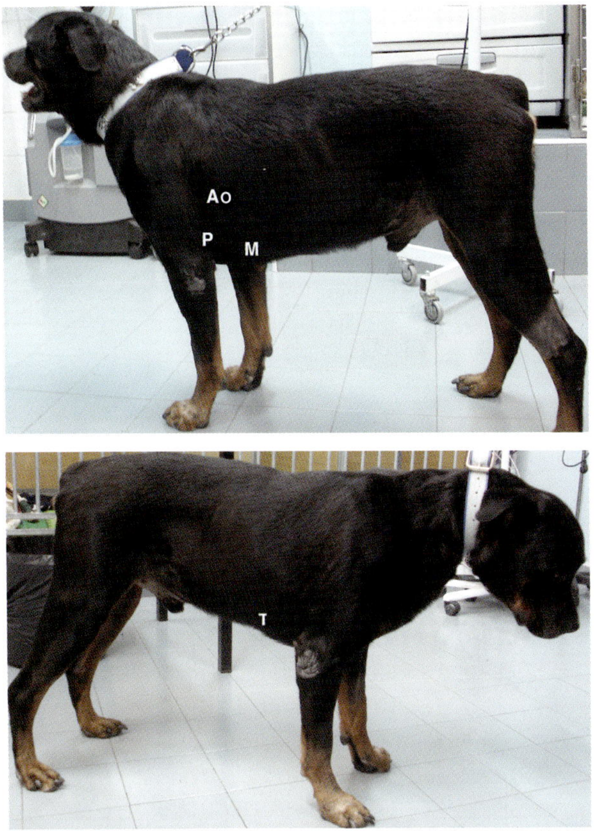

Figure 5.2 (a, b). Images showing the areas of heart auscultation in the dog. Ao, aortic; M, mitral; P, pulmonary; T, tricuspid.

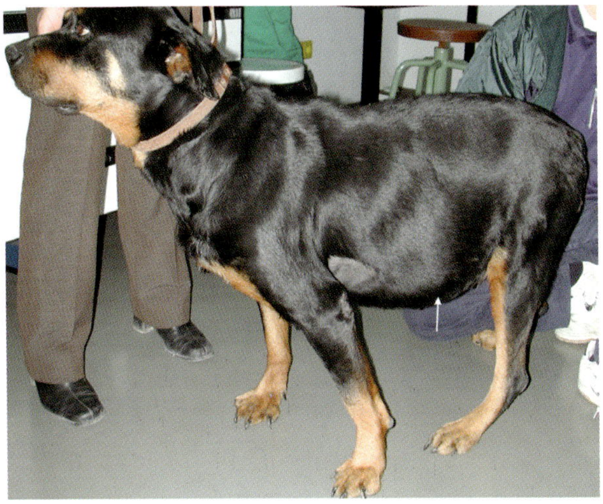

Figure 5.3. Rottweiler with right-sided congestive heart failure due to cardiac tamponade. The image shows an enlarged abdomen (arrow) and ascites.

Aortic valve area. Located over the left heart base, at the level of the 3rd to 4th intercostal spaces. Murmurs caused by aortic stenosis are heard in this area, and in the upper right hemithorax, and radiate towards the ventricular apex.

Pulmonary valve area. This is located over the left heart base, somewhat higher than the aortic area. It is the point of maximum intensity for murmurs due to stenosis and pulmonary insufficiency, which are also heard in the upper right hemithorax.

Tricuspid valve area. This is located over the 4th intercostal space in the right hemithorax, over the costochondral joint. Tricuspid regurgitation murmurs are heard most intensely here.

Other areas:

- Murmurs corresponding to perimembranous ventricular septal defects are heard most intensely over the upper right hemithorax, towards the sternum.
- Murmurs due to patent ductus arteriosus are heard most intensely over the heart base in both hemithoraces, radiating towards the thoracic inlet.

Examination of the abdomen

The abdomen should be examined for ascites or organomegaly, secondary to right-sided congestive heart failure (Figure 5.3); this is usually consistent with a modified transudate or chyle.

In cats, ascites due to cardiac disease is very rare and the list of differential diagnoses should include non-cardiac causes. However, hepatomegaly of the caudate lobe of the liver can be observed in cats with right-sided heart failure.

Examination of the limbs

The limbs should be examined with attention paid to temperature, muscle tone, peripheral oedema and femoral pulse characteristics. Animals with reduced cardiac output or cats with thromboembolism can present with cold extremities.

Femoral pulse

Examination of the femoral pulse provides valuable information on pulse rate, quality, rhythm, synchrony with heartbeat and symmetry in the extremities. The pressure detected by palpation of the pulse corresponds to the difference between arterial systolic pressure and diastolic pressure.

Characteristics of the femoral pulse

Reduced pulse pressure, or a weak pulse, can occur when the systolic ejection volume is reduced, as occurs in patients with heart failure, severe aortic or pulmonary stenosis or reduced peripheral resistance.

Increased pulse pressure, or a bounding pulse, can occur in cases of systemic systolic hypertension, or reduced diastolic pressure (aortic insufficiency), or a combination of both (patent ductus arteriosus).

Pulse deficits can be secondary to tachyarrhythmias, as the ventricles do not fill adequately because diastole is very short.

Paradoxical pulse, or reduced pulse pressure during inspiration and increased during expiration, is typical of pericardial tamponade.

Rectal temperature

A high rectal temperature can suggest infective endocarditis and the opposite, hypothermia, can be a sign of cardiogenic shock and low cardiac output.

Introduction to electrocardiographic diagnosis

The electrocardiogram (ECG) is a graphic record of the electrical activity generated by the heart muscle during each cardiac cycle. Signals are detected by metal electrodes placed on the extremities and the thoracic wall; these are then amplified and captured by the electrocardiogram. Electrocardiographic leads show instantaneous potential differences between the electrodes.

The electrocardiographic trace is recorded on graph paper, with time represented on the horizontal axis and potential difference, shown in millivolts, on the vertical axis (Figure 5.4).

Electrocardiogram measurements

The main clinical indications for an ECG are:

- measuring **heart rate**
- evaluating **heart rhythm** and conduction
- evaluating the effect on the heart of:
  - electrolyte imbalances (hyperkalaemia)
  - medicines (digoxin, anaesthetics)
  - endocrine disorders (hypoadrenocorticism)
- cardiac monitoring of critically ill patients

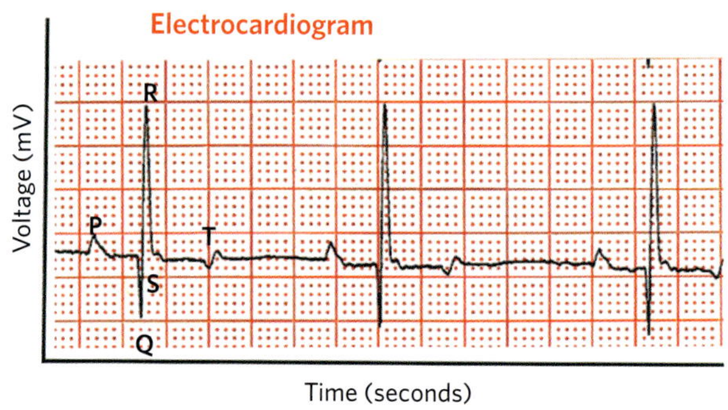

Figure 5.4. Electrocardiographic trace showing electrocardiographic waves: time or duration (s) of waves and intervals on the horizontal axis and voltage on the vertical axis (mV).

- identification of myocardial hypertrophy or enlargement of the heart chambers.

Data obtained from the ECG should be interpreted within the patient's clinical context, along with data from the consultation, physical examination, thoracic radiographs, echocardiography and laboratory analysis, amongst other techniques.

Obtaining the electrocardiographic trace

The standard ECG is taken with the animal in right lateral recumbency on an insulated surface, with the limbs extended perpendicularly to the axis of the body (Figure 5.5). If recumbency is not well tolerated (dyspnoeic animals), the ECG can be taken with the animal standing or in sternal recumbency (especially cats); however, position should be taken into account when interpreting the ECG.

Once the animal is positioned, electrodes are placed at various points on the body surface. Typically, these are attached on the skin under the elbows and knees, using crocodile clips or adhesive discs and applying alcohol or ultrasound gel to improve contact. This detects the difference in potential between two electrodes, one negative and the other positive; each one of these combinations is called a lead.

The **two standard electrode positions** in veterinary medicine are the thorax and the extremities, so that each registers the electrical activity of the heart in different planes.

1. The precordial leads (V1 to V6), which evaluate the heart's electrical activity in the transverse plane, are obtained by placing electrodes on the thorax.
2. The limb leads, which evaluate the heart's electrical activity in the frontal plane, are obtained by placing electrodes on the extremities.

In this chapter the limb leads will be referred to, as they are used most commonly in animals.

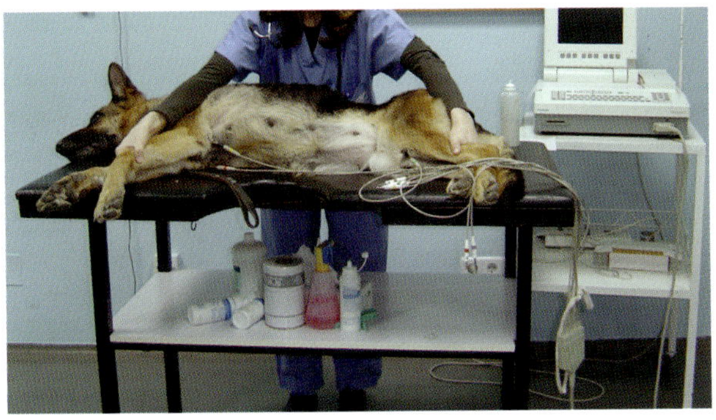

Figure 5.5. The standard position for performing an electrocardiogram in dogs.

Electrodes are placed in the standard position on the extremities as follows.

- Right forelimb (RF).
- Left forelimb (LF).
- Left hindlimb (LH).
- Right hindlimb (RH). This acts as an earth to prevent interference by alternating current from other electrical equipment in the room (Figure 5.5).

The **six leads** that constitute the **hexaxial reference system** used to determine the heart's electrical axis in the frontal plane (Figure 5.6) are obtained as follows.

- Three **bipolar leads.** These form the so-called Einthoven's triangle. They capture electrical activity from the potential difference between each pair of leads.
  - Lead I: potential difference between the electrodes on the left forelimb (positive pole) and the right hindlimb (negative pole).
  - Lead II: potential difference between the electrodes on the right forelimb and the left hindlimb (positive pole).
  - Lead III: potential difference between the left forelimb and left hindlimb.
- Three **unipolar leads.** These use the same electrodes as the bipolar leads, and also measure electrical activity between two of them, but the electrodes that they record are always positive ('a' represents augmented; 'V', vector):
  - aVL: left forelimb
  - aVR: right forelimb
  - aVF: left hindlimb.

The negative terminal corresponds with the average of the other electrodes placed on the extremities and is analogous with the centre of the heart (zero).

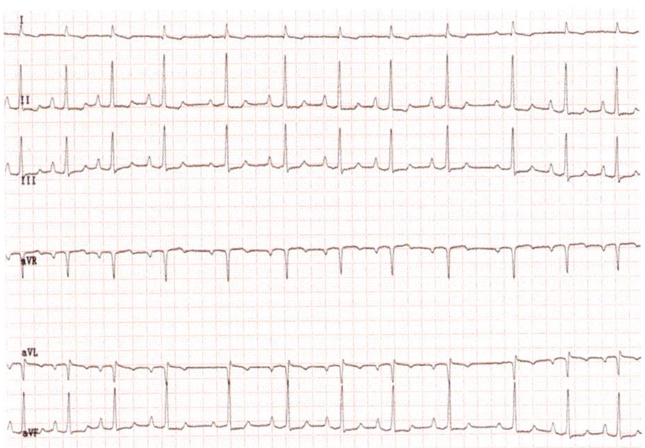

Figure 5.6. Six leads (unipolar and bipolar) from a superficial electrocardiogram in a normal dog showing mild respiratory sinus arrhythmia. 50 mm/s; 1 cm = 1 mV.

Once the electrodes are in place, the following should be selected on the electrocardiograph.

- The **leads**.
- **Paper speed** (mm/s). Paper speed of 50 mm/s is recommended when the heart rate is raised. A speed of 25 mm/s is more appropriate when the heart rate is low.
- **Amplitude** of the waves, based on electrical voltage (millivolts, mV). Standard: 10 mm = 1 mV. If wave voltage is very low, as is the case in cats, sensitivity can be increased (20 mm = 1 mV). If wave voltage is high, sensitivity can be reduced (5 mm = 1 mV), so that the wave trace remains within the margins of the paper and the leads do not overlap.

Electrocardiographic waves

Electrocardiographic waves are generated by propagation of cardiac action potentials through the specialised conduction system and the atrial and ventricular myocardium (Figure 5.4). The electrical impulse generated in the cells of the sinus node moves through the internodal pathways and the atrial myocardium, generating **P waves** on the ECG (representing atrial activation).

When the impulse reaches the atrioventricular node, conduction velocity decreases, which registers as a small isoelectric segment on the ECG trace, contributing to the **PR interval.** The electrical impulse then travels quickly towards the bundle of His and its right and left bundle branches (the left branch is divided into two fascicles: anterior and posterior) to depolarise the ventricles, giving rise to the **QRS complex**, which has several components: the Q wave, R wave and S wave.

Another small isoelectric segment then follows on the ECG, preceding the **T wave** and indicating ventricular repolarisation (the ventricles return to their electrical resting state). The time between onset of the QRS complex and the end of the T wave is the **QT interval**, which represents ventricular depolarisation and repolarisation.

The voltage of each electrocardiographic wave depends on the lead, as shown in Figure 5.6.

Guidelines for ECG interpretation

Once obtained, the ECG should be interpreted systematically.

First, the particular leads used, the quality of the trace, paper speed and calibration should be considered.

Then heart rate, heart rhythm and the mean electrical axis (MEA) are determined and the waves and intervals measured.

Heart rate

Heart rate is very variable, depending on the species and other factors, such as activity level.

- In **dogs**, heart rate ranges between **70 and 160 bpm**.
- In **cats**, it ranges between **120 and 200 bpm**.

Heart rate (number of complexes per minute) can be measured in two ways, as follows.

- If **cardiac rhythm is regular**, heart rate can be determined by measuring the distance between R waves (**RR interval**). If paper speed is 50 mm/s, it is divided by 3000 (60 s × 50 mm/s = 3000), by the RR interval (mm), or by 1500 if paper speed is 25 mm/s.
- If **cardiac rhythm is irregular**, counting the number of **QRS complexes** registered on **15 cm of paper** and **multiplying this by 20** (if trace speed is 50 mm/s), or by 10 (if speed is 25 mm/s) is more appropriate.

Cardiac rhythm

Assessment of cardiac rhythm (the sequence of P-QRS-T waves) should include the following considerations.

1. Is the rhythm (RR intervals) regular or irregular?
2. Are P waves visible?
3. Is a P wave visible before each QRS, and a QRS before each P wave?
4. What is the relationship between P waves and QRS complexes?
5. Are all the QRS complexes equal?
6. Is there a sinus rhythm or ectopic foci (from the atrium, AV junction, ventricle)?
7. What is the heart rate?

Mean electrical axis

The MEA represents the net direction of cardiac depolarisation across the animal's frontal plane.

Normal MEA:

- In dogs, between +40° and +100°.
- In cats, between 0° and +110°.

MEA deviations:

- **Right axis deviation**. Seen in cases of right ventricular hypertrophy or right bundle branch block.
- **Left axis deviation**. Seen in cases of severe left ventricular hypertrophy and partial or complete branch block.

Procedures for measuring MEA

The electrical axis will correspond to the lead perpendicular to the most isoelectric, positive or negative (Figure 5.7).

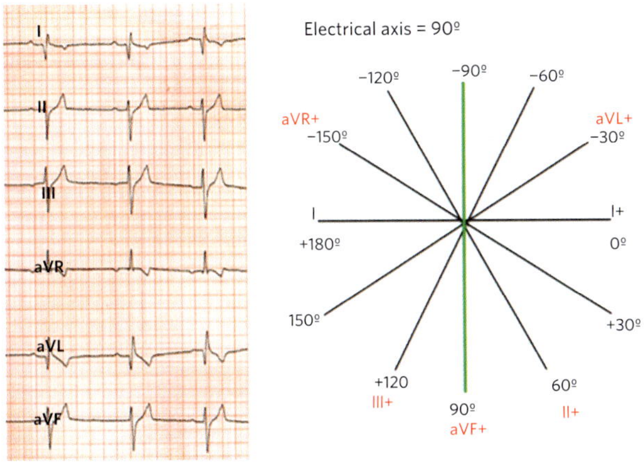

Figure 5.7. Determination of the mean electrical axis of the frontal plane: I is the most isoelectric lead, so the perpendicular lead corresponds to +90° (green line).

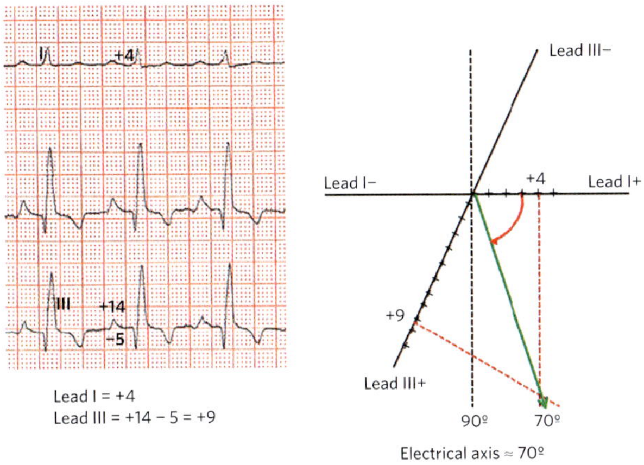

Figure 5.8. Determination of the mean electrical axis in the frontal plane from leads I and III. 50 mm/s; 1 cm = 1 mv.

Table 5.1. Electrocardiographic measurements in healthy dogs and cats (Tilley, 1992).

	Dogs	Cats
Heart rate (bpm)	Large breeds: 60–140 Small breeds: 70–180 Puppies: up to 220	120–240
P wave	Duration: ≤0.04 s Voltage: ≤0.4 mV	Duration: ≤0.04 s Voltage: ≤0.2 mV
PR interval (s)	0.06–0.13	0.05–0.09
QRS	**Duration:** Large breeds: ≤0.05 s Small breeds: ≤0.6 s **R wave voltage:** Large breeds: ≤3.0 mV Small breeds: ≤2.5 mV	Duration: ≤0.04 s R wave: ≤0.9 mV
ST segment	Depression: ≤0.2 mV Elevation: ≤0.15 mV	Without significant depression or elevation
T wave	≤1/4 R wave amplitude	≤0.3 mV
QT interval (s)	0.15–0.25	0.12–0.18
Frontal plane mean electrical axis	+40° to +100°	0° to +160°

In the hexaxial system, the most isoelectric lead is the one in which the voltages of the positive and negative components of the QRS complexes are most similar.

Leads I and III are selected, the negative components of each are added to the positive components, and the resulting values (positive or negative) are transferred to the hexaxial system. Lines are drawn perpendicular to these leads, then a line is traced from the centre of the axes to the point at which they cross the perpendicular lines (Figure 5.8).

Morphology and measurement of waves and intervals

Lead II is used in standard measurement of waves and intervals, preferably at **50 mm/s**.

Each mm on the horizontal axis represents 0.04 s in duration, and on the vertical axis, 0.1 mV amplitude. Normal wave and interval values are listed in Table 5.1.

P wave

P waves represent **atrial depolarisation**. They are positive on leads I, II, III and aVF, and negative on aVR and aVL.

They may be **absent** in cases of atrial fibrillation, atrial standstill or sinus arrest.

Although each P wave is usually followed by a QRS complex, they can also appear in isolation in cases of second- and third-degree AV block. P waves may also be **inverted and retrograde** in cases of supraventricular premature complexes and escape beats.

PR interval

This represents the time that passes between generation of the electrical impulse in the sinus node and its arrival at the atrioventricular node and bundle of His.

Although this interval is usually constant, it can vary in cases of sinus arrhythmia, AV blocks (where it increases) or arrhythmias related to accessory pathways (where it decreases).

QRS complex

This complex represents **depolarisation of the ventricles**. It starts with the Q wave, a negative deflection, continues with the R wave, a positive deflection (I, II, III and aVF) and ends with the negative S wave. **Q and S waves are not always visible** in normal animals. QRS complexes which come from an electrical impulse with a supraventricular origin (sinus node, atrium, AV junction) are narrow because they travel via rapid conduction pathways.

In the case of bundle branch blocks, or electrical impulses originating in the ventricle, the QRS complex lasts longer than normal, appearing wider (Figure 5.9).

QRS and MEA voltages can be disrupted in ventricular hypertrophy, mainly of the right side of the heart (Figure 5.10).

ST segment

This segment represents the end of ventricular depolarisation and the onset of repolarisation.

This can be disrupted in cases of myocardial disease (myocardial ischaemia in dogs with severe obstruction of the ventricular outflow tracts, dilated cardiomyopathy, etc.) and pericardial disease.

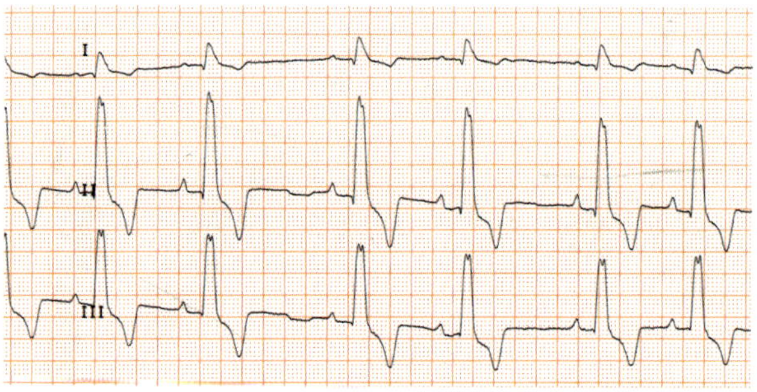

Figure 5.9. Superficial electrocardiogram from a dog with left bundle branch block (QRS width = 0.1 s; normal <0.05 s). 50 mm/s; 1 cm = 1 mV.

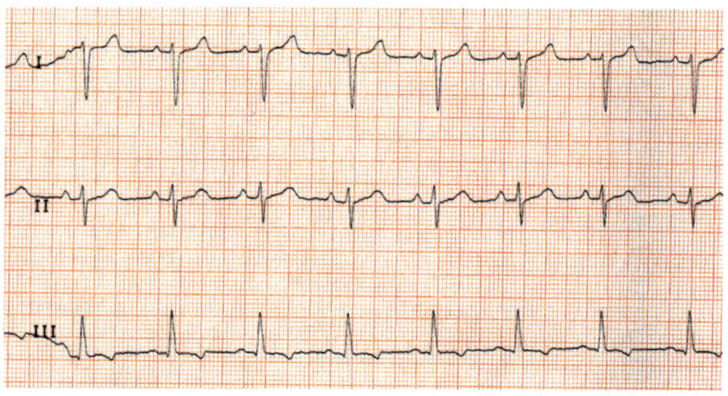

Figure 5.10. Superficial electrocardiogram from a dog with pulmonary stenosis. Right deviation of the electrical axis in the frontal plane (electrical axis = +170°; normal range +40° to +100°). 50 mm/s; 1 cm = 1 mV.

T wave

This wave represents **ventricular repolarisation**. It is very variable in dogs and cats, and can appear to be positive, negative or biphasic.

T waves can be affected in cases of hypoxia, electrolyte imbalance (hyperkalaemia), changes in ventricular conduction and digoxin poisoning.

QT interval

This measures **the time between the onset of the QRS complex and the T wave.** It can be altered in cases of hypo- or hypercalcaemia.

Prolongation of this period can predispose the animal to ventricular arrhythmias.

Cardiac radiology

Introduction

Thoracic radiology is one of the crucial techniques for exploring the cardiorespiratory system, as it enables the **size and shape of the cardiac silhouette**, lung field, pleural space, mediastinum and diaphragm to be assessed. To satisfactorily interpret radiographs, the quality must be good (position of the patient, exposure techniques, etc.) and knowledge of cardiorespiratory anatomy and physiology must be applied.

Radiographic projections

Two views are recommended: lateral (right or left), and dorsoventral (DV) or ventrodorsal (VD) (Figures 5.11 and 5.12).

The characteristics of different radiographic projections in dogs and cats are as follows.

- **Right lateral** is preferable when assessing the **heart**.
- **DV** is tolerated better by **dyspnoeic** patients than VD.
- **DV** enables the **perihilar region** and the inferior pulmonary vessels to be assessed with greater precision.
- VD allows the lung field and **mild pleural effusions** to be better assessed.

Radiograph quality depends on the parameters selected for each patient and correct positioning of the animal.

High kilovoltage (kVp) and **low milliamperage/time (mAs)** are recommended to obtain a satisfactory resolution of **soft tissues** with minimal exposure time, and to prevent interference from movements during breathing. In obese patients, the kVp should be increased to 10% above reference values.

The radiograph should ideally be taken during inspiration to obtain better contrast between pulmonary air

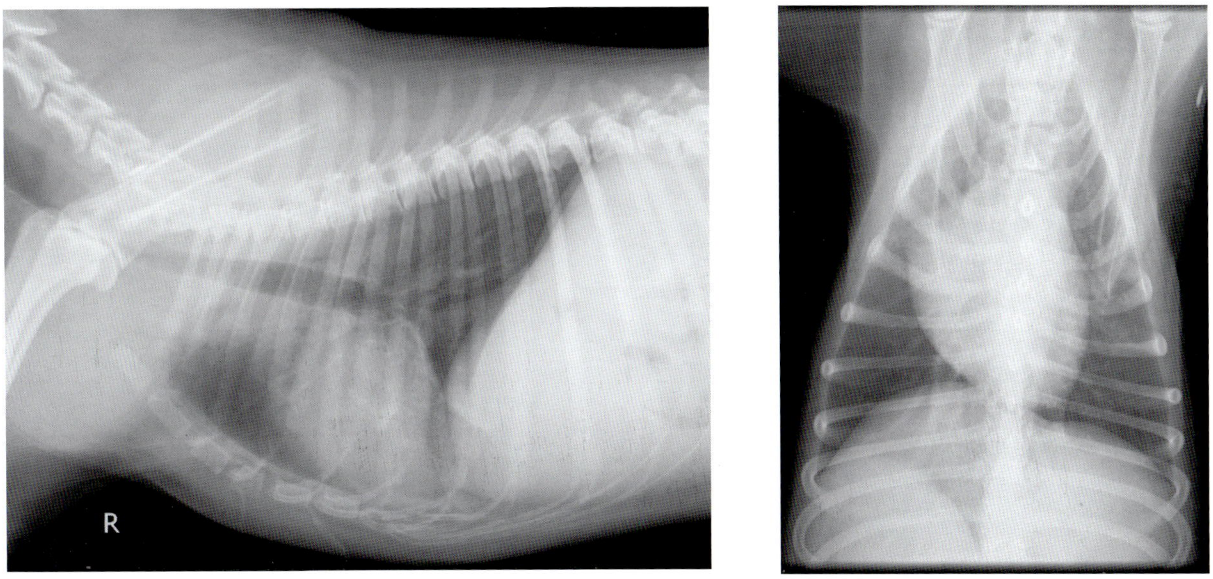

Figure 5.11. Radiographs of a healthy dog: (a) lateral and (b) ventrodorsal.

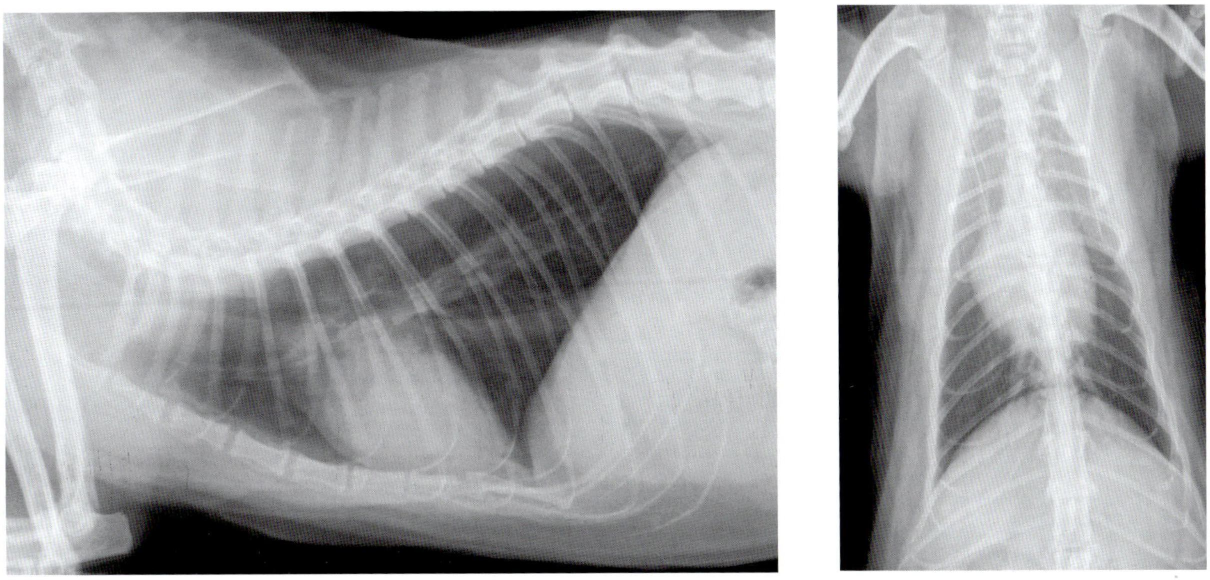

Figure 5.12. Radiographs of a healthy cat: (a) lateral and (b) ventrodorsal.

and soft tissues (cardiac silhouette and large vessels), and better separation of the caudal heart silhouette and the diaphragm.

Patients should be positioned correctly in both lateral projections and DV or VD projections.

- **Lateral projections**: The forelimbs should be in a forward position so they are not superimposed on the cranial thorax; the area between the thoracic inlet and the last rib should be included, in order to observe the cranial abdomen. The sternum and spine should be equidistant from the body axis so that the ribs are aligned and parallel, otherwise the cardiac silhouette can be affected.
- **DV/VD projections**: The spinous processes, vertebral bodies and sternebrae should appear superimposed, the ribs symmetrical and the spine straight.

Interpretation of radiographs

Thoracic radiographs should be interpreted systematically, assessing:

- radiograph quality
- ribcage
- cranial abdomen
- diaphragm
- mediastinum

- trachea and bronchi
- lung field
- pulmonary vessels
- great vessels
- cardiac silhouette.

These factors must be combined with any other tests which complement the examination, such as medical records, physical examination, echocardiography and laboratory analysis that are relevant to the clinical case.

Radiographic anatomy

Lateral projection

In lateral radiographs the heart is an **ovoid shape** that is more pointed towards the apex, especially in cats (Figures 5.11a and 5.12a).

- The **long axis of the heart** (apex–base) is defined by tracing a line from the tracheal bifurcation (carina) to the apex, at an angle of approximately 45° to the sternum. In cats, this angle decreases with age.
- The **short axis** is defined by tracing a line perpendicular to the long axis from the ventral part of the inferior vena cava.

Barrel-chested dogs (Beagle, Lhasa Apso, Bulldog) tend to show more globular silhouettes, with greater contact between the sternum and the cranial silhouette, than deep-chested dogs (Doberman, Setter, Collie) where the heart appears much more vertical in the thoracic cavity. The **dorsal heart border** includes both atria, the pulmonary arteries and veins, the superior and inferior vena cava and the aortic arch. The **cranial border** is made up of the right ventricle and right atrium (auricle), defined as the cranial waist. The **caudal margin** is made up of the left atrium and ventricle, with the atrioventricular junction defined as the caudal waist (Figure 5.13).

The **longitudinal cardiac measurement** (apex–base) occupies approximately 70% of the dorsoventral length of the thoracic cavity. The **craniocaudal cardiac measurement** (short axis) occupies 2.5 intercostal spaces in deep-chested dogs and 3.5 in barrel-chested dogs; in cats it varies between 2 and 2.5 intercostal spaces.

The size of the cardiac silhouette can be assessed more objectively using the **vertebral heart scale**, where the size of the heart is compared to the size of the vertebrae (V). The long and short axes are positioned along the length of the spine, from the cranial edge of the 4th thoracic vertebra, and the total score is the sum of the number of vertebral bodies covered (Figure 5.14). Average scores are as follows.

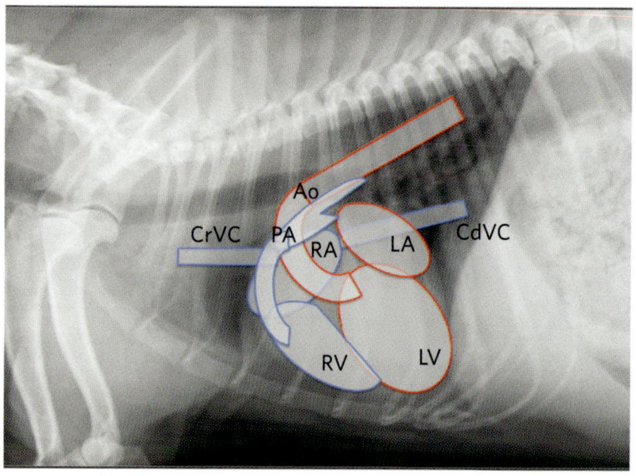

Figure 5.13. Lateral radiograph of the thorax showing the position in which the heart chambers and great vessels can best be interpreted. Ao, aorta; CrVC, cranial vena cava; CdVC, caudal vena cava; LA, left atrium; LV, left ventricle; PA, pulmonary artery; RA, right atrium; RV, right ventricle.

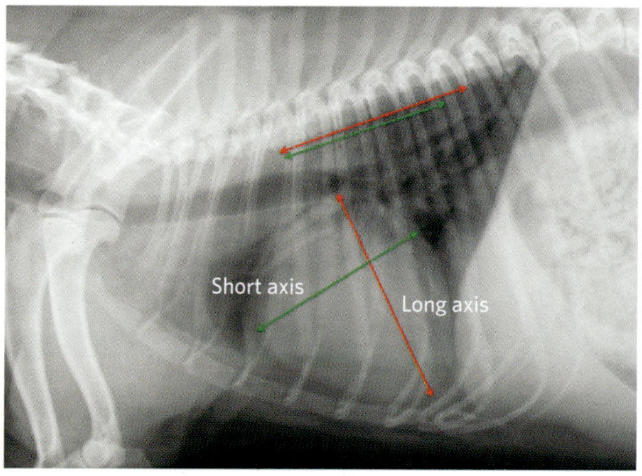

Figure 5.14. Right lateral thoracic radiograph of a healthy dog, showing measurement of the heart using the vertebral heart scale. The lengths of the short and long axis of the cardiac silhouette are placed over the spine, starting from the 4th thoracic vertebra. The total score is sum of the number of vertebral bodies covered by both axes.

- **In dogs**, 9.7 V (range of 8.5–10.5 V); this can be higher in certain breeds (e.g., Boxer, 11.6 ± 0.8 V).
- **In cats**, 7.5 ± 0.3 V; higher in obese animals.

The main pulmonary artery cannot be assessed in a lateral projection. Although the left pulmonary artery can sometimes be seen, dorsally and caudally to the tracheal bifurcation. The **right pulmonary artery** can be seen at the end of the main pulmonary artery, ventral to the carina; this should **not be mistakenly interpreted as a mass**. This image is accentuated in pulmonary hypertension (especially in cases of dirofilariasis).

Pulmonary veins can be identified entering the left atrium at the base of the heart. The arteries are dorsal and the veins ventral to the bronchus. The vessels of

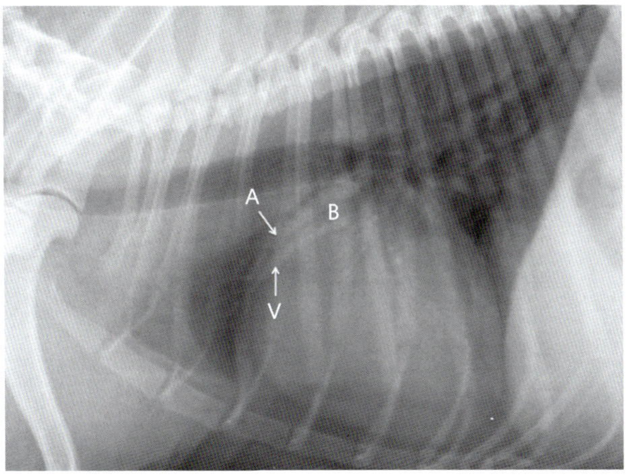

Figure 5.15. Lateral thoracic radiograph of a healthy dog, showing the cranial lobe vessels, artery (A) and vein (V) with the bronchus (B) in between.

the cranial pulmonary lobes **appear in pairs** with their respective bronchus (Figure 5.15). The arteries and veins should be the same size. The width of the vessels as they cross the 4th rib should not exceed the narrowest width of the rib, at its most dorsal part.

Dorsoventral/ventrodorsal projections

Given that the heart is rotated on its axis, the right chambers are orientated to the right and cranially, and the left chambers, to the left and caudally (this rotation is greater in cats).

The **cardiac silhouette in the dog** has an elliptical form on radiographs, with the long axis orientated 30° to the left of the midline (Figure 5.11b). It occupies 60–65% of the width of the thoracic cavity.

In cats, the axis is closer to the midline and occupies 50% of the width of the thoracic cavity during inspiration (Figure 5.12b). The silhouette may be larger in obese cats because of pericardial fat.

The **heart silhouette** includes numerous overlapping structures. **Imagining a clock face**, the cardiac structures are projected as follows (Figure 5.16).

- Aortic arch, 11 o'clock.
- Main pulmonary artery, 1–2 o'clock.
- Left atrium:
  - In cats, 2–3 o'clock.
  - In dogs with atrial dilatation, the auricle is projected at 2–3 o'clock.
- Left ventricle, 2–6 o'clock.
- Right ventricle, 7–11 o'clock.
- Right atrium, 9–11 o'clock.
- The cardiac apex can sometimes appear to be displaced towards the right hemithorax in animals that do not suffer from any cardiopathy.
- In puppies, the thymus can obscure the cranial heart border.

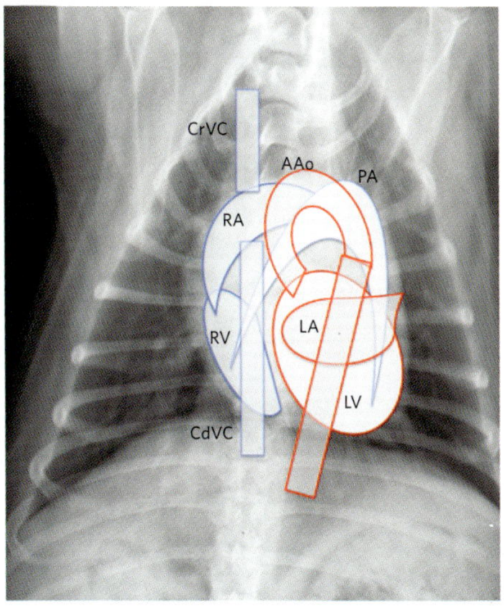

Figure 5.16. Ventrodorsal radiograph of the thorax, showing the positions in which the heart chambers and large vessels can best be identified. AAo, ascending aorta; CrVC, cranial vena cava; CdVC, caudal vena cava; LA, left atrium; LV, left ventricle; PA, pulmonary artery; RA, right atrium; RV, right ventricle.

- The left and right pulmonary arteries originate from the main pulmonary artery.
  - The right pulmonary artery crosses the cranial cardiac silhouette, extending to the right edge at 8 o'clock.
  - The left branch of the PA passes over the caudal part of the left ventricle, extending past the left border, at about 4 o'clock.
- The pulmonary veins can be seen entering the left atrium and are situated more axially than the arteries.
- The descending aorta overlaps the heart and extends caudally, dorsally and medially.
- The caudal vena cava crosses the diaphragm and proceeds cranially to the right of the midline and the right border of the heart.

Evaluation of the cardiac silhouette

Overall enlargement of the cardiac silhouette

Main causes

- Pericardial effusion.
- Left-sided heart diseases with pulmonary hypertension (chronic degenerative mitral valve disease, cardiomyopathies, congenital heart diseases, etc.).
- Pericardial fat.

Radiological signs

Generalised cardiomegaly must be differentiated from severe pericardial effusion with tamponade. In the latter, the heart appears globe-like in shape, with no visible localised chamber enlargement (Figure 5.17).

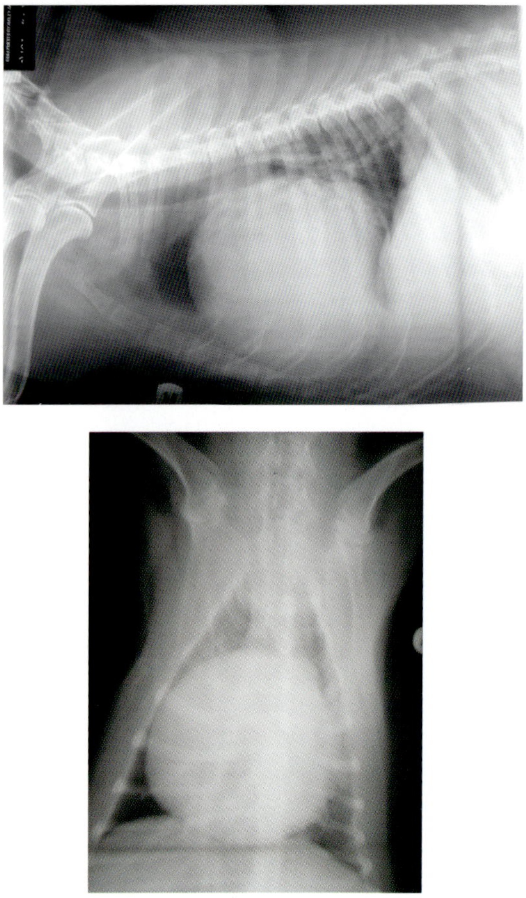

Figure 5.17. (a) Lateral and (b) ventrodorsal thoracic radiographs of a dog showing cardiomegaly secondary to significant pericardial effusion.

Reduced overall size of the cardiac silhouette

Principal causes

Reduced cardiac silhouette size can be due to deficient venous return caused by hypovolaemia (Addison's disease) and is also known as microcardia (Figure 5.18).

Radiological signs

- Pointed heart.
- Apex separated from sternum and diaphragm.
- Pulmonary vessels and inferior vena cava reduced in size.

Enlarged silhouette of the left atrium

Principal causes

- Chronic degenerative mitral valve disease in dogs (Figure 5.19).
- Cardiomyopathies.
- Congenital cardiomyopathies (mitral valve dysplasia, PDA, ventricular septal defect, etc.).

Radiological signs

In lateral projections, dorsal elevation of the trachea, carina and left main bronchus (compression), and loss of the caudal waist can be seen (Figures 5.19 and 5.20).

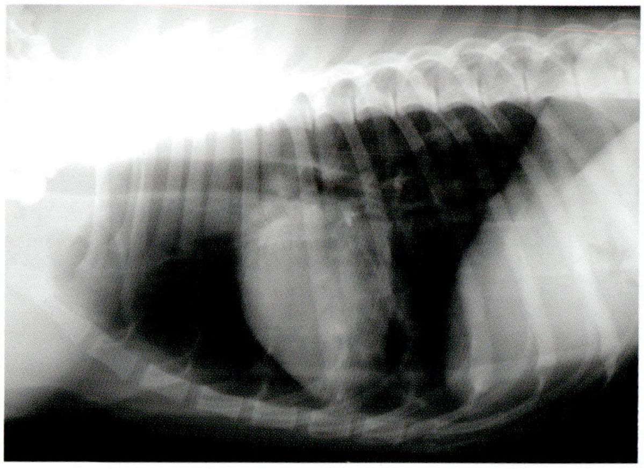

Figure 5.18. Lateral thoracic radiograph of a dog with hypoadrenocorticism, showing microcardia and a small inferior vena cava, secondary to hypovolaemia.

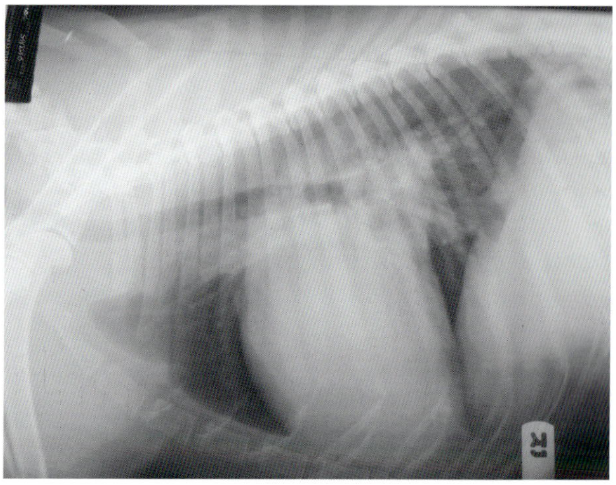

Figure 5.19. Lateral thoracic radiograph of a dog with chronic degenerative mitral valvulopathy, showing dorsal displacement of the trachea, enlarged left atrium and ventricle silhouettes, and perihilar alveolar oedema.

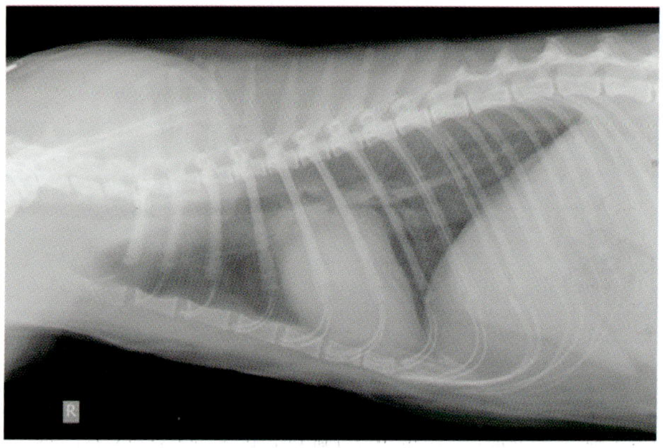

Figure 5.20. Right lateral thoracic radiograph of a cat with hypertrophic cardiomyopathy, showing enlarged left atrium (between 2 and 3 o'clock) and ventricular silhouettes, and interstitial patterns.

In DV/VD projections, enlargement of the left atrial silhouette can be seen at 2–3 o'clock, as well as an increased opacity of the atrial body (between the main bronchi) overlapping the cardiac silhouette. In

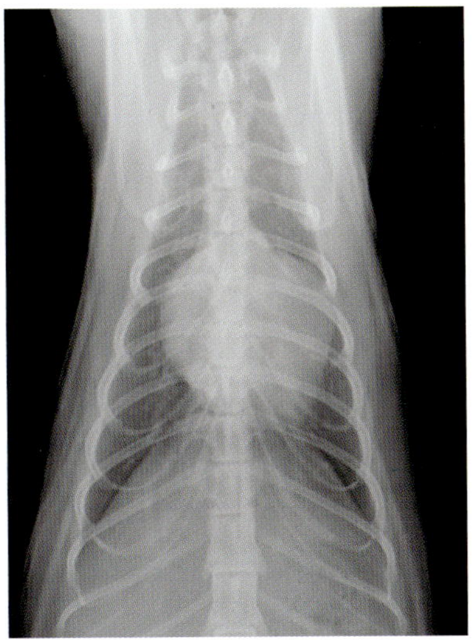

Figure 5.21. Dorsoventral thoracic radiograph of a cat with hypertrophic cardiomyopathy, showing an enlarged left atrium (between 2 and 3 o'clock) and ventricular silhouettes, an image typical of a 'Valentine-shaped' heart, due to atrial enlargement.

cats, dilation of the left atrium is seen as the border of the heart protruding between 2 and 3 o'clock (Figure 5.21).

Enlarged left ventricle

Principal causes

- Chronic degenerative mitral valve disease.
- Cardiomyopathies.
- Congenital heart diseases (mitral valve dysplasia, PDA, ventricular septal defect, aortic stenosis, etc.).
- Anaemia.
- Arteriovenous fistula.
- Hyperthyroidism (cats).

Radiological signs

In **lateral projections** this includes the loss of the caudal waist, a caudal border straighter and more perpendicular than normal, and dorsal displacement of the tracheal bifurcation (in many cases atrial and ventricular enlargement coexists) (Figures 5.19 and 5.20).

In **DV/VD projections** this ventricular border and apex are rounder and enlarged from 2 o'clock to 5–6 o'clock; the apex can sometimes be displaced to the right. In **cats** with cardiomyopathy, it is common to see the classic 'Valentine-shaped' heart silhouette, characterised by a pointed apex and atrial dilation (Figure 5.21).

Enlarged silhouette of the aortic arch and ascending aorta

Principal causes

- Patent ductus arteriosus.
- Aortic stenosis (post-stenotic dilation).
- Systemic hypertension (in cats).

Radiological signs

In **lateral** projections, enlargement of the craniodorsal heart border can be seen.

In **DV/VD projections**, the silhouette of the aortic arch appears enlarged at 11–1 o'clock. In dogs, patent ductus arteriosus causes localised enlargement of the descending aorta, pulmonary artery and left atrium (Figure 5.22).

Right atrial enlargement

Principal causes

- Tricuspid valve dysplasia (Figure 5.23).
- Pulmonary hypertension.
- Cardiomyopathies.
- Atrial neoplasms (haemangiosarcoma).

Radiological signs

In **lateral projections**, elevation of the cranial aspect of the trachea, a pronounced cranial waist and an enlarged silhouette of the cranial border can all be seen, due to enlargement of the atrium (Figure 5.23a).

In **DV/VD projections,** variable degrees of enlargement of the heart silhouette can be seen at 9–11 o'clock (Figure 5.23b).

Enlarged right ventricular silhouette

Principal causes

- Tricuspid valve insufficiency.
- Cardiomyopathy.
- Pulmonary hypertension.
- Congenital heart diseases (pulmonary stenosis, tetralogy of Fallot, tricuspid valve dysplasia, etc.).

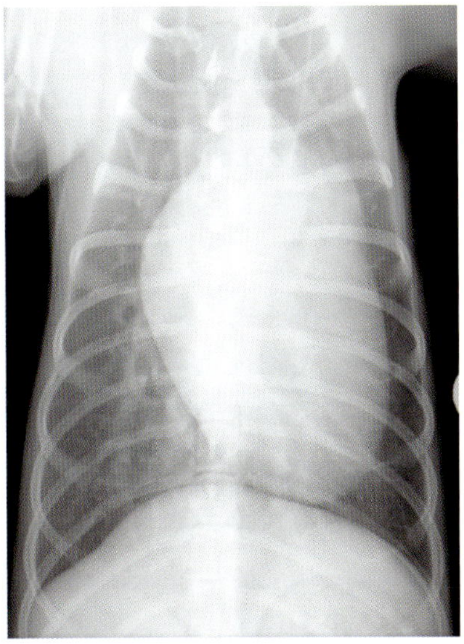

Figure 5.22. Ventrodorsal thoracic radiograph of a dog with patent ductus arteriosus, showing an enlarged cardiac silhouette caused by dilation of the left ventricle, aortic arch and main pulmonary artery. The caudal pulmonary arteries are also prominent, and a diffuse interstitial pattern can be seen.

Radiological signs

In **lateral projections**, variable degrees of enlargement of the cranial heart silhouette and sternal contact can be seen (Figure 5.23a), with elevation of the cardiac apex, overall rounding of the heart silhouette and dorsal elevation of the inferior vena cava.

In **DV/VD projections** it tends to appear as an inverted 'D' shape (Figure 5.23b), with an enlarged silhouette in the 6–9 o'clock area and, in some cases, displacement of the apex towards the right hemithorax.

Enlarged silhouette of the main pulmonary artery

Principal causes

- Pulmonary hypertension.
- Pulmonary thromboembolism.
- Pulmonary stenosis.
- Patent ductus arteriosus.

Radiological signs

In **lateral projections**, enlargement of the craniodorsal heart silhouette can be seen (Figure 5.23a).

In **DV/VD projections**, protrusion of the heart border over the 1–2 o'clock area is common (Figure 5.23b).

Pulmonary vessels: hypercirculatory pattern

Principal causes

- Pulmonary stenosis.
- Tetralogy of Fallot.
- Hypovolaemia.

Radiological signs

Very transparent lungs and small pulmonary arteries can be seen (Figure 5.23).

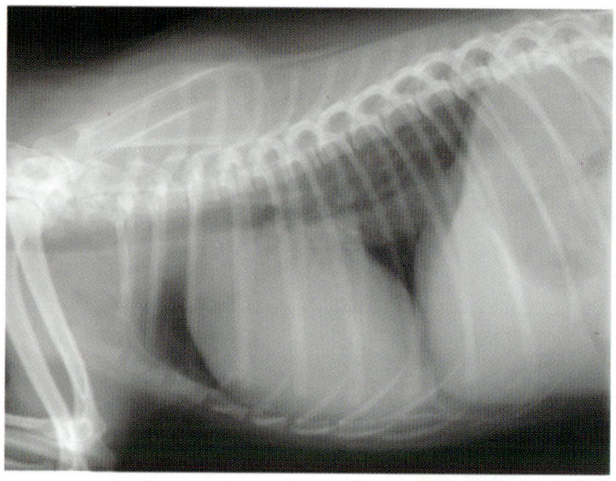

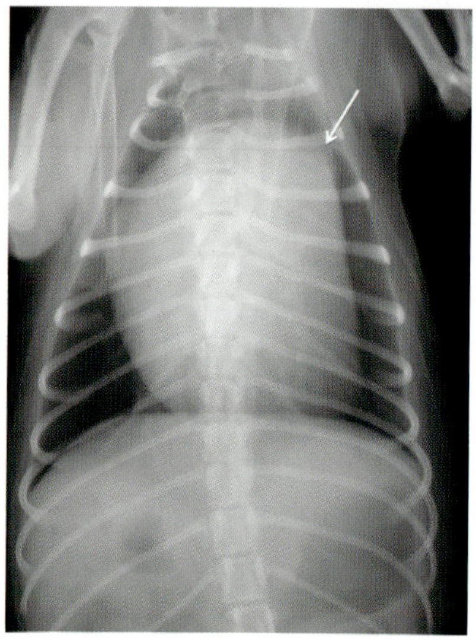

Figure 5.23. (a) Right lateral and (b) ventrodorsal thoracic radiographs of a dog with congenital tricuspid valve dysplasia and pulmonary stenosis. (a) A large part of the heart is resting on the sternum, the right atrial and main pulmonary artery silhouettes are enlarged, and dilation of the inferior vena cava is visible. (b) The silhouette of the right chambers and the projection of the main pulmonary artery (arrow) are also enlarged. Poor pulmonary circulation can be seen in both views.

Pulmonary vessels: hypocirculatory pattern

Principal causes

- Left–right shunt (ventricular septal defect, PDA, atrial septal defect).
- Left-sided heart failure.
- Hypervolaemia.

Radiological signs

Enlargement of pulmonary arteries and veins (pulmonary congestion) and increased lung opacity are seen (Figure 5.22).

Alterations in diameter and position of the inferior vena cava

Only the inferior vena cava (IVC) is visible on plain radiographs.

Principal causes

- Reduced IVC diameter is usually associated with hypovolaemia (Figure 5.18) and reduced venous return.
- Increased IVC diameter suggests raised venous pressure due to cardiac tamponade, right-sided congestive heart failure, constrictive pericarditis or obstruction of the right ventricular outflow tract (Figure 5.23a).

Radiological signs

The diameter is considered to be larger than normal when IVC/aorta >1.5, IVC/length of the vertebra located at the level of the tracheal bifurcation >1.3, or IVC/width of the 4th rib just below the spine is >3.5. The IVC can be dorsally displaced in patients with left ventricular dilation.

Left-sided congestive heart failure

Radiological signs (Figures 5.24 and 5.25)

- Enlargement of the silhouette of the left-sided chambers.
- Pulmonary venous congestion.
- Interstitial or alveolar oedema.
- Pleural effusion.

Pulmonary oedema initially accumulates in the interstitial space surrounding the vessels and bronchi. If it develops, air bronchograms can be seen, and opaque areas appear which gradually join together, making it difficult to see the cardiac silhouette, IVC and pulmonary vessels (Figure 5.24). This cardiogenic oedema is mainly spread throughout the perihilar and dorsal areas.

In cats, the distribution pattern can vary (Figure 5.25).

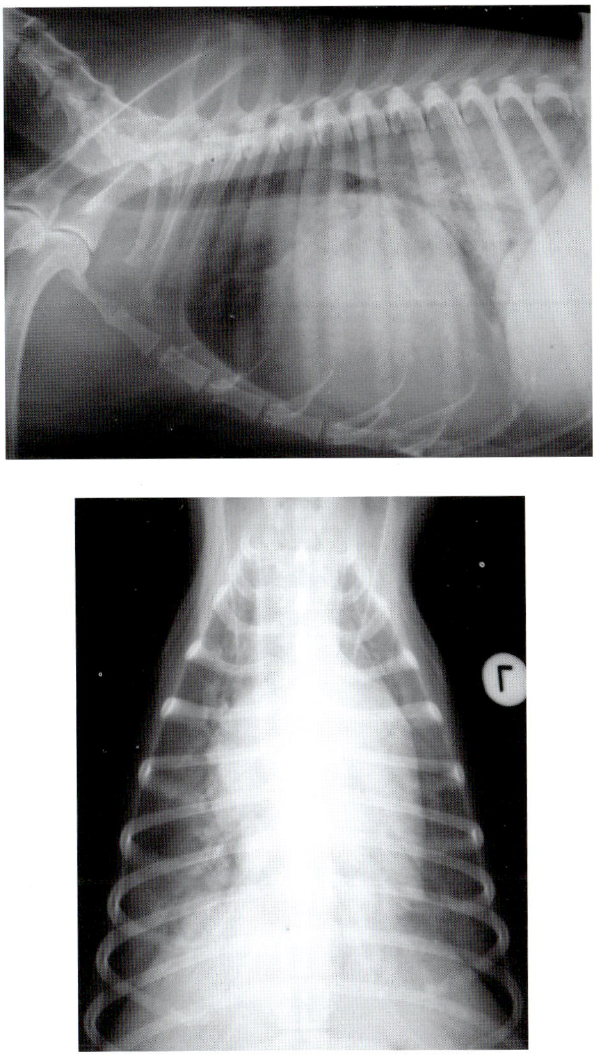

Figure 5.24. (a) Right lateral and (b) ventrodorsal thoracic radiographs of a dog with congestive heart failure. (a) Dorsal displacement of the trachea, cardiomegaly of the left chambers and significant pulmonary alveolar oedema. (b) Enlarged silhouette of the left chambers, pulmonary alveolar oedema and air bronchograms.

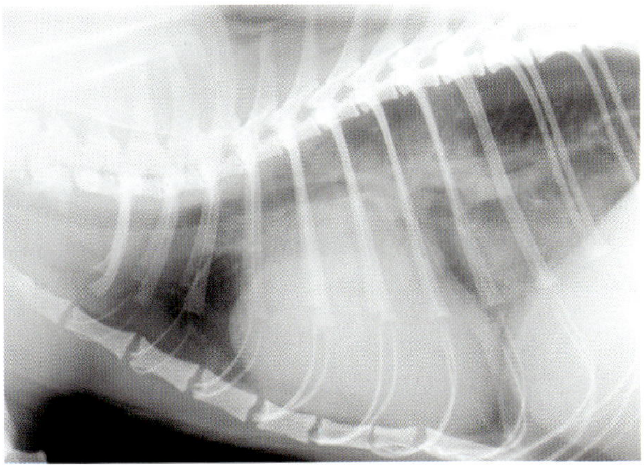

Figure 5.25. Lateral thoracic radiograph of a cat with left-sided congestive heart failure, showing dorsal displacement of the trachea, cardiomegaly of the left-sided chambers and pulmonary alveolar oedema.

In cases of right-sided congestive heart disease, the enlarged silhouette of the right chambers and inferior vena cava can be seen, along with hepatomegaly, ascites and pleural effusion (if left-sided failure is also present).

Echocardiographic imaging modalities and examination protocol

Transthoracic echocardiography (ultrasound) is the main non-invasive imaging technique and has no known side effects. In the majority of cases, it is considered the definitive diagnostic tool.

This technique uses ultrasound waves to create images of the heart in movement, providing information on heart anatomy and function. However, results of the echocardiographic examination should be interpreted within the patient's clinical context, along with the clinical history, physical examination and other diagnostic techniques, such as thoracic radiographs, electrocardiograms, laboratory analysis and measurement of systemic arterial blood pressure.

Guidelines for echocardiographic examination

Echocardiographic examinations are useful in the following situations.

- Examination of patients with symptoms suggestive of cardiac aetiology.
- Assessment of suspected congenital cardiopathy, both in young and adult animals.
- Preliminary assessment of murmurs in patients where there is reasonable suspicion of valvulopathy or structural heart disease.

- Preliminary assessment of suspected endocarditis with positive blood culture or recently occurring murmur.
- Assessment of pericardial diseases: pericardial effusion and constrictive pericarditis.
- Preliminary assessment of known or suspected cardiomyopathy.
- Monitoring patients following diagnosis or treatment of heart disease.

Echocardiographic imaging modalities

Ultrasound is based on reflection of ultrasound waves (above a frequency of 20,000 Hz) from cardiovascular tissues. As the ultrasound waves pass through the tissue, some are reflected, and some are refracted and pass through to deeper tissues. The waves that return to the transducer (reflected) are undergo a special process where they are transformed and reproduced in visual or audible form on the ultrasound scanner's monitor.

The main modes used in routine clinical practice are:

- two-dimensional (2D) echocardiography
- time–motion (M-mode or TM-mode) echocardiography
- Doppler echocardiography.

Two-dimensional echocardiography

This mode enables the heart to be examined in a particular plane, producing a two-dimensional image (Figure 5.26). The anatomy and movement of the cardiac structures can be evaluated, and specific measurements taken which can be used to study heart functionality. It also serves as a guide for the other echocardiographic modes.

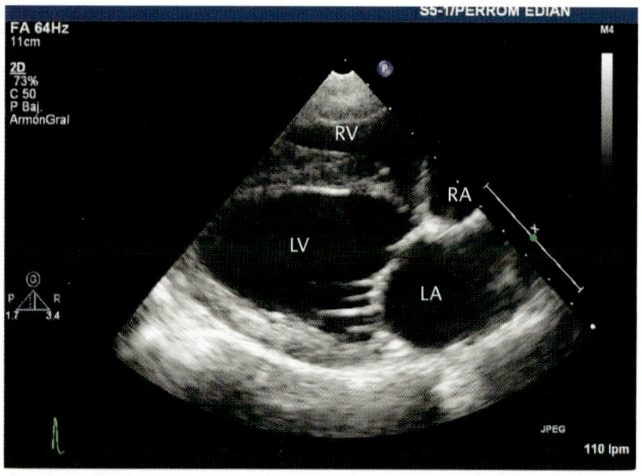

Figure 5.26. Right parasternal long-axis four-chamber 2D echocardiogram of a normal dog: the left chambers appear larger than the right, and the atrioventricular valves are located between the atria and the ventricles. LA, left atrium; LV, left ventricle; RA, right atrium; RV, right ventricle.

Time–motion mode (M-mode or TM-mode) echocardiography

This mode enables the heart to be examined using a single ultrasound beam, producing a one-dimensional image. The depth of the cardiac structures is shown on the vertical axis, and time (movement of the structures during the cardiac cycle) on the horizontal axis (Figure 5.27).

M-mode is mainly used to obtain quantitative data on the size of the cardiac chambers and walls, and the great vessels, and on movement of the cardiac structures.

Doppler echocardiography

Doppler enables normal flow within the cardiac and vascular structures to be evaluated and abnormal flow detected through changes in flow direction and velocity. It also detects and provides information on valvular lesions (stenosis or insufficiency) and abnormal cardiac communications.

Doppler technology is based on changes in the frequency of sound waves when they are reflected by a moving object. When an object moves towards an observer, the frequency increases and, when it moves away, the frequency decreases. With echocardiography, the frequency change in the ultrasound wave is caused by blood cells, which are the moving objects.

Ultrasound waves are emitted at a particular frequency, which is altered on contact with the moving red blood cells, so the return frequency is different from that of the original wave. The difference between the

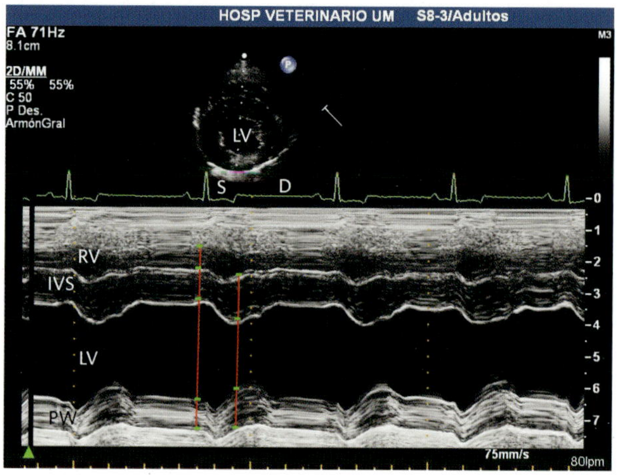

Figure 5.27. Right parasternal short-axis M-mode echocardiogram of the left ventricle of a normal dog. The short axis of the left ventricle (LV) can be seen in the upper part of the 2D ultrasound image, and this serves as a guide as to where to place the cursor in the corresponding M-mode image. The phases of the cardiac cycle can easily be identified on the ECG: systole (S) and diastole (D). Note that the interventricular septum (IVS) and the posterior wall (PW) of the left ventricle (LV) move closer to each other in systole, and draw apart in diastole. Diastolic measurements are made at Q wave level on the ECG, and systolic, where the IVS is at its lowest, from upper border to upper border in both cases.

frequency emitted and frequency reflected is proportional to the velocity of the object against which the signal has 'crashed', in this case, the cells in the blood. This phenomenon was described by Austrian doctor and astronomer, Johann Christian Doppler (1803–1853), and is therefore known as the Doppler effect.

Under normal conditions, blood flows through the cardiovascular structures forming **laminar flows**, which are organised layers of red blood cells with the same alignment and very similar velocity. With **abnormal flow**, however, the red blood cell layers tend to become **disorganised**, creating eddies which change the speed and direction of the layers abruptly, causing turbulent flow patterns. Doppler echocardiography is useful for detecting flow patterns, categorising them as normal or turbulent and quantifying their velocity and pressure gradients.

There are two main types of Doppler echocardiography:

- **spectral Doppler**, which can either be:
  - pulsed Doppler
  - continuous wave Doppler
- **colour Doppler.**

Spectral Doppler

In spectral Doppler, the signal or Doppler spectrum captured by a transducer is displayed on axes where time is represented on the horizontal, and velocity on the vertical (cm/s or m/s). The baseline is zero m/s; 'positive' velocities of flows which approach the transducer are situated above the baseline; 'negative' velocities of flows which are moving away from the transducer are situated below.

Pulsed Doppler

This technique uses a single crystal which both emits and receives the ultrasound signal. The transducer emits a pulse at a certain interval and does not send the next until the response to the previous pulse has returned. This type of Doppler enables measurements to be made in a specific area. The sample volume to be examined with pulsed Doppler is placed over an image in 2D mode. If a colour Doppler scan has already been carried out, areas of abnormal flow can be quickly identified and the sample volume which has been scanned by spectral pulsed Doppler can be superimposed on the abnormality in the colour Doppler image (Figure 5.28).

This type of Doppler has some velocity limits, as it is unable to detect large changes in frequency, usually produced by velocities above 2 m/s. When the difference exceeds the maximum velocity, a phenomenon called 'aliasing' arises, causing artefacts and errors in blood flow direction and velocity. The limit above

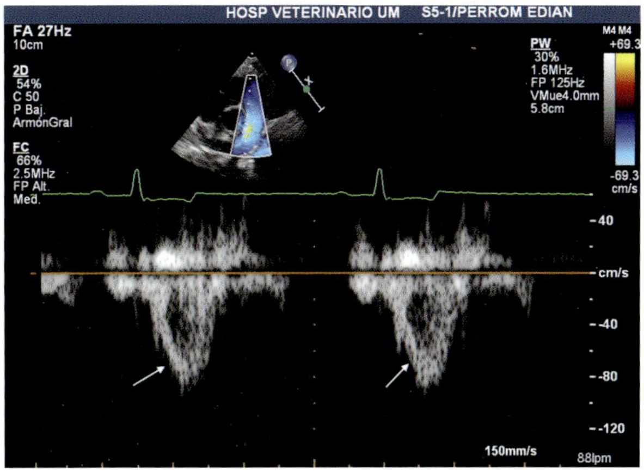

Figure 5.28. Right parasternal short-axis pulsed Doppler echocardiogram of pulmonary blood flow (arrows) in a normal dog. A scale corresponding to the range of velocities is shown to the side.

which aliasing occurs is called the Nyquist limit, and it depends on the ultrasound emission frequency, the distance to the point where velocity is to be measured, and the velocity of the blood at that point. Continuous wave Doppler is used to measure these abnormally high velocities.

Continuous wave Doppler

Continuous wave Doppler employs two piezoelectric crystals: one emits the ultrasound signal and the other receives the reflected ultrasound waves. This type complements pulsed Doppler, as it enables the high velocities which produce aliasing with pulsed Doppler to be measured. Continuous wave Doppler is guided by a cursor, not a sample volume, so it does not allow selection of a specific area, but studies flows along the whole ultrasound beam (Figure 5.29). Continuous wave Doppler does not depend on pulse repetition, so is unaffected by the Nyquist limit and therefore the aliasing phenomenon does not occur.

A haemodynamic study can be carried out, based on the measurement of blood flow velocities (V), and calculating the pressure gradient using the simplified Bernoulli equation.

Equation for the determination of V:

$$V = C \times fd \,/\, 2\,(fo) \times \cos \Delta$$

C: constant corresponding to the velocity of the ultrasound signal in the tissues (approximately 1540 m/s)

fd: difference between the frequency emitted and frequency received

fo: emission frequency

cos Δ: cosine of the angle between the ultrasound beam and blood flow.

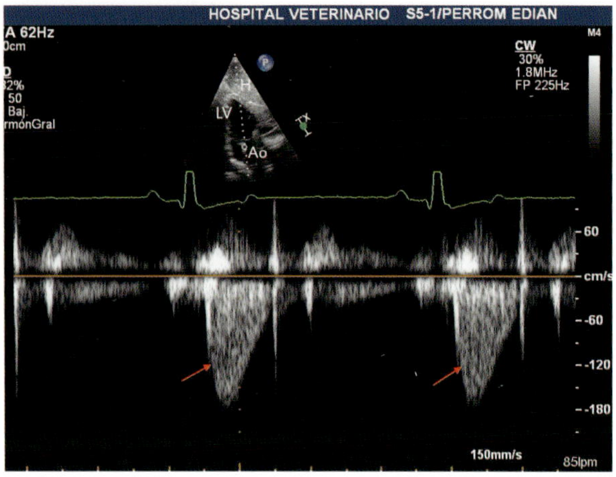

Figure 5.29. Subcostal continuous wave Doppler echocardiogram of aortic blood flow (arrows) in a normal dog. The liver (H) acts as a window for ultrasound waves. Ao, ascending aorta; LV, left ventricle.

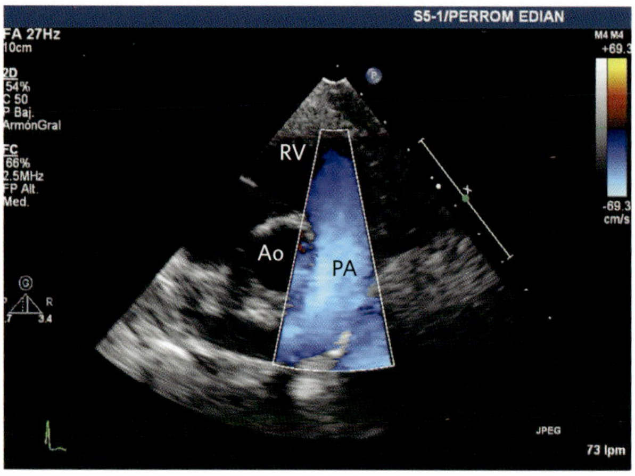

Figure 5.30. Right parasternal short-axis transaortic colour flow Doppler echocardiogram of pulmonary blood flow in a normal dog. A blue-coloured flow can be observed, as it is moving away from the transducer, from the right ventricle (RV) to the pulmonary artery (PA). A colour scale can be seen on the right of the image, numbered according to the pulse repetition frequency which corresponds to the flow velocity to be measured. Ao, ascending aorta.

The **angle of the ultrasound beam** is critical, and should be aligned with blood flow as closely as possible to obtain data on maximum velocity. The greater the angle to the flow, the lower the velocity value. This is because the equation uses the cosine of the angle between the Doppler cursor and the flow and, as this angle increases, the cosine decreases and draws nearer to zero.

Distance is another important parameter, as the further away the point to be measured, the lower the maximum velocity which can be measured by pulsed Doppler.

Transducer frequency also affects Doppler measurements: lower frequencies permit higher velocities to be measured.

Examination of blood flow with Doppler ultrasound requires the **use of an ECG synchronous** with echocardiographic images, enabling the cardiac cycle in which the different Doppler spectra are obtained to be determined and any arrhythmias to be detected.

Colour Doppler

This mode uses both ultrasound applications, a combination of **2D images** and **blood flow** movement (Figure 5.30). The technology used is similar to that used with pulsed Doppler, but differs in that it uses multiple sample volumes along the multiple ultrasound beams exploring a particular area.

Difference in flow velocity and direction are colour-coded: **red corresponds to flow towards** the transducer and **blue represents flow away** from it. The stronger the colour, the greater the flow velocity.

As this technique uses a type of **pulsed Doppler**, it can be affected by aliasing, which registers as colour inversions (turbulent patterns or colour mosaics) when velocities exceed the preset limits. The size of the examination window can also be chosen in colour Doppler; the larger the window, the more chance there is of errors occurring, so the **window should be restricted** to the size of the vessel or area which is being assessed.

Colour Doppler is recommended as a first option and any abnormal flow detected should be studied and quantified using spectral Doppler.

Echocardiographic examination protocol

An echocardiographic examination is an interactive procedure involving the clinician, ultrasound equipment and animal. A perfect interaction between these three components is key to obtaining echocardiographic images and signals which can be used to diagnose and monitor heart disease.

The clinician carrying out the examination should be familiar with:

- the **equipment** and the basic principles of ultrasound physics
- the **anatomy** and physiology of the cardiovascular system
- the **haemodynamic** effects typical of different heart diseases.

The ultrasound equipment should include the following.

- 2D, M-mode and spectral Doppler (pulsed and continuous), and colour flow Doppler modes.
- A system for recording videos and images.
- Specialised software for measurement of cardiac structures and blood flow velocities.

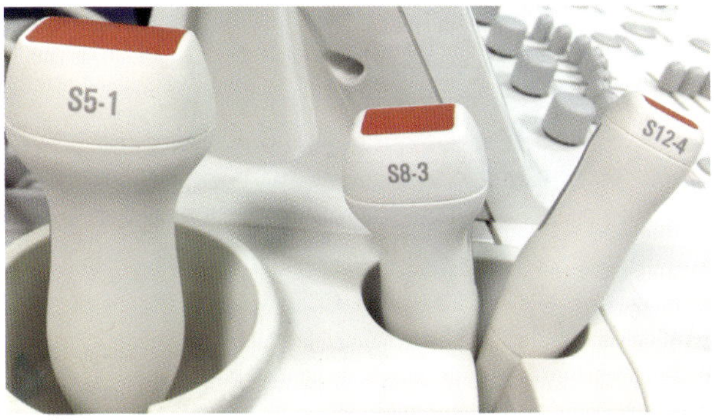

Figure 5.31. Phased array sectorial transducers of various frequencies as used by the author for echocardiographic examination of dogs and cats of different sizes: frequencies of 5-1 for large dogs, 8-3 for small to medium-sized dogs and 12-4 for very small dogs, and cats.

- Phased array sectorial transducers with a frequency suitable for the animal's size. **High frequencies are usually used in small dogs and cats**, and the **lowest frequencies in medium-sized and large dogs** (Figure 5.31). Frequency affects the depth of ultrasound wave penetration and image resolution (the higher the frequency, the greater the penetration and resolution, and vice versa). Body condition should also be considered: obese animals require transducers with lower frequencies. Doppler ultrasound uses low-frequency transducers, as these allow pulse repetition frequency to be increased and higher velocities to be measured without causing aliasing.
- **Synchronous electrocardiograph** to simultaneously record an ECG over the echocardiogram. This allows the cardiac phase corresponding to each image to be measured (particularly important when taking measurements or interpreting spectral Doppler). For this method, three electrodes are connected to the extremities using paediatric adhesive discs, and secured with elastic bandages or clips (Figure 5.32).

Preparation and positioning of the patient

Preparation

An echocardiographic examination is usually well tolerated by the majority of animals. However, puppies and some nervous or stressed animals may require sedation. Although no sedative or combination of medication acts without side effects on the cardiovascular system (altering sympathetic tone, changing blood pressure or disrupting ventricular function), the following are the most commonly used.

- **In dogs**: a combination of acepromazine (0.03 mg/kg) and buprenorphine (0.005–0.0075 mg/kg) IM or IV.
- **In cats**: a combination of acepromazine (0.1 mg/kg) and buprenorphine (0.25 mg/kg) IM or IV.

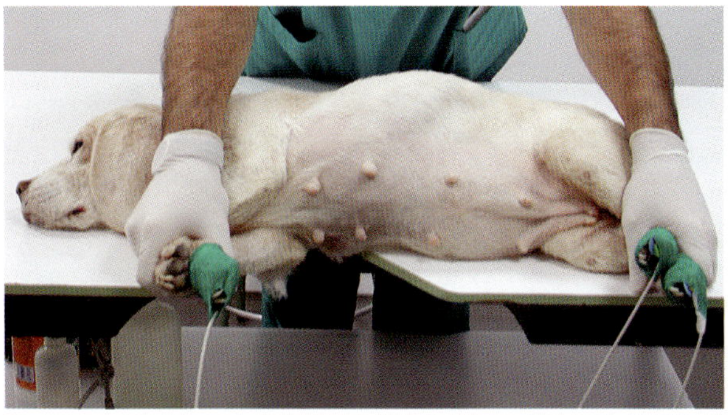

Figure 5.32. Dog positioned in right lateral recumbency ready for the echocardiographic examination; the electrodes for the simultaneous ECG to accompany the echocardiographic images can be seen placed on the dog's pads.

- If acepromazine is contraindicated (patients with right–left shunts, hypertensive animals, etc.) or in patients in critical states, **butorphanol** can be used alone, to reduce anxiety.

In order to improve image quality, hair should be clipped from the area around the heart (from the 3rd to the 6th intercostal space on each side) and the area cleaned with alcohol.

Positioning

The animal should be placed in **lateral recumbency** for the examination (Figure 5.32) on a table with a cut-out corresponding to the cardiac area, so that the transducer can be applied from below to improve access to the heart. If this position is not well tolerated (particularly in dyspnoeic animals), an emergency echocardiograph can be carried out with the animal standing (dog) or in sternal recumbency (cat), although some images are difficult to capture in the latter position.

Basic ultrasound equipment controls

Once the animal is prepared and the ultrasound machine switched on, some basic adjustments can be made to the equipment to obtain a suitable 2D echo image.

- **Field depth**. The image of the cardiac structures to be visualised should occupy most of the image sector in the 2D image. A **scale indicating depth** is displayed at the sides of the image sector; the distance between two points corresponds to 1 cm.
- **Gain**. This is used to control the intensity of the transducer signal over the whole image sector. **Very high gains produce a very white image**, while very low gains give rise to weak signals and a very faint image. The ideal gain allows cardiac structures to be observed clearly, without superimposing ultrasound image sectors.

- **Time gain compensation**. This consists of increasing the gain at different depths to **improve image quality** without losing information in either shallow or deep sectors.
- **Sector size**. Sector width can be adjusted from approximately 120° to 45°; reduced image sector width gives **better image resolution**. This should be established when Doppler mode is used.

Obtaining standard echocardiographic images

Animal position: right lateral recumbency

In this position, the transducer is applied from below, over the **4th–5th intercostal spaces** and **1–5 cm from the sternal border**, with liberal use of ultrasound gel to optimise the passage of the ultrasound waves through the skin.

Once the cardiac structures have been located, the transducer is orientated to obtain standardised images from different projections.

Right parasternal long axis

This projection has two main planes.

- **Four-chamber** (atria and ventricles) (Figure 5.26). The proportions of the four chambers can be seen; the largest are the left-sided chambers, and the atrioventricular valves separate the atria and ventricles.
- **Left ventricular outflow tract** and **ascending aorta**, with the apex towards the left of the image (Figure 5.33).

Various cardiac structures can be seen in movement in these images and the following can be assessed.

- The **appearance and movement** of the chambers, valves, walls, pericardium, left ventricular outflow tract and ascending aorta.
- Flow entering and leaving the atria and ventricles (with colour Doppler), to detect abnormal flow associated with valvular insufficiency or stenosis.
- Size of the left atrium and the systolic and diastolic volumes of the left ventricle in the four-chamber view, using the modified Simpson method (Figure 5.34) from which the ejection fraction can be determined.
- The diameter of the aortic ring and the ascending aorta at various different levels, in the view of left ventricular outflow tract.

Right parasternal short axis

Starting in the previous, long-axis position, the transducer is rotated anticlockwise 90°. This gives cross-sectional images of cardiac structures, from the heart apex towards the base, passing through the papillary muscles of the left ventricle, the chordae tendineae, mitral valve and great vessels.

- **Transventricular** image (Figure 5.35a): the papillary muscles can be seen.
- **Transmitral** image (Figure 5.35b): the mitral valve appears ovoid in shape.
- **Transaortic and left atrial** image (Figure 5.35c): dimensions of the left atrium (LA) and ascending aorta (Ao) are measured to obtain the LA/Ao ratio. LA/Ao <1.6 in dogs; LA/Ao <1.3 in cats.
- **Transaortic and pulmonary artery** image (Figure 5.35d): colour Doppler is used to evaluate flow in the pulmonary artery (Figure 5.30), determining the velocity by pulsed Doppler (placing the sample volume behind the pulmonary sigmoids) (V = 0.8–1.6 m/s) (Figure 5.28) or with continuous wave Doppler if the velocity is very high, as occurs in dogs with pulmonary stenosis.

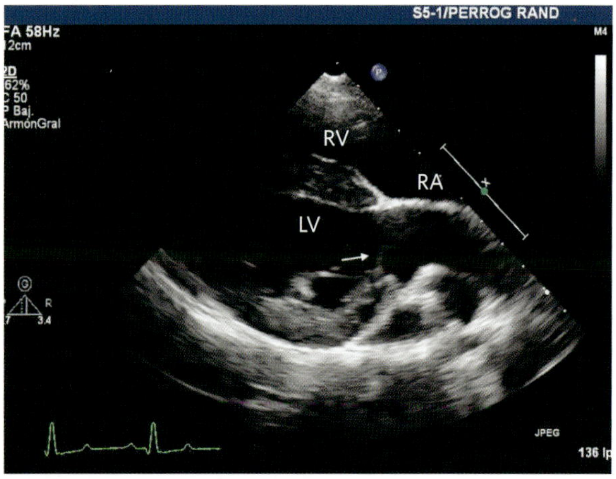

Figure 5.33. Right parasternal long-axis five-chamber 2D echocardiogram of a normal dog, level with the left ventricular outflow tract; the aortic sigmoids (arrow) and ascending aorta (Ao) can be seen. LV, left ventricle; RA, right atrium; RV, right ventricle.

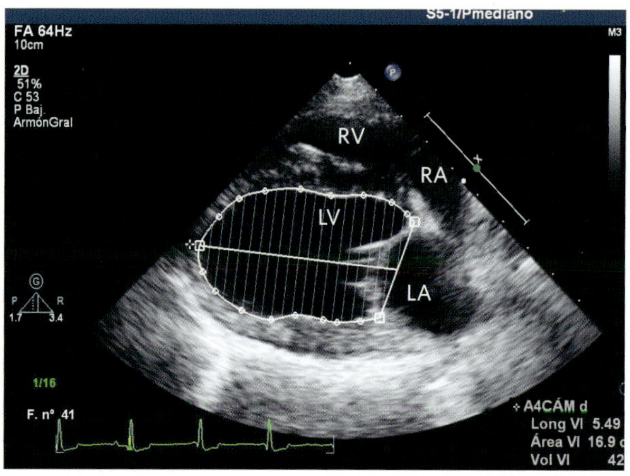

Figure 5.34. Right parasternal long-axis four-chamber 2D echocardiogram of a normal dog, demonstrating the measurement of left ventricular volume. LA, left atrium; LV, left ventricle; RV, right ventricle; RA, right atrium.

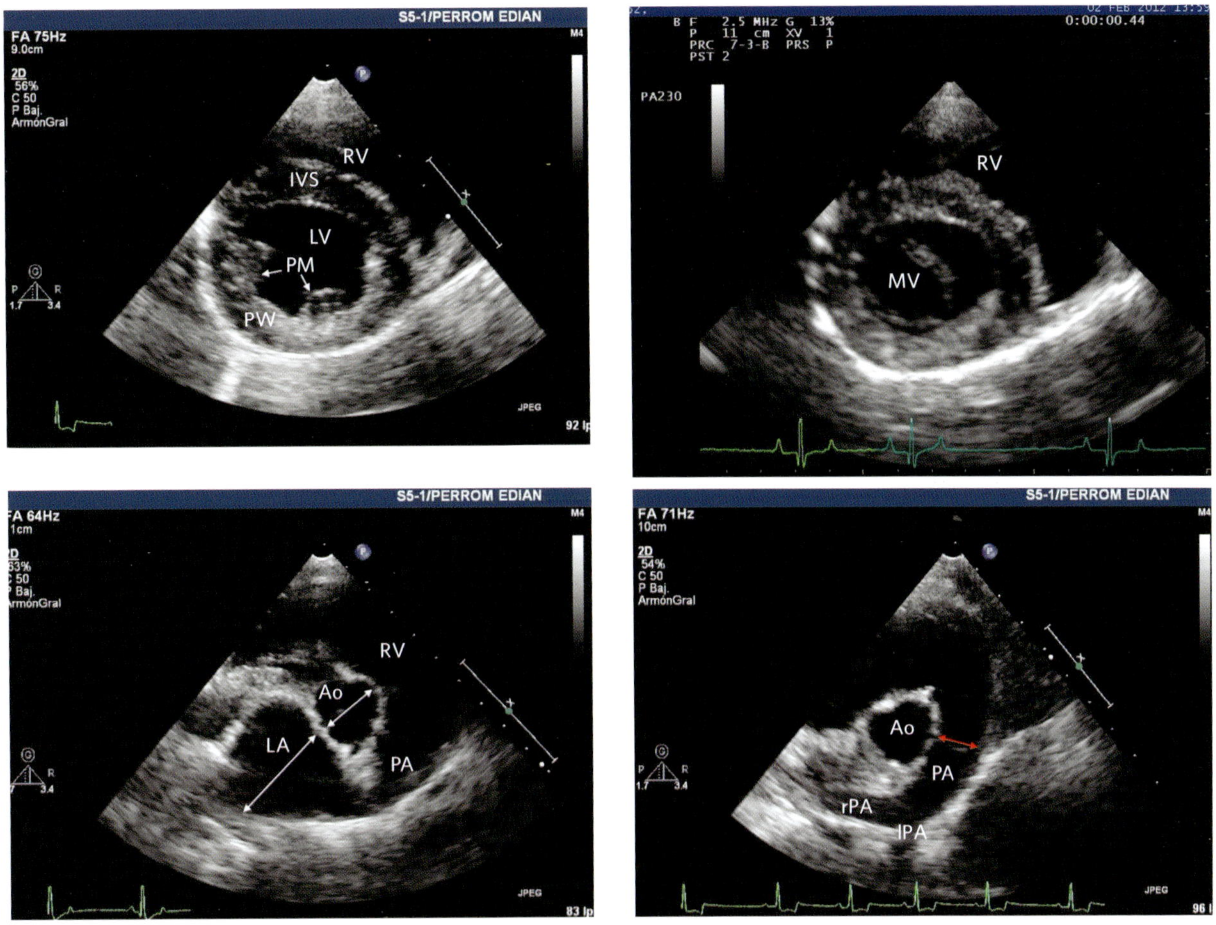

Figure 5.35. Right parasternal short-axis 2D echocardiograms, at different levels. (a) Transventricular, where the left ventricle (LV) can be observed with the papillary muscles (PM) towards the lumen (arrow) and the right ventricle (RV) in the upper part of the image, in a half-moon shape. (b) Transmitral, where the oval shape of the mitral valve (MV) can be seen in the centre of the LV. (c) Transaortic, where the ascending aorta (Ao) can be seen in the centre of the image, surrounded by the left atrium (LA), right ventricle (RV) and the pulmonary artery (PA); measurements of the Ao and LA are shown. (d) Transaortic, more cranially, where the Ao can be seen in the centre of the image, the RV and the PA at the bifurcation; measurement of the PI ring is shown. IVS, interventricular septum; rPA, right pulmonary artery; lPA, left pulmonary artery; PW, posterior wall.

Using the cross-sections mentioned previously, and placing the **M-mode cursor** over the three-dimensional images, standardised views can be obtained in which cardiac structures (walls, chambers and great vessels) can be directly measured (Tables 5.2 and 5.3).

- **Transventricular** level (the chordae tendineae are visible): septal and parietal densities, ventricular cavities in systole and diastole, and left ventricular free wall excursion are measured (Figure 5.27). Indices of functionality, such as the left ventricular shortening fraction (SF), can be calculated from these direct measurements. SF = LVd – LVs/LVd (where LVd and LVs = size of the left ventricle in diastole and systole).
  - **In dogs**: SF = 24–44%.
  - **In cats:** SF = 30–50%.
- **Transmitral** level: the distance between the point of maximum aperture of the mitral valve (E) and the interventricular septum (IVS) can be measured (Figure 5.36). E–IVS < 7 mm in dogs.
- **Transaortic** level: the dimensions of the aorta at the end of diastole and the left atrium at the end of systole are the main measurements taken (Figure 5.37).

Subxiphoid and subcostal projection

With the animal still in right lateral recumbency, a low-frequency (2–2.5 MHz) transducer is selected, allowing for examination of the left ventricular outflow tract and ascending aorta. Aim to obtain a good alignment between the Doppler ultrasound beam and the blood flow, including the high-velocity flow in the aorta (important in dogs with aortic stenosis) (V = 1.7–2.2 m/s) (Figure 5.29).

Animal position: left lateral recumbency

The transducer is placed in two principal positions to record diagnostic images.

Table 5.2. Measurements (M-mode) of the dimensions of the left ventricle, interventricular septum and posterior heart wall in dogs according to body weight (Cornell et al., 2004). LVd/LVs, size of the left ventricle in diastole (d) and in systole (s); PWd, posterior wall in diastole; IVSd, interventricular septum in diastole.

Body weight (kg)	LVd (cm)	LVs (cm)	PWd (cm)	IVSd (cm)
3	2.1 (1.8–2.6)	1.3 (1.0–1.8)	0.5 (0.4–0.8)	0.3 (0.4–0.8)
6	2.6 (2.2–3.1)	1.7 (1.2–2.2)	0.6 (0.4–0.9)	0.6 (0.4–0.9)
9	2.9 (2.4–3.4)	1.9 (1.4–2.5)	0.7 (0.5–1.0)	0.7 (0.5–1.0)
15	3.4 (2.8–4.1)	2.2 (1.7–3.0)	0.8 (0.5–1.1)	0.8 (0.6–1.1)
20	3.7 (3.1–4.5)	2.4 (1.8–3.2)	0.8 (0.6–1.2)	0.8 (0.6–1.2)
30	4.2 (3.5–5.0)	2.8 (2.1–3.7)	0.9 (0.6–1.3)	0.9 (0.7–1.3)
40	4.5 (3.8–5.5)	3.0 (2.3–4.0)	1.0 (0.7–1.4)	1.0 (0.7–1.4)
50	4.8 (4.0–5.8)	3.3 (2.4–43)	1.1 (0.7–1.5)	1.1 (0.7–1.5)
60	5.1 (4.2–6.2)	3.3 (2.6–4.6)	1.1 (0.7–1.6)	1.1 (0.8–1.6)
70	5.3 (4.4–6.5)	3.6 (2.7–4.8)	1.1 (0.8–1.6)	1.1 (0.8–1.6)

Table 5.3. M-mode measurement of the left ventricle, interventricular septum and posterior heart wall in cats (Luis Fuentes, 2010). The heart rate is taken using 2D ultrasound because the cursor passes over the auricle of the left atrium and not over the atrium itself. LVd/LVs, size of the left ventricle in diastole (d) and in systole (s); PWd/PWs, posterior wall in diastole and systole; IVSd/IVSs, interventricular septum in diastole and systole.

Parameter	Value
Weight (kg)	3.2–7.2
Heart rate (bpm)	145–267
IVSd (cm)	≤5
LVd (cm)	11.5–17.8
PWd (cm)	<5
IVSs (cm)	4.4–10.1
LVs (cm)	2.6–10.9
PWs (cm)	5.6–9.5

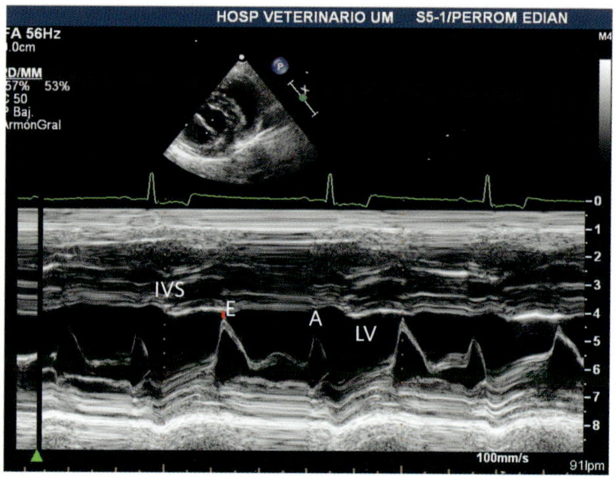

Figure 5.36. Right parasternal transmitral M-mode echocardiogram, showing the 'M'-shaped anterior leaflet and 'W'-shaped posterior leaflet. The distance from the point of maximum excursion of the mitral valve (E) to the interventricular septum (IVS) is shown. LV, left ventricle.

Caudal or apical left parasternal projection

The transducer is placed over the 5th–7th left intercostal spaces, orientated dorsally towards the heart base.

- **Four-chamber image.** The transmitral flow spectrum, consisting of two peaks, can be obtained from this view: E (V = 0.5–1 m/s) and A (V = 0.3–0.6 m/s) (Figure 5.38).
- **Three- and five-chamber image.** Aortic flow can be measured if it is impossible to measure it via the subcostal window (V = 0.8–1.7 m/s) (Figure 5.39).
- **Two-chamber image**, from the apical position and with the ultrasound beam parallel to the long axis of the heart. The left ventricle (LV), left atrium (LA) and auricles can be seen, separated by the mitral valve (Figure 5.40). This image allows the auricle to be

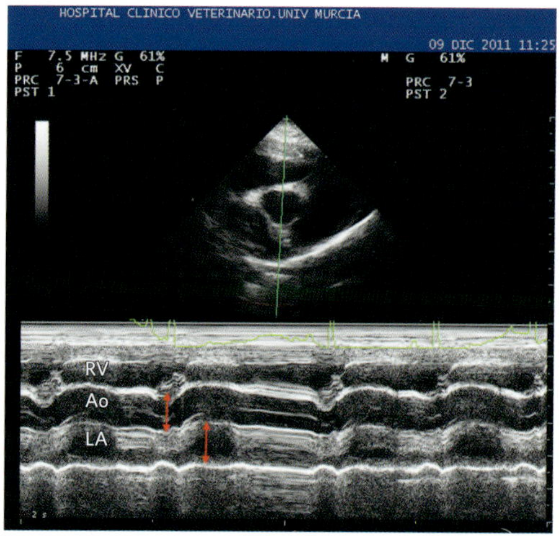

Figure 5.37. Transaortic M-mode echocardiogram, where measurement of the ascending aorta (Ao) at the end of diastole and the left atrium (LA) in systole are shown. RV, right ventricle.

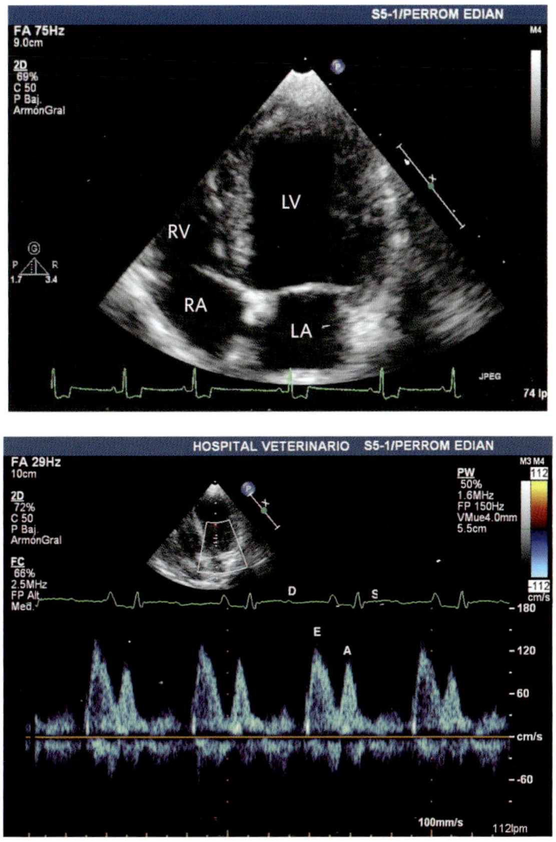

Figure 5.38. Left apical parasternal four-chamber 2D echocardiogram (a) and pulsed Doppler (b) in a normal dog. (a) In this plane the left-sided chambers are seen as larger than the right. (b) The transmitral flow spectrum can be seen: peak E corresponds with the initial diastolic phase and peak A, with a lower velocity, to the final phase or atrial systole. LA, left atrium; LV, left ventricle; RA, right atrium; RV, right ventricle.

visualised, which is important in cats with suspected thromboembolism.

Left cranial parasternal projection

The transducer is placed further cranially, over the 3rd–4th intercostal spaces between the sternum and the costochondral joints, producing long- and short-axis images.

Long-axis images

- Image of the left ventricular outflow tract, aortic valve and ascending aorta (Figure 5.41a).
- Oblique view of the left ventricle, right atrium, inferior vena cava inlet, tricuspid valve and right ventricular inflow tract with the auricular appendix; this view is important for visualisation of neoplasms, such as haemangiosarcomas, in dogs with pericardial effusion (Figure 5.41b).
- Image of the left ventricle and the right ventricular outflow tract, the pulmonary valve and main pulmonary artery. This image is important for visualisation and measurement of patent ductus arteriosus (Figure 5.41c).

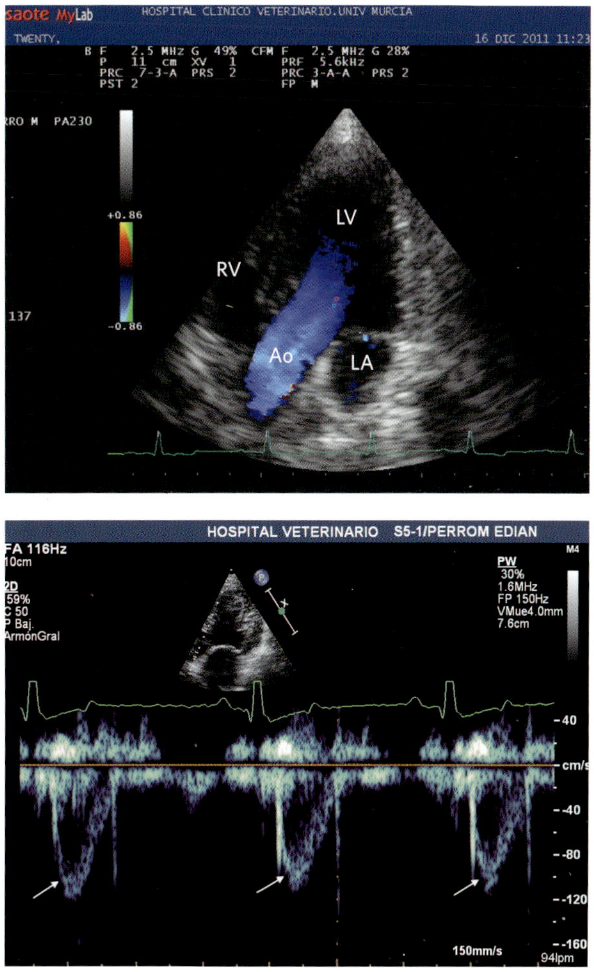

Figure 5.39. Left apical parasternal three–five-chamber colour (a) and pulsed (b) Doppler echocardiograms in a normal dog. (a) Aortic flow is coloured blue, as it moves away from the transducer, from the left ventricle (LV) towards the aorta (Ao). LA, left atrium; RV, right ventricle.

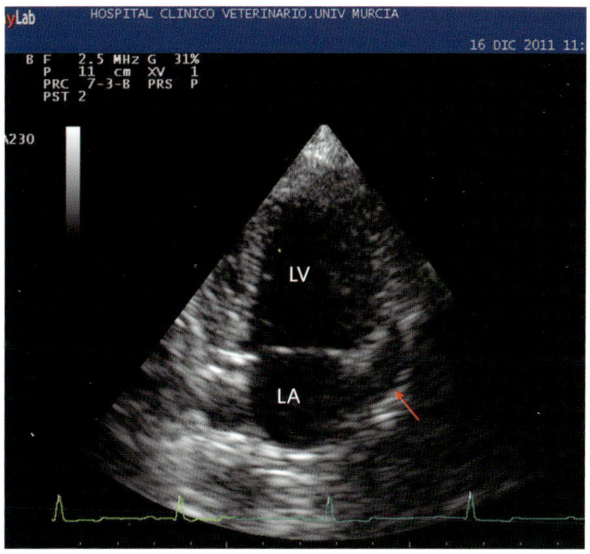

Figure 5.40. Right apical parasternal two-chamber 2D echocardiogram, showing the left ventricle (LV), left atrium (LA) and auricle (arrow).

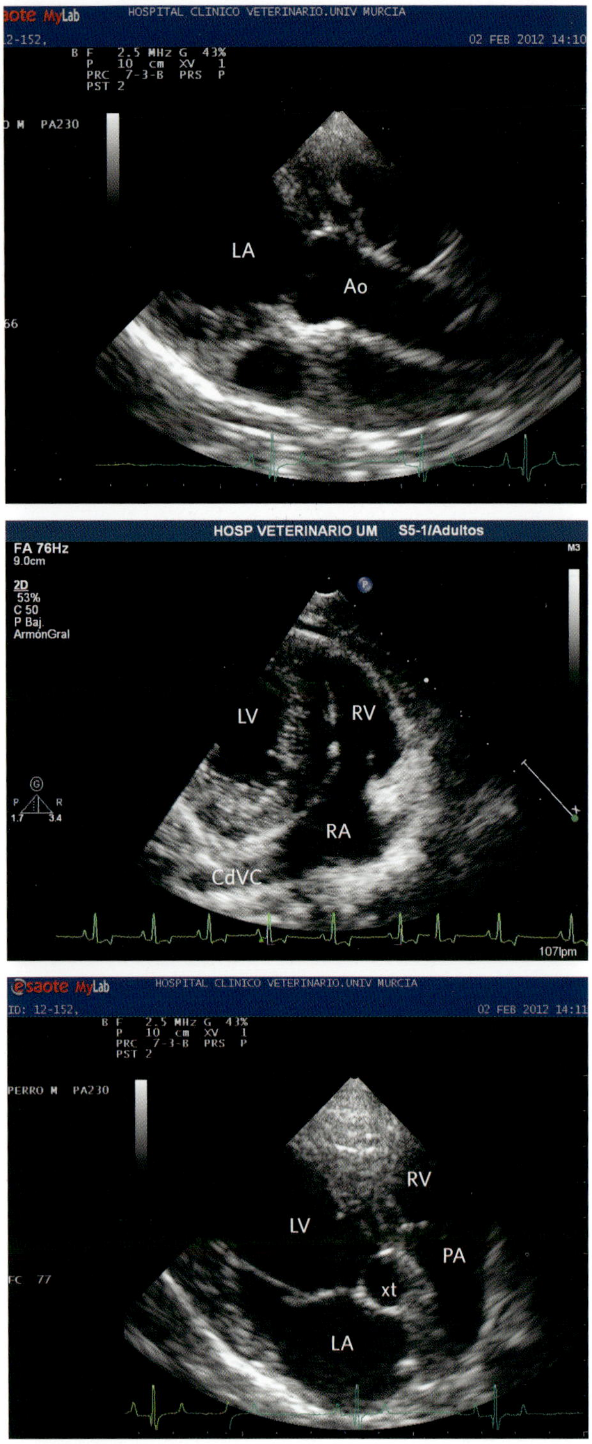

Figure 5.41. Left cranial parasternal long-axis 2D echocardiograms. (a) The left ventricular outflow tract, left atrium (LA) and pulmonary artery with sigmoids can be seen. (b) The right ventricle (RV), tricuspid valve, right atrium (RA) with the auricle and the inferior vena cava inlet (IVCi) are shown. (c) The left and right ventricles (LV, RV), left atrium (LA) and pulmonary artery (PA) can be observed.

Short-axis image

Start with a long-axis image and rotate the transducer 90° anticlockwise to give the short-axis image, with the aortic root in the centre surrounded by the structures on the right side of the heart (right atrium, tricuspid valve, right ventricular outflow tract and main pulmonary artery with the bifurcation) (Figure 5.42).

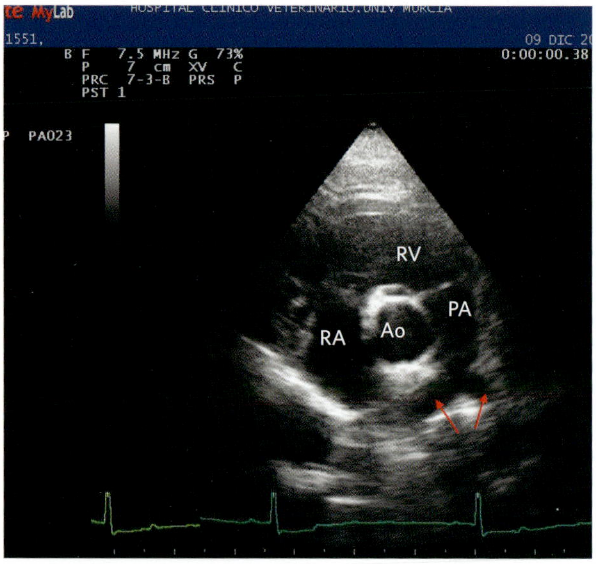

Figure 5.42. Left cranial parasternal short-axis 2D echocardiogram showing the aorta (Ao) in the centre of the image, surrounded by the right atrium and ventricle (RA and RV) to the left, and the main pulmonary artery (PA) with the bifurcation (arrows) to the right of the picture.

Heart failure

Definitions

Heart disease

Heart disease is defined as any structural or functional abnormality of the heart which may or may not cause heart failure. Many animals with heart disease, and particularly those in the early stages, are asymptomatic because cardiac functionality and neurohormonal activity are minimally affected, or not affected at all.

Heart failure

Heart failure is a progressive, complex clinical syndrome which can arise from any functional or structural abnormality that modifies the capacity of the ventricles to fill or eject blood flow according to tissue requirements at the time (including when venous filling pressures are normal).

Congestive heart failure

Congestive heart failure is an oedematous state secondary to a combination of excessive sodium and water retention, and a failing heart. Raised atrial pressures increase hydrostatic pressure and fluid accumulation in the interstitial spaces (pulmonary oedema) and body cavities (pleural effusion or ascites).

Aetiopathogenesis

There is no one specific cause of heart failure, as the syndrome is triggered by multiple heart diseases and characterised by cardiac, haemodynamic, renal, neurohormonal and cytokine disturbances. The causes of heart diseases can be classified by their aetiology when this is known, but many are genetic or idiopathic. Classic physiopathological classification includes systolic and diastolic dysfunction, and haemodynamic overload (pressure or volume).

The anatomical location of the disease is a useful aid to morphological diagnosis. Problems can be located in the pericardium, myocardium, endocardium, valves, systems responsible for formation and conduction of the electrical impulse and the blood vessels.

In dogs, the most common heart diseases are:

- chronic degenerative mitral valve disease (CDMVD)
- dilated cardiomyopathy (genetic or idiopathic)
- pericardial effusion (idiopathic, neoplastic)
- congenital abnormalities
- arrhythmias (atrial fibrillation, ventricular tachycardia, atrioventricular blocks, etc.).

In cats, cardiomyopathies are the most common cardiac diseases.

The causative agent or trigger for heart failure damages cardiac structures, causing loss of myocyte functionality, and disrupts the ability of the myocardium to generate force, impeding normal heart contraction. This trigger can act suddenly (myocardial infarction) or gradually (pressure or volume overload).

Most patients remain asymptomatic or minimally symptomatic for a long time. As heart disease develops, a series of **compensatory mechanisms** are activated in response to the damage or reduced cardiac output. These seem to modulate ventricular function within a homeostatic/physiological range, maintaining the patient's functional capacity. However, when the patient passes into the symptomatic phase, sustained activation of neurohormonal and cytokine systems give rise to a series of systemic and myocardial changes, collectively known as **cardiac remodelling**.

Neurohormonal mechanisms

Activation of the sympathetic nervous system (adrenergic)

This occurs in the early stages of heart failure, as the reduced cardiac output stimulates pressure receptors in the aortic arch and the carotid sinus, causing the release of norepinephrine, levels of which increase two- or threefold in late stages. This mechanism contributes to increased myocardial contractility and cardiac output, and increases peripheral vasoconstriction, all of which consume a large amount of energy and oxygen, which can in turn cause arrhythmias and myocardial damage over time.

Activation of the renin–angiotensin–aldosterone system (RAAS)

The **RAAS** is activated in the **late stages of heart failure**. This activation is considered to be due to renal hypoperfusion secondary to the drop in cardiac output, reduction in sodium filtered at the macula densa level in the distal tubule, and sympathetic activation. This causes production of renin by the juxtaglomerular apparatus, contributing to the formation of angiotensin I from hepatic angiotensinogen. Angiotensin I is transformed into angiotensin II (AgII) by pulmonary angiotensin-converting enzyme (ACE). AgII can also be synthesised by other means than renin, from the transformation of angiotensinogen into angiotensin I by kallikrein and cathepsin C. AgII is also formed in tissues by routes that are independent of ACE (chymase activation).

In the short term, AgII is important for maintaining homeostasis; however, in the long term, it **causes fibrosis** of the heart, kidneys and other organs. AgII can also exacerbate neurohormonal activation, increasing norepinephrine release and aldosterone production by the adrenal cortex. Like AgII, aldosterone also supports circulation in the short term, improving sodium reabsorption and potassium elimination in the distal tubule of the nephron. In the long term, aldosterone activation also leads to hypertrophy and fibrosis of the myocardium and blood vessels, reducing compliance, and causes ventricular stiffness and endothelial dysfunction. This results in oxidative stress and tissue inflammation.

Neurohormonal disruption of renal function

One of the main neurohormonal effects on renal function is the **retention of salt and water** by the kidneys due to reduced effective arterial blood volume, which activates the RAAS and the sympathetic nervous system. Renal sympathetic stimulation causes liberation of the hormone **arginine vasopressin** by the pituitary gland, reducing free water excretion and exacerbating peripheral vasoconstriction, and increasing endothelin production.

In order to counteract all the adverse effects caused by the vasoconstrictor systems, a series of neurohormonal systems are activated, such as metabolites of vasodilator **prostaglandins (PGE2)**, **prostacyclins (PGI2)** and **natriuretic peptides (ANP and BNP)**. Prostaglandins tend to increase renal sodium excretion and modulate the action of arginine vasopressin. Once vasoconstrictor neurohormonal systems are activated, atrial and/or myocardial distension occurs due to increased venous volume, and then natriuretic peptides are activated. The action of these peptides in the kidney is centred on maintaining homeostasis by increasing sodium and water elimination. However, as heart disease progresses, these systems become ineffective.

Neurohormonal changes in peripheral vessels

Complex interactions between the **autonomic nervous system** and local autoregulatory mechanisms in patients with heart failure maintain circulation to the brain and heart, and reduce blood flow to the skin, skeletal muscles, splanchnic organs and kidneys. Activation of the **sympathetic nervous system** in the peripheral arteries and increased circulating concentrations of vasoconstrictors (norepinephrine, endothelin, AgII, urotensin II, thromboxane A2, etc.) contribute to arteriolar vasoconstriction and maintenance of arterial pressure. In the venous system, sympathetic stimulation increases tone, helping maintain return, ventricular filling and cardiac function according to Starling's law of the heart.

Ventricular remodelling

Ventricular remodelling includes complex changes in **myocyte biology** (volume of myocytes and other components) and in ventricular **geometry and architecture**.

Changes in myocyte biology

There is a gradual loss of contractile function and loss of myofilaments from cardiac myocytes due to disruption of the cytoskeleton, alterations in excitation–contraction coupling and desensitisation to β-adrenergic signals.

Myocardial hypertrophy

There are two patterns of cardiac hypertrophy which occur in response to haemodynamic overload (Figure 5.43).

- **Hypertrophy** caused by **pressure overload** (subaortic stenosis, systemic hypertension) or concentric hypertrophy: increased systolic pressure in the heart wall causes sarcomeres to be added in parallel and gives rise to an increased cross-sectional area of myocytes, causing parietal thickening and reducing the ventricular lumen.
- **Hypertrophy** caused by **volume overload** or eccentric hypertrophy: the increase in diastolic pressure in the heart wall causes myocytes to lengthen by adding sarcomeres in series, giving rise to ventricular dilation.

Changes to excitation–contraction coupling

In patients with heart failure, the cascade of events that starts with the potential for the event and ends with myocyte contraction is disrupted, so that the potential for the event is prolonged and cardiac contractions are disrupted and diminished in the late stages of heart failure.

Contractile and regulatory protein abnormalities

In patients with heart failure, there are changes in atrial and ventricular myosin light chains and the troponin–tropomyosin complexes. In the late stages, concentrations of foetal isoforms, such as cTnT1, are also elevated.

Cytoskeletal protein abnormalities

The **myocyte cytoskeleton** is made up of actin, desmin, titin and tubulin. A loss of cytoskeletal integrity and links between the sarcomere, the sarcolemma and the extracellular matrix are responsible for contractile dysfunction, both in the myocyte and myocardium in patients with heart failure.

Myocardial changes in patients with heart failure

These can be divided into two types:

- changes to the volume of myocytes
- changes to the composition of the extracellular matrix.

Where there are volume changes, there is a progressive loss of myocytes by phenomena such as necrosis.

Changes in the extracellular matrix (composed of a basement membrane, fibrous collagen network around the myocytes, proteoglycans, glycosaminoglycans and biologically active molecules) include changes in synthesis and degradation of the collagen fibrils, and alterations in the connections between collagen and myocytes.

In both cases, expression of the embryonic genes which cause cellular disruption, and eventual contractile dysfunction, increases (Figure 5.43). Apoptosis and autophagic cell death start to occur, and all of these contribute to progressive cardiac dysfunction and ventricular remodelling.

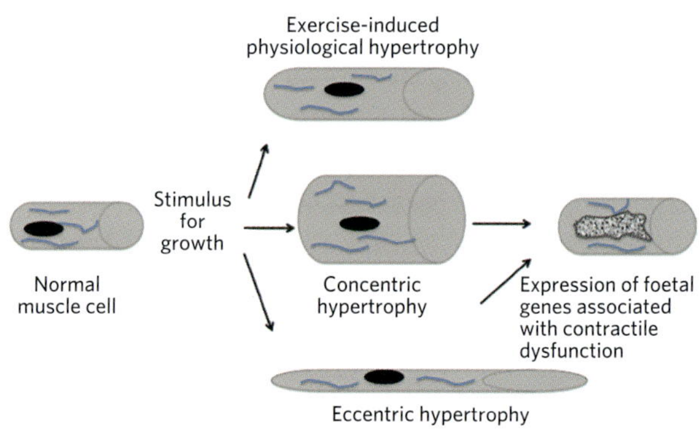

Figure 5.43. Diagram showing myocardial changes in diseases accompanied by pressure overload (concentric hypertrophy) and volume overload (eccentric hypertrophy).

Ventricular changes

The main changes are in ventricular size and shape. In advanced stages of heart failure, the left ventricle becomes more spherical and less elliptical, with increased blood volume and energy consumption. In addition to this volume increase at the end of ventricular diastole, there is also thinning of the ventricular wall. These changes contribute to an afterload mismatch and reduced ventricular ejection volume.

Increased parietal stress contributes to gene activation (expression of AgII, endothelin and tumour necrosis factor [TNF]), **ventricular hypertrophy** and reduced subendocardial perfusion, contributing to **myocardial dysfunction**. Ventricular dilation also causes poor positioning of the papillary muscles, leading to mitral valve incompetence and valvular regurgitation, and reducing ventricular ejection volume, increasing ventricular preload (volume at the end of diastole) and raising atrial pressures. All of these changes promote loss of ventricular function, regardless of the neurohormonal status of the patient.

Inflammatory mediators

Proinflammatory cytokines (IL-1 and TNF) are produced locally in the myocardium as heart failure develops and these contribute to cardiac remodelling in both the myocytes and the extracellular matrix. High levels of these cytokines indicate a poor prognosis in patients with heart failure.

Clinical signs

The terms **'left-sided heart failure'** and **'right-sided heart failure'** are used to characterise the clinical signs presented by patients with cardiac insufficiency. Given that cardiac output from both ventricles should be the same, bilateral heart failure is common.

Clinical signs of left-sided heart failure

Pulmonary oedema is the main symptom. This is induced by raised hydrostatic capillary pressure, secondary to elevated pulmonary venous pressure. There is then transudation from the capillary to the interstitial space, and signs of pulmonary oedema occur when lymphatic drainage is overwhelmed.

Signs of **respiratory dysfunction** can be due to:

- pulmonary oedema (interstitial and/or alveolar)
- pleural effusion compressing the lung and causing atelectasis
- dilation of the left atrium compressing the main left bronchus
- pulmonary fibrosis induced by chronic oedema
- pulmonary hypertension (dyspnoea and tachypnoea caused by complex mechanisms).

Clinical signs associated with **low cardiac output and tissue perfusion** include:

- weakness during exercise
- exercise intolerance
- pallor
- syncope.

Clinical signs associated with **pulmonary oedema and pleural effusion** include:

- tachypnoea
- dyspnoea
- orthopnoea
- fatigue
- pulmonary crepitation
- cough
- haemoptysis
- cyanosis.

Clinical signs of right-sided heart failure

Right-sided heart failure is characterised by **systemic venous distension**, congested abdominal organs (liver) and **effusion** in the serosal cavities (ascites; effusion in the subcutaneous tissue of the deteriorated parts is also common in large dogs). This is due to elevated capillary and venous pressures, secondary to failure of right ventricular drainage, and sodium and water retention in the kidney, causing an increase in plasma volume.

Ascites is caused by elevated venous pressure in the hepatic sinusoids (less dense than the pulmonary capillaries). Formation of protein-rich hepatic lymph through the walls of the sinusoids and within the interstitial space of the liver is increased during passive hepatic congestion.

This fluid accumulates in the liver capsule before passing into the peritoneal space and when fluid formation overwhelms the lymphatic drainage system, ascites results (usually with the characteristics of a modified transudate).

Development of **pleural effusion** involves mechanisms similar to those described previously, although somewhat more complex. It is more common when the haemodynamic consequences affect both ventricles, or when left ventricular failure causes pulmonary hypertension and secondary right ventricular failure.

Clinical signs associated with **low cardiac output** include:

- exercise-related weakness
- exercise intolerance

- pallor
- syncope.

Signs related to **systemic venous congestion** include:

- enlargement of the liver and, occasionally, the spleen
- mild pericardial effusion
- pleural effusion (leading to pulmonary atelectasis, tachypnoea, respiratory distress and cyanosis)
- peritoneal effusion (ascites)
- distension of cutaneous veins
- subcutaneous oedema in large-breed dogs.

Signs of bilateral heart failure

Clinical signs presented by these patients include signs of both left-sided and right-sided heart failure.

Diagnosis

Factors to consider when diagnosing heart failure are as follows.

- **Epidemiology and risk factors** of certain age and breed groups for certain heart diseases.
- **Physical examination**: particular attention should be paid to arterial and venous pulse, thoracic auscultation (pulmonary and cardiac) and abdominal palpation.
- **Thoracic radiographs** help establish a diagnosis of heart failure and exclude thoracic or bronchopulmonary disease.
- **Doppler and 2D echocardiography** enable structural, haemodynamic and functional changes to be identified.
- **Electrocardiogram**: despite being non-specific for diagnosing heart diseases, the electrocardiogram is crucial when evaluating changes in heart rhythm. Holter 24-hour electrocardiographic monitoring may be necessary in certain patients with transitory arrhythmias.
- **Systemic arterial pressure** does not usually cause heart failure but can contribute to deterioration of other heart diseases.
- **Laboratory analysis**: complete blood count, biochemistry and urinalysis help evaluate renal functionality, and tests for natriuretic peptides (NT-proBNP) are useful for monitoring the evolution of heart diseases.

Functional classifications

New York Heart Association (NYHA)

Extrapolated from human medicine, this functional classification of patients with heart failure is based on the signs and symptoms of heart disorders and the capacity for exercise.

- **Class I**: objective signs of heart disorders and normal capacity for exercise.
- **Class II**: objective signs of heart disorders and clinical evidence of cardiac failure on exercise or with intense activity.
- **Class III**: objective signs of heart failure on minimal exercise or sometimes at rest, for example, nocturnal orthopnoea.
- **Class IV**: dyspnoea while at rest.

International Small Animal Cardiac Health Council (ISACHC)

Developed for veterinary patients and more appropriate in practical terms.

- **Class I**: no sign of heart failure (NYHA Class I).
- **Class II**: the animal presents some degree of exercise intolerance (NYHA Classes II and III).
- **Class III**: signs of heart disease evident at rest (NYHA Class IV).

American College of Cardiology and American Heart Association, accepted by the European Society of Veterinary Cardiology and the American College of Veterinary Internal Medicine study group.

These institutions have developed a classification based on the progressive nature of heart failure, which can be adapted to canine patients as follows.

- **Class A**: dogs without structural changes to the heart but with a high risk of them developing (Cavalier King Charles Spaniels, chronic degenerative mitral valve disease; Dobermans, dilated cardiomyopathy).
- **Class B**: dogs with structural changes to the heart but which have not yet developed clinical signs of heart failure (small-breed dogs with mitral regurgitation murmur, Boxers with many ventricular premature complexes [VPCs] on Holter monitoring).
- **Class B1**: no cardiomegaly on thoracic radiology or echocardiography.
- **Class B2**: signs of cardiomegaly on thoracic radiology or echocardiography.
- **Class C**: dogs with past or current clinical signs of heart failure, including those which are asymptomatic with treatment.
- **Class D**: dogs in the late stages of the disease, with clinical signs refractory to standard therapies for heart failure (diuretics, ACE inhibitors, digoxin, pimobendan).

Treatment

Treatment of heart failure should be based on **precise diagnosis** of the aetiology, the clinical state of each

patient and the current clinical signs, considering as patients all those who are asymptomatic, those who present with pulmonary oedema, cardiogenic shock or arrhythmias, chronic patients, and those with complications (renal disease).

Patient monitoring and **periodic re-evaluation** are essential to assess the response to treatment and evaluate the need to adjust dosage and add or substitute medication.

Only general guidelines and the medications most commonly used to treat heart failure are covered in this section; treatments for specific heart diseases are explained in the relevant sections.

Specific corrective therapy

Recommended for heart diseases which can be corrected/minimised by surgery (closure of the patent ductus arteriosus), catheterisation (balloon valvuloplasty in congenital pulmonary stenosis) or pacemaker implantation (complete atrioventricular block, sick sinus syndrome, etc.) and pericardiocentesis (pericardial tamponade), amongst others.

Exercise restriction

Restricting exercise is advisable, especially in patients in late stages of heart failure, to avoid overloading the heart. However, light, regular exercise can be beneficial.

Dietary management

Development of heart failure causes a reduced appetite in many patients, leading to cardiac cachexia, which is seen as a sign of a poor prognosis. Insufficient nutrition has many adverse effects, so the primary objective of dietary management is ensuring that the animal keeps eating, and it is preferable not to introduce any dietary changes that may lead to food rejection.

Dietary recommendations are listed below.

- Restricting salt intake. Gradual introduction of a commercial diet for animals with heart failure is recommended in symptomatic patients.
- Omega-3 fatty acid supplements. These reduce production of the cytokines responsible for reduced appetite, and prevent cardiac cachexia developing.
- Taurine and L-carnitine supplements. For use in patients with a deficiency, such as cats with dilated cardiomyopathy caused by taurine deficiency, or American Cocker Spaniels and Boxers with dilated cardiomyopathy.

Drug therapy

Diuretics

These are essential for the treatment of congestive heart failure, along with restricted sodium.

Furosemide, a potent diuretic which acts along the ascending part of the loop of Henle, is the drug of choice for treating oedemas associated with heart failure. *Guide: 1–6 mg/kg, IV, SC or PO*, depending on whether the treatment is administered in an emergency situation or long term.

Torasemide is a loop diuretic that is up to ten times more potent than furosemide, with a longer duration of action, and causes less potassium loss. The maximum peak of diuresis is estimated at 2–4 hours and it lasts for 12 hours. Studies in dogs with chronic degenerative mitral valve disease have shown that it is well tolerated and has a good efficacy when administered orally every 12 or 24 hours.

Dosage: Dogs: *0.2–0.3 mg/kg/12–24 h PO*. Cats: *0.1–0.2 mg/kg/12–24 h PO*.

Spironolactone, a mild, potassium-sparing diuretic which acts on the collecting tubule, is administered with furosemide in long-term therapy for heart failure. Dosage: *1–3 mg/kg/24 h PO*.

Hydrochlorothiazide, a diuretic used in some clinical cases of refractory oedema or ascites, acts on the distal convoluted tubule. Dosage: *1–2 mg/kg/24 h*.

ACE inhibitors and vasodilators

These are crucial in the treatment of heart failure. At a dose of *0.5 mg/kg/12–24 h* **ACE inhibitors** (benazepril, enalapril, ramipril, lisinopril) have discrete vasodilatory effects, but reduce AgII and aldosterone levels, protecting cardiac muscle and improving patient survival and quality of life. Their main adverse effects include reducing arterial pressure and causing an increase in potassium levels.

Direct vasodilators include cutaneous **nitroglycerine**, sodium nitroprusside (*0.5–5 μg/kg/min*) and sildenafil (*1.0–3 mg/kg/8–12 h, PO*). Nitrates increase nitric oxide, causing systemic vasodilation and sildenafil inhibits phosphodiesterase 5, leading to vasodilation of the pulmonary arteries, which is particularly important in patients with severe pulmonary hypertension. **Amlodipine** (*0.05–0.1 mg/kg/12 h PO*) is a selective vascular calcium channel blocker used in dogs with heart failure combined with arterial hypertension. Its use requires arterial pressure to be monitored frequently.

Positive inotropes

This group includes the catecholamines (dobutamine, dopamine), digoxin and pimobendan.

Dobutamine (*2.5–10 μg/kg/min*) is used in dogs in cardiogenic shock (administered in a 5% dextrose solution for 24–48 h).

Digoxin (*0.005–0.0075 mg/kg/12 h PO*) is a mild positive inotropic drug, which is also used to reduce heart rate. Digoxin is mainly indicated in dogs with advanced heart failure and atrial fibrillation, where potentiation of vagal tone helps to slow atrioventricular conduction frequency, improving baroreceptor sensitivity. Adverse effects (anorexia, vomiting, diarrhoea, depression and cardiac arrhythmias) can be prevented by monitoring serum drug levels (adequate between 0.8 and 1.2 ng/ml).

Pimobendan (*0.2–0.3 mg/kg/12 h PO*) is a potent positive inotropic drug with vasodilatory properties as it is a calcium sensitiser and phosphodiesterase 3 inhibitor.

β-blockers

Carvedilol, metoprolol and **atenolol** are mostly used by some clinicians to protect cardiac muscles during long-term treatment of dogs with dilated cardiomyopathy (DCM) and cats with hypertrophic cardiomyopathy (HCM). These should not be used in patients with congestive heart failure, because of their negative inotropic properties.

Antiarrhythmics

These are not specifically used to treat patients with heart failure but are used in arrhythmias such as atrial fibrillation, ventricular arrhythmias and specific cardiac rhythm disruptions. Atrial fibrillation can be controlled with a combination of digoxin and diltiazem (starting with a dose of *0.5 mg/kg/8 h* and increasing to *2 mg/kg/8–6 h PO*); if the preparation is long-acting, *6 mg/kg/24 h* can be administered.

Treatment of ventricular arrhythmias during congestive heart failure is difficult. **Lidocaine** (used in bolus form [*2–4mg/kg IV to 8 mg/kg*] in hospitals) and **mexiletine** (not available in most European countries) are the best alternatives for long-term treatment. **Sotalol** is a potassium channel blocker with β-blocking properties and is widely used to treat ventricular arrhythmias where there is no congestive heart failure. **Amiodarone** (potassium channel blocker) is also used as an antiarrhythmic (*10 mg/kg/24 h PO initially, for 2 weeks, and thereafter at 4–6 mg/kg*).

Specific treatment guidelines: asymptomatic patients

There is considerable controversy over whether treatment in the early stages of the main acquired heart diseases in dogs and cats delays the onset of clinical signs. In dogs with chronic degenerative mitral valve disease, administration of ACE inhibitors has not been conclusive. Preliminary results from the European Prospective Investigation into Cancer and Nutrition (EPIC) study, which includes administration of pimobendan in asymptomatic dogs, indicates prolongation of this state and longer survival than the control group given the placebo. It has also been demonstrated that pimobendan delays the onset of symptoms and improves survival in Dobermans in the preclinical phase of DCM. No benefits have been demonstrated from the use of medication in the preclinical stage in studies on asymptomatic cats with HCM.

Patients with acute pulmonary oedema

In this difficult situation, parenteral administration of furosemide, nitroglycerine or sodium nitroprusside, oxygen therapy and sedation with butorphanol constitute the treatment options of choice during hospitalisation. An initial dose of *2 to 4 mg/kg furosemide IV* should be administered and revised after 30 minutes, with the aim of reducing the dose to *2 mg/kg every 4, 6 or 8 hours* depending on progression of the oedema. Monitoring respiratory frequency helps evaluate these patients' progress.

Sodium nitroprusside is indicated for use in patients with severe pulmonary oedema and haemoptysis; arterial pressure should be monitored carefully for safe use. Administration of **pimobendan IV** is also beneficial at this stage.

Patients in cardiogenic shock

These patients are characterised by **severe hypotension (<80 mm Hg)** and signs of low cardiac output (pallor, depression, hypothermia and elevated blood lactate). Dogs and cats with dilated cardiomyopathy are more susceptible. In addition to the treatment described for patients with pulmonary oedema, cardiac output, arterial pressure and renal perfusion must be raised via the administration of **dobutamine in continuous infusion**.

Patients undergoing long-term treatment

Most of these dogs are maintained with treatment based on sodium restriction, furosemide, ACE inhibitors, spironolactone and pimobendan. Long-term treatment in cats depends on the type of cardiomyopathy (see the specific topic).

Prognosis

The prognosis for patients with heart failure depends on the cause, severity and response to treatment. For example, dogs in the early stages of heart failure secondary to chronic degenerative mitral valve disease can live several months or years asymptomatically, while complications are frequent and the prognosis is poor in later stages of the disease. Causes of death from congestive heart failure include arrhythmias, which can often lead to sudden death, hypoxia from pulmonary oedema and pleural effusion, pulmonary or aortic embolism (cats) and kidney failure.

Canine and feline cardiomyopathies

Introduction

The cardiomyopathies are a heterogeneous group of myocardial diseases associated with mechanical and/or electrical dysfunction, which manifest with inappropriate ventricular hypertrophy or dilation.

Aetiology

Aetiology may be very varied, difficult to identify at an individual level, and often genetic.

In 2006, the American Heart Association classified cardiomyopathies as follows.

- **Primary**. When myocardial changes are the main abnormality, as in hypertrophic cardiomyopathy (HCM).
- **Genetic**. HCM and arrhythmogenic right ventricular cardiomyopathy (ARVC).
- **Acquired**. Dilated cardiomyopathy (DCM) and myocarditis.
- **Mixed**. Cardiomyopathies with both genetic and acquired components (DCM) and restrictive cardiomyopathy (RCM).
- **Secondary**. Cardiomyopathies associated with hyperthyroidism (cats), systemic hypertension (cats and dogs), and doxorubicin toxicity (cancer treatment).

Canine cardiomyopathies

Canine cardiomyopathies are the most common acquired heart diseases in large-breed dogs. These include DCM and ARVC.

Dilated cardiomyopathy

Definition

DCM is a primary disease of the myocardium, characterised by ventricular dilation and systolic dysfunction with eccentric hypertrophy; remodelling makes the left ventricle lose its elliptical shape and appear very rounded.

A clear predisposition to primary DCM is evident in certain breeds, with an **autosomal dominant** transmission model of familial distribution with incomplete and age-dependent penetrance. The following breeds are most commonly affected.

- **Giant breeds**: Irish Wolfhound, Great Dane, Newfoundland, Saint Bernard, Spanish Mastiff and Neapolitan Mastiff.
- **Large breeds**: Doberman, Boxer, Schnauzer, Weimaraner, Dogue de Bordeaux, Golden Retriever, Labrador Retriever and German Shepherd.
- **Medium-sized breeds**: American Cocker Spaniel, English Cocker Spaniel and English Springer Spaniel.
- **Others**: Portuguese Water Dog.

Aetiopathogenesis

Aetiology is unknown. There are various hypotheses, including genetic, familial, metabolic, nutritional, toxic factors, etc., which are difficult to identify on an individual level. Macroscopic examination of the heart shows marked dilation of the left chambers, or of the whole heart. Two main patterns of disease symptoms have been described.

- In most giant-breed dogs attenuation of the wavy fibres with minimal inflammation or fibrosis predominates.
- **Dobermans and Boxers** characteristically have myocardial infiltration by adipocytes and fibrosis. The right ventricle is the most commonly affected in the latter (similar to human patients with ARVC). Ultrastructural examination in Boxers has revealed the fact that the desmosomes are affected by this disease.

The final phenotype is very similar, regardless of the cause.

Ventricular remodelling occurs in the early stages, with changes to the structure and function of the myocytes and the extracellular matrix. The **cardiomyocytes become elongated** and attenuated, causing dilation of the heart chambers and systolic dysfunction. These changes reduce cardiac output, and neurohormonal mechanisms are activated, causing sodium and water retention and systolic and diastolic dysfunction, which together lead to left-sided or bilateral congestive heart failure.

In DCM, there is also marked parietal ventricular stress, associated with dilation of the chambers, wall thinning and elevated filling pressures, which predisposes the animal to deficient coronary perfusion and ventricular arrhythmias.

Clinical signs

There are a great variety of clinical signs, depending on the breed and particular stage the animal is in. These patients can vary from asymptomatic to showing signs of congestive heart failure.

- **Syncope** can affect dogs with arrhythmia before signs of congestive heart failure appear. It is usually associated with exercise or agitation and can be indicative of a risk of sudden death.
- **Weight loss**, exercise intolerance, variable degrees of dyspnoea and tachypnoea (due to pulmonary oedema

and pleural effusion), coughing and ascites; in some dogs, subcutaneous oedema also appears in the lower thorax and abdomen.

- **Physical examination**: pale mucous membranes, increased capillary refill time, weak or irregular pulse, or a pulse that does not coincide with heartbeat (especially in auricular fibrillation), lung crepitations, systolic murmur (mitral and tricuspid regurgitation through dilation of the rings around both atrioventricular valves), gallop (S3) and changes to cardiac rhythm (extrasystoles, atrial fibrillation, ventricular tachycardia, etc.). In cases of severe systolic dysfunction, systolic arterial pressure may be reduced.
- In **Boxers with ARVC**, the predominant clinical sign is syncope and sudden death is the only manifestation of the disease in some cases. Only a small percentage of dogs develop signs of left-sided congestive heart failure.

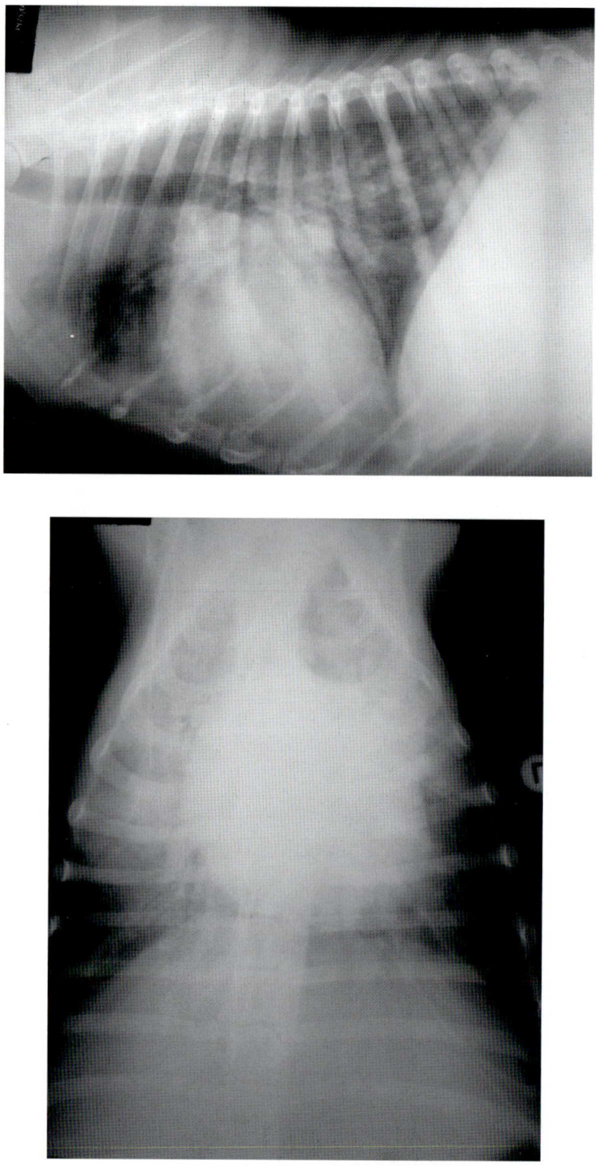

Figure 5.44. (a) Lateral and (b) ventrodorsal thoracic radiographs of a dog with left-sided congestive heart failure secondary to DCM. Cardiomegaly of the left chambers, alveolar pulmonary oedema and air bronchograms can be seen.

Diagnosis

Differential diagnoses include other cardiac and systemic causes which give rise to similar ventricular morphology.

Thoracic radiographs

In most symptomatic dogs, the silhouette of the **left heart chambers is enlarged** to some degree and is accompanied by venous congestion and pulmonary oedema (Figure 5.44). Pleural effusion, congestion of the abdominal organs and ascites can also occur in later stages.

Electrocardiogram and Holter monitoring

The ECG may be normal or show **wide P waves** and **high QRS** voltage, or supraventricular and ventricular premature complexes (Figure 5.45), atrial fibrillation (Figure 5.46), ventricular tachycardia, etc. Ventricular arrhythmias can be seen in Boxers and Dobermans before any sign of congestive heart failure; 24-hour Holter monitoring of cardiac rhythm is therefore the technique of choice in these cases (Figure 5.47).

The risk of DCM has been classified according to the number of VPCs/24 h.

- **>50 VPCs/24 h** suggests DCM in **Dobermans**.
- **>100 Vs/24 h**, in the absence of other predisposing causes, suggests DCM in **Boxers**.

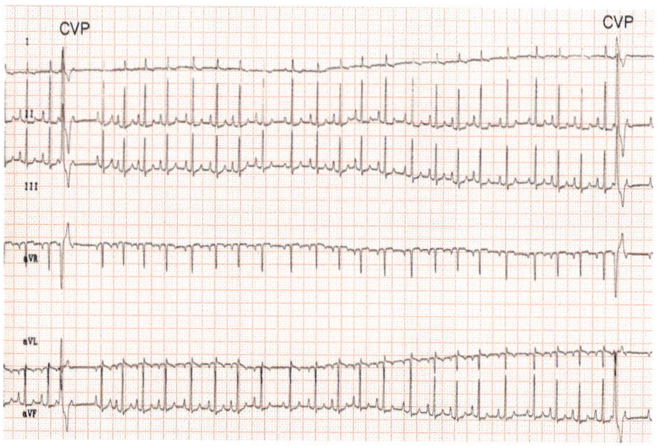

Figure 5.45. Superficial electrocardiogram of a Boxer with arrhythmogenic right ventricular cardiomyopathy where two ventricular premature complexes (VPC) originating in the right ventricle can be seen. 25 mm/s; 1 cm = 1 mV.

Echocardiography

This enables a diagnosis to be confirmed and other congenital or acquired heart diseases to be excluded.

The main echocardiographic signs are as follows.

- **Left ventricular dilation**. Increased normal ventricular systolic and diastolic diameters for breed and body weight, and loss of elliptical shape (Figure 5.48).

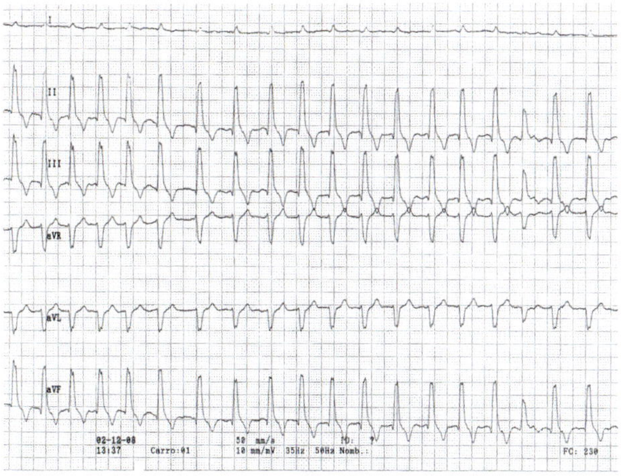

Figure 5.46. Superficial electrocardiogram of a dog with DCM where no P waves can be seen, and rhythm is irregular. Consistent with atrial fibrillation. 50 mm/s; 1 cm = 1 mV.

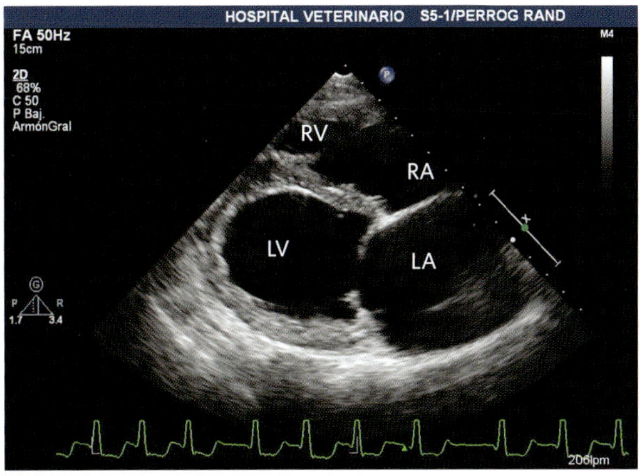

Figure 5.48. Right parasternal long-axis four-chamber 2D echocardiogram, showing dilation of all four chambers and thinning of the left ventricular walls. LA, left atrium; LV, left ventricle; RA, right atrium; RV, right ventricle.

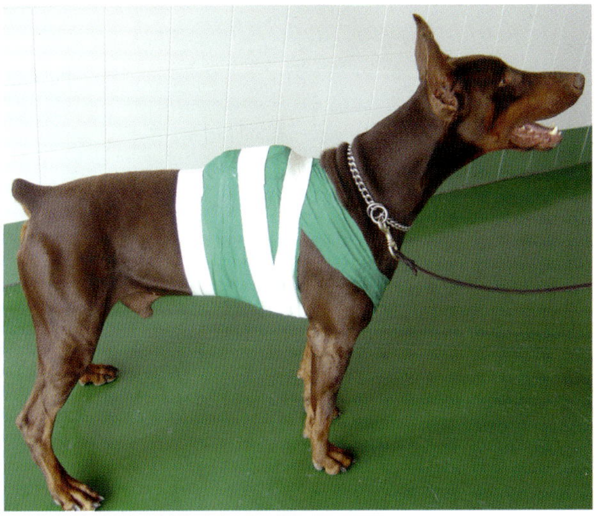

Figure 5.47. Doberman with a history of syncope, wearing a Holter monitor to evaluate cardiac rhythm for 24 hours and determine whether arrhythmias are occurring.

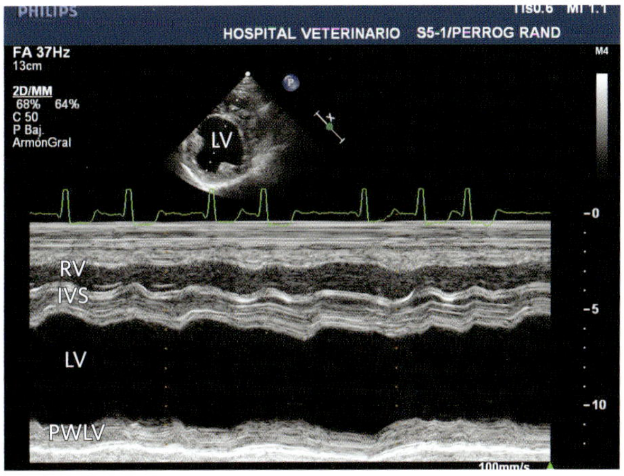

Figure 5.49. Right parasternal transventricular short-axis M-mode echocardiogram, showing hypokinesia of both the interventricular septum (IVS) and the left ventricular free wall. LV, left ventricle; RV, right ventricle; PWLV, posterior wall of LV.

- Disruption of systolic and diastolic functions. **Reduced fractional shortening** (<20%) (Figure 5.49) and ejection fraction. A restrictive transmitral flow pattern is a sign of poor prognosis.
- Variable degrees of left atrial dilation: **LA/Ao ratio >1.6**.
- Mitral and tricuspid regurgitation due to dilation of the corresponding valve rings.
- In Boxers with ARVC, the **echocardiogram can be normal**.

Blood tests

A complete blood count and biochemistry are **usually normal**, except in congestive heart failure, where hepatic enzymes and urea levels can be high due to low renal perfusion.

Hypothyroidism must be excluded in certain breeds, as deficiency of thyroid hormones can contribute to systolic dysfunction. **Blood biomarkers**, such as troponin I and natriuretic peptides, can be elevated even in preclinical stages. They can also be used to **monitor** treatment.

Early detection

An investigatory examination with echocardiography and 24-hour Holter monitoring should be considered in susceptible breeds (Doberman, Boxer), to detect the disease at an early stage and collaborate with breeders to eradicate the disease.

Treatment

Treatment for DCM is merely palliative. The following objectives should be considered:

- reduction of clinical signs
- improved quality of life
- increased survival time.

Treatment should be based on clinical state:

- high-risk breeds
- preclinical DCM (no clinical signs)
- moderate heart failure
- severe congestive heart failure
- refractory heart failure.

Patients with preclinical disease

Treatment of Dobermans in preclinical phases with **pimobendan** has been demonstrated to **delay the onset of the clinical phase** and improve survival. Dogs with significant arrhythmias should be treated appropriately.

Patients with mild to moderate heart failure

The standard treatment includes oral *furosemide* (*1–2 mg/kg/12–24 h*) or *torasemide* (*0.1–0.2 mg/kg/12–24 h*), an *ACE inhibitor*, *pimobendan* (*0.1–0.3 mg/kg/12 h*), *spironolactone* (*0.5–1 mg/kg/12–24 h*) and digoxin alone or with diltiazem if there is atrial fibrillation.

Patients with severe congestive heart failure

In cases of acute pulmonary oedema, oxygen and *furosemide IV* (*1–2 mg/kg/1–2 h* until respiration rate decreases to 40 breaths per minute) are administered, avoiding stress (under sedation if necessary) and pleural and abdominal effusions are drained if impeding respiration. Administration of a potent positive inotrope, such as *pimobendan IV* or dobutamine in continuous infusion, may be necessary in patients with severe systolic dysfunction and cardiogenic shock. **Fluids should be avoided** in these animals, despite the hypotension.

Patients with refractive congestive heart failure

It can be difficult to control the clinical signs as heart failure progresses, as intestinal congestion impedes the absorption of drugs and nutrients, and ascites contributes to hypoproteinaemia and cachexia. **Thoracocentesis** is indicated in dogs with pleural effusion, and **abdominocentesis** when abdominal fluid hinders respiration.

In general, treatment options consist of the following.

- Increasing the dose of furosemide, or even changing PO to SC, or replacing furosemide by torasemide if the initial response is inadequate.
- Increasing the ACE inhibitor dose every 12 hours.
- Diuretic dose of spironolactone (1–2 mg/12–24 h).
- Digoxin (even in sinus rhythm).

Nutraceuticals, such as taurine and carnitine, have proven beneficial in some Boxers and Cocker Spaniels. The antioxidant properties of omega-3 fatty acids (fish oil) can also benefit dogs with cachexia (due to the release of TNF-α, other cytokines and interleukins during heart failure).

Treatment of cardiomyopathy in Boxers

Antiarrhythmics are recommended in Boxers with severe ARVC and arrhythmia. Lidocaine for sustained ventricular tachycardia, and sotalol- or atenolol-based oral treatment combined with mexiletine has proven effective in long-term therapy.

Feline cardiomyopathies

Hypertrophic, dilated, restrictive, arrhythmogenic right ventricular and unclassified cardiomyopathies have all been described in cats.

Hypertrophic cardiomyopathy

Definition

HCM is the most significant feline cardiomyopathy and shows the widest phenotypic variation. It is defined as **left ventricular hypertrophy** without apparent cause (so no systemic hypertension, aortic stenosis or hyperthyroidism). Hypertrophy can affect the septum, the posterior wall or both; the papillary muscles can appear markedly thickened.

Epidemiology

Although cats with HCM are mostly young adults, this condition can affect kittens under 6 months old and cats over 10 years old. Breeds such as the Maine Coon, Persian, Ragdoll and Cornish Rex are particularly susceptible.

Aetiopathogenesis

The aetiology appears to be related to sarcomere protein mutations, as in humans, but it is still not clear in many cases. Genetic mutations in myosin binding protein C have been discovered in Maine Coons and Ragdolls.

Physiopathologically, HCM is characterised by abnormal relaxation of the left ventricle and increased myocardial stiffness. This causes diastolic dysfunction and disrupts ventricular filling, increasing atrial pressures and causing left-sided congestive heart failure.

Dynamic obstruction of the ventricular outflow tract, caused by abnormal movement of the anterior mitral valve leaflet (systolic anterior movement) towards the ventricular outflow tract during systole, instead of normal closure, is common in some animals.

Clinical signs

Some cats with HCM are asymptomatic or when the cardiomyopathy is discovered they may present a murmur, gallop and, occasionally, arrhythmias. When congestive heart failure develops it is usually severe and acute, with pulmonary oedema and pleural effusion, manifested with varying degrees of dyspnoea and tachypnoea. The first clinical sign in some cats is paralysis of the hind quarters or of some other extremity, due to thromboembolism.

Diagnosis

Radiology

Thoracic radiographs of asymptomatic cats can be normal, or the silhouette of the left chambers may be enlarged ('valentine-shaped' heart), and alveolar patterns and even pleural effusion present.

Electrocardiography

ECG can be normal or show increased R wave voltage, ventricular or supraventricular premature complexes and, when the left atrium is very dilated, atrial fibrillation.

Echocardiography

Diagnosis of HCM by echocardiography is made when the diastolic thickness of the posterior wall and/or **interventricular septum is >6 mm** (Figure 5.50a). In some cases, significant thickening of the papillary muscles, with a septal and parietal thickness of >5.5 mm, is highly suggestive of HCM. The thickness of the myocardium must be evaluated in various 2D images, as the extent of the hypertrophy can be very variable. The left atrium can appear very dilated in severe cases.

Obstruction of the left ventricular outflow tract is visible on colour or spectral Doppler echocardiography (Figure 5.50b), as well as diastolic dysfunction (transmitral flow and flow in the pulmonary veins characteristic of abnormal relaxation).

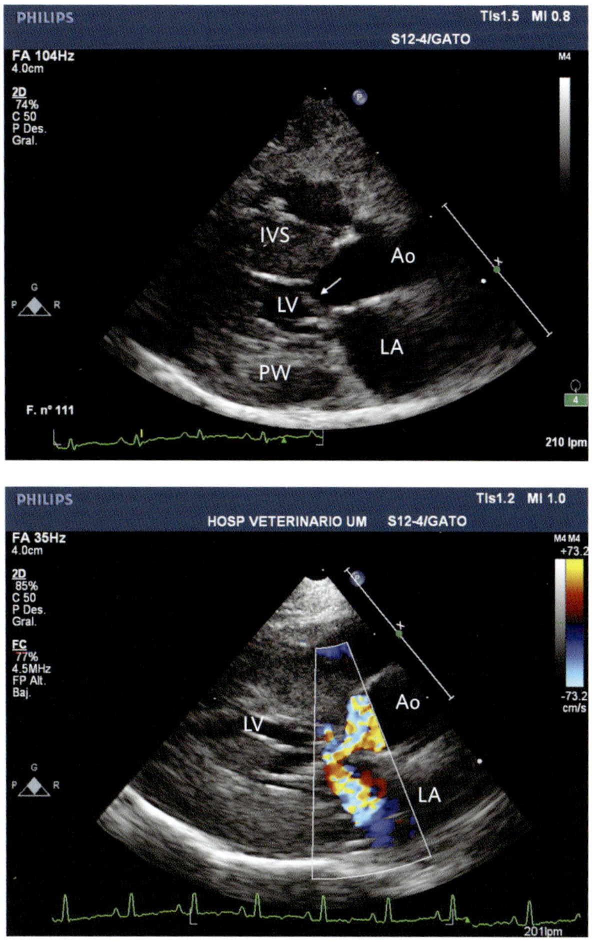

Figure 5.50. (a) Right parasternal long-axis four-chamber 2D echocardiogram and (b) colour Doppler, showing hypertrophy of both the interventricular septum (IVS) and the posterior wall (PW) of the left ventricle (LV), and systolic anterior movement of the mitral valve towards the IVS (arrow). (b) Turbulent flow can be seen in the left ventricular outflow tract, due to the obstruction, and mitral regurgitation in the left atrium (LA). Ao, ascending aorta.

Dilated cardiomyopathy

Definition

DCM is characterised by dilation of the four chambers, parietal thinning and systolic dysfunction.

Epidemiology

DCM affects adult and elderly cats. It has become uncommon since taurine began to be added to commercial pet foods in the 1980s.

Aetiopathogenesis

Aetiology is currently unknown in most cases. DCM has been described in cats fed with dog food, meat that has been cooked for a long time, or a vegetarian diet, but it can also be the final stage of other cardiomyopathies, or the result of immune-mediated or viral factors, amongst others. Systolic dysfunction reduces cardiac output and increases ventricular refill pressures, causing left-sided congestive heart failure.

Clinical signs

When present, the most common clinical signs are varying degrees of dyspnoea and tachypnoea, related to **low cardiac output** (hypotension) and left-sided congestive heart failure. Aortic thromboembolism is also common.

Diagnosis

Echocardiography reveals dilation and increased sphericity of the left ventricle and reduced shortening and ejection fractions. **Dilation of the four chambers** and pericardial effusion are sometimes seen.

Restrictive cardiomyopathy

Definition

RCM is characterised by **abnormal diastolic filling** associated with ventricular stiffness. Ventricular function and dimensions are more or less normal.

Epidemiology

RCM mostly affects elderly cats.

Aetiopathogenesis

Aetiology is unknown in most cases of RCM. Two forms have been described.

- **Endomyocardial**. Associated with fibrosis which affects even the mitral valve.
- **Myocardial**. Fibrosis extends through the myocardium.

Severe dilation of the left atrium is typical of both forms.

Clinical signs

Clinical signs are the same as in biventricular congestive heart failure, arrhythmias and possible thromboembolic disease.

Diagnosis

Diagnosis is made by echocardiography.

- In the endomyocardial form of RCM, the typical image shows fibrosis of the endocardial border and **severe dilation of both atria**.
- In the myocardial form of RCM, the myocardium appears almost normal, or with hypertrophy in some segments, and severe **dilation of the left atrium** can also be observed.

Spectral Doppler of transmitral flow shows a restrictive fill pattern due to ventricular stiffness and high atrial pressures.

Arrhythmogenic right ventricular cardiomyopathy

Definition

ARVC is characterised by infiltration of the right ventricular myocardium by fibrosis and fat.

Clinical signs

The clinical picture in cats is typical of right-sided congestive heart failure, and the arrhythmia causes syncope.

Diagnosis

The characteristic signs on echocardiography are dilation of the right atrium and ventricle, and tricuspid regurgitation.

Unclassified cardiomyopathies

Definition

These include myocardial diseases with unknown aetiology which cannot be classified as any of the other forms, but which present characteristics of DCM and RCM, the final result being varying degrees of left-sided congestive heart failure.

Treatment guidelines for cats with cardiomyopathies

Emergency treatment in decompensated cats

It is not particularly important to establish which type of cardiomyopathy is presented by a dyspnoeic cat before commencing treatment, but it is important to determine if the cat is presenting with congestive heart failure (pulmonary oedema, pleural effusion). Treatment should be tailored to each individual animal.

Some guidelines are listed below.

- Oxygen therapy: oxygen boxes are a good option.
- Sedation with *butorphanol (0.25 mg/kg IM)*, for example, is recommended if stress is to be avoided, as is often the case.
- *Furosemide: 2 mg/kg IV*, repeated hourly at a dose of 1 mg/kg until dyspnoea is under control.
- Transdermal nitroglycerine: for its vasodilator effects.
- Thoracocentesis in cases of pleural effusion, which greatly relieves dyspnoea.

Where there are signs of systolic dysfunction and low cardiac output, such as apathy, reduced body temperature, arterial pressure and azotaemia, administer dobutamine.

- **Fluid therapy should be avoided** in cats with congestive heart failure. However, when there are signs of low cardiac output without congestive heart failure, small doses of fluids can be administered (0.45% NaCl or 5% dextrose in water supplemented with potassium) to improve arterial pressure and renal perfusion.

Cats with **aortic thromboembolism** are difficult to treat and animals that recover are **predisposed to further episodes**. Treatment regimes in these cases include analgesia (butorphanol), monitoring electrolyte and acid–base abnormalities, and preventing the formation of new thrombi (*heparin, 100–200 IU/kg, then 100 IU/kg/6 h*) or the spread of existing ones.

Maintenance therapy in cats with cardiomyopathy

Objectives and guidelines are as follows.

- **Eliminate fluid retention** and modulate neurohormonal activity. Administer *furosemide orally*

(1 mg/kg/12–24 h) to control oedema and prevent azotaemia. *ACE inhibitors* should be administered at lower doses than in dogs, to help control congestive heart failure and modulate neurohormonal activation.
- **Optimise haemodynamic function**. Reducing heart rate and improving diastolic function in cats with HCM is recommended. Some studies carried out in cats and humans suggest that *diltiazem (30 mg/12–24 h PO)* improves diastolic function by relaxing the ventricle. In cats with dynamic obstructions, *atenolol (6.25–12.5 mg/12–24 h)* reduces left ventricular outflow tract gradients, although this seems to have **no effect on survival**. Pimobendan improves clinical signs.
- **Prevent thromboembolism**. Administer *aspirin (81 mg/72 h)* or *clopidogrel (18.75 mg/24 h)*. The latter has performed better than aspirin in preventing relapses.
- Supplement cats with DCM secondary to taurine deficiency with **taurine (250–500 mg/12 h PO)**.

In cats with arrhythmogenic cardiomyopathy, treat ventricular arrhythmias. *Sotalol 2–4 mg/kg/12 h PO* can be used.

There is **no evidence** that **treating asymptomatic cats** with HCM delays the appearance of clinical signs. The appropriate parameters should be measured periodically to monitor oedema, arterial pressure, renal function, electrolytes and coagulation.

Prognosis in cats with cardiomyopathy

A survival time of 596–732 days is reported in cats with HCM which are still alive after 24 hours' hospitalisation following an episode of congestive heart failure.

Indicators of poor prognosis

- **Troponin cTn1 concentrations >0.7 ng/ml** are a predictor of cardiac death in cats with HCM, regardless of the presence of congestive heart failure and/or atrial dilation.
- **Aortic thromboembolism**. Survival of cats which have overcome an episode of aortic thromboembolism is around 184 days.
- **Other cardiomyopathies**, such as degenerative, restrictive and ARVC.
- In general, a **heart rate above 200 bpm**.
- Syncope.
- Arrhythmias.

Myocarditis

Definition

Myocarditis is a type of **myocardial disease** characterised by myocardial necrosis or **degeneration and inflammation**. A type of atrial myocarditis has been described.

Aetiopathogenesis

Myocarditis has a variety of causes: physical, chemical and infectious (Chagas disease, leishmaniasis, toxoplasmosis, parvovirus, blastomycosis, etc.). The resulting tissue damage and inflammation cause dilation of the heart chambers, similar to that observed in DCM. These myocardial changes also predispose the animal to severe atrial and/or ventricular arrhythmias.

Diagnosis

High plasma concentrations of troponin 1 (cTn1) suggest myocardial damage and aid diagnosis.

Acquired valvular heart disease (dogs)

Introduction

The most common acquired valvular heart diseases are **chronic degenerative valvular disease** and **infective (bacterial) endocarditis**. These lesions cause inadequate closure of the valve leaflets, leading to regurgitation, and congestive heart failure in later stages.

Chronic degenerative valvular disease

Definition

Chronic degenerative valvular disease, previously known as endocardiosis, is the **most common acquired cardiopathy** in dogs. It is a degenerative myxomatous process mainly affecting the mitral valve (in CDMVD) and, less frequently, the tricuspid valve.

Epidemiology

Although **small-breed dogs** seem to be most commonly affected (Cavalier King Charles Spaniel [CKCS], Poodle, Chihuahua, Pekingese, Fox Terrier, mongrels), it is also diagnosed in some large-breed dogs (Boxer, Pointer, German Shepherd, etc.).

The disease becomes apparent from 6–7 years old in most dogs, apart from the CKCS, where it can be detected from 1 year old.

Males are more likely to be affected than females (ratio 1.5:1).

Aetiopathogenesis

The **aetiology** of degenerative valvular disease is **unknown**. One of the factors involved is thought to be a **defect in the connective tissue** (ground substance) in the valve. The genetic basis is not well understood, although it has been shown to be **hereditary in CKCS** and Dachshunds (polygenic inheritance model). There are currently thought to be alterations in the **valvular serotonin receptors** (local serotonin mediates the patterns of expression of the degenerative myxomatous protein in valves with biomechanical volume overload).

The degenerative process starts with subendothelial deposition of glycosaminoglycans **and fibrosis of the valve leaflets and the chordae tendineae**, resulting in their gradual thickening (Figure 5.51), difficulty closing and valvular regurgitation.

In the early stages, the regurgitant volume delivered to the left atrium is small, but marked **dilation of the left atrium** occurs as the disease progresses, with increased atrial pressures and congestion of the pulmonary veins, followed by **pulmonary oedema** (interstitial at first, then alveolar). The reduced volume ejected into the aorta because of the mitral regurgitation activates the **neurohormonal systems** (sympathetic system, and renin–angiotensin–aldosterone and arginine–vasopressin systems) and causes **peripheral vasoconstriction**. These mechanisms help maintain cardiac output and arterial pressure, but eventually increase cardiac effort, cardiovascular volume and fluid retention, causing clinical signs in the long term. Valvular regurgitation and fluid retention also cause cardiac remodelling, with **dilation of the left atrium** and eccentric hypertrophy of the left ventricle. In later stages, these mechanisms cause **left-sided congestive heart failure**. Pulmonary hypertension and bilateral congestive heart failure can occur secondary to the above-mentioned issues in many dogs.

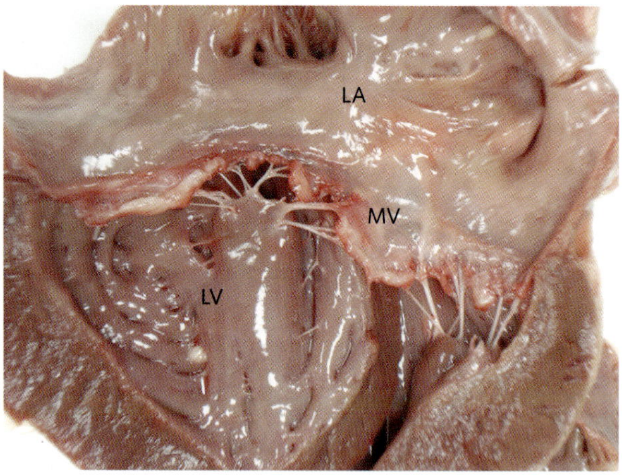

Figure 5.51. Macroscopic image of the mitral valve in a dog with chronic degenerative valvular disease, showing myxomatous degeneration. LA, left atrium; MV, mitral valve; LV, left ventricle.

Clinical signs

The disease is usually chronic and develops slowly.

One of the first clinical findings is auscultation of a **murmur** caused by valvular regurgitation, which develops from protosystolic in the early stages to holo/pansystolic in the more advanced stages, and from 1–4/6 to 5–6/6 degrees of intensity (with left-sided precordial fremitus). **The intensity of the murmur is correlated with the severity** of regurgitation and disease. The point of maximum murmur intensity is over the left apex, radiating irregularly towards the right hemithorax. If the tricuspid valve is involved, or the condition develops into pulmonary hypertension, a holo/pansystolic murmur can be heard in the tricuspid area of the right hemithorax. The period between detection of a low-intensity murmur in asymptomatic animals and clinical signs appearing is very variable (months or years). Auscultation of changes in cardiac rhythm caused by atrial and/or ventricular arrhythmias is common in advanced stages.

Compression of the main left bronchus by cardiomegaly of the left chambers, especially the left atrium, predisposes the animal to **coughing**, one of the first clinical signs that leads to consultation. Owners describe the cough as 'if the animal is trying to clear something from its throat'.

Exercise intolerance and varying degrees of dyspnoea appear in later stages, caused by left-sided congestive heart failure.

Inspiratory crepitations can be auscultated in animals with pulmonary oedema. If pulmonary hypertension develops, varying degrees of right-sided congestive heart failure and ascites can occur.

Diagnosis

Signalment

The signalment, clinical history and physical examination usually indicate the presence of CDMVD and dictate which additional diagnostic tests are necessary to evaluate the severity of the disease and prognosis.

Electrocardiogram

This may be normal at the onset of the disease. **Heart rate is raised** in later stages, and waves and intervals may be disturbed, suggesting **enlargement of the left chambers** (mitral P wave >0.04 s and R wave >2.5 mV in DII) (Figure 5.52), and **atrial and ventricular arrhythmias** (ventricular premature complexes and episodes of ventricular tachycardia) (Figure 5.53).

Thoracic radiographs

Radiographic findings depend on the stage of the disease. In early stages there are few changes (Figure 5.54), but variable degrees of **dorsal displacement of the trachea** and compression of the left main bronchus can be observed as the condition develops; the **left chambers appear as enlarged** silhouettes, with congested

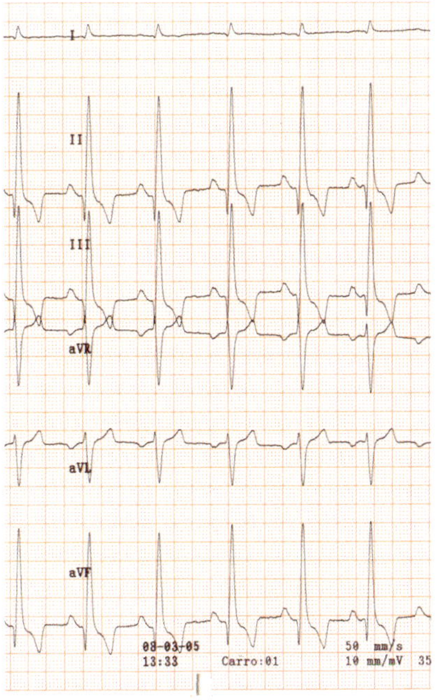

Figure 5.52. Electrocardiogram of a dog with chronic degenerative mitral valve disease, showing sinus tachycardia and mitral P wave.

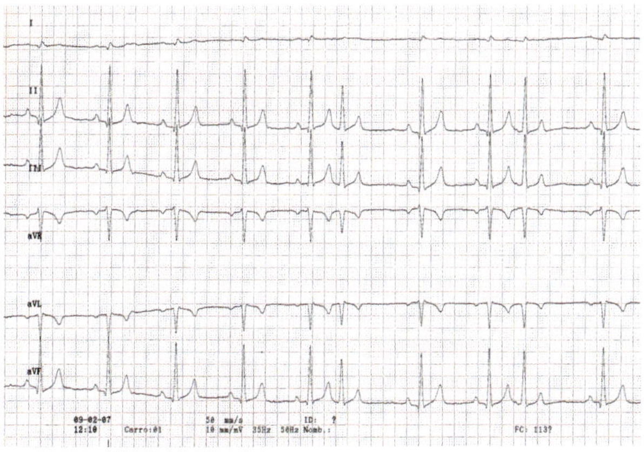

Figure 5.53. Electrocardiogram of a dog with chronic degenerative mitral valve disease, showing supraventricular premature complexes (complexes 6 and 9).

pulmonary veins and varying degrees of pulmonary oedema (interstitial at first, then alveolar) (Figure 5.55).

Echocardiography

This helps confirm the diagnosis and assess the degree of valvular disruption, chamber remodelling and cardiac functionality.

In the **early stages** of the disease, mild thickening of the valve leaflets, valvular prolapse and mild dilation of the left chambers can be observed, or the left chambers may not be visible. **Colour Doppler** reveals little mitral regurgitation.

In **late stages**, the valve leaflets appear thickened, and part of one of the valve leaflets may even be seen inside the left atrium when one of the chordae is broken (Figure

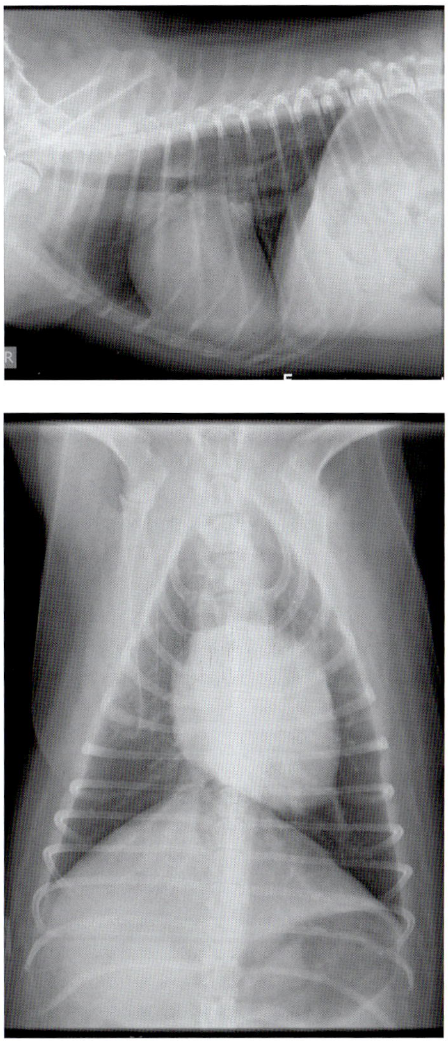

Figure 5.54. (a) Right lateral and (b) dorsoventral thoracic radiographs of a dog with chronic degenerative mitral valve disease in stage B2, showing mild cardiomegaly.

5.56). The left chambers present varying degrees of dilation (Figure 5.57) and the mitral regurgitation area may eventually occupy most of the left atrium (Figure 5.58).

The right chambers appear dilated when pulmonary hypertension is established (Figure 5.56) and tricuspid regurgitation (Figure 5.58) is >2.8 m/s due to the increased pressure in the pulmonary arteries.

Treatment

Treatment is focused on correcting the clinical signs caused by congestive heart failure. Treatment should be adjusted to each individual patient, based on their clinical state. The most widely accepted classification system and treatment guidelines are currently those of the American College of Veterinary Internal Medicine Consensus Statement (2001). This classification is based on the fact that heart failure is an evolving process.

- **Stage A**: High-risk dogs (CKCS, old dogs).
- **Stage B**: Asymptomatic dogs with murmurs.

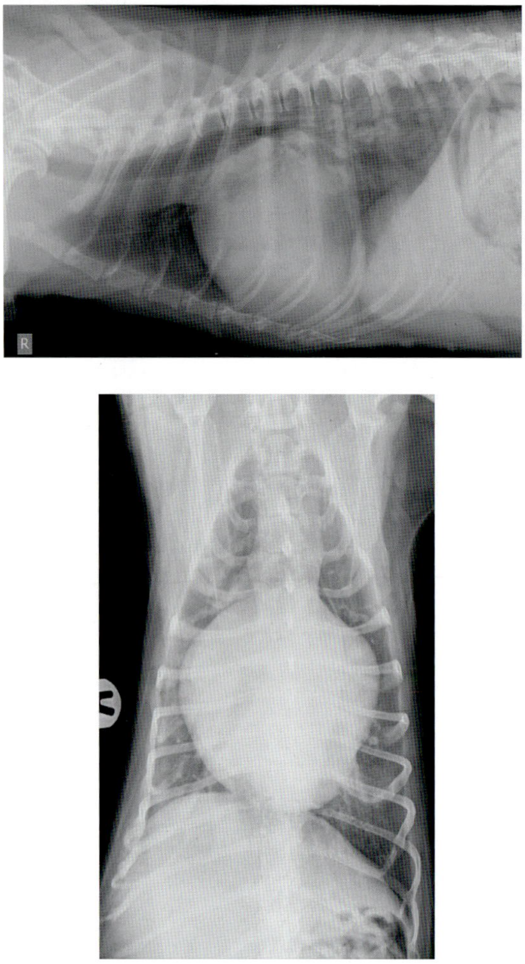

Figure 5.55. (a) Right lateral and (b) dorsoventral thoracic radiographs of a dog with chronic degenerative mitral valve disease in stage C, showing dorsal displacement of the trachea, left main bronchus collapse, significant enlargement of the left atrium and ventricular silhouette, and alveolar pulmonary oedema.

- B1: no cardiomegaly.
- B2: ± cardiomegaly (radiograph, echocardiography).
- **Stage C**: Symptomatic dogs.
- **Stage D**: Dogs refractory to conventional therapy.

Treatment is provided according to clinical stage, as described below.

Stage A

No treatment is required. Periodic monitoring (yearly) is required.

Stage B1

No treatment (either pharmaceutical or nutritional) has been shown to delay the appearance of clinical signs. Annual monitoring (more frequent in large-breed dogs) is required.

Stage B2

Although there is no consensus, most experts consider that administration of an ACE inhibitor is beneficial where cardiomegaly is present. In this stage it has been shown that only **pimobendan can delay the onset of clinical signs** with respect to the placebo group (EPIC study).

Stage C

Hospital based therapy

- **Control anxiety** and agitation with butorphanol or buprenorphine–acepromazine if necessary.
- Administer **oxygen** therapy.
- Administer *furosemide IV at 2 mg/kg (1–4 mg/kg)* and monitor heart rate to determine efficacy. If heart rate

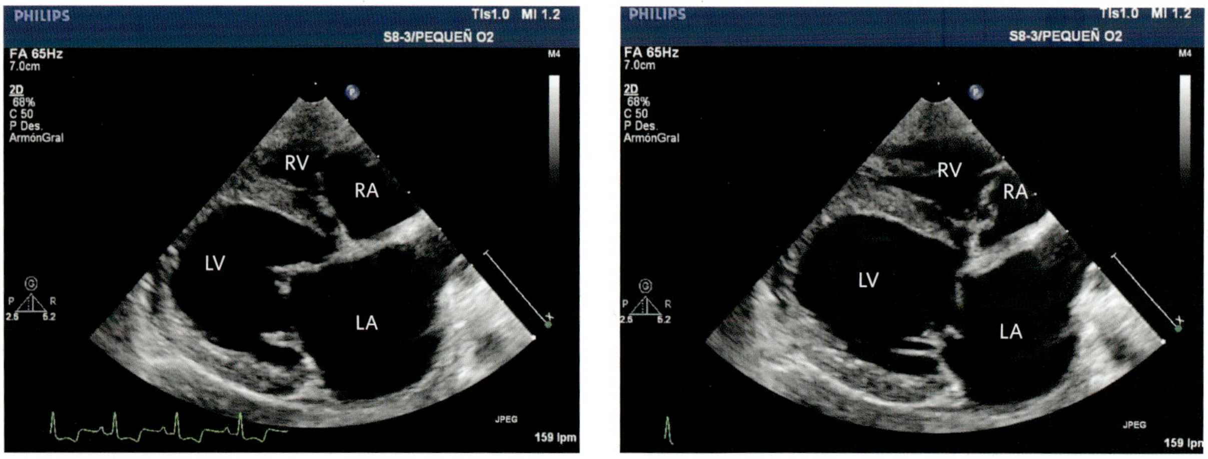

Figure 5.56. Right parasternal long-axis four-chamber 2D echocardiogram, taken in (a) diastole and (b) systole. Significant dilation of the left chambers and moderate dilation of the right chambers can be observed, and the mitral valve is thickened. Tricuspid valvular prolapse and some ruptured mitral valve chordae in the left atrium (LA) can be seen in image (b). LV, left ventricle; RA, right atrium; RV, right ventricle.

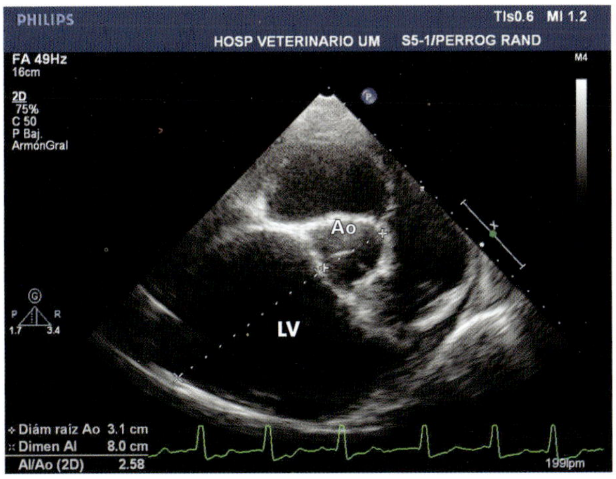

Figure 5.57. Right parasternal short-axis 2D echocardiogram level with the aorta (Ao) and left atrium (LA), showing considerable dilation of the latter (LA/Ao ratio, 2.4; normal LA/Ao <1.6).

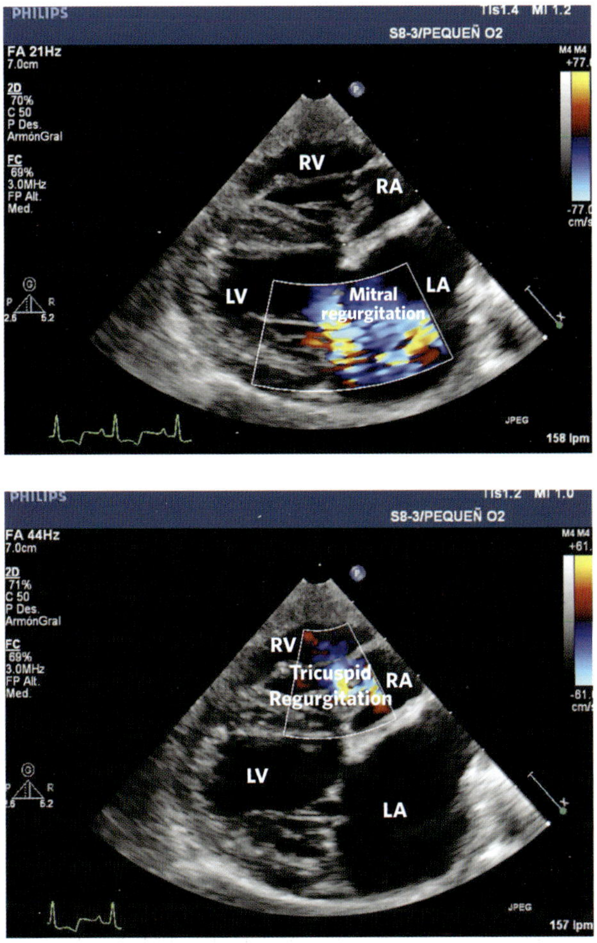

Figure 5.58. Right parasternal long-axis four-chamber colour Doppler echocardiograms showing (a) moderate mitral regurgitation (MR), and (b) mild tricuspid regurgitation (TR). LA, left atrium; LV, left ventricle; RA, right atrium; RV, right ventricle.

does not slow, repeat after 1 hour, then every 2 hours, depending on the response (reduction in oedema). If there is no response to furosemide, administer nitroprusside in continuous infusion.

- Water ad libitum.
- Administer *pimobendan IV: 0.15 mg/kg in a single dose.*
- **Abdominocentesis** should be performed if abdominal effusion is severe and impedes respiration.

There is no consensus on the use of ACE inhibitors or nitroglycerine during hospital treatment.

Home based therapy

- Oral *furosemide: 1–2 mg/kg/8–12 h* or oral *torasemide: 0.1–0.2 mg/kg/12–24 h.*
- Start or continue with **ACE inhibitor** administration.
- *Pimobendan: 0.25–0.3 mg/kg/12 h.*
- *Spironolactone.*
- In cases of **atrial fibrillation** administer *digoxin: 0.005 mg/kg/12 h.*
- Maintain calorific intake, restrict dietary sodium levels and monitor potassium levels.

Stage D

Hospital based therapy

This is similar to hospital treatment for stage C. In some cases, the following adjustments may be necessary.

- Increase the dose of pimobendan.
- Administer **dobutamine** in continuous infusion if arterial pressure is low.
- Administer **sildenafil** if there is significant pulmonary hypertension.

Home based therapy

- Furosemide SC or PO split into three doses.
- ACE inhibitor.
- Pimobendan.
- Spironolactone.
- Low-sodium diet.
- Digoxin in cases of atrial fibrillation.

Infective endocarditis

Definition

Infective endocarditis (IE) is a complex disease caused by **microorganisms** which colonise the **valve endothelium**, causing proliferative or erosive lesions and **valvular insufficiency**.

Epidemiology

Although the prevalence of IE is considered low in dogs (0.04–0.13% of the canine clinical population), the diagnosis is difficult and the clinical signs tend to be non-specific. A lack of post-mortem examinations would suggest the actual prevalence is probably higher than reported.

The **mitral and aortic valves** are most widely affected and middle-aged, medium- or large-breed dogs are particularly at risk.

Aetiopathogenesis

Bacteraemia of any origin (discospondylitis, pneumonia, urinary infections, pyoderma, catheters, etc.) can predispose the patient to IE. However, other factors such as structural heart diseases (subaortic stenosis, patent ductus arteriosus) or immunosuppressive therapy (corticosteroids) can do the same.

The trigger for IE is adhesion ofbacteria to the surface of the damaged valve endothelium due to mechanical (subaortic stenosis) or inflammatory lesions. Extracellular matrix proteins, thromboplastin and tissue factor trigger coagulation when the endothelium is damaged. A clot containing fibrinogen, fibrin and platelet proteins is formed, which is extremely attractive to bacteria.

Some of the main bacteria involved (Table 5.4) escape the immune system because they remain inside the endothelial cells. The bacteria produce enzymes which destroy valve tissue and promote proliferation of valve vegetations. These **fibrinous vegetations isolate the bacteria** from the blood flow, creating a significant **obstacle to antibiotic penetration**.

The **valve vegetations** cause valvular insufficiency and increase ventricular diastolic pressure and atrial and pulmonary capillary pressure, causing cardiogenic pulmonary oedema.

Patients with bacterial endocarditis tend to develop raised antibody titres against the circulating bacteria and immune complexes. Deposition of these immune complexes can damage other organs, such as the kidney (destruction of the glomeruli), joint capsules and dermis.

Clinical signs

Lameness is the most common medical history and symptom in dogs, followed by **non-specific signs** such as lethargy, anorexia, respiratory abnormalities, weakness and collapse; less common are signs of fever (trembling and chills).

The most common cardiopulmonary signs include **respiratory distress** secondary to pulmonary oedema (50% of patients), **systolic or diastolic murmurs** (depending on the valve affected), supraventricular and ventricular arrhythmias and (complete AV block). **Thromboembolism** (septic or aseptic) occurs in over 70% of dogs, with infarcts in the kidneys, spleen, myocardium, brain and systemic arteries. Immune-mediated processes, such as polyarthritis and glomerulonephritis, are also common.

Table 5.4. Bacteria most frequently involved in infective endocarditis.

Bacteria
Staphylococcus aureus
Streptococcus canis
Bartonella spp.
Escherichia coli
Pseudomonas spp.

The most common laboratory findings include leucocytosis, neutrophilia and monocytosis. **Thrombocytopenia and mild anaemia** are observed in 50% of cases. Blood biochemistry can reflect hypoalbuminaemia, elevated hepatic enzymes, acidosis and, in some cases, azotaemia. Urine culture and analysis is essential to reveal possible **urinary infections** responsible for the bacteraemia. The protein/creatinine ratio in the urine should be evaluated in any dog with proteinuria, to reveal any possible glomerulonephritis.

Diagnosis

Blood culture

Accurate diagnosis of IE is based on blood culture before antibiotic treatment, so that the most appropriate antibiotic can be chosen.

- Three or four blood samples are taken every 30–60 minutes (5–10 ml) to culture for aerobes and anaerobes.

For *Bartonella* spp. culture, the blood should be collected aseptically in EDTA tubes and frozen at −70°C until its culture in specific media. Cultures are negative in most patients; this, combined with the fact that the majority are already undergoing treatment with antibiotics, reduces the likelihood of a positive blood culture considerably.

Echocardiography

This enables diagnosis by **visualisation of the valve vegetations**. These appear as hyperechoic (or even calcified) structures which move independently of the valve and are visible on the atrial surface of the mitral valve and the ventricular surface of the aortic valve (Figure 5.59). These lesions must be differentiated from those which appear during mitral endocardiosis.

Colour and spectral Doppler enables the severity of valvular insufficiency and the resulting haemodynamic effects to be evaluated. These include eccentric hypertrophy of the left ventricle and dilation of the left atrium.

Diagnostic criteria

The criteria that indicate a diagnosis of IE are based on modified Duke criteria for human medicine (Table 5.5).

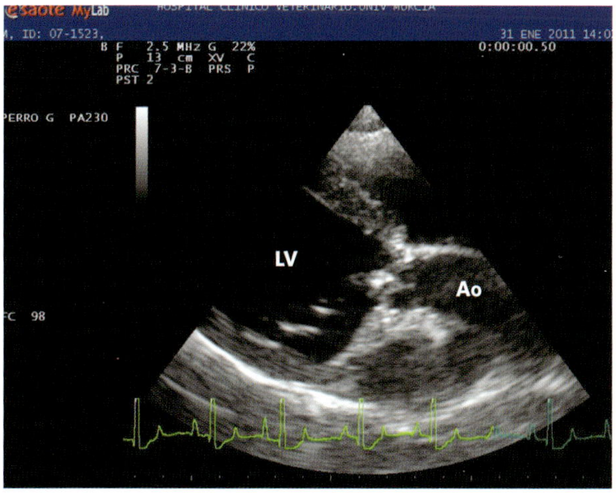

Figure 5.59. Right parasternal long-axis 2D echocardiogram, showing the left ventricular outflow tract and the ascending aorta, with vegetation of the ventricular surface of the aortic valve. Ao, aorta; LV, left ventricle.

Table 5.5. Criteria suggested for the diagnosis of infective endocarditis in dogs.

Major criteria	Minor criteria	Diagnosis
Positive echography		**Definitive**
Vegetative or erosive lesion, abscess	Fever Medium-sized/large dogs Subaortic stenosis	Valvular histopathology 2 major criteria 1 major criterion and 2 minor
Recent valvular insufficiency	Thromboembolic disorder	**Possible**
Aortic insufficiency without subaortic stenosis or annuloaortic ectasia	Immune-mediated disorder (polyarthritis, glomerulonephritis)	1 major criterion and 1 minor 3 minor criteria
Positive blood culture	Positive culture not meeting the major criteria shown in the table	**Impossible**
≥2 positive blood cultures ≥3 if skin is contaminated	*Bartonella* spp. serology ≥1:1024	Diagnosis of other diseases Resolution of the valvular insufficiency or abnormality within 4 days after treatment No histopathological evidence of endocarditis on post-mortem

Treatment

Treatment aims to eradicate the focus of infection and treat secondary complications. To be successful, treatment should be based on early diagnosis and long-term, aggressive treatment (**at least 6–8 weeks**). Only antibiotics which **penetrate fibrin** should be considered, and the minimum bactericidal concentration should exceed that corresponding to the interval between doses.

Ideally, the specific antibiotic indicated by blood culture results should be used; while this is being determined, treatment can be started with another intravenous antibiotic (the *β-lactam imipenem*), *for 1–2 weeks*, and an aminoglycoside such as amikacin (this can be replaced by enrofloxacin for long-term treatment). Patients with congestive heart failure should be treated with furosemide, ACE inhibitors, pimobendan, digoxin (if there is atrial fibrillation) and antiarrhythmics for any possible ventricular arrhythmias.

Monitoring the response to treatment 1–2 weeks after it commences and 2–4 weeks after it finishes, using echocardiography and blood and urine analysis, is recommended. Serology should be repeated in patients infected with *Bartonella* spp. and treatment with antibiotics should be continued if titres remain high.

Prevention

Prevention of IE in susceptible patients consists of antibiotic treatment (β-lactams or cephalosporins) before and after invasive procedures (surgery, catheterisation, etc.) which may be accompanied by bacteraemia.

Prognosis

The **prognosis is poor for patients with IE** and survival rates are low.

Congenital heart disease

Definition

Congenital heart diseases (CHDs) are structural or functional cardiac abnormalities that are **present at birth** and are **inherited** (and therefore transmissible) or **acquired during the foetal stage** (not transmissible).

Epidemiology

The real prevalence of CHD is difficult to determine in veterinary medicine because many animals die before diagnosis.

In dogs, it ranges between **0.5 and 1% of the clinical population**, with pulmonary stenosis (PS), patent ductus arteriosus (PDA) and subvalvular aortic stenosis (SAS) being the most common defects.

In cats, CHDs are less common than in dogs, and atrioventricular valve dysplasias are the most common, followed by atrioventricular septal defects. The most common congenital heart diseases (PS, CAP, SAS) will be discussed in this section.

Aetiology

Heart malformations are thought to be due to the interaction between environmental and genetic factors, although in many cases the causative agent cannot be identified on an individual level. Several studies have revealed breed predispositions to certain types of CHD in dogs, and discovered models of heritability for these disorders. CHDs are mainly, but not exclusively, disorders of young animals, as mild defects allow the animal to live for several years without clinical signs.

Classifications

CHDs are classified as follows.

- **Valvular malformations**: Pulmonary stenosis, aortic stenosis, atrioventricular valve dysplasia.
- **Cardiac shunts**: Patent ductus arteriosus and atrial and ventricular septal defects.
- **Malformations characterised by cyanosis**: Tetralogy of Fallot and Eisenmenger's syndrome.
- **Anomalous venous connections**: Persistent left superior vena cava.

Clinical evaluation

This focuses on two aspects: **detection and identification of the CHD**. Detection is usually easy, as most CHDs are accompanied by a **murmur**. Pathological murmurs must be differentiated from so-called innocent murmurs, which can be auscultated in some puppies but have no clinical significance.

Innocent murmurs are of low intensity (lower than 3/6), more audible over the left heart base and vary with body position and heart rate. However, murmurs of any degree that persist beyond 16 weeks of age in dogs should be assessed to determine their aetiology and significance.

Identification of CHDs is based on a complete assessment, including background and clinical history, physical examination, thoracic radiographs, electrocardiography and echocardiography, in the same way as for acquired heart diseases. Doppler echocardiography is required for definitive diagnosis in many cases, and cardiac catheterisation and angiocardiography less frequently.

Aortic stenosis

Introduction

Obstructions of the left ventricular outflow tract (LVOT) can be located at supravalvular, valvular or subvalvular level. The latter, subvalvular aortic stenosis or subaortic stenosis, is more common in dogs (rare in cats).

Epidemiology

Large-breed dogs, such as the Newfoundland, Golden Retriever, Rottweiler, Boxer, German Shepherd and Samoyed, are most commonly affected by this defect.

Aetiopathogenesis

This lesion consists of a fibrous or fibromuscular ring located below the aortic sigmoids. It can vary in size from small nodules to a band surrounding the whole LVOT. In some dogs, it coexists with a mitral valve abnormality, while others have a dynamic form of stenosis as well as the static form, due to upper septal hypertrophy combined with systolic anterior movement of the mitral valve. The hereditary nature of the abnormality has been demonstrated in Newfoundlands.

Obstruction of the LVOT causes **chronic pressure overload** to which the ventricle responds with **myocardial hypertrophy**, without increasing capillary density, so less blood and oxygen flow to the myocardium. The papillary muscles and subendocardial regions are most affected by the myocardial ischaemia, predisposing them to **ventricular arrhythmias and syncope**. Left ventricular hypertrophy and ischaemic lesions can also reduce ventricular compliance and diastolic dysfunction. Aortic regurgitation is common, associated with damage to the sigmoids from the high-velocity flow through the stenosis.

Although cardiac output is normal at rest, the fixed obstruction impedes the normal increase in ejection volume in response to requirements for exercise, leading to reduced exercise tolerance and syncope. The elevated pressures in the left ventricle can also trigger the mechanoreceptors, causing neurally mediated reflex responses such as **bradycardia, hypotension and syncope**. Severe forms of subaortic stenosis tend to develop into systolic dysfunction and congestive heart failure, reducing aortic velocity and pressure gradients.

Clinical signs

Patients with mild forms of SAS are usually asymptomatic. The most common clinical sign in dogs with moderate or severe forms is **exercise-induced syncope** and, occasionally, sudden death. The clinical picture can develop into congestive heart failure in dogs with some severe forms of SAS.

A **systolic murmur** can be heard on auscultation (crescendo–decrescendo), with the point of maximum intensity over the left heart base and in the cranial right hemithorax; intensity usually corresponds to the severity of the obstruction. The femoral pulse can be normal in mild forms and weak in the most severe forms.

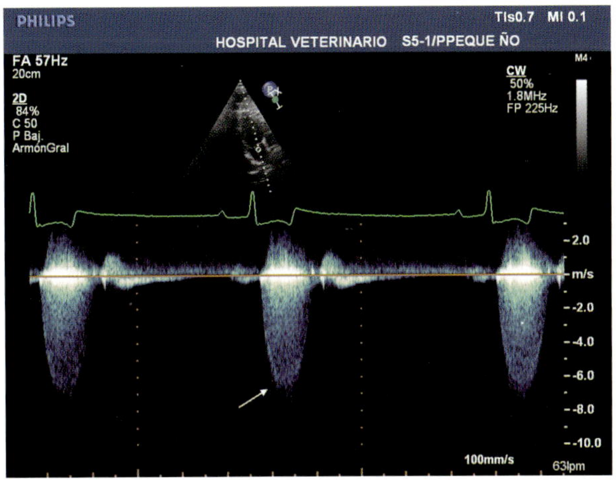

Figure 5.61. Continuous Doppler echocardiogram, subcostal view, of a dog with SAS, showing high-velocity flow in systole due to the obstruction.

Diagnosis

Electrocardiography

The ECG is normal in most dogs. Signs of left ventricular enlargement, depression of the ST segment on exercise, and ventricular arrhythmias can appear in severe forms.

Radiology

The most common radiological findings in dogs with severe SAS include varying degrees of enlargement of the apex–base dimension of the heart, and post-stenotic dilation (prominent aortic arch). Thoracic radiographs are normal in mild forms.

Echocardiography

2D echocardiography enables moderate to severe obstructions, such as a hyperechoic or fibromuscular band below the aortic sigmoids, to be visualised (Figure 5.60). Mild forms can be difficult to see. In severe cases, left ventricular hypertrophy and hyperechoic areas of subendocardial fibrosis can be observed.

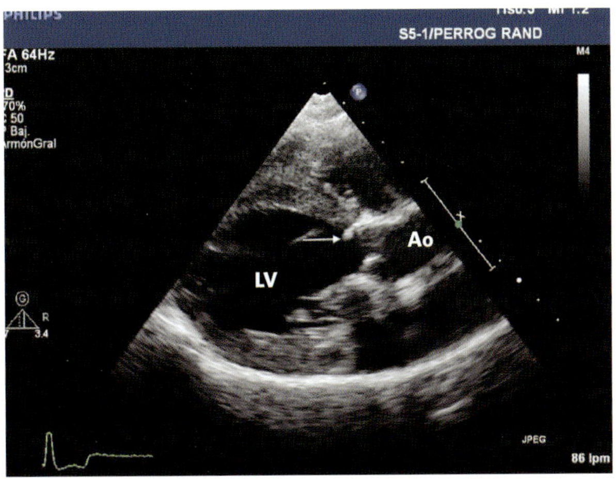

Figure 5.60. Right parasternal long-axis 2D echocardiogram of a dog with SAS, where obstruction of the left ventricular outflow tract below the sigmoids can be seen (arrow). Ao, ascending aorta. LV, left ventricle.

Diagnosis is confirmed by **Doppler echocardiography**.

In the absence of conditions which increase systolic ejection volumes, such as patent ductus arteriosus or a hyperdynamic state, maximum aortic velocities above 2.35 m/s, obtained from the subxiphoid view, are indicative of obstruction of the LVOT (Figure 5.61).

The transvalvular Doppler pressure gradient (DPG) classifies SAS as mild (DPG <40 mm Hg), moderate (DPG 40–80 mm Hg) or severe (DPG >80–100 mm Hg). A colour mosaic typical of high-velocity turbulent flow through the LVOT obstruction can be seen on colour flow Doppler.

Treatment

This focuses on limiting exercise and eliminating the obstruction. Reducing the obstruction by balloon catheter can reduce its severity in extreme cases, in the short term at least. However, long-term results have not been satisfactory.

Medical treatment in dogs with severe forms of SAS is based on the use of β-blockers (atenolol) to improve diastolic filling and left ventricular function, and reduce the severity of the LVOT obstruction. β-blockers also have direct antiarrhythmic effects, reducing the incidence of syncope and sudden death.

Prognosis

Prognosis in symptomatic dogs with high-intensity murmurs, ST segment depression and/or ventricular arrhythmias on ECG, and DPG >80 mm Hg tends to be serious.

Prophylaxis

Antibiotic treatment should be considered to prevent bacterial endocarditis when there is a potential risk of haematogenous spread of infectious microorganisms (such as dental cleaning or surgical procedures).

Pulmonary stenosis

Introduction

The most common obstruction of the right ventricular outflow tract (RVOT) is the **valvular form**, although both subvalvular and supravalvular forms of PS have been described.

Epidemiology

Predisposed dog breeds include the English Bulldog, Boxer, Mastiff, Fox Terrier, Samoyed, Miniature Schnauzer, Cocker Spaniel and West Highland White Terrier.

Aetiopathogenesis

The valvular form of RVOT obstruction, also called valvular dysplasia, consists of varying degrees of fusion, hypoplasia and thickening of the pulmonary sigmoids, or a combination of these. In English Bulldogs and Boxers, PS can be associated with an abnormal coronary artery surrounding the pulmonary trunk just below the valve, causing subvalvular stenosis. Pulmonary atresia is the extreme form of RVOT obstruction.

PS can occur as an isolated defect or associated with others, such as tricuspid dysplasia, PDA, SAS, ventricular septal defect or forming part of the tetralogy of Fallot. A hereditary form of PS has been described in Beagles and Boykin Spaniels.

RVOT obstruction increases ejection resistance and causes a corresponding increase in ventricular systolic pressure, giving rise to right-sided ventricular hypertrophy, interventricular septal deviation towards the left and a pressure gradient across the pulmonary valve. Turbulent flow through the pulmonary valve is associated with systolic murmurs and post-stenotic dilation of the pulmonary artery.

Clinical signs

Animals with mild isolated PS are asymptomatic. Severe cases present signs related to low cardiac output, such as exercise intolerance and syncope, and frequently **right-sided heart failure (ascites)**.

Chest auscultation reveals a systolic murmur (crescendo–decrescendo) in the pulmonary valve area which radiates dorsally. In cases of tricuspid valve regurgitation, a holosystolic murmur can be auscultated in the tricuspid area (right hemithorax).

Diagnosis

Electrocardiography

The ECG is normal in mild stenosis. In moderate to severe forms, the electrical axis deviates towards the right in the frontal plane (>120°), and signs of right ventricular hypertrophy such as deep S waves on leads I, II, III and aVF, high-voltage T waves (Figure 5.62) and right bundle branch block can be seen.

Radiology

Thoracic radiographs are normal in mild forms. In severe forms, varying degrees of enlargement of the right ventricular silhouette, a prominent main pulmonary artery, and pulmonary hypoperfusion can be observed (Figure 5.63).

Echocardiography

Echocardiography enables visualisation of the type of obstruction.

In cases of valvular fusion, valve cusps appear to be fused at their edges, and appear domed during systole (Figure 5.64a). In other cases, the sigmoids can appear thickened and hypoplastic with little movement, and

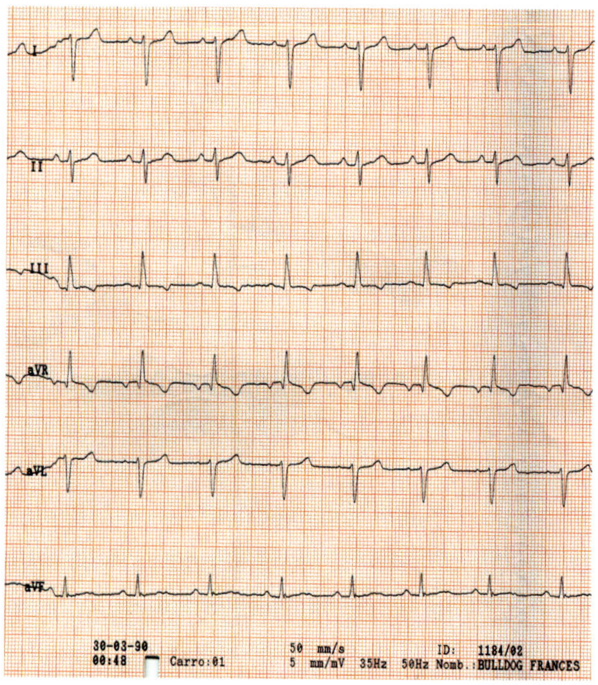

Figure 5.62. Electrocardiogram of a dog with PS, showing deep S waves on leads I and II, typical of right ventricular hypertrophy.

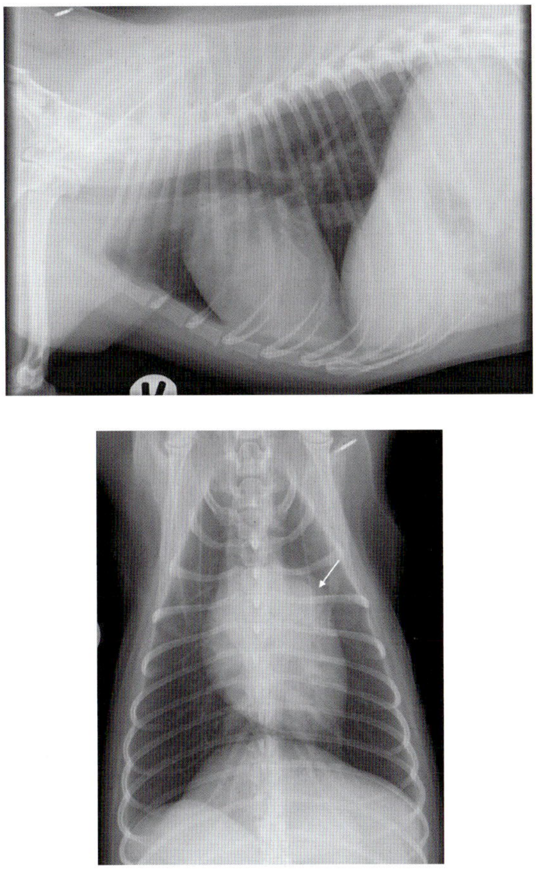

Figure 5.63. (a) Right lateral and (b) dorsoventral radiographs of a dog with PS, showing a mildly enlarged silhouette of the right chambers, prominent main pulmonary artery (arrow) and poor pulmonary circulation.

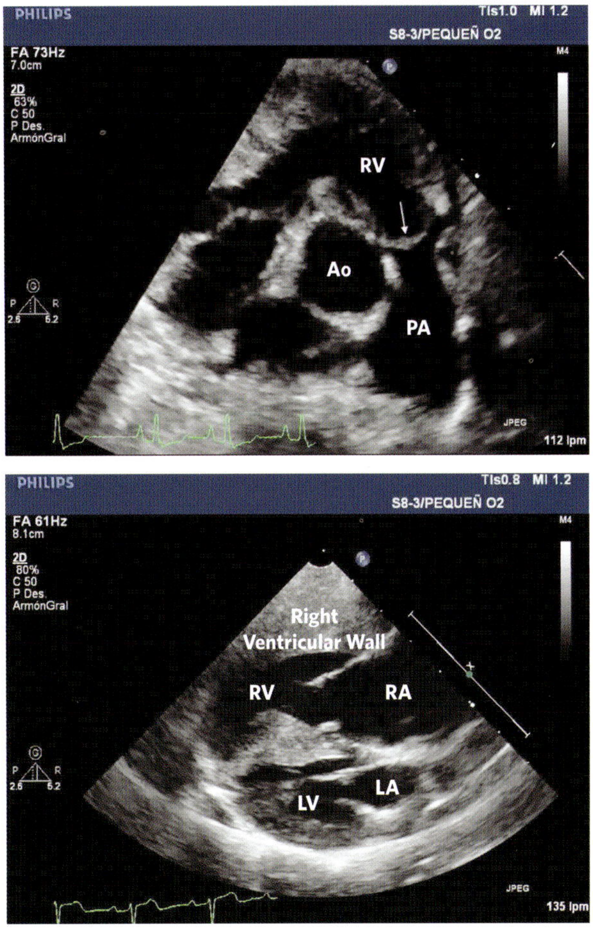

Figure 5.64. Right parasternal 2D echocardiograms of a dog with PS. (a) Short-axis view, at the level of the ascending aorta (Ao) and pulmonary artery (PA). The sigmoids are seen to be fused in the shape of a dome during systole (arrow). (b) Long-axis four-chamber view, showing concentric hypertrophy of the right ventricular free wall (RVW) and reduced size of the left chambers. LA, left atrium; LV, left ventricle; RA, right atrium; RV, right ventricle.

even the valvular ring appears narrow and hypoplastic. The main haemodynamic effects of moderate to severe PS can be seen on the echocardiogram in the form of concentric right ventricular hypertrophy, paradoxical septal movement and reduced left atrial and ventricular size (Figure 5.64b). Dilation of the main pulmonary artery can be seen distally to the obstruction, near the bifurcation (Figure 5.64a).

Doppler echocardiography shows increased flow velocity in the pulmonary artery (Vmax >1.6 m/s) and, frequently, pulmonary insufficiency. DPG <50 mm Hg through the stenosis is indicative of mild PS. Gradients between 50 and 80 mm Hg correspond to moderate PS, and gradients >80 mm Hg are associated with severe PS.

Treatment

Balloon valvuloplasty is the procedure of choice in severe PS where the sigmoids are fused. However, results are more variable where there is hypoplasia of the pulmonary ring and thickening of the sigmoids. Although there have been no long-term controlled studies, it seems that animals with severe stenosis, but which are asymptomatic, can benefit from the use of β-blockers.

Prognosis

Prognosis is favourable in mild to moderate forms. However, it is poor in severe forms without correction of the defect.

Patent ductus arteriosus

Introduction

In the foetus, the ductus arteriosus connects the flow of the pulmonary artery to the descending aorta to ensure oxygenation in the placenta, ventilating the lungs. After birth, the increased oxygen tension causes local prostaglandin inhibition, which leads to functional closure

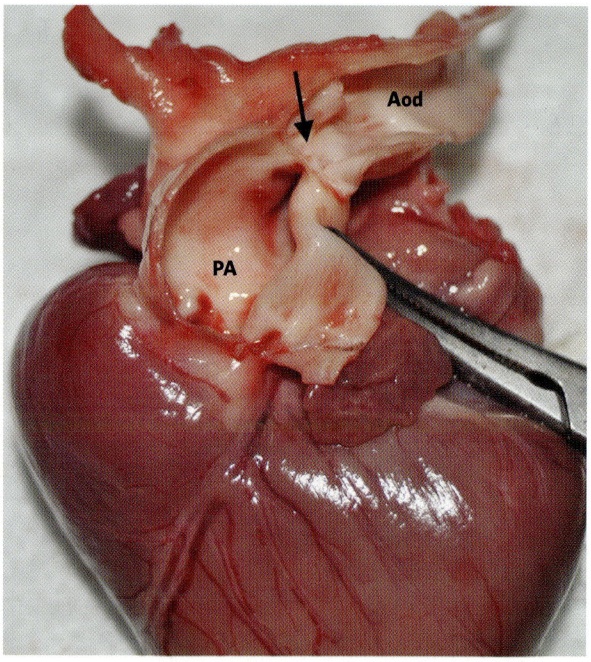

Figure 5.65. Macroscopic image of a dog's heart, showing the ductus arteriosus (arrow) between the pulmonary artery (PA) and the descending aorta (Aod).

of the ductus, followed by anatomical closure, usually during the first week of life. If duct closure fails (Figure 5.65), the blood flows from the descending aorta to the pulmonary artery, and an excess of blood flows to the lungs.

Epidemiology

This defect is relatively common in certain breeds of dog, such as the Poodle, German Shepherd, Collie, Pomeranian, Shetland Sheepdog, Maltese, English Springer Spaniel, Keeshond and Yorkshire Terrier. The inheritance pattern has been identified in Poodles.

Females are more likely to be affected than males (ratio 3:1).

Aetiopathogenesis

The effects of the persistent duct depend mainly on its diameter, and on systemic and pulmonary resistance. When pulmonary resistance is normal, flow is deviated from the descending aorta to the pulmonary artery (left–right shunt) because the pressure in the aorta is higher than in the pulmonary artery, both in systole and diastole. This increases pulmonary blood flow, and also flow to the pulmonary veins, left atrium and left ventricle. The volume overload of the left chambers causes atrial dilation, eccentric hypertrophy of the left ventricle and mitral insufficiency secondary to mitral ring dilation. The end result is **left-sided congestive heart failure**. In some animals with large diameter ducts, the large volume of blood flowing to the lungs can cause reactive changes in the pulmonary arteries, reducing the arterial lumen and causing pulmonary hypertension, usually before 6 months of age. As pulmonary resistance increases, the shunt from the aorta to the pulmonary artery decreases and even inverts (Eisenmenger's syndrome), leading to differential cyanosis (affecting the animal's hind quarters).

Clinical signs

The clinical picture depends on duct size, and systemic and pulmonary resistance. Large-breed dogs with significant shunts can present with delayed growth and develop left-sided congestive heart failure and even bilateral heart failure. The most obvious clinical signs on physical examination are a hyperkinetic femoral pulse and continuous murmur, with maximum intensity over the heart base, usually accompanied by fremitus, which

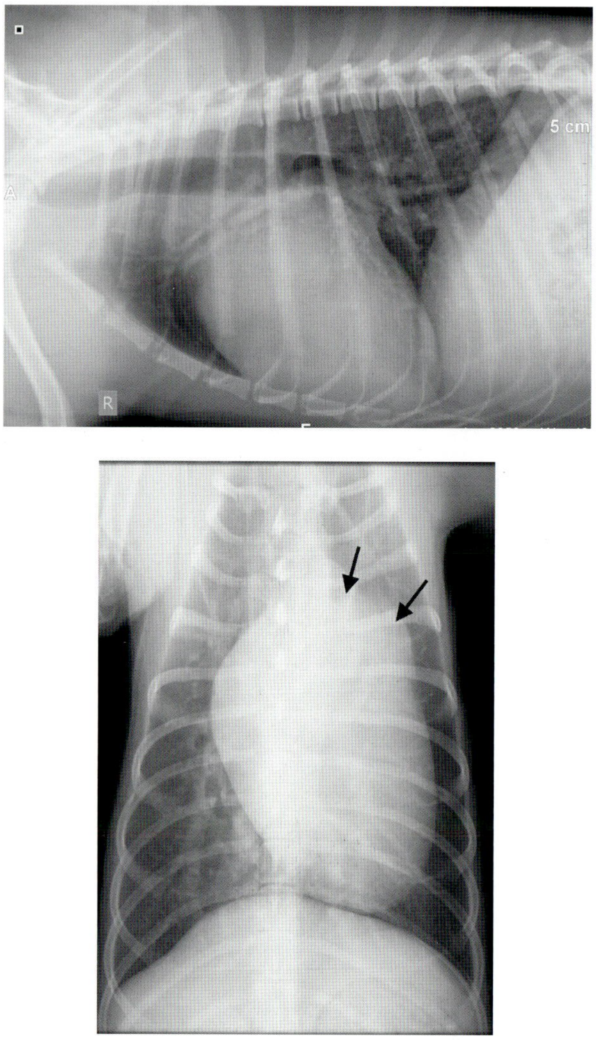

Figure 5.66. (a) Lateral and (b) dorsoventral radiographs of a dog with PDA, showing poor pulmonary circulation, elongated silhouette of the left chambers, and protrusion of the aortic arch and main pulmonary artery (arrows) due to persistence of the duct.

can radiate cranially towards the manubrium and the right heart base. A systolic murmur can often be auscultated over the left apex, due to mitral regurgitation secondary to dilation of the ring.

Diagnosis

Electrocardiography

The most characteristic electrocardiographic findings include wide P waves and increased Q and R wave voltages from leads I, II, III and aVF. Large-breed dogs with congestive heart failure can present with **atrial fibrillation**.

Radiology

Thoracic radiographs usually show poor pulmonary circulation and dilation of the left atrium and ventricle, main pulmonary artery and descending aorta (Figure 5.66).

Echocardiography

Echocardiography can be used to verify the diagnosis, assess severity (by measuring the size of the duct) and exclude other coexisting defects (Figure 5.67a). Spectral Doppler shows a characteristic continuous flow with maximum velocity through the defect of 5 m/s (Figure 5.67b). Lower velocities suggest development of pulmonary hypertension or myocardial failure.

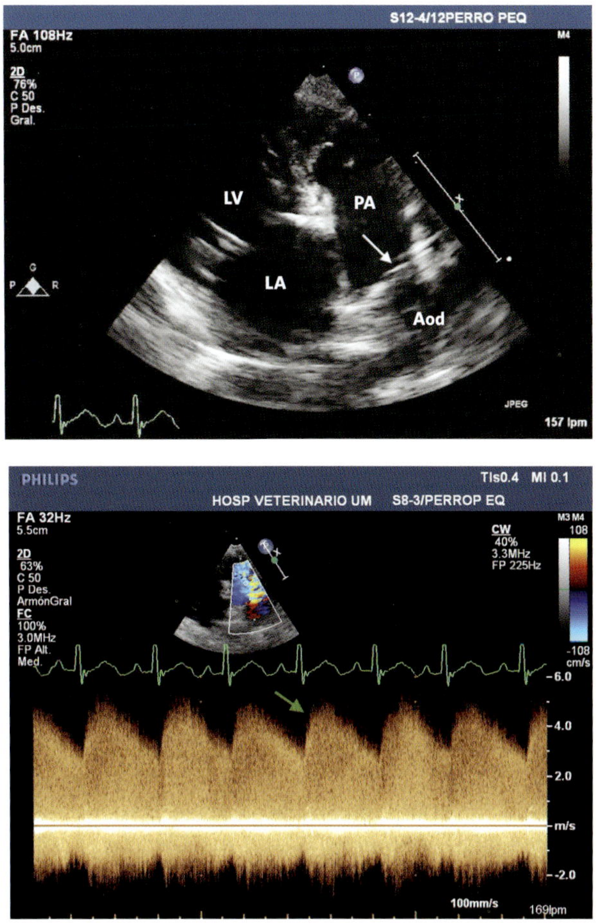

Figure 5.67. Cranial left parasternal long-axis echocardiograms of a dog with PDA. (a) 2D image showing the ductus arteriosus (arrow) connecting the pulmonary artery (PA) with the descending aorta (Aod). (b) Continuous Doppler image showing the continuous flow spectrum of the duct (both in systole and in diastole) (arrow). LA, left atrium; LV, left ventricle.

Treatment

Closure of the duct is recommended in all cases of left–right shunt, as soon as a diagnosis is made. It has been estimated that if the PDA is not closed, over 50% of animals are likely to die in the year following diagnosis.

Some dogs live with small deviations for years, asymptomatically or with medical treatment. Closure can be accomplished by surgical ligature or by provoking embolism of the duct with coils or the Amplatzer duct occluder using catheterisation.

Cardiac arrhythmias

Introduction

A cardiac arrhythmia is a disruption to the sequence of heart contraction and relaxation, altering rhythm, frequency and conduction of electrical impulses.

Aetiopathogenesis

Arrhythmias can be primary cardiac electrical system disorders or secondary to structural damage, metabolic or systemic disturbance, or the cause may be extracardiac (e.g., medication).

The **mechanisms** causing arrhythmias are complex and difficult to determine clinically. In general, they can be divided into two categories, and a combination of both.

- **Changes in cardiac automation** (formation of the electrical impulse): these can be due to abnormal automation or the activity of an electrical trigger.
- Disturbances in the sequence of myocardial activation or electrical conduction: blocks or re-entry.

Clinical signs

Arrhythmias which do not produce haemodynamic alterations are sometimes asymptomatic. However, the bradyarrhythmias and severe tachyarrhythmias can produce clinical signs, such as weakness, lethargy, syncope and sudden death.

Patients can also present with pale mucous membranes, tachypnoea, ataxia, a weak femoral pulse and progressive or refractory congestive heart disease.

Diagnosis

Diagnosis of arrhythmias includes detection, characterisation and determination of their aetiology.

- **Detection**. The clinical history enables identification of events triggering arrhythmias, such as stress and exercise, and family history of heart disease and sudden death. The physical examination and, more specifically, chest auscultation and palpation of the femoral pulse, can detect heart rate and rhythm disruptions, and heartbeat and pulse mismatches.
- **Characterisation**. Superficial electrocardiography is the most sensitive and specific technique to characterise and classify the arrhythmias, although an intracavity ECG may be required in the case of complex arrhythmias. When arrhythmias are infrequent, 24-hour Holter monitoring and monitoring events increases the probability of determining causes, and associating them with the clinical signs.
- **Determination of aetiology**. First, the arrhythmia has to be classified as primary or secondary to structural cardiac damage or extracardiac disorders. Clinical history, physical examination and ECG can all be used, and it may be useful to add thoracic radiographs, echocardiograms and laboratory tests (complete blood count and biochemistry, urinalysis, measurement of thyroid hormones, gases, etc.).

Classification

Arrhythmias are classified according to heart rate as:

- bradyarrhythmias
- tachyarrhythmias.

They are also classified according to their location as:

- supraventricular (atrial and at the atrioventricular junction)
- ventricular.

Bradyarrhythmias

These are arrhythmias with a ventricular frequency which is below normal for the species, breed, age and activity level of the animal. In general, bradyarrhythmias can be considered when the frequency is:

- **in dogs**: <60 bpm
- **in cats**: <140 bpm.

Bradyarrhythmias can be classified as follows.

- **Physiological**. Those occurring secondary to extracardiac disruption, for example of systemic arterial pressure, body temperature, intracranial pressure or gastrointestinal distension. These are mostly mediated by **increased vagal tone** or reduced sympathetic tone.
- **Iatrogenic**. Caused by the **administration of drugs** which reduce discharge from the sinus node, AV conduction or both (opioids, α2-agonists, β-blockers, diltiazem, digoxin, etc.).
- **Pathological**. The most common are sick sinus syndrome, persistent atrial standstill, atrioventricular blocks and neurocardiogenic bradycardias.

The **atropine test** is recommended to evaluate sinus node function and differentiate physiological bradyarrhythmias from pathological ones. The test consists of injecting *0.04 mg/kg atropine SC* and evaluating heart rate after 30 minutes. In normal dogs it will be elevated to over 160 bpm. A partial response (100 bpm) or no response can be interpreted as sinus node dysfunction.

Sick sinus syndrome

This is an arrhythmia where there is intermittent failure of normal discharge from the sinus node, causing clinical signs such as weakness, lethargy and syncope. In some cases, the subsidiary pacemaker cells do not function adequately and there are long pauses. Although the aetiology is unknown, the increased susceptibility to this syndrome of Miniature Schnauzers, Boxers, Dachshunds, West Highland White Terriers and Cocker Spaniels suggests a genetic component in these breeds.

ECG abnormalities include sinus bradycardia, sinus arrest (normal P waves and QRS complexes, but lasting more than twice as long as the normal RR interval), sinoatrial block, supraventricular tachycardia, AV block and other disruptions to the conduction system (Figure 5.68). Due to the intermittent nature of this arrhythmia, 24-hour Holter monitoring may be required to identify it.

Persistent atrial standstill

Persistent atrial standstill is characterised by an absence of atrial depolarisation despite normal sinus node discharge. This is due to muscular dystrophy caused by infiltration of the myocardium by inflammatory cells, resulting in fibrosis. This arrhythmia should be differentiated from transitory failure of atrial depolarisation

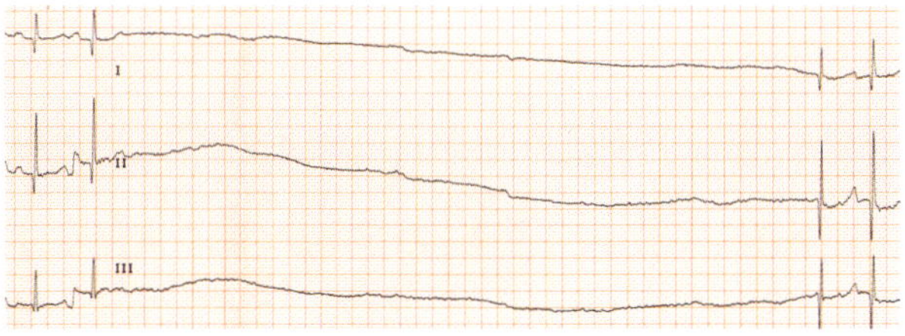

Figure 5.68. Electrocardiogram of a dog with a history of syncope, showing significant sinus arrest followed by an escape complex. 50 mm/s; 1 cm = 1 mV.

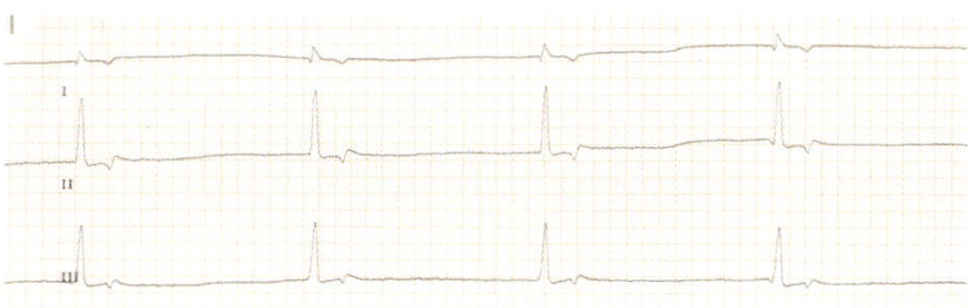

Figure 5.69. Superficial electrocardiogram from a Springer Spaniel showing no P waves, and an escape rhythm from the atrioventricular junction, consistent with persistent atrial standstill. 50 mm/s; 0.5 cm = 1 mV.

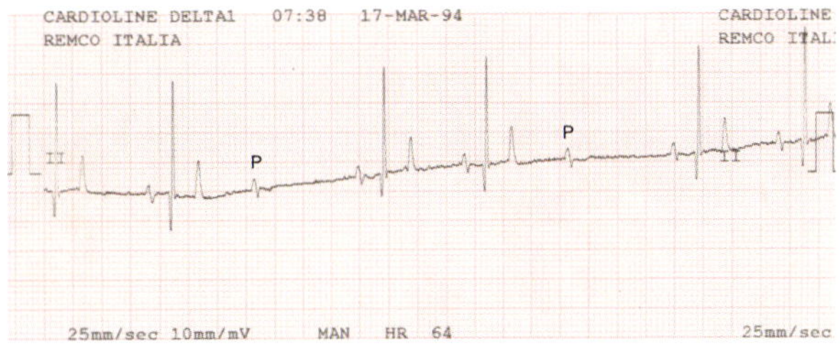

Figure 5.70. Electrocardiogram of a dog with second-degree Mobitz type II atrioventricular block where several P waves can be seen which are not followed by QRS complexes. 25 mm/s; 1 cm = 1 mV.

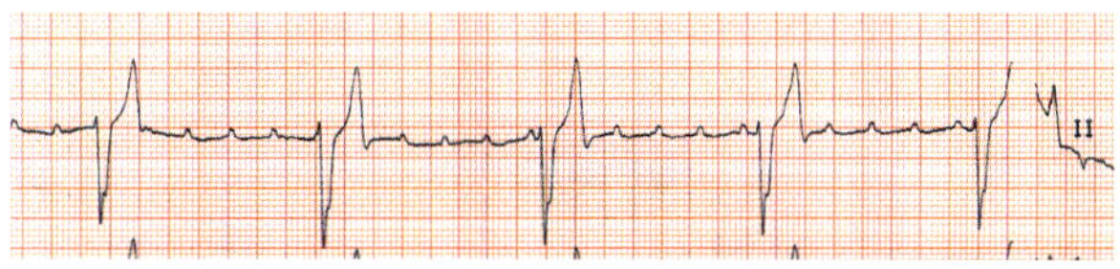

Figure 5.71. Electrocardiogram of a dog with complete atrioventricular block, showing P waves which are not followed by a QRS complex, and a ventricular escape rhythm is also visible. 25 mm/s; 0.5 cm.

in cases of hyperkalaemia, digitalis poisoning or hypothermia. Persistent atrial standstill has been described in cats and also in young adult Springer Spaniels and Labradors. The ECG shows a low ventricular frequency, an absence of P waves, and escape rhythms from the AV junction or ventricles (Figure 5.69).

Atrioventricular blocks

These are arrhythmias characterised by failure in the transmission of the electrical impulse from the atria to the ventricles. They can be classified into three types.

- **First-degree or partial AV block**. Characterised on an ECG by a prolonged PR interval that does eventually lead to the ventricles.
- **Second-degree AV block**. Not every P wave is followed by a QRS complex. These can be further divided into:
  - **Mobitz type I** (Wenckebach). A gradually increasing PR interval, culminating in non-conduction.
  - **Mobitz type II**. Characterised by a constant PR interval (Figure 5.70). Mobitz type II AV block can develop into a complete block.
- **Third-degree or complete AV block**. Characterised by the absence of P wave conduction through the AV node (AV dissociation) and nodal or ventricular escape rhythms (Figure 5.71). In dogs, the ventricular escape rhythm varies between 30 and 60 bpm; and in cats, between 120 and 140 bpm.

Neurally mediated bradyarrhythmias

Neurally mediated bradycardias are the result of **reflex activation of the parasympathetic nervous system** and suppression of the sympathetic nervous system and are accompanied by reduced peripheral vascular tone (hypotension) and syncope. **Vasovagal syncope** is believed to be caused by stimulation of the ventricular receptors which activate the vasodepressor areas of the brainstem medulla (Bezold–Jarisch reflex). These episodes can be triggered by stimuli such as coughing, excitement and sudden exercise. In some Boxers with ventricular arrhythmia, episodes of sinus arrest have been reported as responsible for the syncope.

Supraventricular tachyarrhythmias (SVTs)

SVTs are arrhythmias originating in one or various ectopic foci in the atrial tissue or the AV junction, and are characterised by a frequency above 180–200 bpm. These must be differentiated from sinus tachycardias, which are usually physiological and caused by anxiety, fever, anaemia, pain, drugs, etc.

The most common SVTs in clinical practice are:

- atrial fibrillation
- atrial flutter
- atrial tachycardia.

Atrial fibrillation

This is the **most common persistent arrhythmia in dogs**, associated with severe atrial dilation (structural cardiopathy) and potentiation of autonomic tone. It can also occur in large-breed dogs with no detectable pathology. It can be seen in **cats with cardiomyopathies and severe left atrial dilation**. Electrocardiographic criteria include the absence of P waves from more than two

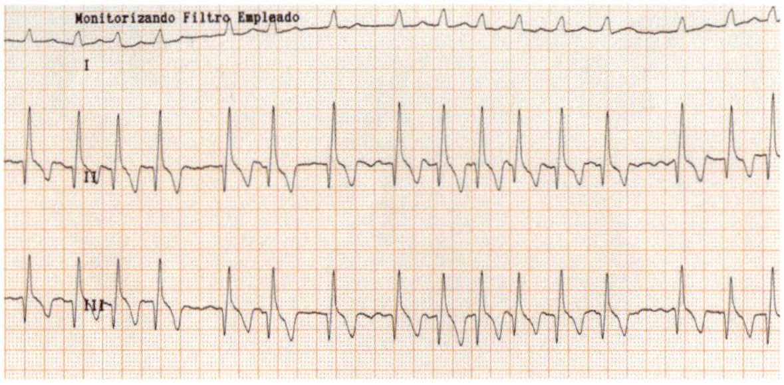

Figure 5.72. Electrocardiogram of a dog where no P waves can be seen and rhythm is irregularly irregular, characteristic of atrial fibrillation. 50 mm/s; 1 cm = 1 mV.

leads (sometimes small baseline waves can be seen), an irregularly irregular rhythm and elevated ventricular frequency (Figure 5.72).

Atrial flutter

Also called **macroreentrant atrial tachycardia**, this is an arrhythmia that results in a very wide circuit of the right atrium (and sometimes the left). The most common type is characterised by **P waves with a sawtooth morphology**, and a frequency of >300 bpm. Ventricular frequency and RR intervals depend on AV conduction (2:1, 3:1).

Atrial tachycardia

Defined as an arrhythmia with **multiple consecutive supraventricular complexes which originate from very rapid ectopic foci in the atria**. The electrophysiological mechanisms include abnormal automaticity, re-entry and triggered activity. Atrial tachycardias can be classed as focal (the most common) and multifocal. These are usually **narrow QRS arrhythmias** with organised auricular activity, and where a superficial ECG shows visible P waves which are usually distinct from the sinus waves, separated by an isoelectric line. The frequency is very high:

- **in dogs**: >180 bpm
- **in cats**: >240 bpm.

Atrioventricular junction tachycardias

The AV node can be involved in the development of these arrhythmias, which can arise without any structural cardiopathy. The most commonly described in dogs are:

- **AV reciprocating (orthodromic) tachycardia**, which involves the ventricles, accessory pathways (usually right heart), atria and AV-His-Purkinje system.
- **AV junctional tachycardia (focal)**, caused by rapid discharge of the distal part of the AV node and bundle of His.

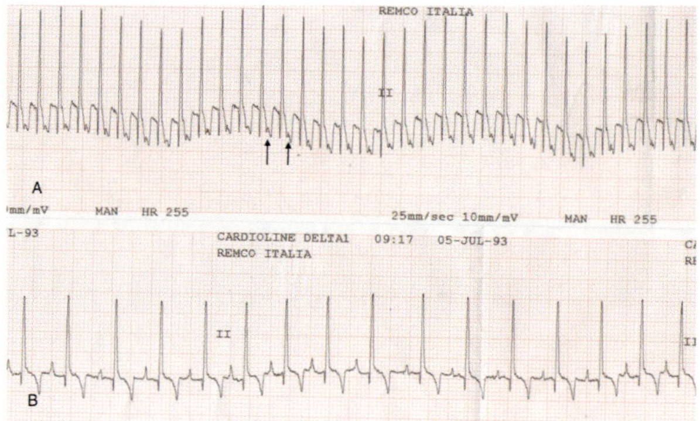

Figure 5.73. (a) An ECG from a dog with supraventricular tachycardia of the atrioventricular junction, in which P waves can be seen in the TS segment (arrows). (b) ECG from the same dog, showing sinus rhythm after vagal manipulation (pressure on the carotid sinus) for several seconds. 25 mm/s; 1 cm =1 mV.

Electrocardiographic characteristics include **narrow QRS complexes** (except when ventricular conduction is disrupted) and P waves which are not always visible, and may be positive, negative or located at the start of the T wave. They are usually regular, paroxysmal arrhythmias with sudden onset (Figure 5.73).

Ventricular tachyarrhythmias

These are ectopic rhythms originating in the ventricular myocardium. They include ventricular premature complexes (VPCs) (Figure 5.74), ventricular tachycardia and ventricular fibrillation.

Ventricular tachycardia

Ventricular tachycardia is a tachyarrhythmia which consists of a series of three or more consecutive VPCs originating from rapid ventricular ectopic foci (Figure 5.75). **QRS complexes are wide** with **tall T waves in**

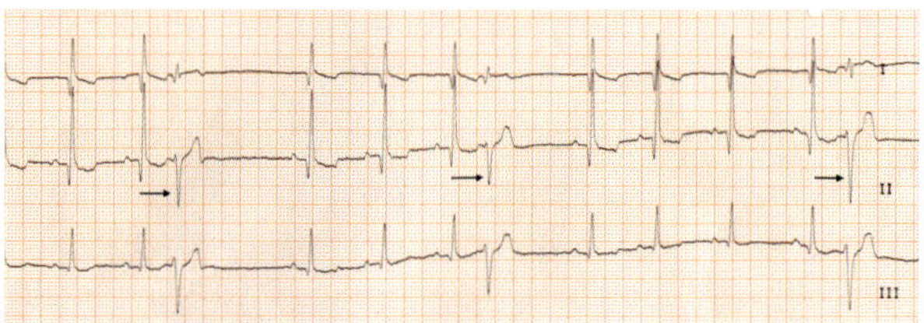

Figure 5.74. ECG from a dog showing isolated ventricular premature complexes (arrows). 50 mm/s; 1 cm = 1 mV.

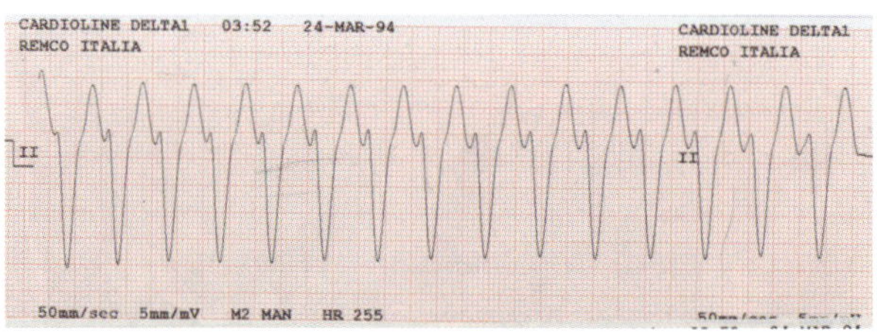

Figure 5.75. Superficial electrocardiogram of a dog showing ventricular tachycardia. 50 mm/s; 0.5 cm = 1 mV.

the opposite direction to the QRS. This arrhythmia arises suddenly, interrupting sinus rhythm and without any association with P waves. Morphology can be variable and depends on the origin of the ectopy, which may be monomorphic or multiform (polymorphic). Ventricular tachycardia can be paroxysmal or sustained (>30 s). It can be caused by heart diseases or systemic problems (splenic neoplasms, gastric dilation–torsion, etc.).

Ventricular fibrillation

Ventricular fibrillation is a disorganised, irregular rhythm which does not give rise to organised ventricular contraction and **requires defibrillation to terminate**. The ECG shows deflections in the voltage baseline and variable duration, during which no normal electrocardiographic waves (P, QRS, T) can be seen.

Treatment of cardiac arrhythmias

Physical manipulation

Applying pressure to the eyeballs and carotid sinus is a technique that increases vagal tone, reducing discharge from the sinus node, prolonging AV nodal conduction time and refractoriness. These techniques can terminate phenomena associated with re-entrant atrioventricular tachycardia by blocking conduction in a pathway involved in the re-entry circuit (Figure 5.73). This method can therefore be used to differentiate between wide complex supraventricular tachycardia and ventricular tachycardia.

Drug therapy

Drugs which reduce automaticity and prolong the refractory period are used. Examples are included here according to the Singh–Vaughan Williams classification, based on their main physiological effect.

Class I

These are drugs which block the sodium channels responsible for rapid responses in atrial and ventricular tissues.

Class IA

These drugs (quinidine and procainamide) depress normal and abnormal automaticity, conduction velocity and refractory period in atrial and ventricular tissues. They are used in the treatment of both supraventricular and ventricular tachyarrhythmias.

Class IB

These drugs (lidocaine and mexiletine) depress normal and abnormal automaticity in Purkinje fibres and reduce the duration of the action potential in tissues that depend on rapid responses. They have minimal effect on automaticity and conduction velocity in the sinus node, atrioventricular node and atrial myocardium. The main indication for this group of drugs is for the **treatment of ventricular arrhythmias**.

Class IC

These drugs (flecainide) significantly depress normal and abnormal automaticity, and conduction velocity.

Class II (β-blockers)

These drugs (atenolol, esmolol and metoprolol) block the β-adrenergic receptors. Atenolol PO is the most widely used in the **treatment of ventricular arrhythmias**, and esmolol IV is also common.

Class III (potassium channel blockers)

These drugs (amiodarone and sotalol) prolong atrial and ventricular action potentials by interfering with repolarisation (potassium, sodium and calcium channels).

They are used to **treat atrial flutter and fibrillation**, and ventricular tachycardia and fibrillation. Sotalol is also a β-blocker, and it is successfully used to treat symptomatic ventricular arrhythmias in Dobermans and Boxers.

Class IV

Diltiazem belongs to this group of calcium channel blockers which impede calcium entry into the slow-response myocardium and the smooth muscle of the vessels, depressing normal or abnormal and vasodilator automaticity, respectively. It is used in dogs to **control ventricular frequency during atrial fibrillation** (in combination with digoxin) and other supraventricular arrhythmias.

Drugs with antiarrhythmic effects not included in other classifications

These include digoxin, adenosine, anticholinergics and sympathomimetics. Digoxin is a cardiac glycoside which inhibits sodium–potassium ATPase pump activity, causing accumulation of intracellular calcium (positive inotropic effect). It is therefore responsible for increased central parasympathetic tone, which slows conduction at the AV level and prolongs refractoriness, reducing ventricular response during atrial fibrillation.

Other therapies

When vagal manipulation and drugs cannot control and terminate significant arrhythmia, or in the case of ventricular fibrillation, **defibrillation and cardioversion** are used.

Radiofrequency catheter ablation is an alternative that can be used to treat certain arrhythmias (atrial tachycardias) and consists of irreversibly damaging the part of the atrial tissue involved in a fixed re-entrant circuit or an automatic focus with a low-frequency energy current.

Atrial and ventricular pacemakers are indicated for patients with pathological bradycardias.

Treatment guidelines

Before treating a patient with a cardiac arrhythmia, the following basic questions should be answered.

- **Which arrhythmia is the patient presenting?** It is essential to identify the arrhythmia, whether it be via superficial ECG or 24-hour Holter monitoring in the case of transitory arrhythmias.
- **What is causing the arrhythmia?** Identification of non-cardiac causes of the arrhythmia is essential, as many of these can be resolved by treating the primary cause.
- **What are the consequences of treating the arrhythmia?**

The decision to treat an arrhythmia can be difficult and each case should be approached individually, taking the following into account:

- The antiarrhythmic therapy must be justified as being able to relieve symptoms, improve quality of life and extend survival.
- Suppression of symptomatic or asymptomatic arrhythmia does not always reduce mortality.
- Antiarrhythmic drugs can have proarrhythmic effects.
- Two of the most important factors determining the arrhythmia's potential for mortality are the degree and nature of the ventricular dysfunction.
- There are no controlled studies on treatments for many of the arrhythmias in dogs and cats, so treatment has been extrapolated from human medicine.
- Consider the role of the arrhythmia in the context of the clinical case, as it is the patient that should be treated, not the ECG. Holter monitoring may be necessary to associate the clinical signs (syncope) with the arrhythmia.
- Arrhythmias which do not usually cause haemodynamic instability or clinical signs (isolated premature complexes, idioventricular rhythms, low-grade first- and second-degree AV blocks) do not require specific treatment. However, symptomatic arrhythmias which cause haemodynamic disruption need antiarrhythmic therapy and/or treatment of the causative condition.
- Which treatment can best control the arrhythmia?

Guidelines for the treatment of bradyarrhythmias

Bradyarrhythmias are treated when they are **associated with clinical signs**, such as syncope, lethargy, depression or congestive heart failure.

If the response to atropine is positive, therapy can be initiated with anticholinergics (propantheline) or sympathomimetics (theophylline or terbutaline) to potentiate sinus mode and AV conduction (sinus bradycardia, sinus arrest and second-degree AV block). High-grade second-degree AV blocks, complete AV block and permanent AV standstill are treated by implantation of a permanent pacemaker (Figure 5.76) when they cause symptoms.

In cats, complete AV block can be transitory or with a high ventricular escape rhythm (100–120 bpm), so they are often asymptomatic; a pacemaker is the treatment of choice when the escape rhythm fails.

Treatment guidelines for supraventricular tachyarrhythmias

1. **Compression of the carotid sinus** should be attempted initially in all cases of SVT, as some AV junctional SVTs can terminate rapidly in response to vagal manipulation.
2. If there is no response, drug therapy for specific SVTs is as follows.
   - **Sustained focal atrial tachycardia.** Conversion can be attempted using procainamide, sotalol or amiodarone. β-blockers and diltiazem help maintain ventricular frequency.
   - **Focal AV junctional tachycardia.** β-blockers (esmolol) and diltiazem can be useful to attempt conversion and maintain ventricular frequency.
   - **Reciprocating atrioventricular tachycardia.** Drugs such as procainamide, lidocaine, esmolol, sotalol, amiodarone and diltiazem can be used to convert to

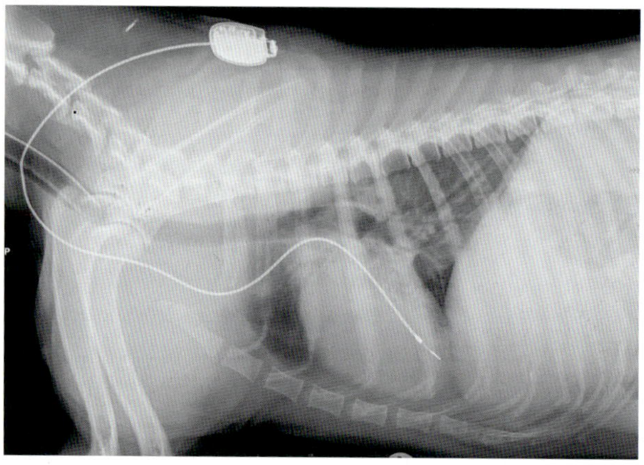

Figure 5.76. Right lateral thoracic radiograph of a dog with complete atrioventricular block, showing the implanted pacemaker (the cable in the right ventricle and the battery, placed dorsally).

sinus rhythm. β-blockers and diltiazem help maintain ventricular frequency.

When SVTs do not respond to drug therapy, electrical cardioversion or radiofrequency ablation may be the only alternatives.

Guidelines for the treatment of atrial fibrillation

Treatment of atrial fibrillation (AF) depends on whether it is recent-onset or chronic.

- **Acute AF**, with no sign of heart failure, can be converted to sinus rhythm spontaneously, by the use of drugs or electrical cardioversion. The longer the AF has been established, the harder it is to convert. The drugs most commonly used for conversion include lidocaine (for vagally mediated AF), amiodarone and flecainide.
- **Chronic AF** is usually caused by structural heart diseases and is less likely to convert to sinus rhythm as atrial distension and electrical remodelling cause changes in the atrial myocardium which promote its perpetuation. The aim of treatment in these cases is to control ventricular frequency.
  - **In dogs**, *digoxin (0.005 mg/kg/12 h)* is the drug of choice, due to its parasympathomimetic properties, as it reduces AV conduction velocity. Although the optimum resting ventricular frequency is unknown, most authors consider it to be <140 bpm. Some studies have demonstrated that treatment with a combination of digoxin and diltiazem controls ventricular frequency better than either alone.
  - **In cats**, the first choice is *atenolol (6.25–12.5 mg/24 h)*; if this does not control ventricular frequency, sotalol (20 mg/12 h) or diltiazem can be used. In cases of eccentric hypertrophy (ventricular septal defects or dilated cardiomyopathy), *digoxin (0.01 mg/kg/48 h)* can be useful, alone or with atenolol.

Guidelines for the treatment of ventricular tachyarrhythmias

Ventricular tachyarrhythmias are usually treated when they cause **haemodynamic compromise** (very rapid ventricular frequency, causing hypotension) or there is a risk of ventricular fibrillation or sudden death (very frequent VPCs, polymorphs or R-on-T phenomenon).

In dogs:

1. The drug of choice to treat ventricular tachycardia is *lidocaine IV*, administered in an initial *bolus of 1 to 2 mg/kg to a maximum of 8 mg/kg in 10 min*. Once this has an effect, it is administered in a continuous infusion (as it has a short half-life), at *25–80 µg/kg/min for continuing treatment*.
2. If there is no response, procainamide is the second option, administered in a bolus of 8–20 mg/kg, and then in a continuous infusion at 25–55 mg/kg/min.
3. If there is still no response, sotalol, β-blockers or amiodarone may be the next choice.
4. For long-term maintenance of ventricular arrhythmias in Boxers, oral administration of sotalol or atenolol with mexiletine is recommended.

In cats:

- Treatment with lidocaine is recommended for sustained ventricular tachycardias with ventricular frequency of >280 bpm, hypotension or syncope; atenolol or sotalol are also good choices in cats with ventricular arrhythmias and hypertrophic cardiomyopathy.

Monitoring of treatment of ventricular arrhythmia should include 24-hour Holter monitoring before and 7–10 days after initiating therapy, to evaluate the change in severity of the ventricular arrhythmia. An adequate response is considered to be a 75% reduction in episodes of ventricular arrhythmias and a 90% reduction in episodes of ventricular tachycardia.

Pericardial disorders

Introduction

The pericardium is the structure wrapped around the heart and the exit of the great vessels. It is made up of two layers (visceral and parietal) which include nerves, blood and lymph vessels.

This structure has active and passive functions (it prevents over-distension of the ventricles, helps balance cardiac output, protects the heart from contiguous infections, etc.).

Diseases affecting the pericardium in dogs and cats can be:

- congenital:
  - peritoneal–pericardial diaphragmatic hernia
- acquired:
  - pericardial effusions
  - constrictive pericarditis
  - cardiac/pericardial tumours.

Peritoneal–pericardial diaphragmatic hernia

Definition

This is a congenital, **persistent communication between the peritoneal and pericardial cavities** which allows abdominal structures to pass through the ventral part of the diaphragm. **In cats**, the hernia typically contains **fat and some hepatic lobules**, while **in dogs** it is more common to find **intestinal loops**.

Clinical signs

Although the hernia is present at birth in the majority of cases, clinical signs can present at any age, or not appear at all. It is often discovered by accident, on thoracic radiograph or during necropsy.

In symptomatic animals, the clinical **signs are gastrointestinal** (vomiting, diarrhoea, weight loss), **respiratory** (exercise intolerance, dyspnoea–tachypnoea and coughing) and, less frequently, cardiac tamponade. Attenuated or displaced heart sounds can be auscultated if the effect is widespread.

Diagnosis

Radiography

Changes in radiographic density (Figure 5.77) in the caudoventral pericardial space may raise suspicions of this defect.

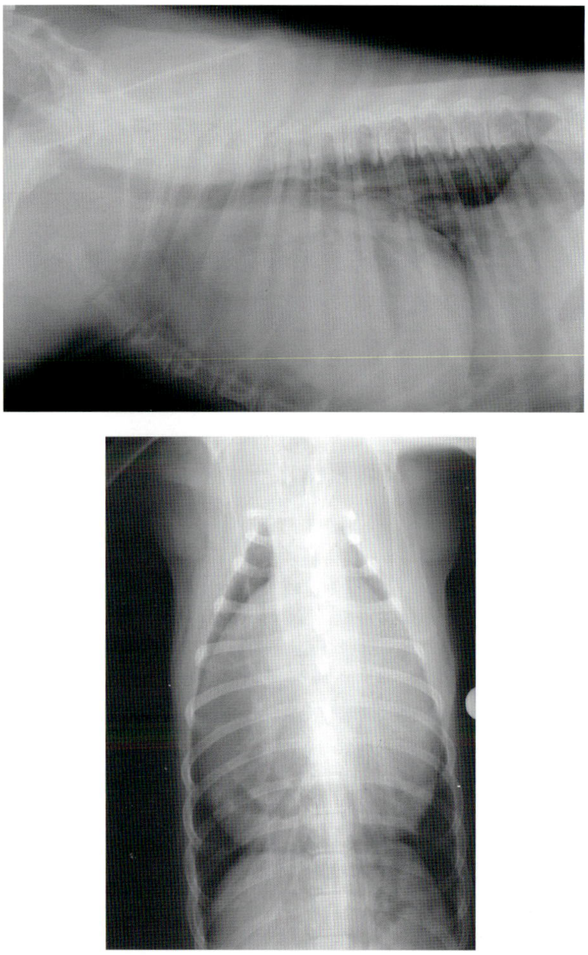

Figure 5.77. (a) Lateral and (b) dorsoventral thoracic radiographs of a dog with peritoneal–pericardial diaphragmatic hernia, showing overall cardiomegaly and irregular radiopacity of the cardiac silhouette.

A persistent mesothelial remnant can appear ventrally to the superior vena cava, indicative of the dorsal edge of the hernia.

Coexisting sternal abnormalities have also been described.

Echocardiography and barium contrast

Echocardiography (Figure 5.78) and barium contrast (if intestinal loops are present) **enable a diagnosis** to be made.

Treatment

Treatment for this hernia is surgery. However, the necessity of surgery must be evaluated in adult animals diagnosed incidentally, with no clinical signs present.

Pericardial effusion/cardiac tamponade

Definition

This refers to an **increase in the volume of fluid inside the pericardial sac**. Tamponade is caused by haemodynamic disruption of the heart due to the increased intrapericardial pressure, caused by the accumulation of a large amount of liquid inside the pericardial space. Pericardial effusion is the most **common acquired pericardial disorder in dogs**, but it is infrequent in cats.

Aetiopathogenesis

The nature of the fluid in the pericardial sac varies and may consist of any of the following.

- **Transudate**. In patients with peritoneal–pericardial diaphragmatic hernias, right-sided congestive heart failure, hypoalbuminaemia or increased vascular permeability. It does not usually interfere

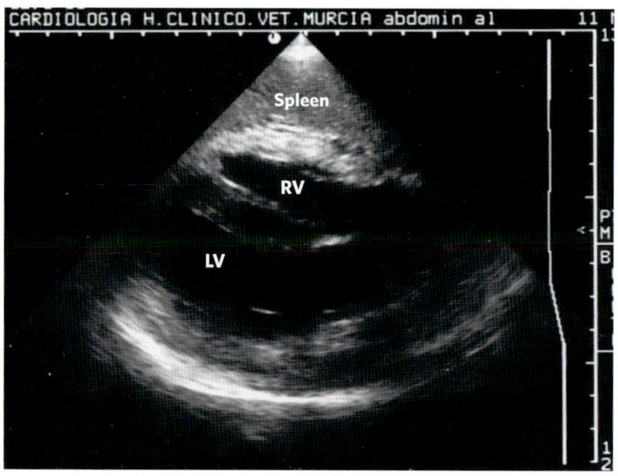

Figure 5.78. Right parasternal long-axis 2D echocardiogram of the dog in Fig. 5.77, showing a homogeneous, echogenic structure between the chest wall and heart, consistent with the spleen. LV, left ventricle; RV, right ventricle.

with heart function, except in patients with tumours of the heart base which cause lymphatic compression.

- **Exudate**. This can be secondary to infective pericarditis (nocardiosis, coccidioidomycosis and perforating foreign bodies) or non-infective pericarditis. Idiopathic and sterile (inflammatory) pericarditis can occur in dogs secondary to recurrent idiopathic haemorrhage; and in cats, as polyserositis with feline infectious peritonitis virus.
- **Haemorrhage**. The idiopathic form is the most common in dogs. The secondary form can be caused by neoplasms of the pericardium (mesothelioma), heart (haemangiosarcoma in dogs, lymphosarcoma in cats) or the heart base (chemodectoma, ectopic thyroid carcinoma). Other causes of intrapericardial haemorrhage include atrial wall rupture in dogs with mitral regurgitation, chest injury, cardiac perforation and coagulopathies.
- **Chyle**. This is very uncommon in animals.

From a physiopathological perspective, pericardial effusions can induce **four functional states**.

1. Slow production of fluid.
2. Effusion without cardiac compression.
3. Sufficient effusion to cause cardiac compression but controlled by compensatory mechanisms.
4. Cardiac tamponade. Pericardial effusion increases the pressure inside the pericardial sac higher than the pressure in the right chambers, causing haemodynamic disorders. If this occurs, right atrial and ventricular collapse restrict cardiac filling and therefore reduce preload and cardiac output.

In cases of **acute pericardial effusion** (acute bleeding in patients with right atrial haemangiosarcoma or rupture of the left atrium in dogs with mitral valve endocardiosis) a sudden increase in intrapericardial pressure occurs. This prevents appropriate distension and adaptation of the fibrosa, causing an abrupt reduction in cardiac output, accompanied by hypotension, collapse and syncope.

In cases of **chronic pericardial effusion**, the pericardial sac can accommodate a larger volume of fluid due to the capacity of the pericardium for greater distension. However, the elevated systemic venous pressure combined with activation of the neurohormonal compensatory mechanisms (caused by reduced cardiac output), lead to fluid retention and signs of congestive heart failure (ascites, hepatomegaly, jugular distension/pulsation and, occasionally, pleural effusion).

Clinical signs

Patients may present with a **history of syncope**, signs of cardiovascular collapse or right-sided congestive heart failure.

The combination of jugular vein distension and/or pulsation, changes in arterial pressure with respiration (pulsus paradoxus) and attenuation of heart sounds on auscultation is fairly indicative of significant pericardial effusion.

Diagnosis

Electrocardiography

Although electrocardiographic findings are **not specific** to patients with pericardial effusion, reduced R wave voltage (Figure 5.79) and electrical alternation (due to the periodic oscillation of the heart in the effusion) or elevated ST segments (due to epicardial damage) may be seen in some patients.

Thoracic radiography

Thoracic radiographs can be normal with small effusions, but **generalised cardiomegaly** with **loss of heart contours** is typical of large volumes (Figure 5.80). Heart base tumours usually cause displacement of the trachea dorsally and to the right.

Echocardiography

Echocardiography is the **most sensitive and specific technique** to detect pericardial effusions, enabling the volume to be estimated and, in many cases, the cause to be determined. Fluid accumulation can be seen as a hypoechogenic space extending from the apex to the base in the image (Figure 5.81).

Visualisation of diastolic collapse of the walls of the right chambers is an indication of elevated intrapericardial pressure with tamponade (Figure 5.81). **Tumours** can be seen inside the chambers, infiltrating the myocardium, or surrounding the great vessels at the heart base (Figure 5.82).

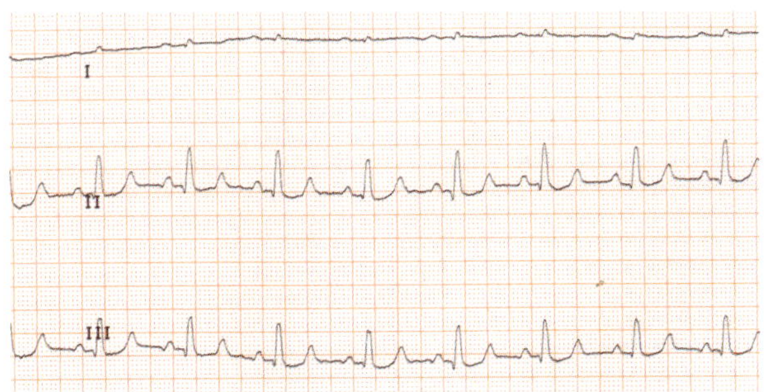

Figure 5.79. Electrocardiogram of a dog with significant pericardial effusion, showing sinus rhythm and low R wave voltage. 50 mm/s; 1 cm = 1 mV.

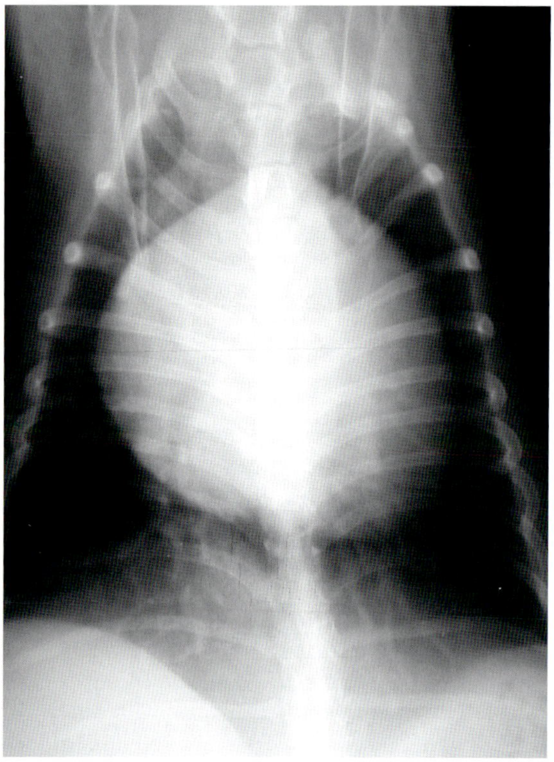

Figure 5.80. Ventrodorsal radiograph of the thorax of a dog with idiopathic pericardial effusion, showing severe cardiomegaly and the globular shape of the heart.

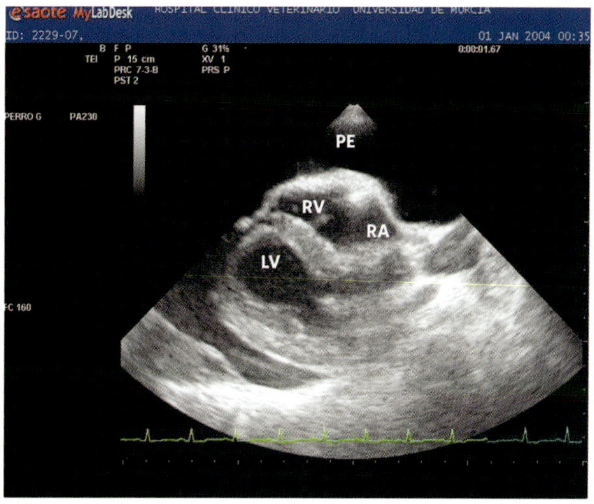

Figure 5.81. Right parasternal long-axis four-chamber 2D echocardiogram of a dog with cardiac tamponade, showing pericardial effusion (PE) and collapse of the right atrium (RA) during diastole. LV, left ventricle; RV, right ventricle.

Mesotheliomas affecting the pericardium are very difficult to diagnose *in vivo*.

Laboratory analysis

Laboratory analysis can **reflect the cause of the effusion**.

- Increased **leucocyte levels** may indicate inflammation, infection or haemorrhage.

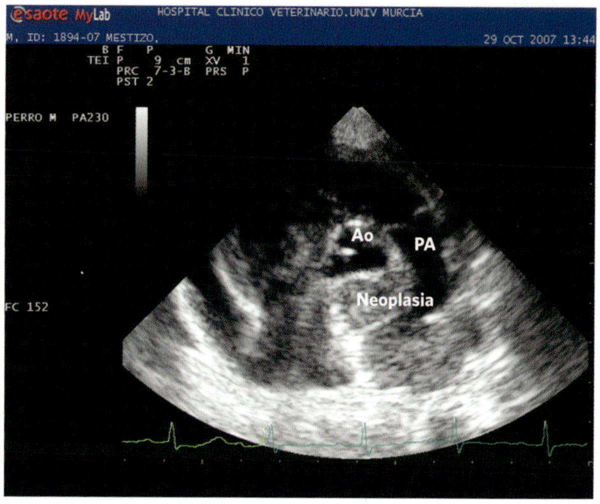

Figure 5.82. Right parasternal short-axis 2D echocardiogram at the level of the heart base, of a dog with tumours of the heart base, specifically, a chemodectoma. PA, pulmonary artery; Ao, ascending aorta.

- Increased circulating **nucleated erythrocytes** have been described in splenic and cardiac haemangiosarcomas.
- Analysis of the effusion usually **indicates its nature** (transudate, exudate or chyle).
- **Bacterial cultures** and blood analysis for fungi and viruses (cats) from the effusion can be positive in cases of pericarditis.
- Raised concentrations of **blood troponin cTn1** have been detected in dogs with haemangiosarcoma, compared to dogs with idiopathic effusion.
- Examination of **cells** from the effusion provides little information on the cause of the effusion, except in patients with lymphoma or septic inflammation.
- **The pH** of the effusion has also not proved conclusive in determining the neoplastic character of the effusion.

Treatment

Although it depends on the aetiology, the first step in cases of cardiac tamponade is to stabilise the patient by performing **pericardiocentesis** and extracting most of the fluid (except where there is left atrial rupture or coagulopathy).

Diuretics and vasodilators are contraindicated as they reduce ventricular filling, predisposing the animal to hypotension, syncope and renal failure. Low doses of furosemide can be administered after pericardiocentesis in patients with signs of right-sided congestive heart failure, to promote the elimination of ascites.

Surgical treatment is by **partial pericardiectomy** below the phrenic nerve, and is indicated in dogs with recurrent idiopathic haemorrhagic effusions or slow-growing tumours of the heart base. Appropriate therapy to treat the specific cause of effusion should also be administered.

Constrictive pericarditis

Definition

This pericardial disorder causes a **disruption to diastolic filling** due to the inability of the thickened pericardium to distend, and significant adhesion between the leaflets. The amount of fluid in the pericardial sac is usually small.

Aetiopathogenesis and clinical signs

Pericardial effusion constriction usually appears secondary to chronic inflammation, recurrent haemorrhage or neoplasia (mesothelioma). As the pericardial space is much reduced and the heart is encased in a rigid sac which prevents distension, the ventricles are also unable to distend, reducing cardiac output and causing signs of right-sided or biventricular heart failure.

Diagnosis

Doppler echocardiography can be useful in establishing a diagnosis, as significant differences in atrioventricular inflow related to the phases of respiration (reduction in transmitral flow velocities during expiration) can be seen.

Treatment

The treatment of choice to correct the constriction is **surgical removal of the pericardium**, including the visceral layer, by decortication of the epicardium.

Pericardial/cardiac neoplasms

Epidemiology

Neoplasms affecting the heart are **rare in dogs and cats** (0.19% of the clinical population).

The latest publications indicate that **primary tumours are more common in dogs** than metastases and that haemangiosarcomas are the tumours most frequently diagnosed, followed by chemodectomas. Other less common types include undifferentiated sarcomas, myxomas, ectopic thyroid carcinomas, fibromas, fibrosarcomas, rhabdomyosarcomas, chondrosarcomas and mesotheliomas.

In cats, the most common types are lymphomas, chemodectomas, metastatic haemangiosarcomas, fibrosarcomas and mammary gland carcinomas.

Clinical signs

Clinical signs depend more on the anatomical location of the tumours and the haemodynamic disruptions they cause than on their histological type. They can be responsible for severe pericardial effusions, ventricular dysfunction, cardiac arrhythmias and obstruction of the ventricular outflow and atrioventricular inflow tracts.

Diagnosis

Two-dimensional echocardiography constitutes the diagnostic procedure of choice to identify tumours and masses in the heart (Figure 5.82), although magnetic resonance imaging (MRI) or computed tomography (CT) and a biopsy may be required in some cases.

Treatment

Treatment for cardiac neoplasms depends on the type of tumour and is usually complex. It is based on a **combination of surgery and chemotherapy**.

Cor pulmonale

Definition

Cor pulmonale is a **right heart cardiopathy**, secondary to pulmonary vascular or parenchymal diseases.

Epidemiology

Common in **brachycephalic** dog breeds with **obstructed airways** (nasal stenosis, collapse of the trachea and bronchi, or chronic bronchitis). Isolated cases have been described in equines.

Aetiopathogenesis

The main causes **in dogs** are as follows.

- **Primary pulmonary disorders:** chronic obstructive disease (bronchitis) and pulmonary fibrosis being the most common.
- **Pulmonary vascular obstruction** secondary to dirofilariasis, thromboembolism or compression by neoplasms.
- **Obesity** which restricts the movement of the chest walls, resulting in insufficient inspiration and hypoxaemia.
- **Chest deformations** such as pectus excavatum.
- Pulmonary disorders cause hypoxia, pulmonary hypertension and right-sided congestive heart failure.

Clinical signs

The disease can be **acute or chronic**.

Severe cases can present with **respiratory distress** and abdominal respiration, cyanosis or sudden death.

Moderate cases can present with **syncope**, anorexia, weakness, depression, whistling, dyspnoea, panting, cough and signs of congestive heart failure (ascites, jugular distension, hepatomegaly, etc.). A satisfactory differential diagnosis must be made as pulmonary disease coexists with chronic mitral valve degeneration in many dogs, and these animals sometimes present with dyspnoea and coughing.

Physical examination

Chest auscultation can reveal abnormal lung sounds depending on the pulmonary disease (e.g., crepitation in pulmonary fibrosis and bronchitis) and can also detect fluid secretion. Heart sounds may be normal or the second tone may be split, or a murmur heard if tricuspid regurgitation is significant.

Diagnosis

The patient's **clinical history** and physical examination may indicate an underlying disease likely to cause cor pulmonale, and certain tests help confirm right-sided heart failure.

Thoracic radiographs and CT can show signs of pulmonary disease and an enlarged silhouette of the **right chambers** (Figure 5.83) and inferior vena cava.

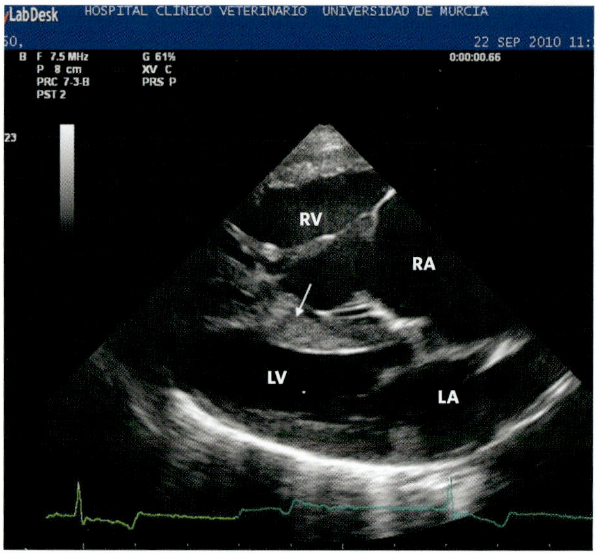

Figure 5.84. Right parasternal long-axis four-chamber 2D echocardiogram of a dog with pulmonary thromboembolism and hypertension, showing severe dilation of the right chambers, reduced size of the left chambers and flat interventricular septum. LA, left atrium; LV, left ventricle; RA, right atrium; RV, right ventricle.

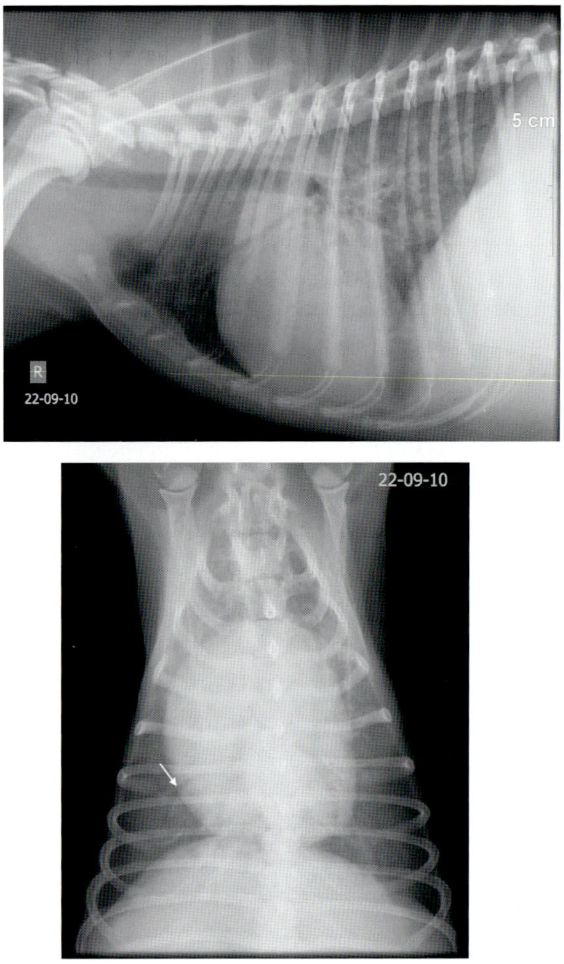

Figure 5.83. (a) Right lateral and (b) dorsoventral thoracic radiographs of a dog with pulmonary thromboembolism, showing an alveolar pattern, air bronchograms and enlarged silhouette of the right chambers.

Laboratory analysis enables evaluation of the level of hypoxaemia and the existence of dirofilariasis. ECG may be normal or show signs of right chamber enlargement (P pulmonale and deep S wave in DI and DII).

The **echocardiogram** may reveal varying degrees of **dilation of the right chambers** and main pulmonary artery in most cases, accompanied by a reduction in size of the left chambers (Figure 5.84). In dogs with a high parasite load, adult *Dirofilaria* can be seen in the main pulmonary artery and the right chambers.

In cases of pulmonary thromboembolism, thrombi can be seen at the bifurcation of the main pulmonary artery and its branches. **Spectral Doppler** is used to measure tricuspid regurgitation velocity (V), enabling the Doppler pressure gradient, which is indicative of pressure in the pulmonary arteries, to be determined ($DPG = 4V^2$). This enables the severity of pulmonary hypertension (systolic arterial pressure >30 mm Hg) to be determined.

Treatment

Treatment should be focused on treating the **underlying disease** causing the cor pulmonale, and improving right ventricular oxygenation and function. In many cases, the disease causing the pulmonary hypertension is so advanced that treatment **options are limited**.

Oxygen administration

Oxygen is administered because it is a potent vasodilator.

Treatment of underlying disease

- If there is a risk of thromboembolism, **anticoagulants** are used.
- In cases of **chronic bronchitis**, treat with bronchodilators (terbutaline, butorphanol and corticosteroids).
- Treatment for **dirofilariasis**, etc.

Treatment to alleviate the symptoms of right ventricular dysfunction

To **prevent ascites**, ACE inhibitors and diuretics (furosemide, spironolactone) are used. To **reduce pressure in the pulmonary arteries**, treat with sildenafil, as it has been proven to improve quality of life in patients with severe pulmonary hypertension.

Prognosis

The prognosis depends on the cause, although **it is reserved** in cases of severe pulmonary hypertension.

Systemic arterial hypertension

Definition

Systemic arterial hypertension (SAH) is defined as sustained elevated systemic arterial pressure (SAP), above the range considered normal in the species.

Although there is some disagreement around the subject, repeated **systolic SAP values of >160 mm Hg** and or diastolic values of >100 mm Hg using consistent measuring procedures, in calm dogs and cats, are consistent with SAH.

Epidemiology

The true prevalence of SAH in dogs and cats is unknown, as measurements of SAP are not included in routine tests in all clinics and hospitals. Animals with SAH can be asymptomatic for months or years.

Aetiopathogenesis

SAH has been classified into three main types, according to their aetiology.

- SAH due to the **'white coat effect'**.
  - This is considered secondary to the measurement process, usually due to alterations in autonomic tone, which is itself an effect of anxiety on the higher centres of the central nervous system. This type of hypertension is resolved when the cause is removed (e.g., by measuring SAP at home).
- **Primary, essential or idiopathic SAH.**
  - Considered as such until the cause of the sustained increase in SAP is determined. Diagnosis is usually made based on normal values for complete blood counts, biochemistry and urinalysis. As many subclinical systemic disorders, or those in early stages, can be difficult to identify, complementary diagnostic tests such as abdominal ultrasonography, laboratory testing, etc. should be included in borderline cases.
- **SAH secondary to other diseases** or to drug administration.
  - This is when there is a known cause. The main disorders which cause SAH in dogs and cats are:
    - chronic renal disease
    - hyperadrenocorticism
    - diabetes mellitus
    - primary hyperaldosteronism
    - pheochromocytoma
    - obesity (small effect in dogs and unknown in cats)
    - hypothyroidism in dogs (rare) and hyperthyroidism in cats.

The most common type in both dogs and cats is **SAH secondary to kidney disease**.

SAH secondary to chronic kidney disease is thought to affect more than **50% of dogs and cats**. Arterial hypertension can be the result of any type of kidney disease: acute or chronic; mild, moderate or severe; vascular, tubulointerstitial or glomerular. In dogs, glomerulonephritis is a well-documented common cause of SAH.

The pathogenesis of SAH secondary to nephropathy is **multifactorial**: reduced sodium excretion capacity and vasodilator (prostaglandin) activity, increased renin production (causing stimulation of angiotensin II) and production of norepinephrine, increased cardiac output and total peripheral resistance. Activation of the renin–aldosterone system causes hypertension due to a combination of excess volume and vasoconstriction mechanisms.

Nitric oxide deficit and the action of endothelin-I, a potent vasoconstrictor found in the endothelial cells and smooth vascular muscles, are other substances which can promote the development or maintenance of arterial hypertension during renal insufficiency. **In cats** it is possible that SAH is associated with mechanisms that depend on renin production, which could have significant implications for treatment.

SAH can occur at **any stage of chronic kidney disease**, and whether blood creatinine concentrations are directly related to the SAP value has not been documented.

In hypertensive cats the only parameter related to survival is the **urinary protein/creatinine ratio**.

Clinical signs

Hypertensive animals can remain asymptomatic for months or years, until tissue damage is evident and **clinical signs related to the target organs** (cardiovascular, central nervous, urinary and ocular systems) appear, all of which cause significant arteriolar tissue vascularisation.

SAH is diagnosed by clinical signs related to these organs in most cases.

Cardiovascular effects

The most common effect of SAH on the cardiovascular system in dogs and cats is **left ventricular concentric hypertrophy**. This is a response to the chronically increased afterload and to parietal stress. Although ventricular stiffness reduces ventricular filling and raises diastolic filling pressure, it is uncommon for hypertensive animals to suffer from congestive heart failure, except when there is an underlying cardiopathy.

The most common clinical signs in dogs and cats with SAH include systolic murmurs, gallop sounds and cardiomegaly. Using echocardiography, varying degrees of concentric hypertrophy have been documented in nearly all studies, with a prevalence between 70% and 91%. Varying degrees of dilation of the ascending aorta and aortic regurgitation have also been seen.

Ocular effects

Effects of SAH in the eyes are common, both in cats and dogs. As in other microvascular beds, once the upper limit for autoregulation has been exceeded, any further increase in flow and pressure in the choroidal arterioles and capillaries causes plasma extravasation with associated **oedema, haemorrhage and retinal detachment**.

This syndrome is known as hypertensive **retinopathy or choroidopathy**. Other ocular lesions include tortuous retinal vessels, vitreal haemorrhage, hyphaemia, glaucoma and, in late stages, retinal degeneration.

Effects on the central nervous system

Autoregulation of the central nervous system blood flow within an appropriate pressure range is mediated by smooth arteriolar muscle, which is capable of causing vasoconstriction in response to increased SAP. When the autoregulatory limit is exceeded, an increase in pressure and blood flow is produced within the microcirculation, altering Starling's forces across the capillary wall.

The subsequent increases in capillary hydrostatic pressure increase transcapillary filtration, promoting interstitial **oedema within the cerebral parenchyma**.

This involves an increase in intracranial pressure which, in turn, causes neurological dysfunction, known as **hypertensive encephalopathy**. The associated clinical signs include disorientation, ataxia, stupor, convulsions and coma.

Effects on the kidney

The contribution of SAH to the **progression of kidney disease** has been documented, due to the unique characteristics of renal microcirculation (the glomerular capillary bed is preceded and continued by afferent and efferent arterioles, respectively).

If the kidney is critically damaged, production of renin and its associated angiotensin II (systemic or local) increases. This raises cardiac output and peripheral resistance, **increasing the effects of hypertension**. As a result, the afferent arteriole dilates and angiotensin II causes vasoconstriction of the efferent arteriole, leading to increased intraglomerular pressure. Sustained high arterial pressure above 160 mm Hg causes irreversible vascular damage and **nephron death**, contributing to the progression of kidney disease.

Diagnosis

Diagnosis of SAH is based on **multiple measurements** of SAP and consideration of the clinical signs related to the target organs and the disorders which can cause secondary hypertension.

Measurement of SAP

Although measuring SAP appears to be a simple procedure, it is one of the least reliably executed, with scant compliance with recommendations.

The difficulties involved in measuring the SAP in an animal, which make the results unreproducible, are caused by **three different factors**.

- High variability, as SAP is modified by many external and internal factors.
- Limited precision of indirect measurements, the observer being the main source of inaccuracy.
- Iatrogenic pressure modification due to the 'white coat effect'.

Arterial pressure can be measured directly, by puncturing an artery (of little use in routine medicine), or indirectly (non-invasively), by **Doppler or oscillometry**.

1. **Doppler method**
   This is based on the use of a probe containing a piezoelectric crystal that emits high-frequency (8–10 MHz) ultrasound waves which, on collision with moving blood cells, are reflected at a different

frequency from that emitted (Doppler deviation). This change in frequency is amplified by the detector and heard by the person measuring the pressure. This means systolic arterial pressure can be measured in dogs and cats (Figure 5.85). The main disadvantage of this method is that **diastolic arterial pressure is difficult to measure**.

2. **Oscillometry**
   This is based on detection of fluctuations in the pressure produced by the pulse on the cuff. It enables automatic measurement of systolic and diastolic arterial pressure, average SAP and pulse frequency. Recently developed high-definition oscillometry means that sensitivity and quality of the technique have improved, and reliable values for SAP can be obtained as the pressure curve can be visualised on a computer screen (Figure 5.86). Movement of the animal, elevated heart rate, arrhythmias, low SAP or incorrect positioning of the cuff have negative effects on the precision of measurements determined by oscillometry.

In **both methods**, Doppler and oscillometry, measuring the SAP requires a **suitable cuff** to be fitted (width should be 40% of the diameter of the limb (radius, metatarsal) or the tail) and acclimatisation of the patient. Optimum measurement of SAP is the **average of 5–7 measurements** obtained from a **calm animal**. It is useful to note the heart rate in order to interpret the result appropriately.

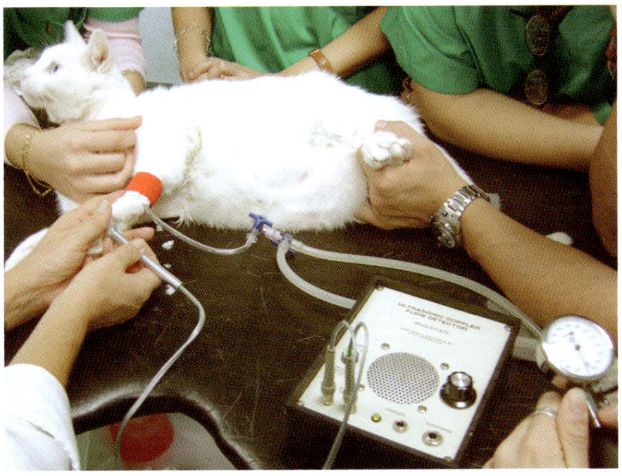

Figure 5.85. Measurement of systemic arterial pressure in a cat by the Doppler method.

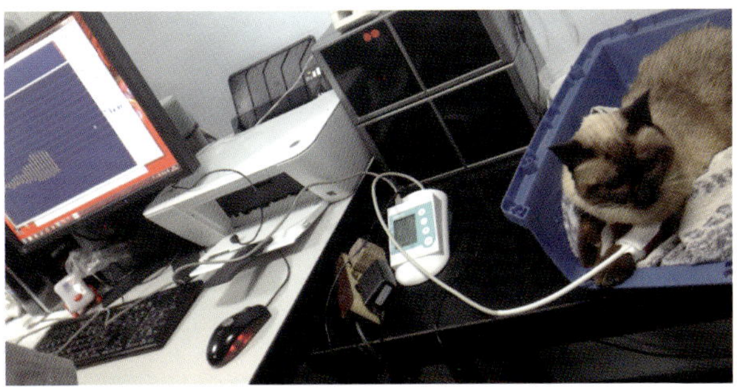

Figure 5.86. Measuring arterial pressure in a cat by high-definition oscillometry.

This is why consistency, and the protocol followed in each laboratory (clinic), is as important as the method used to obtain the SAP.

SAP values should be interpreted in the context of the clinical case, considering the animal's stress levels, the medications administered, cardiovascular function, etc. Variations in breed, age and sex tend to be small except in Greyhounds (increased by 10–20 mm Hg).

Four categories of SAP have been established to identify, evaluate and treat dogs and cats with SAH.

Category I or minimum risk:

SAP <150/95 mm Hg

These SAP values are considered to cause minimum risk of damage to target organs, so animals with these levels do not require antihypertensive therapy. These figures are also a goal to aim for when treating animals with higher SAP values.

Category II or low risk:

SAP 150–159/95–99 mm Hg

Several studies in normal animals have indicated that these SAP values are normal, although it is difficult to know whether they are real or due to the 'white coat effect'. These patients are considered to be low risk and treatment is not recommended.

Category III or moderate risk:

SAP 160–179/100–119 mm Hg

Most animals in this category, particularly those with damage to target organs or secondary hypertension, are candidates for antihypertensive therapy, which can reduce progression of the disease in patients with chronic kidney disease.

Animals with SAP levels in the low part of this range and those without effects on the target organs but where the 'white coat effect' cannot be excluded, do not require treatment.

Category IV or high risk:

SAP >180/120 mm Hg

The aim of treating animals in this category is to limit the degree of damage to target organs. At least two measuring sessions are recommended to verify these elevated SAP values, except when there is ocular damage or severe compatible neurological lesions. These animals are candidates for antihypertensive treatment and treatment for possible disorders caused by SAH.

Treatment

The main objective of antihypertensive treatment is to reduce SAP and the progression of damage to the target organs.

The **general guidelines** for treatment of hypertense patients are listed below.

- Identify, where possible, and **treat the causes** of SAH, although resolution of these does not always resolve the SAH.
- Decide **whether or not to treat** the animal based on the category it fits into.
- **Inform the owner** of what a hypertensive animal means (risk of damage to target organs, prolonged treatment, periodic revisions) and that controlling SAP does not mean that the disorder is resolved, or the animal cured.
- Administer the **preferred treatment** once a day and use as few medications as possible.
- Reduce SAP progressively and persistently (therapeutic objective).
- If an antihypertensive agent is only partially effective, increase the dose or add another drug.
- **Monitor SAP frequently** (every 1–3 days) after commencing treatment in patients with severe SAH and damage to target organs. Any change in treatment should be monitored after 7–10 days. Monitoring after varying periods of 1 to 4 months is recommended in long-term therapy with stable SAP.

Remember that antihypertensive therapy includes both dietary management and drug administration.

Diet

There is controversy over the restriction of sodium in the diets of hypertensive patients, as there is no evidence that this measure reduces SAP. It is therefore recommended to adapt diets to the underlying disorders, taking palatability into account and avoiding or replacing high-sodium diets.

Pharmaceutical agents

ACE inhibitors

These are the first drugs used in the treatment of canine hypertension secondary to kidney disease, based on inhibition of the renin–angiotensin–aldosterone system. They also reduce intraglomerular pressure and therefore proteinuria.

Renal function should be assessed before administration, as ACE inhibitors can exacerbate pre-existing azotaemia. It is unlikely that ACE inhibitors will reduce SAP values sufficiently in dogs with very high SAP and damage to target organs, so administration of other drugs may be necessary.

ACE inhibitors are less effective in cats than dogs and do not reduce SAH sufficiently as monotherapy in cats.

Angiotensin receptor antagonists

Telmisartan (1 mg/kg body weight) is licensed for use in cats and is a specific angiotensin II receptor antagonist. Studies have shown that it reduces SAP and also proteinuria.

Calcium channel blockers

Amlodipine (besylate) is the most widely used and belongs to the dihydropyridine group *(0.05–0.2 mg/kg/24 h in dogs; 0.625–1.25 mg/24 h in cats)*. It acts by blocking the flow of calcium for contraction of smooth muscle and reducing systemic vascular resistance. Its action is prolonged and gradual, so one dose per day is sufficient. It is the most widely used drug to control SAH in cats.

β-blockers

These are used in cats and dogs when the drugs described above have not reduced SAP. *Atenolol* is most commonly used *(0.25–1 mg/kg/12–24 h in dogs; 6.25–12.5 mg/12–24 h in cats)*.

Atenolol has been used in combination with amlodipine to treat SAH associated with hyperthyroidism in cats.

Other drugs

In patients with severe SAH and damage to target organs (encephalopathy or hypertensive retinopathy), parenteral agents such as sodium nitroprusside in continuous infusion (causing arterial and venous vasodilation) or esmolol, etc. can be used. In these cases, arterial pressure must be monitored frequently, as a sudden reduction can compromise cerebral perfusion.

Bibliography

Atkins, C., Bonagura, J., Ettinger, S., Fox, P., Gordon, S., Haggstrom, J., Hamlin, R., Keene, B., Luis-Fuentes, V. and Stepien, R. (2009) Guidelines for the diagnosis and treatment of canine chronic valvular heart disease. *Journal of Veterinary Internal Medicine*, 23, 1142–1150.

Boon, J.A. (2011) *Veterinary Echocardiography*, 2nd edn. Wiley-Blackwell, Iowa.

Brown, S., Atkins, R., Bagley, A., Carr, A., Cowgill, L., Davidson, M., Egner, B., Elliott, J., Henik, R., Labato, M., Littman, M., Polzin, D., Ross, L., Snyder, P., Stepien, R.; American College of Veterinary Internal Medicine (2007) Guidelines for the identification, evaluation, and management of systemic hypertension in dogs and cats. *Journal of Veterinary Internal Medicine*, 21, 542–558.

Bruce, G.K. and Moise, N.S. (2014) Bradyarrhythmias. In: Bonagura, J.D. and Twedt, D.C. (eds) *Kirk's Current Veterinary Therapy XV*. Elsevier Saunders, St Louis, MO, pp. 731–736.

Buchanan, J.W. (1992) Causes and prevalence of cardiovascular disease. In: Kirk, R.E. (ed.) *Current Veterinary Therapy XI*. WB Saunders, Philadelphia, PA, pp. 647–655.

Coté, E. (2014) Feline cardiac arrhythmias. In: Bonagura, J.D. and Twedt, D.C. (eds) *Kirks Current Veterinary Therapy XV*. Elsevier Saunders, St Louis, MO, pp. 748–755.

Fernández del Palacio, M.J. (2010) Evaluación de la presión arterial. In: Cortadellas, O. (ed.) *Manual de nefrologia y urologia clinica canina y felina*. Servet Diseño y Comunicación, SL, Zaragoza, Spain, pp. 109–116.

Fernández del Palacio, M.J. (2010) Tratamiento de la hipertensión arterial sistémica. In: Cortadellas, O. (ed.) *Manual de nefrologia y urologia clinica canina y felina*. Servet Diseño y Comunicación, SL, Zaragoza, Spain, pp. 189–198.

Fernández del Palacio, M.J. (2014) Ecocardiografía: modalidades de imagen y protocolo de examen. In: Agut, A. (ed.) *Diagnóstico por Imagen en pequeños animales*. Multimédica Ediciones Veterinarias, Barcelona, Spain, pp. 503–520.

Fernández del Palacio MJ. (2014) La ecocardiografia en la evaluación de las principales afecciones cardiacas. In: Agut, A. (ed.) *Diagnóstico por Imagen en pequeños animales*. Multimédica Ediciones Veterinarias, Barcelona, Spain, pp. 521–532.

Gómez, A., Fernández del Palacio, J., Latorre, R., Henry, R.W., Sarriá, R. and Albors, O.L. (2012) Plastinated heart slices aid echocardiographic interpretation in the dog. *Veterinary Radiology and Ultrasound*, 53, 197–203.

Häggström, J., Boswood, A., O'Grady, M., Henry, R.W., Sarriá, R. and Albors, O.L. (2008) Effect of pimobendan or benazepril hydrochloride on survival times in dogs with congestive heart failure caused by naturally occurring myxomatous mitral valve disease: the QUEST study. *Journal of Veterinary Internal Medicine*, 22, 1124–1135.

Keene, B.W. and Bonagura, J.D. (2014) Management of heart failure in dogs. In: Bonagura, J.G. and Twedt, D.C. (eds) *Kirk's Current Veterinary Therapy XV*. Elsevier Saunders, St Louis, MO, pp. 772–784.

Luis Fuentes, V. (2010) Echocardiography. In: Luis Fuentes, V., Johnson, L.R. and Denis, S. (eds) *BSAVA Manual of Canine and Feline Cardiorespiratory Medicine*, 2nd edn. BSAVA, Gloucester, UK, pp. 79–97.

Oyama, M.A., Kraus, M.S. and Gelzer, A.R. (2014) *Rapid Review of ECG Interpretation In Small Animal Practice*. CRC Press, London, UK.

Oyama, M.A. and Reynolds, C.A. (2014) Ventricular arrhythmias in dogs. In: Bonagura, J.D. and Twedt, D.C. (eds) *Kirk's Current Veterinary Therapy XV*. Elsevier Saunders, St Louis, MO, pp. 745–747.

Pariaut, R., Santilli, R.A. and Moise, N.S. (2014) Supraventricular tachyarrhythmias in dogs. In: Bonagura, J.D. and Twedt, D.C. (eds) *Kirk's Current Veterinary Therapy XV*. Elsevier Saunders, St Louis, MO, pp. 737–744.

Pox, P.R., Sisson, D. and Moise, N.S. (1999) *Textbook of Canine and Feline Cardiology: Principles and Clinical Practice*, 2nd edn. WB Saunders, Philadelphia, PA.

Shaw, S.P. and Rush, J.E. (2007) Canine pericardial effusion: diagnosis, treatment, and prognosis. *Compendium: Continuing Education For Veterinarians*, 29, 405–411.

Schrope, D.P. (2015) Prevalence of congenital heart disease in 76,301 mixed-breed dogs and 57,025 mixed-breed cats. *Journal of Veterinary Cardiology*, 17, 192–202.

Thomas, W.P., Gaber, C.E., Jacobs, G.J., Kaplan, P.M., Lombard, C.W., Moise, N.S. and Moses, B.L. (1993) Recommendations for standards in transthoracic two-dimensional echocardiography in the dog and cat. Echocardiography Committee of the Specialty of Cardiology, American College of Veterinary Internal Medicine. *Journal of Veterinary Internal Medicine*, 7, 247–252.

Tilley, L.P. (1992) *Essentials of canine and feline electrocardiography*, 3rd edn. Lea Febiger, Philadelphia, PA.

Treggiari, E., Pedro, B., Dukes-McEwan, J., Gelzer, A.R. and Blackwood, L. (2017) A descriptive review of cardiac tumours in dogs and cats. *Veterinary and Comparative Oncology*, 15, 273–288. doi: 10.1111/vco.12167.

Ware, W.A. (2011) *Cardiovascular Disease in Small Animal Medicine*. Mason Publishing, London, UK.

Test

1. Which of the following statements is false concerning cardiopathies in dogs and cats?

A) They form a significant part of the clinical population of dogs and cats.
B) Chronic degenerative mitral valve disease is the most common cardiopathy in small-breed dogs.
C) Dilated cardiomyopathy has not been diagnosed in cats.
D) Coughing is a common sign of heart disease in dogs.

2. In cats with congestive heart failure, which of the following is not a clinical sign?

A) Dyspnoea.
B) Frequent dry cough.
C) Orthopnoeic position.
D) Exercise intolerance and anorexia.

3. Which of the following statements is false concerning heart murmurs?

A) Not all murmurs are indicative of a cardiopathy.

B) In cats, murmurs can be auscultated better over the sternum.

C) Patients with grade 4/6 murmurs present with precordial fremitus.

D) Continuous murmurs are characteristic of a patent ductus arteriosus.

4. A dog that has fewer pulsations than heartbeats suggests:

A) Atrial fibrillation.

B) Sinus tachycardia.

C) Pulmonary thromboembolism.

D) A wandering pacemaker.

5. Which of the following is true concerning the evaluation of cardiac size on lateral thoracic radiographs?

A) The vertebral heart scale measurement system is based on comparing the size of the heart with that of the first thoracic vertebra.

B) The cardiac size obtained using the vertebral scale for measurement is greater in cats than in dogs.

C) On a lateral radiograph in cats, a prominent aortic arch is always indicative of a congenital pathology.

D) Dogs with a patent ductus arteriosus generally present with an enlarged silhouette of the left-sided chambers, the aortic arch and the main pulmonary artery.

6. Which of the following statements about echocardiography is false?

A) Ultrasound is based on the use of high-frequency sound waves.

B) M-mode examines the heart using a linear beam.

C) Doppler echocardiography is based on the change in frequency which ultrasound waves experience when they hit blood cells.

D) Colour Doppler allows the speed of blood flow to be measured.

7. Which of the following statements concerning congestive heart failure is true?

A) It is uncommon in dogs with right-sided cardiopathies.

B) In cats, a pleural effusion is a common consequence of congestive heart failure.

C) Natriuretic peptides and cytokines are responsible for the signs of heart failure.

D) The sympathetic nervous system maintains cardiac function, particularly in advanced stages of the disease.

8. With respect to patent ductus arteriosus, which of the following is false?

A) It is only diagnosed in small-breed dogs.

B) It can be diagnosed in both large- and small-breed dogs.

C) Is characterised by a hyperkinetic pulse.

D) The murmur can be auscultated on both sides of the thorax.

9. Regarding canine dilated cardiomyopathy, which of the following statements is correct?

A) Pekinese and Yorkshire Terriers are particularly predisposed to the condition.

B) In Dobermans the long-term prognosis is good.

C) In Boxers thoracic radiographs may be normal.

D) Standard treatment includes a diuretic, negative ionotropic and antiarrhythmic.

10. Which medication is most suitable for the treatment of sustained ventricular tachycardia in dogs?

A) Digoxin.

B) Lidocaine.

C) Atropine.

D) Propranolol.

11. Furosemide can be used in the treatment of:

A) Pericardial effusion.

B) Stage B heart failure.

C) Stage C heart failure.

D) Chylothorax.

12. Which of the following is true regarding chronic degenerative mitral valve disease in dogs?

A) Detection of a systolic murmur in the mitral region is essential for a diagnosis.

B) Coughing is a pathognomonic clinical sign of the disease.

C) The information obtained through an electrocardiogram is essential to prescribe a treatment.

D) The clinical state of the animal does not influence treatment.

13. Which of the following is a predisposing factor for the development of bacterial endocarditis?
   A) Subaortic stenosis, interventricular defects and immunosuppressive agents.
   B) Dilated cardiomyopathy.
   C) Cardiac arrhythmia.
   D) Systemic treatment with fluoroquinolones.

14. Pericardial tamponade occurs when:
   A) The ventricles cannot distend in diastole due to arrhythmias.
   B) The pressure in the pericardial space is greater than the diastolic pressures of the right atrium and ventricle due to the accumulation of fluid.
   C) Pulmonary hypertension occurs.
   D) The inspiratory phase of respiration is very long.

15. Which of the following statements is correct regarding cor pulmonale (CP)?
   A) Pulmonary fibrosis is one the most common causes of CP in dogs.
   B) Chronic degenerative mitral valve disease is a common cause of CP in dogs.
   C) Echocardiographic examination is normal in the majority of cases.
   D) Generally, CP does not require treatment.

16. Which of the following regarding systemic arterial hypertension is false?
   A) It is very common in cats with chronic renal insufficiency.
   B) One of the clinical signs is blindness, both in dogs and cats.
   C) Calcium channel blockers are contraindicated as a treatment.
   D) Congestive heart failure is uncommon.

Answers on page 254

Clinical case 1

Signalment: Mixed-breed dog, 12 years old, 8 kg.

Reason for consultation: Coughing for several months, but this has become worse over the last 2 weeks and the dog has difficulty going up stairs. The dog has been treated with antibiotics over the last week without a satisfactory response.

Physical examination: Slightly pale mucous membranes with a capillary refill time of 2 seconds, and a weak, irregular pulse which does not always coincide with the heartbeat. Expiratory dyspnoea when being handled during the examination, with a respiratory rate of 70 breaths/minute.

Thoracic auscultation: Inspiratory crepitations are present in both hemithoraces. There is an irregular heart rate (160 bpm); grade 5/6 pansystolic murmur with a point of maximum intensity over the 5th intercostal space on the left side of the thorax towards the sternum; and grade 4/6 systolic murmur with a point of maximum intensity over the 4th–5th intercostal space on the right side of the thorax.

Complete blood count and blood biochemistry: Values within reference ranges.

Thoracic radiographs

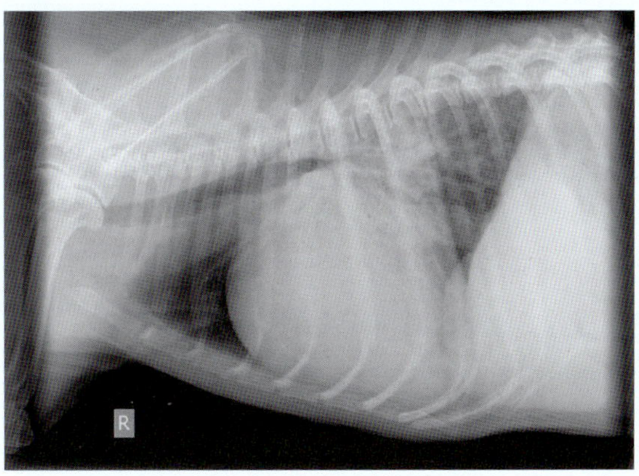

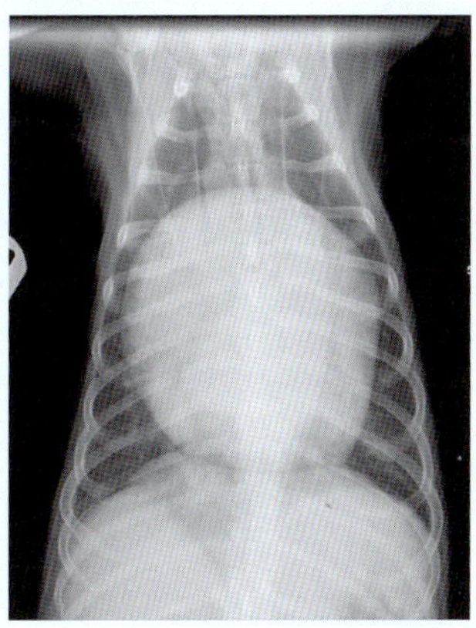

Electrocardiogram: 50 mm/s; 1 cm = 1 mV.

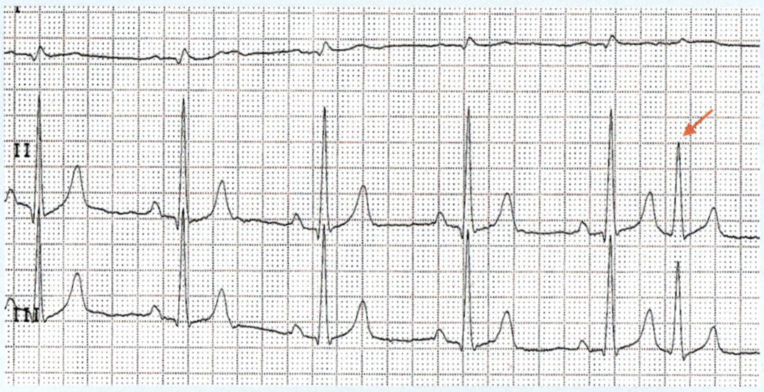

Echocardiography

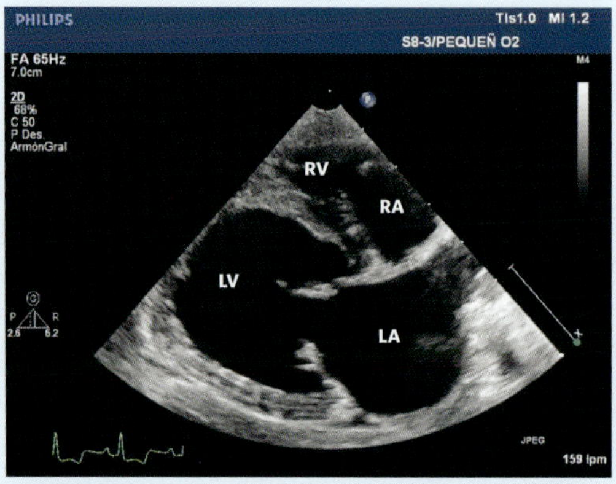

1. **Based on the signalment and history, which is the most likely cause of the cough in this dog?**
   A) Chronic tracheobronchitis.
   B) Pulmonary neoplasia.
   C) Pleural effusion.
   D) Cardiopathy.
2. **Which is the most likely cause of the murmur in this dog?**
   A) Innocent murmur.
   B) Physiological murmur.
   C) Dilated cardiomyopathy.
   D) Chronic degenerative mitral valve disease.
3. **The cardiac rhythm seen on the ECG is caused by:**
   A) Premature ventricular complexes
   B) Premature supraventricular complexes
   C) Atrial fibrillation
   D) Sinus arrhythmia.
4. **Which is the following is true of the thoracic radiographs?**
   A) Tracheal collapse and a bronchial pattern can be seen.
   B) The most obvious finding is overall cardiomegaly, compatible with pericardial effusion.
   C) Dorsal displacement of the trachea with compression of the main bronchi due to enlargement of the left atrium and perihilar oedema can be seen.
   D) An increase in the size of the silhouette of the right-sided chambers and an interstitial pattern can be seen, compatible with pulmonary fibrosis.
5. **The 2D electrocardiogram (right parasternal access on the long axis, four chambers) is compatible with:**
   A) Dilated cardiomyopathy
   B) Chronic degenerative mitral valve disease with possible pulmonary hypertension
   C) Patent ductus arteriosus
   D) Bacterial endocarditis.
6. **What is the most appropriate treatment for this dog?**
   A) Furosemide, digoxin and an ACE inhibitor.
   B) ACE inhibitor, furosemide and pimobendan.
   C) Atenolol, ACE inhibitor and pimobendan.
   D) Pimobendan, furosemide and spironolactone.

Answers on page 254

Clinical case 2

Signalment: Persian cat, 6 years old and weighs 3.5 kg.

Reason for consultation: Fatigue since the day before.

History and clinical signs: Since last week, when the cat was taken to the hairdresser, it has been less active and has less appetite. It is up to date with vaccinations and worming treatments and lives indoors.

Physical examination: Dyspnoeic respiratory pattern in the consultation, with tachypnoea (respiratory rate 60 breaths per minute). Very weak femoral pulse, which does not coincide with the heartbeat.

Thoracic auscultation: Dull heart and respiratory sounds. Heart rate = 190 bpm; irregular rhythm.

Electrocardiogram: 50 mm/s; 1cm = 1 mV.

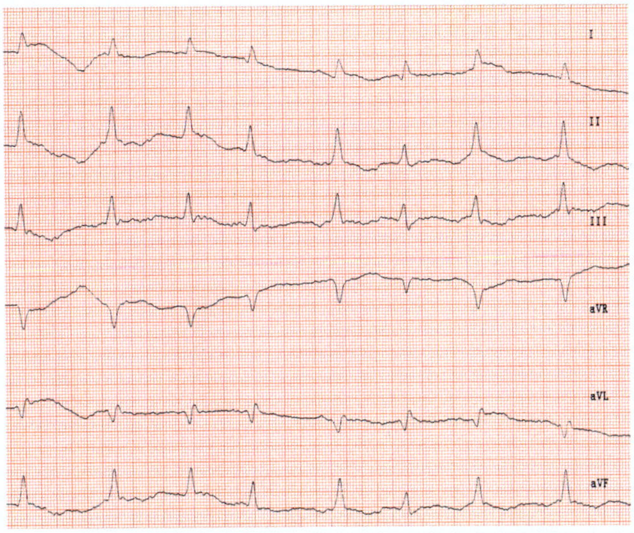

Echocardiography

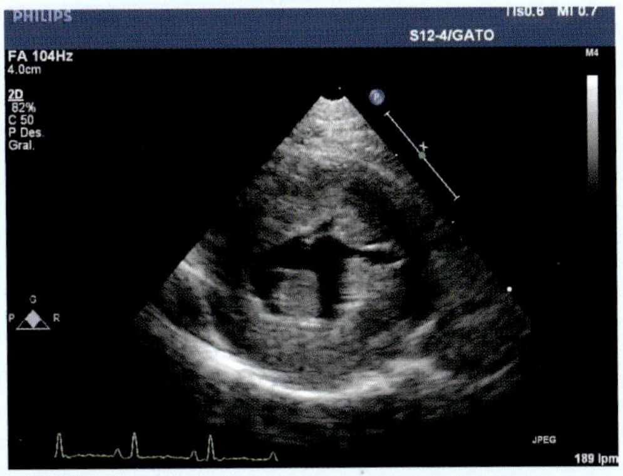

Thoracic radiographs

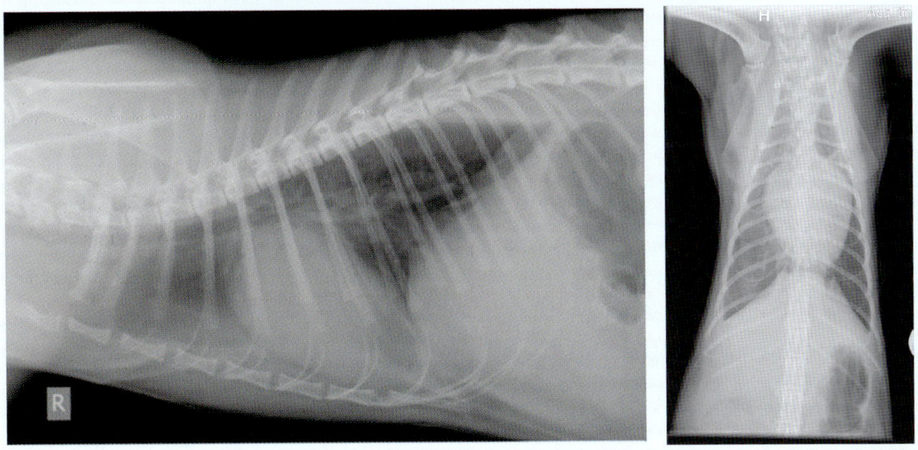

1. **Based on the history and physical examination, which is the most likely cause of the respiratory problem in this cat?**
   A) Congenital cardiopathy.
   B) Pulmonary neoplasia.
   C) Pleural effusion.
   D) Feline asthma.
2. **What is the most appropriate way to stabilise this cat?**
   A) Administer oxygen and perform thoracocentesis.
   B) Administer intravenous furosemide.
   C) Sedate and administer subcutaneous furosemide.
   D) Administer a bronchodilator.
3. **Which cardiac rhythm could be seen on the electrocardiogram?**
   A) Sinus rhythm.
   B) Sinus arrhythmia.
   C) Atrial fibrillation.
   D) Ventricular tachycardia.
4. **After stabilising the cat, which of the following is the most characteristic sign seen on radiographs?**
   A) Mild pleural effusion and cardiomegaly.
   B) Interstitial and bronchial pattern, characteristic of feline asthma.
   C) Mediastinal mass.
   D) Diaphragmatic hernia.
5. **Considering information from all of the tests, which is the most likely cause of the disease in this cat?**
   A) Chronic bronchial disease.
   B) Hypertrophic cardiomyopathy.
   C) Patent ductus arteriosus.
   D) Mediastinal lymphoma.
6. **Which medications should be used to treat this cat in the short term?**
   A) Furosemide, atenolol and benazepril.
   B) Mannitol, diltiazem and benazepril.
   C) Furosemide and nitroglycerine, with oxygen as an inpatient.
   D) None is necessary as it is breathing much better.

Correct answers

Test

1. C	7. B	13. A
2. B	8. A	14. B
3. C	9. C	15. A
4. A	10. B	16. C
5. D	11. C	
6. D	12. A	

Clinical case 1

1. **Based on the signalment and history, which is the least likely cause of the cough in this dog?**
   C. Pleural effusion.
2. **Which is the most likely cause of the murmur in this dog?**
   D. Chronic degenerative mitral valve disease.
3. **The cardiac rhythm seen on the ECG is caused by:**
   B. Premature supraventricular complexes.

4. **Which of the following is true of the thoracic radiographs?**
   C. Dorsal displacement of the trachea with compression of the main bronchi due to enlargement of the left atrium and perihilar oedema can be seen.
5. **The 2D electrocardiogram (right parasternal access on the long axis, four chambers) is compatible with:**
   B. Chronic degenerative mitral valve disease with possible pulmonary hypertension.
6. **What is the most appropriate treatment for this dog?**
   B. ACE inhibitor, furosemide and pimobendan.

Clinical case 2

1. **Based on the history and physical examination, indicate which is the most likely cause of the respiratory problem in this cat.**
   C. Pleural effusion.
2. **What is the most appropriate way to stabilise this cat?**
   A. Administer oxygen and perform thoracocentesis.
3. **Which cardiac rhythm could be seen on the electrocardiogram?**
   C. Atrial fibrillation.
4. **After stabilising the cat, which of the following is the most characteristic sign seen on radiographs?**
   A. Mild pleural effusion and cardiomegaly.
5. **Considering information from all of the tests, which is the most likely cause of the disease in this cat?**
   B. Hypertrophic cardiomyopathy.
6. **Which medications should be used to treat this cat in the short term?**
   C. Furosemide and nitroglycerine, with oxygen as an inpatient.

Reproductive system disorders

6

Simón Martí Angulo and Cintia García Echarri

Chapter summary

It is a sad truth that many a veterinarian's only experience of canine or feline reproduction is when faced with an emergency caesarean section. However, the field of reproductive medicine is far wider and more sophisticated than merely fire-fighting when something goes wrong.

This chapter takes a detailed look at all aspects of reproductive medicine, ranging from the hormones of pregnancy to predictors of labour; from pregnancy diagnosis to neonatal physiology. The aim is to provide the practitioner with the knowledge necessary to promote successful pregnancies, eliminate unnecessary complications and attain healthy litters for our feline and canine patients.

Key learning points

- Understand the endocrinology of pregnancy, and the relevance of monitoring for a successful pregnancy.
- Learn about neonatal physiology, how this differs from that of the adult and its impact on their care.
- Calculate gestational age from an ultrasound examination, for an accurate prediction of the birthing date.
- Troubleshoot common causes of infertility in the dog and cat.
- How to resuscitate and support neonates to increase their survival.

Pregnancy and gestation in the dog and cat

Definition

The **gestation period** is defined as:

> The time elapsed between fertilisation of the female's ovum and the birth of offspring.

Gestation period in the bitch

- Canine gestation period 57–71 days from mating. Gestation can be calculated most accurately by identifying the date when progesterone levels increase from 0 to >1.5 mg/ml, which also coincides with a peak in luteinising hormone (LH) level.
- 67% of births occur between 64 and 66 days of this peak.
- 100% of births occur 62–88 days post-peak LH levels.

Gestation period in the queen

- Feline gestational period 59–69 days from mating.

A wide gestational range of 52–74 days is considered normal, because in felines coitus does not always induce ovulation and so fertilisation may be delayed. A narrower gestation range, of 63–66 days, can be calculated by knowing the date of the rise in blood progesterone levels, which indicates that ovulation has taken place.

In both the dog and cat, as pregnancy progresses the mother undergoes a variety of endocrine, physical and behavioural changes, which we consider in detail.

The endocrinology of pregnancy

A complex interplay of reproductive hormones is necessary to maintain a healthy pregnancy.

In the bitch

The bitch is monoestrous, with a complete reproductive cycle lasting approximately six months (subject to wide variability).

Progesterone

Progesterone can be described as the hormone of pregnancy.

It has various important functions which serve to maintain pregnancy. These include:

- inhibition of the action of oestrogen on the uterus, which would otherwise cause uterine contractions
- promotion of endometrial differentiation
- maintenance of the integrity of the endometrium
- promotion of placental attachment.

In the pregnant dog, serum progesterone concentrations continue to rise over the next 15–25 days to reach a peak. After this, levels slowly decline but remain raised above non-pregnant levels. A sharp decrease in progesterone, when levels drop to below 2 ng/ml, occurs 48 hours before birth. This is due to a sudden increase in prostaglandin F2-alpha.

It is important to know that blood progesterone levels are the same in pregnant and non-pregnant females. This is because although the production of progesterone by the corpus luteum is significantly increased during pregnancy, metabolism and faecal excretion of the metabolites also increase.

Progesterone monitoring

Adequate progesterone levels are required to **maintain a healthy pregnancy**, and a gradual decrease will result in the commencement of parturition. Therefore, it is advisable to monitor progesterone levels during pregnancy.

Since the **corpus luteum** is responsible for the majority of **progesterone production**, destruction of the former results in falling progesterone levels. If this takes place too soon, it will result in failure of the pregnancy and abortion. This inappropriate fall in progesterone levels can be caused by nutritional, environmental, traumatic and inflammatory factors.

Prolactin

Prolactin and LH regulate progesterone levels. Prolactin is the main luteotropic hormone, but is not diagnostic of pregnancy.

Prolactin levels rise in the second half of pregnancy to remain high through the remainder of gestation and lactation. However, prolactin levels vary significantly between individuals, by the day and due to external factors such as the environment. These can also be raised in non-pregnant bitches with pathologies such as pseudo-pregnancy. For these reasons, prolactin levels are not diagnostic of pregnancy.

Luteinising hormone

The role of **LH** is to stimulate the production of progesterone; however, the means by which this happens is not clear. For example, it has been shown that inhibition of LH by the action of anti-LH antibodies does not affect the secretion of progesterone or the function of the corpus luteum. Therefore the role of LH appears to be more luteotrophic than luteotropic.

Relaxin

Relaxin levels rise and become detectable 21–24 days after the LH surge. Levels remain raised until just before birth, at which point they drop dramatically but remain detectable for 30 days after whelping.

At days 40–50 of gestation, blood relaxin levels are between 4 and 5 ng/ml. This is the only hormone associated with pregnancy that is not present in the non-pregnant female, and therefore it is reliably used as an indicator of pregnancy. It is variably detected in the dog and cat:

- relaxin detectable on day 35 after the LH peak in the bitch
- relaxin detectable on day 20 after mating in the queen.

The role of relaxin in pregnancy is not fully understood. In some species relaxin regulates the production of prolactin, whilst in others it has been shown to stimulate progesterone secretion and, indirectly, an increase in prolactin.

Follicle-stimulating hormone (FSH)

From the start of gestation until day 35 after the LH peak, high concentrations of **FSH** are detectable.

High levels of FSH (>150 ng/ml) on days 16–18 post mating are a reliable indicator of pregnancy. These raised levels drop suddenly immediately after birth.

In non-pregnant dogs FSH levels never reach 150 ng/ml.

Oestrogen

In pregnant dogs an increase in **urine oestrogen** levels can be detected approximately 21 days after mating. This does not occur in non-pregnant females.

Fibrinogen

Fibrinogen levels begin to increase when embryos implant, and continue to rise between days 30–50 reaching levels of 280 mg/dl. Other pathologies that cause inflammation can also cause a rise in fibrinogen, so this is not a reliable indicator of pregnancy.

Reactive C protein

In pregnant females the levels of **Reactive C protein** rise 20–25 days after ovulation, and decrease dramatically should resorption or abortion occur.

In the queen

Cats are seasonal, poly-oestrus breeders. Ovulation is induced by the stimulation caused by the male penis in the vagina, rather than being a spontaneous event as in the dog. It is coital stimulation that causes the release of gonadotrophic-releasing hormone (GnRH), which results in a surge of LH 15 minutes after mating. A critical level of LH is necessary for ovulation, which can mean that multiple matings are required for conception.

Typically, in mid-oestrus, the amount of LH released by mating results in ovulation in only around 50% of cats. Generally, four to five matings on alternate days are required to ensure ovulation, as this causes accumulating waves of LH.

Once optimal LH levels are reached, ovulation occurs 24 hours later.

Fertilisation

Fertilisation is defined as:

> The fusion of the female pronucleus of a mature secondary oocyte, with the male pronucleus of the spermatozoid. This results in a single cell, with a single nucleus, which will form the embryo.

In the bitch

Fertilisation in the bitch has differences that are unique to canines.

1. **Late maturation of the oocyte**: This occurs 2–3 days after ovulation, and 60 hours after the LH peak. This means that maturation takes place at any point between the end of pro-oestrus and the middle of oestrus. In practical terms, this means that if the female is covered by several males, puppies in the same litter may have different fathers.
2. **Luteinisation**: This takes place before ovulation from the middle to end of pro-oestrus. Findings that back this up include the following.
   A) **Endocrine system**: increased preovulatory serum progesterone is seen.
   B) **Morphological changes** occur, with the presence of small patches on the inner wall of the follicles.
   C) **Oocytes remain viable for a further 3–5 days**. After ovulation, it is possible for fertilisation to take place up to 6–8 days later. In other words, fertilisation can occur 10–11 days after the preovulatory peak in LH.
3. **Late implantation of the blastocysts**: In the normal bitch, ovulation of primary oocytes occurs two days after the peak in LH. These then require a further 2 to 3 days to reach final maturity. These morulas develop in the distal oviduct and give rise to blastocysts, which enter the uterus 10–12 days after the LH surge and do not attach until days 18–20.

Pregnancy diagnosis

In the bitch

The most appropriate method of pregnancy diagnosis varies depending on the stage of gestation.

Abdominal palpation

Embryonic vesicles are palpable 17–22 days after ovulation. However, the optimal time to palpate the uterus is **35–45 days**.

There can be problems detecting pregnancy manually in the dog that tenses her abdomen, or large and giant dogs with few foetuses, often located far cranially.

Abdominal palpation should always be done with care.

Laboratory diagnosis

Laboratory diagnosis of pregnancy relies on the detection of high plasma **concentrations of relaxin**, which peak at **4–5 ng/ml**.

Relaxin is produced from week 3, around days 20–30 of pregnancy. False negatives can occur if the test is performed on day 21, because relaxin production has not yet occurred. It is therefore wise to repeat the test 7–10 days later in order to confirm the result.

Radiography

From day 21 after ovulation, an enlarged uterus may be evident radiographically but it is not until days 43–46 that one can identify puppy skulls and spines (Figure 6.1).

Radiological landmarks:

- day 21 onwards: enlarged uterus
- days 43–46 onwards: foetal skulls and spines
- days 58–63: foetal teeth become evident, 3–8 days prior to birth.

In addition, radiological studies prior to birth can provide information about the positioning of the puppies and whether it is correct. This facilitates decision making about whether a caesarean may be necessary.

Ultrasound

Ultrasound is preferred as the most reliable method of pregnancy diagnosis. However, it is not 100% reliable in detecting the number of foetuses.

Ultrasound can identify foetal pathologies such as anasarca or detect signs of foetal distress (Figure 6.2). In addition, measurement of the biparietal diameter or the

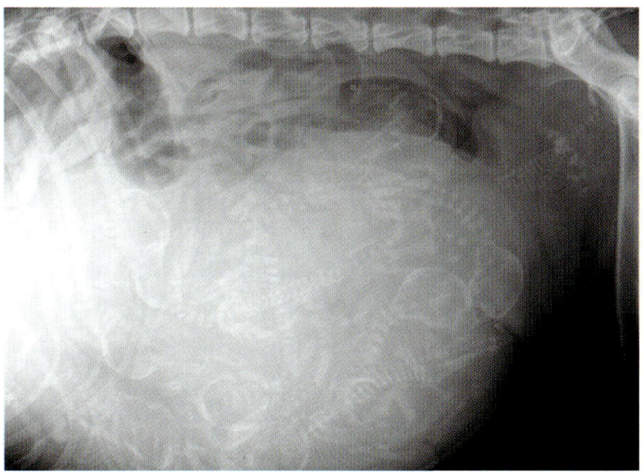

Figure 6.1. Abdominal radiography to determine litter size by counting the number of skulls and spines.

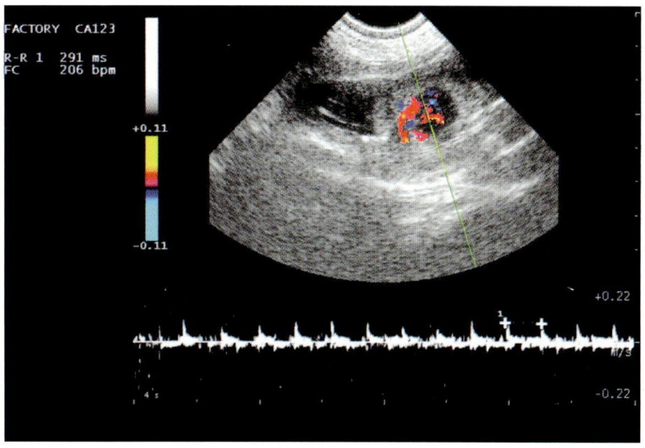

Figure 6.2. Ultrasonography for the detection of foetal distress.

external diameter of the chorionic cavity aids in calculation of the anticipated parturition date.

The following can be visualised using ultrasound:

- day 21: embryonic vesicles
- days 23–25: foetal heartbeats
- days 30–39: foetal movements
- days 57–63: foetal intestine.

Canine foetal heart rate:

- >220 bpm normal
- 180–220 bpm moderate foetal distress
- <180 bpm serious or severe foetal distress.

In the queen

Abdominal palpation

In the queen the ideal time to detect pregnancy with abdominal palpation is **21–35 days post-LH peak**.

Foetal vesicles measure approximately 2.5 cm in diameter. Uterine palpation should be performed with great care, especially in early gestation.

Radiography

Radiography of the foetal skeleton makes detection of pregnancy possible from days 36 to 45.

Ultrasound

Ultrasound is a quick and non-invasive method of pregnancy diagnosis.

The embryo is detectable from days 14–16, with foetal organs visible after day 30. In addition, there is an established correlation between gestational age and the following foetal measurements: abdominal, biparietal and gastric (see Table 6.1). A **foetal heart rate >193 bpm** indicates that everything is **normal**.

Maintenance of pregnancy in the dog

In the pregnant dog, progesterone levels are much higher compared to the non-pregnant dog.

Table 6.1. The relationship between gestational age and foetal measurements.

Days from mating	Abdominal diameter (cm)	Biparietal diameter (cm)	Gastric diameter (cm)
30	1.32	1.12	0.36
35	1.57	1.35	0.47
45	1.84	1.53	0.62
50	2.81	1.93	0.85
60	3.83	2.60	1.18

To maintain a pregnancy, progesterone levels must remain >15 ng/ml. In the second half of gestation, progesterone levels gradually drop, which causes a corresponding rise in prolactin. High levels of progesterone have an inhibitory effect on milk let-down. The fall in progesterone associated with parturition allows for prolactin to trigger milk release.

Around the time of parturition, prostaglandins produced at the site of foeto-placental units give rise to luteolysis, causing a sharp decline in prostaglandins to <2 ng/ml, which is a trigger for parturition.

Key events in pregnancy

Fertilisation: Takes place on day 3 after the peak in LH. The primary oocytes enter the oviduct but do not reach the uterus until day 11.

From day 20: The embryo begins to grow.

From day 22: The embryo implants in the endometrium. This is also when embryos become detectable on ultrasound.

Day 26: A rise occurs in serum relaxin and acute phase proteins.

Day 30: There is a significant increase in the weight of the embryos. This coincides with an increase in prolactin secretion, which is the likely trigger for a rise in progesterone secretion.

Day 42: The size of the embryo exceeds that of the placental band.

Physiological changes during pregnancy

Pregnancy induces various physiological changes which the clinician should consider akin to pathological changes. These changes have implications for how the patient responds to anaesthesia or medications, such as antibiotics. Therefore, it is appropriate to make modifications to day-to-day anaesthetic protocols and/or pharmacological treatments.

These physiological changes include the following.

- *Days 30–35 approximately*: A **normocytic, normochromic anaemia** occurs. This reflects an increased plasma volume, with a haematocrit of 30–40% expected around the 7th–9th week of gestation.
- *Weeks 3–5*: An **increase in plasma cholesterol** levels occurs.
- *From day 55*: There is an increase in **insulin resistance**.
- *From day 56 to birth*: Blood **calcium levels drop**.
- Although not routinely assessed, reactive C protein and fibrinogen **levels rise**.
- Also raised are cholesterol and lactate dehydrogenase.
- **Protein levels**, blood urea nitrogen (BUN) and cholesterol are **reduced**.

Calculation of gestational age in the dog

In the dog, mating is not a reliable reference for the date of conception. However, in cases where only one mating took place and the pregnancy is uncomplicated, birth should occur between days 58 and 68.

The first studies looking at a more exact way to calculate gestation were published in 2003 by Kutzler et al. They reached the following conclusions.

- 100% of births occur 65 ± 3 days from the peak in LH.
- 90% of births occur 65 ± 2 days from the peak in LH.
- 67% of births occur 65 ± 1 days from the peak in LH.

The timing of the LH peak can be determined when blood progesterone concentrations rise above the baseline of ≥1.5 ng/ml or when baseline levels double.

In cases where the exact day of ovulation is unknown, various methods can be used to calculate gestational age. These are of great importance to establish a predicted parturition and spot problems relating to birth.

Methods of calculation of gestational age

Vaginal smear

Vaginal smears are not a precise technique, since vaginal changes occur variably 6–11 days after the LH peak. However, what can be checked is whether the transition from oestrus to di-oestrus has occurred – typically 7–9 days after the peak in LH, which is approximately 57 days before birth.

Ultrasound

The diameter of the uterus can give an indication of the length of gestation (Table 6.2):

- days 22–24 after LH peak: 1 cm
- day 32 after LH peak: 3 cm.

Useful sonographic landmarks include:

- days 28–30: foetal heartbeat can be detected
- days 40–42: length of the embryo exceeds the width of the placental band.

Ultrasonographic features, both non-foetal and foetal, can reliably be used to determine gestational age (Table 6.3).

Between **45 and 25 days before birth**, the most accurate ultrasound measurement for prediction of the anticipated whelping date is the **inner diameter of the chorionic cavity** (Figure 6.3).

The chorionic cavity is an anechoic structure within the uterus, with clearly defined spherical margins. The measurement is made using two diameters at a 90° angle from one side of the decidual trophoblastic reaction to the other.

The accuracy of the calculation is dependent on neither the gender nor size of the litter, but the breed (Table 6.2). In small breeds, the calculation is accurate to ±1 day in 77% of cases; in medium and large breeds, to ±2 days in 88 and 85% of cases, respectively.

In the **final 25 days of pregnancy**, the **biparietal diameter** is the most accurate measurement with which to predict when birth will occur (Figure 6.4). This is taken in longitudinal section when the parietal bones of the skull are parallel, measuring the distance between them.

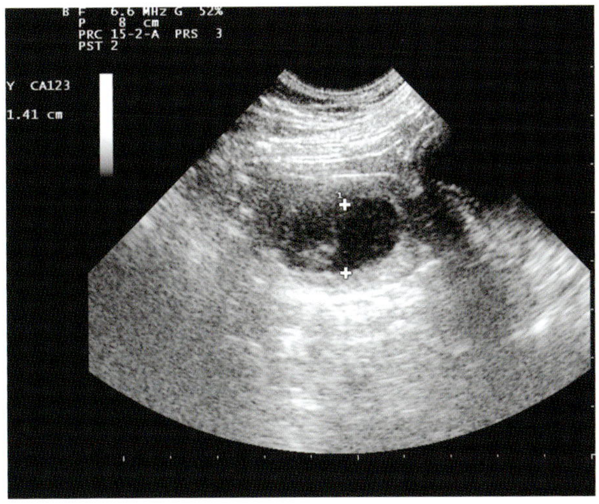

Figure 6.3. Ultrasound: measurement of the internal diameter of the embryonic vesicle.

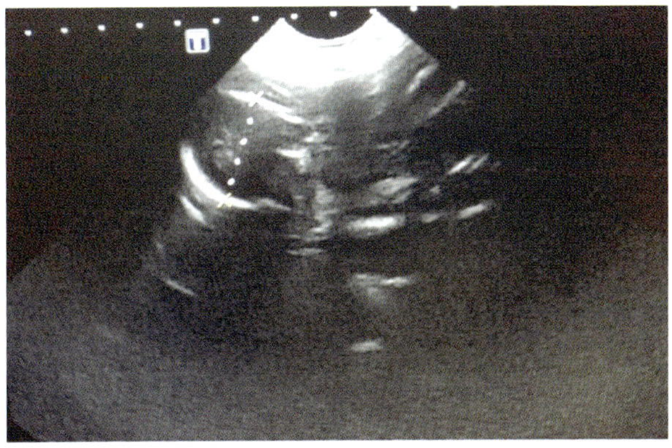

Figure 6.4. Ultrasound: measurement of biparietal diameter.

The accuracy of this calculation for the date of birth (±1 day) is 75–63% in small and medium-size breeds, with a variation of ±2 days in 88 and 81% of cases, respectively.

Table 6.2. Calculation of gestational age based on biparietal and chorionic cavity diameter.

Parameter	Breed size	Formula (days until birth)
Diameter of the chorionic cavity (mm)	Small	68.68/1.53
	Medium	82.12/1.8
Biparietal diameter (mm)	Small	25.11/0.61
	Medium	29.18/0.7

Table 6.3. Other features that can be observed with ultrasound depending on gestational age.

Foetal features on ultrasound	Day(s) of gestation when first observed
Uterine vesicle	19
Embryo first detectable	23
Foetal heartbeat	24
Limbs	33–35
Eyes, kidneys and liver	39–47
Skull and spine	47–49
Intestine	57–63
Teeth	58–63

Nutritional management

Gestation can be described as a state of accelerated starvation, due to the metabolic demands that must be met by the mother. Inadequate and irregular food intake has a strong negative impact on pregnancy and embryonic survival.

It has been demonstrated that good nutrition during pregnancy has a positive influence on the size, weight and survival of puppies at birth. Therefore, it is essential to provide appropriate and controlled nutrition throughout the whole reproductive process.

A balanced diet during pregnancy should include essential fatty acids as well as vitamins and trace elements. These have a direct influence on ovarian hormone production and foetal development.

Pregnant females that are underweight may show signs of abnormal foetal development, and difficulty in maintaining pregnancy and lactation, whilst obese females are at an increased risk of dystocia and neonatal death.

The Association of American Feed Control Officials (AAFCO) has established minimum requirements for dietary components in feeds intended for reproduction. Recommendations for these diets are:

- **proteins of animal origin**: 29–32% for both pregnant and lactating females
- **fats**: at least 18%, and managing the proportions of omega-3 and omega-6 fatty acids
- **carbohydrates**: 20–30%.

It should be noted that the established recommendations are minimum levels, not optimal ones. Also, it should be recognised that the quality, quantity and composition of the foodstuffs are of great importance.

It is relevant to remember that the mother's weight, as well as calorie requirements, increase during pregnancy, especially during the last trimester.

- **Calorie requirements** may increase by 50%.
- **Body weight increases** at a constant rate from the 4th to 7th weeks of pregnancy.
- **Appetite drops** during the last 2 weeks, but maternal weight continues to increase due to foetal growth and mammary development.

Care of the pregnant dog

All necessary vaccines should be given before mating and conception, except that for canine herpesvirus where the first dose should be administered on the first day of mating and the second (and last) dose 1 week before birth.

At the start of pregnancy, it is the owner's responsibility to monitor their dog's activity levels, behaviour, weight and physical appearance. Should the owner be uncertain as to whether changes are normal or not during pregnancy, they should seek the advice of a veterinarian.

It is beneficial to keep a pregnant female in her regular daily routine. Only unusually nervous or active bitches should have their usual activities restricted.

Previously mentioned clinical tests are beneficial for monitoring the clinical development of the pregnancy. This is especially important in young, old or nervous dogs, and those with a history of previously problematic pregnancies or birth.

A care plan should be developed for the owner or care-giver, advising the following:

- environmental conditions:
  - temperature: 29.4°C
  - humidity: 55–65%
- disinfection of the whelping box to avoid diseases and pathologies of both the mother and puppies
- privacy is of high importance, along with a good supply of materials for nesting such as clothes and towels.

Complications of pregnancy

Embryonic resorption

Assessing embryonic resorption can be difficult, since often the female is not known to be pregnant when resorption occurs or dead foetuses expelled.

Resorption can be diagnosed radiologically, by the presence of gas in the uterus and the abnormal position of the foetus (Figure 6.5).

The causes of foetal death can be maternal or **foetal**. In the latter, both **genetic** defects and abnormal development of foetal organs can cause resorption or abortion, depending on the stage of gestation.

Maternal causes include a variety of factors: reproductive or non-reproductive systemic disease, trauma, primary or secondary stress, etc.

The most important **infectious agents** are:

- bacteria: *Brucella canis*, *Salmonella* spp., *Campylobacter* spp., *Escherichia coli* and *Streptococcus* spp.
- viruses: canine herpesvirus, canine distemper and canine adenovirus
- parasites: *Toxoplasma gondii*.

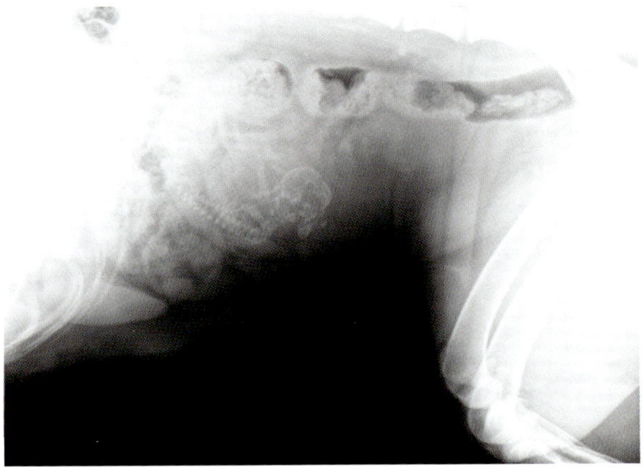

Figure 6.5. In this radiograph a dead puppy can be seen within the uterus.

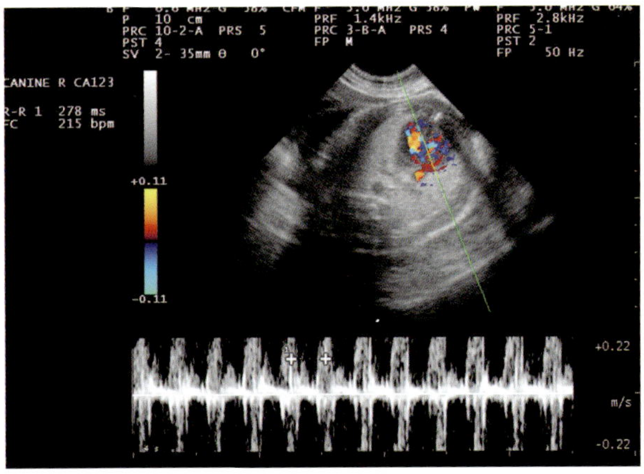

Figure 6.7. Ultrasound measurement of foetal heartbeats. Rates higher than double that of the mother, as in this case, indicate that there is no foetal distress.

When one of these cases presents in a consultation, it is important to conduct a foetal necropsy and take both serological and vaginal exudate samples from the mother, for laboratory investigation.

Endocrine diseases such as **progesterone deficiency** and **hypothyroidism** can also influence embryonic resorption.

Radiography and ultrasound

Radiography (Figure 6.6) and ultrasound (Figure 6.7) are useful techniques in monitoring the progress of pregnancy.

Tocodynamometry

Tocodynamometry is the use of an external device, transmitting data via wi-fi, to monitor and record uterine activity and foetal heartbeats.

This information makes it possible to identify and assess foetal distress and to differentiate between eutocia and dystocia before it becomes clinically evident. This is relevant because early intervention decreases mortality in both mother and foetuses.

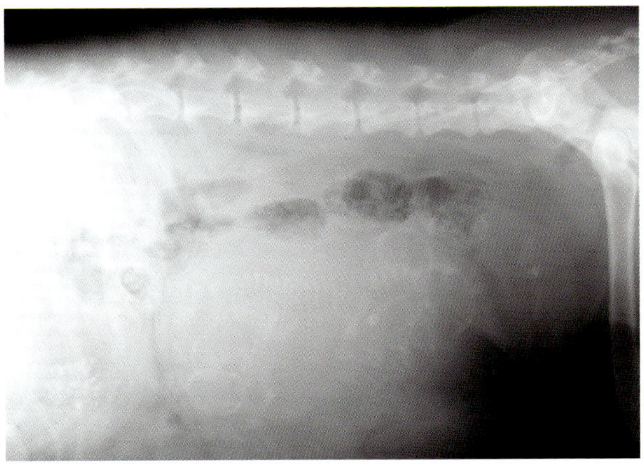

Figure 6.6. Radiography prior to parturition allows establishment of the exact number of puppies, by counting their skulls and/or spines.

Causes of pregnancy complications

Pregnancy complications can be due to factors such as contagious infectious disease, maternal health and inherited genetic factors. Also, serious maternal disease can result from changes associated with pregnancy, the most notable being:

- toxaemia
- diabetes mellitus
- eclampsia
- hypertension
- hypoluteinism.

Toxaemia

Toxaemia represents a significant pregnancy complication in the dog.

Toxaemia is caused by inappropriate nutrition during the final stage of pregnancy, and mainly affects pregnant females carrying more than three foetuses. It causes serious disorders in the mother's ability to metabolise carbohydrates and volatile fatty acids.

In a state of calorie deficit due to inadequate nutrition, the body uses fats and certain amino acids to supply energy. This results in ketone body formation, and the condition known as pregnancy toxaemia.

Diabetes mellitus

Clinical signs of diabetes mellitus are not specific and include polydipsia and polyuria. Diabetes can be differentiated from toxaemia by the presence of glycosuria, with or without an associated ketonuria. Gestational diabetes can be life-threatening to both mother and the litter.

Hypertension

Vascular changes occur as a consequence of pregnancy. If this results in abnormal hypertension, it can affect the growth and survival of the foetuses or neonates.

Hypoluteinism

This occurs when the corpus luteum produces insufficient progesterone. Hypoluteinism can be either **primary** (when the problem originates within the ovary) or **secondary** (due to changes in hormone secretion by the pituitary gland).

The accurate diagnosis of hypoluteinism requires identification of LH concentrations <2 ng/ml in di-oestrus.

Treatment consists of administration of oral progesterone at a dose of 0.88 mg/kg/day, until between 7 and 2 days prior to the expected birth date, based on the LH peak. Side effects have been described, such as the masculinisation of female foetuses and a decrease in milk production by the mother, although the latter is usually transient.

Hypoluteinism has not been described in the cat.

Birth in the dog and cat

Introduction

To recognise a dystocic birth, it is first necessary to understand the progression and stages of a natural (eutocic) delivery.

The mechanisms that trigger normal parturition are still largely unknown. However, studies in both the dog and cat, along with data from other species, provide information about the most important physiological and endocrinological changes involved in the progression of a normal birth.

The endocrinology of birth

From an endocrinological perspective, parturition can be defined as:

> A sequence of events that occur due to a reduction in inhibitory factors (progesterone and relaxin) and an increase in stimulatory factors (prostaglandins and oxytocin), along with an increase in uterine activity.

Before birth, an increase in **foeto-maternal cortisol** due to the maturation of the foetal pituitary–adrenal axis causes an increase in **maternal prostaglandin, PGF2**. This also causes luteolysis and therefore a decrease in serum progesterone concentrations (from 10 to 4 ng/ml 2 days prior to birth and <2 ng/ml 24 hours before birth).

In addition, **prostaglandins** stimulate uterine contractility which, together with the decrease in progesterone, triggers placental detachment.

Oxytocin is released in response to pressure on the neck of the uterus, and also stimulated by uterine contractions.

Relaxin, which is released by the placenta throughout the whole of gestation, drops sharply at birth but can be detected up to 9 weeks afterwards; it is responsible for the physiological delay in canine uterine involution.

The reduction in serum progesterone concentrations causes prolactin levels to rise after birth; both processes are responsible for the onset of milk production.

Prediction of birth

Certain physiological parameters develop prior to parturition, which give clues to its imminent progression. These include changes in body temperature and blood progesterone levels.

The day before parturition, body temperature drops by 1 °C. This is triggered by the rapid fall in progesterone levels and reliably occurs 12–24 hours pre-partum. Therefore, 1 week before the expected date of birth, it is helpful to record the dog's rectal temperature on a daily basis.

Around 24 hours before birth, levels of blood progesterone decrease to <3 ng/ml, dropping to <1 ng/ml as parturition begins. This is a reliable indicator, as higher serum progesterone concentrations are indicative that gestation has not yet reached full term.

However, there is an exception: In pregnancies where there is only one puppy, levels may not drop to 2 ng/ml.

Progesterone levels can be helpful in detecting abnormally prolonged pregnancy and possible dystocia, or in choosing the correct time to perform a caesarean section.

Stages of labour

It is during the second and third stages of labour that decisions about intervention are most likely to be needed.

Stage one: dilation

The first stage of birth can be identified when there is a drop in rectal temperature to 36.9 °C and regular uterine contractions begin, alongside a complete dilation of the cervix.

During first-stage labour, contractions increase progressively in both frequency and intensity but there is no effort to expel the foetuses by the dog.

The duration of stage one is generally 6–12 hours (somewhat shorter in the queen than the bitch), but may be as long as 36 hours in first-time mothers whilst in some multiparous bitches it can go undetected.

Generally, once the female begins to feel uterine contractions, she will exhibit the following behavioural changes.

- The bitch becomes restless, loses interest in food, pants and shakes.
- The queen may become vocal, restless, tachypnoeic and purr strongly.
- Nesting behaviour increases: Some females look for dark isolated areas to give birth and others look for somewhere close to the owner.

It is important to be familiar with the habits of each individual female to avoid poor management, which can result in the voluntary inhibition of birth.

Changes in foetal position take place in the first stage of labour – foetuses rotate around their axis and extend their head, neck and limbs to adopt the normal birth position; if this does not occur it may affect the expulsion phase, giving rise to a dystocia of foetal origin.

Stage two: expulsion

Uterine contractions begin, which move the foetuses closer to the cervix. When the first foetus enters the cervix, this causes dilatation that initiates the Ferguson reflex. This causes an increase in oxytocin secretion and, as a consequence, more intense contractions.

In both the bitch and the queen, the position of the foetus may be anterior or posterior, depending on which body part enters the birth canal first. 60% of neonates are born in an anterior presentation and 40% in a posterior presentation, which is not considered dystocic although it can predispose to a problematic birth due to inadequate cervical dilation.

Position, the orientation of the foetus in relation to the longitudinal axis of the birth canal, can be either dorsal (normal posture), ventral or lateral.

Normal foetal posture is with the head completely extended, the forelimbs extended forwards and hind limbs extended backwards. The initial impetus for change in position is due to uterine contractions and the movement of foetal fluids; however, the foetus itself is primarily responsible for the change in posture.

As the foetus approaches the pelvis, the chorioallantoic membrane (the most outer layer of the foetal membranes) reaches the vulva and breaks either spontaneously or because the mother bites it, releasing liquid. The amniotic sac, which is stronger, enters the vagina and contains a large volume of fluid, which helps vaginal dilation.

At this point the foetus has turned and extended in the birth canal. The rotation and extension from the foetal *in utero* position (resting on its back with head and limbs flexed) is essential for a normal birth. If the head does not extend, the foetal muzzle does not fit correctly into the birth canal. If the occipital region enters first, this can cause an obstruction.

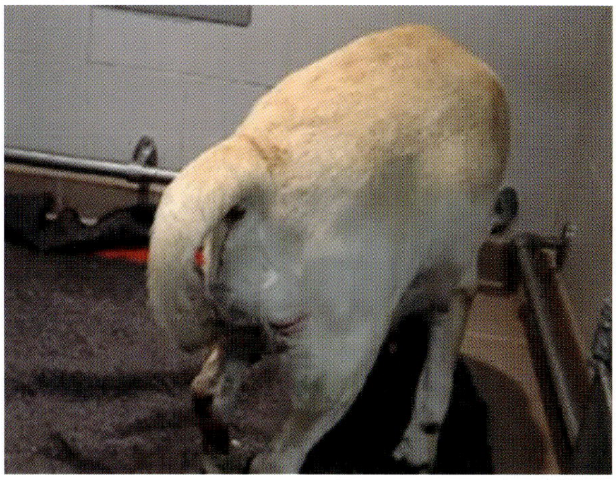

Figure 6.8. Expulsion phase.

A foetus which dies before reaching the birth canal invariably remains in the foetal position.

When the head of a foetus in an anterior presentation fully enters the birth canal, the pressure causes triggering of a simple neural reflex, the pelvic reflex. This causes voluntary abdominal contractions which advance the head and the shoulders through the pelvis. Once these have passed, the rest of the foetus is narrower and expelled easily (Figure 6.8).

When the head of the foetus appears through the vulva, the mother bites and breaks the amniotic membrane, cleans the snout of the neonate and licks the membranes free. Normally, the mother breaks the umbilical cord by biting it with her premolars.

Sometimes the mother needs some assistance to break the foetal membranes. Occasionally, it is necessary to remove the liquid from the puppy's respiratory tract to allow it to breathe.

Once the neonate is free from the foetal membranes, any liquid in the nasal orifices and pharynx should be carefully aspirated (using a syringe). The puppy should be rubbed dry energetically with a towel, which also stimulates breathing. Once the neonate is breathing, the umbilical cord should be ligated and disinfected with povidone iodine or chlorhexidine.

At the same time, the neonate should be inspected for any congenital anomalies such as cleft palate, the absence of limbs, hernias, etc. The litter should then be moved to a warm place (around 32°C) and encouraged to suckle as soon as possible, to ensure colostrum intake.

It has been demonstrated that there is expulsion of neonates in alternate sequence between uterine horns, with the horn containing the greater number of foetuses initiating the process. The presence of a dead foetus may alter this mechanism.

The duration of second-stage labour varies markedly depending on breed and litter size, along with variations between individuals.

In a normal birth

Bitches: Four hours after the start of the expulsion phase, the first puppy is born. The rest of the litter follow at intervals of less than two hours. Many bitches deliver two puppies with only a few minutes between births. It may take up to 6–12 hours to expel the entire litter, although some females finish in just 2–4 hours.

Queens: Often have their first kitten in the hour after the start of second-stage labour, followed by kittens every 10–60 minutes, although this is variable.

During the second stage of birth, the rectal temperature returns to normal.

Stage three: placental expulsion

In this stage, uterine contractions expel the placenta and the remainder of any retained foetal membranes (Figure 6.9).

This normally occurs in the 15 minutes following the birth of each puppy, with the foetal membranes of each neonate expelled at the same time, or a little after, the previous individual. However, there may be a delay of up to 24 hours. As expulsion of the foetuses located in each uterine horn tends to alternate, two foetuses can be born before their respective placentae are expelled or the expulsion of a placenta can accompany the following neonate.

The detachment of the placenta is accompanied by a greenish vaginal discharge. This colour is due to **uteroverdin**, a pigment formed by the products resulting from ruptured erythrocytes in marginal haematomas during the separation of the placenta.

The mother usually eats the placenta, and this may cause her to vomit.

During parturition, an increase in the plasma concentrations of fibrinogen, fibronectin and Von Willebrand factor can be seen.

A normal post-partum scenario is depicted in Figures 6.9 and 6.10.

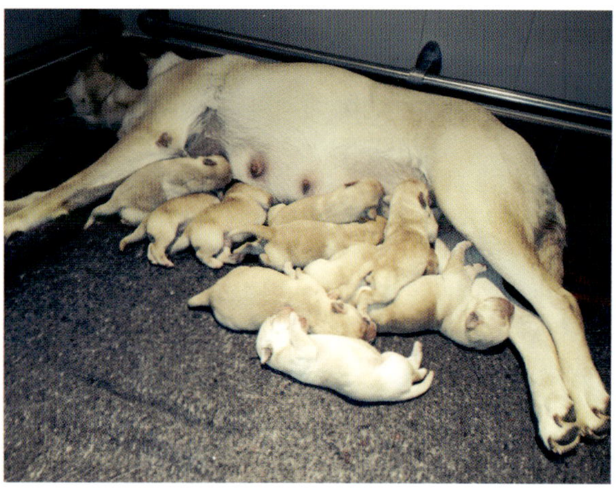

Figure 6.9. Once parturition has finished, the bitch and her puppies should be calm and relaxed.

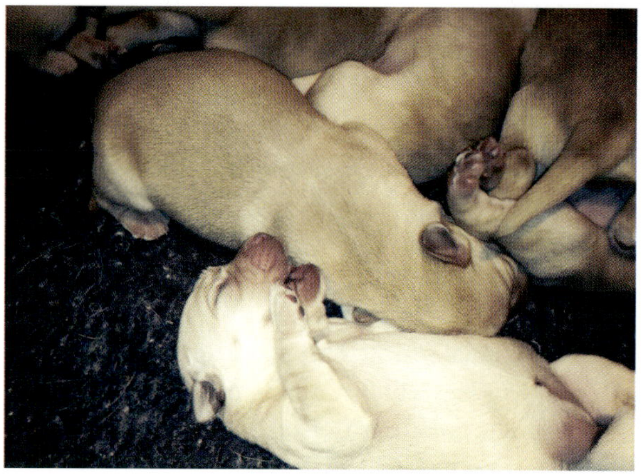

Figure 6.10. Relaxed, calm puppies after suckling.

Eclampsia

Definition

Eclampsia, or **puerperal tetanus**, is a syndrome caused by the development of **hypocalcaemia** during birth and lactation, and is life-threatening if not treated promptly. Eclampsia represents around 23% of peripartum emergencies.

Aetiology

It is thought that the cause is a maternal loss of calcium due to mineralisation in the foetuses and calcium lost during lactation. This condition is therefore related to litter size. However, there are predisposing factors such as an inadequate diet or atrophy of the parathyroid gland resulting from excess calcium supplementation.

Epidemiology

Eclampsia is more common in:

- small-breed, primiparous females
- large-breed females with large litter sizes.

Clinical signs

Eclampsia generally **develops 2–4 weeks** post-partum.

- *In bitches*: **Hyperthermia**, **rigid** shuddering, muscular fasciculation, convulsions, tachycardia, panting and hyperthermia are seen; 20% of cases demonstrate atypical signs such as vomiting, diarrhoea or behavioural changes.
- *In queens*: **Hypothermia**, hyper-excitability, hypersensitivity and also flaccid paralysis.

Diagnosis

Clinical suspicion of eclampsia is raised by the history and physical examination.

Total calcium levels can be analysed, but ionised calcium is more sensitive. An ionised calcium level of < 0.8 mmol/l is diagnostic of eclampsia.

Treatment

Treatment requires a combination of intravenous (IV) fluid therapy and IV calcium gluconate (10%).

The IV fluids are used to treat the fever, dehydration and tachycardia. In addition, calcium gluconate (10%) should be administered immediately by slow infusion. This requires constant monitoring of cardiac function, to detect the onset of bradycardia or arrhythmias (if these appear, treatment should be stopped).

In the bitch, if treatment is required for hyperthermia it should be noted that once the tremors cease, body temperature falls sharply.

Once the condition is under control, calcium carbonate should be administered orally (100 mg/kg/day) during lactation; 20% of cases relapse despite supplementation, and therefore early weaning of neonates is recommended.

Calcium should never be supplemented before birth. However, once parturition has taken place, supplementation is recommended in at-risk animals or those with a history of eclampsia.

Birth and the owner

Fundamental information should be conveyed to the owner regarding how a normal birth progresses and the possible problems that may occur.

The five key points prior to the onset of parturition are shown below.

- House the dog in a **calm environment**.
- Control the **ambient temperature** and **humidity**.
- Prepare the **whelping box** away from any noise. It is important that there are sides to provide protection and avoid puppies being squashed, particularly in large breeds.
- Use a whelping box made from a **safe material** both for the mother and the puppies.
- Position the whelping box in a place which is **accessible to the owner**, taking into account the fact that the animals will be there for several weeks until weaning.

In principle, females are usually able to give birth on their own. However, it is advisable to have someone present (provided the dog is not upset by this) with adequate knowledge to intervene should an emergency arise during the birth, Problems during birth usually occur in stage 2 and result in dystocia.

Embryonic death in the first weeks of pregnancy results in foetal resorption that does not cause any consequences at the uterine level. Late foetal death from day 41 after the peak in LH causes expulsion of the foetus. Complications during birth or infections can cause neonatal death.

Infertility in the bitch

There are numerous causes of reproductive failure in the bitch. In order of frequency:

- poor reproductive management
- changes in the reproductive cycle
- uterine disease
- changes in male semen quality
- failures at the time of mating
- infectious diseases.

Causes of infertility according to changes in the reproductive cycle in the female can be classified as:

- females that do not have heats
- females with persistent heats
- females with shortened cycles
- females that cycle normally.

Prolonged anoestrus

Definition

Anoestrus is defined as the stage in the reproductive cycle where there is no ovarian activity taking place.

An abnormally prolonged anoestrus may be:

- **primary**: in females older than 24 months that have not come into oestrus
- **secondary**: in pubertal females that have not cycled again in the 16–20 months since their last heat.

Differential diagnoses

The most frequent causes are:

- silent heats
- ovarian pathologies
- non-reproductive causes
- other causes.

Treatment

The primary disease should be treated and the reproductive situation reassessed. In bitches with normal annual cycles, oestrus can be induced with prolactin inhibitors such as cabergoline.

Silent heats

Based on clinical experience, approximately 17% of cases of infertility are false diagnoses, due to silent heats.

A silent heat is when follicular development and ovulation take place in the absence of physical signs of a heat (such as vulvar oedema and secretion of a sero-sanguinous discharge).

A diagnosis can be made by:

- **weekly vaginal cytology**, which allows the detection of the onset of pro-oestrus
- **monthly** measurement of **serum progesterone concentrations**: a concentration >2 ng/ml indicates ovarian activity, and >10 ng indicates that ovulation has occurred.

Bitches covered appropriately during a silent heat are **fertile**.

Ovarian pathologies

Various conditions affecting the ovaries exist, such as **luteal cysts**, **aplastic ovaries** and immune-mediated **oophoritis**, which alter normal ovarian function and interrupt the hormonal axes necessary for oestrus to occur.

Luteal cysts

Single or multiple luteal cysts can be present, composed of luteinised cells that secrete progesterone. These may be located either uni- or bilaterally. These cysts cause a prolonged di-oestrus as opposed to a prolonged anoestrus. Older females are more susceptible (Figure 6.11).

Diagnosis is based on the following findings:

- vaginal cytology characteristic of di-oestrus: parabasal cells, neutrophils, basal cells and Signet cells (Figure 6.12)

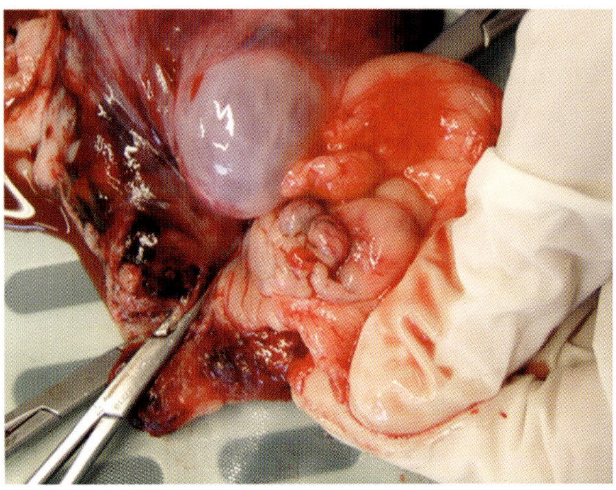

Figure 6.11. Luteal ovarian cysts.

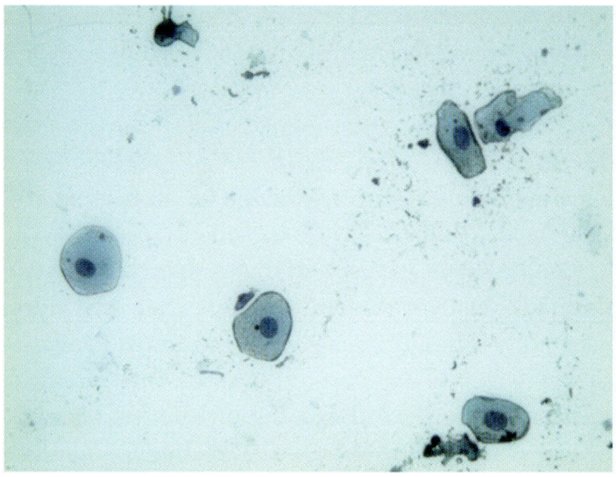

Figure 6.12. Cytology during di-oestrus.

- **progesterone** levels **2–5 ng/ml** for >9–10 weeks
- **hypo-echoic** structures on ultrasound of the affected ovaries
- Improvement after luteinic treatment, consisting of the administration of PGF2-alpha at a dose of 30–100 mg/kg SC every 12 hours over 4 days.

A definitive diagnosis of luteal ovarian cysts is made by biopsy.

Ovarian cysts

The mass of **non-functional ovarian cysts**, such as epithelial or reteovarii cysts, suppresses ovarian function. In these cases there will be **no increase** in blood progesterone or oestrogen levels. Diagnosis can be made using **ultrasound** and confirmed with a tissue biopsy.

Non-reproductive causes of anoestrus

Not all abnormalities of the female reproductive cycle are due to reproductive pathologies and, from the beginning, non-reproductive causes should be included in the diagnostic plan.

First, a complete and thorough patient history should be taken, which allows the following non-reproductive causes of anoestrus to be assessed.

- *Dietary imbalances*. Malnourished bitches in a stressed state due to intense exercise or high levels of training may not cycle.
- *Pharmacological treatments*.
- *Environmental alterations*. Bitches living with dominant females or in locations where there are few hours of daylight may suffer endocrine changes that delay the onset of puberty or oestrus.
- *Ovariohysterectomy*. This may have been performed previously without the current owner's knowledge. Previous **ovariohysterectomy** may be diagnosed

by palpation or the presence of a ventral abdominal midline scar or via an exploratory laparotomy. In spayed dogs, serum concentrations of gonadotropins, LH and FSH are high due to a lack of negative feedback.

- *Systemic diseases*: specifically Cushing's syndrome hypothyroidism or diabetes mellitus.
  - In the case of **Cushing's syndrome**, dogs tend to present with symmetrical alopecia, a pendulous abdomen, polydipsia and polyuria.
  - **Hypothyroidism** is associated with a primary anoestrus, irregular inter-oestrus intervals, small litter size and general infertility. Non-reproductive signs are lethargy, weight gain and symmetrical bilateral alopecia of the trunk.

Other causes

Less commonly seen causes of primary anoestrus include anomalies of sexual differentiation such as **hermaphroditism**. This can be classified in three forms:

- *true hermaphroditism*, where both testicular and ovarian tissue are present
- *masculine pseudo-hermaphroditism*, where the external genitalia are ambiguous, such as the presence of testicles and external female genitalia
- *feminine pseudo-hermaphroditism*, where the dog has both ovaries and external male genitals.

Diagnosis of sexual differentiation abnormalities often requires an exploratory laparotomy and histopathological examination of the excised sexual tissue.

Prolonged heats

An abnormal reproductive cycle should be suspected when vaginal bleeding (typical of pro-oestrus) lasts for more than 28 consecutive days (during this time the bitch may or may not be receptive to mating). This prolonged bleeding is generally the result of abnormally sustained oestrogenic activity.

Epidemiology

The average length of a full female reproductive cycle is 7 months. In some breeds such as the Basenji, and in dingo- and wolf-dog hybrids, it is annual and this is considered normal.

Differential diagnosis

The most common causes of persistent heats include:

- hypothyroidism (diagnosed using serological tests)
- uterine disease
- ovarian cysts
- ovarian tumours, most common in females over 5 years of age, the most frequent types being:
  - cystadenomas
  - adenocarcinomas
  - granulosa cell tumours
  - thecal cell tumours.

Uterine disease

Dogs with cystic endometrial hyperplasia (CEH) or subclinical uterine infections may release prostaglandins from the endometrium, causing premature luteolysis and increasing the frequency of cycles.

CEH can be seen ultrasonographically as a thickening of the uterine wall. Due to the relative inaccessibility of the canine uterus, uterine infection is usually better diagnosed by culture of the anterior chamber in oestrus.

Ovarian cysts

Cystic ovarian disease in dogs is usually caused by a lack of ovulation from a cystic follicle. Persistent secretion of oestrogens manifests clinically as persistent oestrus (Figures 6.13 and 6.14).

Although a persistently high serum oestrogen concentration is diagnostic, tests to evaluate oestrogens are difficult, can be unreliable and are not always available.

However, the identification of corneous vaginal epithelial cells over a period of 6 weeks or more is diagnostic of persistently elevated oestrogen levels. The diagnosis of ovarian follicles as a cause of persistent heats can be based on vaginal cytology in 90% of cases.

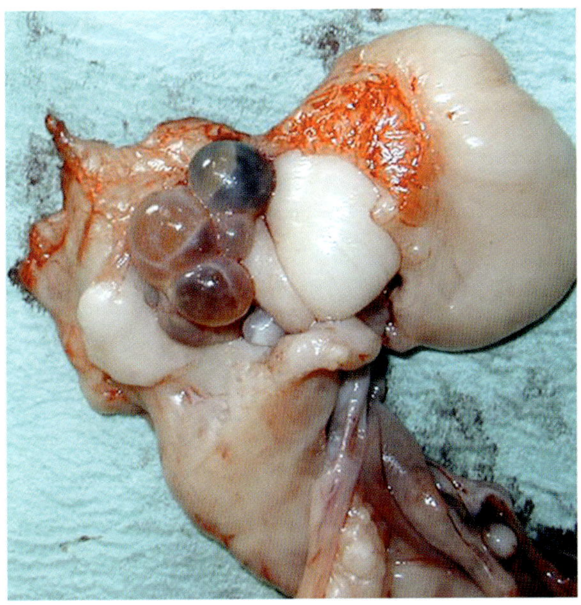

Figure 6.13. Follicular ovarian cysts in a female with persistent heats.

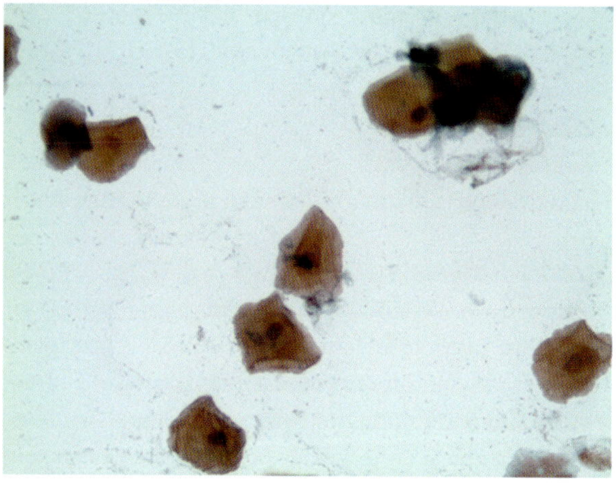

Figure 6.14. Cytology of oestrus.

Ovarian follicular cysts may be visible on abdominal ultrasound, but these are often difficult to visualise.

Cornified cells are present whilst follicular cysts are active.

A sustained increase in oestrogen levels causes secondary effects, such as bone marrow suppression, leading to aplastic anaemia, leukopenia and thrombocytopenia.

It should be noted that certain ovarian pathologies will decrease circulating levels of oestrogen in the blood. This means even though oestrus is occurring, it may be 'silent' or without outward physical signs.

Medical treatment of luteinised follicles utilises human chorionic gonadotrophic hormone, whilst surgical ovariohysterectomy is appropriate for females not used for breeding. As is the case for most ovarian pathologies, ovariohysterectomy resolves the pathology.

Granulosa cell tumours

Functional granulosa cell tumours may manifest clinically as persistent oestrus. They may be palpable as a mass in the cranial abdomen or visible on radiographs or ultrasound. The treatment of choice is ovariohysterectomy.

Shortened cycles

Epidemiology

In some breeds it is normal to see a shorter than average (7 months) interval between cycles, i.e. the German shepherd, Rottweiler and Basset Hound.

Differential diagnosis

The following can cause the inter-oestrus period to differ from the normal:

- short anoestrus syndrome
- split heats
- anovulatory cycles
- hypoluteinism.

Short anoestrus syndrome

This is characterised by normal oestrus (where ovulation and luteinisation take place) that occurs earlier than it should.

The uterus needs an average of **130–150 days to involute** following oestrus. Therefore, heats that occur after less than four months are **infertile**. Even if fertilisation of the ovum takes place, the uterus is not prepared for implantation of the embryo to maintain pregnancy.

Aetiology

Short anoestrus syndrome often occurs secondary to immaturity of the reproductive apparatus. Short anoestrus periods can be considered as normal until the female is approximately 3 years of age.

The cause is believed to be an imbalance in **dopamine levels relative to prolactin**, or an alteration in the hormonal axis that shortens anoestrus.

Epidemiology

There appears to be an **inheritability of 35%** for this pathology in breeds such as the German Shepherd, Rottweiler, Bassett Hound, Cocker Spaniel and Labrador Retriever.

Diagnosis

Routine cytological monitoring and/or measurement of progesterone will be within normal limits for female dogs. This helps differentiate short anoestrus syndrome from hypoluteinism and split heats.

Treatment

Progesterone treatments, such as megestrol acetate, during the first three days of pro-oestrus have been described. However, their use increases the risk of pyometra and other uterine pathologies.

Split heats

A split heat can be defined as pro-oestrus activity for one to two weeks followed by an absence over an average of 1 month, when a resumption of normal ovulatory heat occurs.

The female presents with a first cycle of serosanguinous discharges typical of pro-oestrus, which lasts approximately five to seven days, followed by a short period of time with a normal oestrus cycle. The second cycle generally occurs at 2 to 3 weeks, but may occur up to 2 months after the first heat.

The split heat is not associated with infertility, unless the bitch is forcefully mated during the anovulatory part of the split heat.

Aetiology

These types of cycles are common in young females. In an individual this may happen either as a one-off or repetitively.

It is thought that when ovulation does not occur in the first cycle, inadequate levels (or duration) of progesterone are present and therefore normal anoestrus is not stimulated. Therefore, a short time later a second reproductive cycle breaks through, which is not necessarily abnormal.

Diagnosis

Split oestrus is diagnosed by monitoring vaginal cytology and/or progesterone levels during the intermediate period of anoestrus, a serum **progesterone concentration <2 ng/ml** indicates that **ovulation** has not occurred.

After the second phase of oestrus activity, a serum progesterone concentration >2 ng/ml indicates that ovulation has taken place.

During the first 'cycle' with the onset of bleeding, a typical cytology for pro-oestrus can be seen because follicular activity has begun. When bleeding stops, parabasal cells reappear. This first 'cycle' is anovulatory, so progesterone levels do not usually exceed 3.5–6.0 ng/ml.

The second 'cycle' is fertile; hormonal changes unfold normally and with the associated cytological changes.

Treatment

No treatment is required, due to the normality of the second 'cycle'.

Anovulatory cycles

An anovulatory cycle is defined thus:

> Because a normal peak in LH does not occur, follicles do not burst and the uterine horns do not release oocytes to be fertilised.

Progesterone never exceeds 3.5–6.0 ng/ml, so di-oestrus is shortened and the subsequent cycle occurs sooner that is normal.

Aetiology

There are different hypotheses about the aetiology of this aberration:

- insufficient GnRh from the hypothalamus
- failure of the ovaries' oestrogenic signal to boost LH production
- failure of the pituitary gland to secrete sufficient LH
- failure of the ovary to correctly interpret the LH signal.

Each of these causes means that the progesterone concentrations necessary to ensuring the development of a normal cycle are not reached.

Epidemiology

Anovulatory cycles are not a common condition, and are seen in approximately 1.2% of dogs intended for breeding.

Diagnosis

The main diagnostic method is to measure progesterone levels during di-oestrus, which will be low.

Vaginal cytology is not a reliable tool in this case, as interpretation is complex. Vaginal cytology tends to be normal from oestrus towards di-oestrus.

Treatment

Generally, no treatment is required. Split heats tend to be isolated events and the female can be successfully mated at the next heat.

If the cause is a low LH peak, this can be treated with human chorionic hormone; however, because the risk of pyometra and persistent heat development is high, it is not recommended.

Hypoluteinism

In hypoluteinism, serum concentrations of progesterone drop to <2 ng/ml during or at the end of oestrus (day 65 after the peak in LH).

Although it has not been studied directly, it is assumed that this decline in serum progesterone levels causes an abnormally short anoestrus. As progesterone levels drop, di-oestrus finishes and the female enters anoestrus.

All of this means that the next cycle occurs before it should, when the endometrium is not yet ready for implantation to occur. Another implication is that this condition may cause foetal resorption or abortion, since progesterone is necessary for the maintenance of pregnancy.

Aetiology

Hypoluteinism is due to a decrease or lack of production of prolactin, resulting in a lack of progesterone and therefore an insufficiency of the corpus luteum.

Epidemiology

This condition is more common in some breeds, i.e. German Shepherd and Rottweiler.

Diagnosis

This condition should be considered in females that have unusually short cycles or do not conceive when everything is apparently normal.

Given that alteration in progesterone levels can occur from the end of oestrus to the end of di-oestrus, it is necessary to monitor progesterone levels every week to determine whether these decrease prematurely.

Treatment

Whether or not to treat this condition, once definitively diagnosed, is controversial.

Progesterone administration before days 34–36 of gestation can result in pyometra and masculinisation of female foetuses; therefore, there are protocols which recommend treatment only in at-risk pregnancies of >50 days' duration.

The protocol is based on the administration of 2 mg/kg of progesterone in oil every two days, stopping the treatment at day 61 of the pregnancy to allow progesterone levels to drop, and therefore, on day 63, birth can occur naturally. This does not always happen, and in these cases a caesarean section should be performed on day 65 (although this is unusual).

It is important to know that there is frequently a delay in prolactin secretion, so preparation should be made for correct feeding of the puppies by hand if necessary, whilst at the same time they should be allowed to suckle to help stimulate prolactin secretion.

Apparently normal cycles

Differential diagnosis

The most frequent causes are:

- poor reproductive management
- delayed LH peak
- hypoluteinism and anovulatory cycles; these changes can cause both abnormal cycles and those which appear normal.

Poor reproductive management

In a bitch not suffering from illness or reproductive tract changes, and mated to a male with normal semen quality, failure of pregnancy is due to poor reproductive management.

The most common cause of apparent fertility is mating at an inappropriate time. Reproductive management is optimised by determining when ovulation occurs, by measuring serum progesterone levels. On the day of ovulation, these are 5–8 ng/ml. The ideal time for mating is 2 days after ovulation.

Delayed LH peak

A delayed peak in LH is possibly one of the commonest causes of infertility in veterinary practice. Rather than progesterone levels rising after ovulation, they stagnate at preovulatory levels (2.1 ng/ml) for approximately 3 days.

Ovulation may occur and go undetected by the usual methods, so reproductive management becomes difficult.

Aetiology

The causes are believed to be similar to those of anovulatory cycles, such as:

- a delay in ovarian oestrogen signals that would enhance LH production
- slow or low intensity secretion of LH from the pituitary gland
- delayed follicular response to the peak in LH.

Diagnosis

This is done by monitoring progesteronaemia. Analysing serum LH levels as pro-oestrus/oestrus develops can confirm the suspicion.

Other causes of infertility

Other common causes of infertility include:

- canine herpesvirus
- canine brucellosis
- uterine pathologies: endometritis or cystic endometrial hyperplasia/pyometra (Figures 6.15 and 6.16)
- use of medications
- anatomical abnormalities in the genital tract
- abnormal sexual behaviour
- systemic diseases.

Canine herpesvirus

Canine herpesvirus causes foetal death and loss of pregnancy, and stillbirths and neonatal death in the advanced stages of pregnancy.

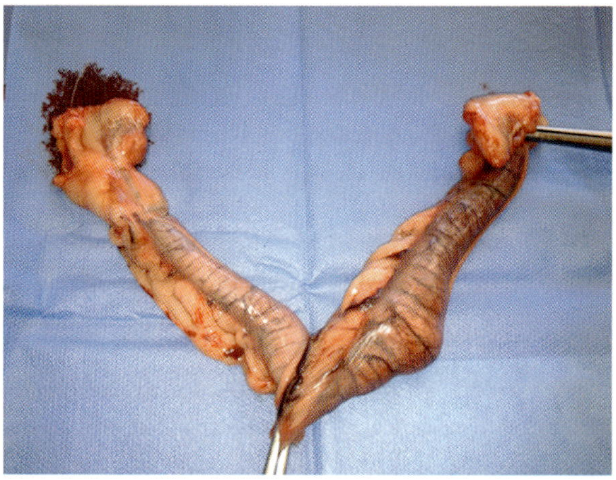

Figure 6.15. Hyperplasic cystic endometrial pyometra complex in a bitch after the first heat.

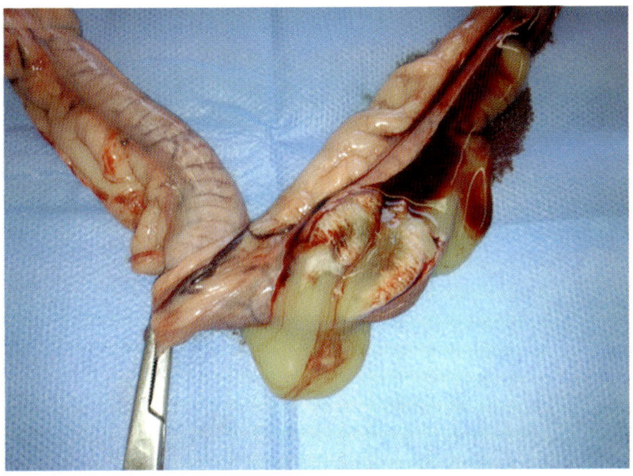

Figure 6.16. Hyperplasia of the endometrium; purulent contents will be noted.

Dogs infected in the final 3 weeks of gestation and puppies infected in the first 3 weeks of life are most likely to show clinical signs. Bitches infected before or after the last 3 weeks of gestation tend to be asymptomatic.

In general, most bitches do not lose more than one litter due to canine herpesvirus. They form sufficient memory cells for an adequate immune response if they are re-exposed. Because the virus results in low antigen levels, titres in dogs are elevated only at the point when they lose the pregnancy.

Canine brucellosis

Infection with *Brucella canis* is characterised by late-stage pregnancy loss. Puppies born alive to infected mothers often have a low birth weight and show poor weight gain.

Infected bitches may have chronic vaginal discharge. Infected male dogs may display epididymitis and reduced semen quality. Both male and female dogs infected with brucellosis may be asymptomatic.

Serological testing for brucellosis is commonly used. Agglutination tests are a good screening test that is sensitive and almost never gives false-negatives. Agglutination tests are available in two forms: tubes that give a numerical titre and slides or cards that give a simple yes/no answer. However, agglutination tests are not specific, so positive results should be re-evaluated with agar gel immunodiffusion.

Brucellosis is not curable in dogs, but antibiotic treatment and sterilisation of the affected animal help to reduce titres and the dissemination of the *Brucella* organism.

Infertility in the queen

The queen is a seasonal poly-oestrus breeder with her cycle heavily influenced by environmental conditions. Recent research has led to protocols for reproductive management in the queen, thereby making the study of infertility in the feline species more relevant.

When dealing with a case of infertility, in addition to studying the female, infertility of male origin should be assessed plus an overview taken of the adequacy of reproductive management protocols.

Anoestrus

As a seasonal poly-oestrus breeder, a shortened photoperiod can induce long periods of anoestrus. But it should be remembered that in addition to the environment, other factors influencing anoestrus include stress (which blocks the onset of oestrus) and the particular breed.

Examples of the part played by breed are the Persian cat, which has only one or two oestrus cycles per year, and the Siamese, which tends to cycle all year round.

Similarly to the bitch, it should be determined whether anoestrus is primary or secondary. The causes of secondary anoestrus are varied and include the following.

Differential diagnosis for the causes of anoestrus

The following entities should be considered:

- environmental factors
- silent heats
- ovarian pathologies
- previous ovariohysterectomy
- iatrogenic factors
- endocrine factors
- nutritional factors
- systemic illness.

Systemic illnesses such as diabetes mellitus, or chronic conditions such as vomiting, can result in fewer cycles. Anoestrus is also recognised in queens infected with feline leukaemia virus. Also, medications previously administered, such as those to suppress oestrus or terminate pregnancy, may have a future effect on fertility.

The above factors should be evaluated by taking a full history, and the relevant tests performed to confirm the diagnosis.

Environmental causes

An investigation into anoestrus requires a thorough evaluation of both social and environmental factors. In some cases this means modifying the female's environment to determine whether this alleviates the trigger.

Environmental examples include the following.

- **14-hour photoperiod**: Expose the cat to 14 hours of daylight all year round. An absence of sufficient day length can induce prolonged anoestrus.
- **Keep her in the company of other on-heat females**.
- **Keep alongside an entire male**: Queens that live alongside male cats, or are regularly exposed to males, are more likely to show signs of oestrus. These signs include behavioural changes that are more obvious to the owner.
- **Reduce stress levels**.

Protocols for pharmacological induction are available, but should be used only after all other possible causes have been ruled out.

Silent heats

Silent heats are defined as:

> Normal ovarian follicular development in the absence of heat-related behaviour.

This is more common in queens low down in their social hierarchy.

Serial vaginal cytology taken every three days allows for the detection of the cornified vaginal epithelial cells associated with oestrus.

Queens diagnosed as being in oestrus by cytology usually allow mating and are fertile. In addition, raised levels of progesterone can be used to assess whether ovulation has occurred (levels >2 ng/ml indicate ovulation).

Ovarian pathologies

Although infrequent, pathologies such as cysts or progesterone-producing ovarian tumours can occur in the queen.

A diagnosis is made by assessing blood progesterone levels in the non-pregnant female. If concentrations are >2 ng/ml and therefore above basal levels, these pathologies should be included as differential diagnoses.

Previous ovariohysterectomy

An assessment of previous ovariohysterectomy can be made through the history, palpation, observing an ovariohysterectomy scan on the flank or midline, or by exploratory laparotomy.

In both sterilised dogs and cats, serum concentrations of LH and FSH are elevated due the lack of negative feedback to the pituitary gland.

Persistent heats

Due to the reproductive characteristics of the queen, short intermittent heats can be confused with persistent oestrus. In some queens, particularly the Siamese, it can be normal to have a period of 1 to 2 days between anovulatory oestrus cycles.

One cause of persistent heat is follicular cysts, which are common in queens and become more frequent with age.

Diagnosis

Persistent heat can be confirmed by:

- serial cytology performed on a daily basis; this fails to show vaginal cytology consistent with interoestrous period
- progesterone <2 ng/ml
- oestradiol >20 pc/ml, indicating a lack of ovulation
- ultrasound, as indicated by cysts of diameter >4 mm and which do not disappear with the other follicles.

Treatment

Treatment is based on inducing ovulation. This can be done by manual vaginal stimulation with a swab, several times a day over a number of days, or by the administration of ovulation-inducing medications.

Anovulatory cycles

The queen is an induced ovulatory, with sexual stimulation triggering a sufficient increase in LH to cause ovulation.

However, in the early stage of heat it is not unusual for ovulation not to occur even though mating has taken place. Serial mating on alternate days may be required, to trigger a cumulative rise in LH. Also, sedative drugs can impact ovulation.

Test progesterone levels five days after mating, to assess whether ovulation did in fact take place.

Disruption of implantation

In the queen, as in the bitch, uterine and endometrial diseases affect implantation and maintenance of pregnancy, causing infertility.

Loss of pregnancy mid-way through gestation may not be clinically evident because the cat may reabsorb foetal tissues. Resorption in the second half of gestation is usually accompanied by the secretion of fluids or foetal tissue from the vulva, although some cats in advanced stages of gestation may resorb completely with no clinical signs of pregnancy.

Differential diagnosis

Causes of pregnancy loss in the queen include:

- luteal insufficiency
- bacterial infection
- protozoal infection
- viral infection
- panleukopenia: can cause abortion, stillbirth or cerebellar hypoplasia of kittens infected *in utero*, with or without classic gastrointestinal signs in the mother.
- feline herpes virus (FHV)
- feline infectious peritonitis (FIP)
- feline leukaemia virus (FeLV).

Luteal insufficiency

Abnormally low serum progesterone concentrations will lead to abortion in felines.

Causes of low progesterone include insufficiency of the corpus luteum and inadequate placental progesterone. Serum progesterone levels >2 ng/ml are necessary to support pregnancy. Should levels not reach this concentration or fall too early, then abortion or premature birth will ensue.

However, routine progesterone supplementation is not recommended during pregnancy since an excess of progesterone leads to:

- masculinisation of female foetuses
- prevention of expulsion of non-viable foetuses
- potential induction of diabetes mellitus
- potential triggering of mammary pathologies such as hyperplasia.

If progesterone concentrations fall too rapidly during gestation, after day 55 of pregnancy oral megestrol acetate at a dose of 2.5 mg on alternate days can be used for supplementation.

Infectious causes

Bacterial infection

Bacterial infection of the uterus and subsequent loss of pregnancy is uncommon in healthy queens living in clean environments.

Cats that abort due to uterine infections with *E. coli* or certain species of *Staphylococcus* and *Streptococcus* tend to display anorexia, depression, fever and a foul-smelling vaginal discharge that is yellow–brown in colour.

A sample of the vaginal discharge should be cultured. Whilst the results are pending, an empirical treatment with amoxicillin (22 mg/kg/12 hours PO) is appropriate.

Radiography or ultrasound may be necessary to ensure that the complete expulsion of uterine contents has occurred.

In cats infected with FeLV, bacterial infection and abortion can occur as a result of viral immunosuppression.

Protozoal infection

The main protozoal cause of abortion in the cat is toxoplasmosis.

The majority of cats infected with toxoplasmosis are asymptomatic carriers. However, those with systemic disease can abort and display dyspnoea, lethargy, diarrhoea, lymphadenopathy or central nervous system changes. Abortion is secondary to the debilitating disease in the mother.

FHV

Abortion secondary to FHV tends to occur at 5–6 weeks of gestation. This is most likely the result of a non-specific reaction caused by infection of the upper respiratory tract, since the virus has not been found in placental tissues or aborted foetuses in cats infected with FHV.

This virus is easily preventable by vaccination. The intranasal vaccine can be administered safely in kittens as early as 3 weeks of age.

FIP

Abortion as a result of FIP infection occurs towards the end of gestation and is often associated with prolonged vaginal bleeding. It is difficult to diagnose the disease with serological tests because the titres of the coronavirus which causes FIP are indistinguishable from those of the non-pathogenic enteric coronavirus. Inbreeding increases the susceptibility to infection with FIP.

FeLV

This virus has been described as causing abortion from the third week of gestation through to term. As viral spread requires close contact between animals, testing and elimination of infected animals is an effective method of control.

Panleukopenia

Can cause abortion, stillbirth and cerebellar hypoplasia of kittens infected *in utero*, with or without the classic gastrointestinal signs in the mother.

Canine and feline neonatology

Neonatal physiology

Key to optimal care of the neonate (first four weeks of life) is to stop thinking of it as a small adult. Instead, understand the transitions which take place during the neonatal period and assess each individual's unique physiological state.

Cardiovascular system

The neonate's cardiovascular system undergoes drastic changes: as the foetal–maternal circulation is lost, its heart takes over the regulation of circulatory homeostasis.

Outline of the circulatory system of the neonate:

Low blood pressure + low volume + decrease in peripheral resistance = increased heart rate + increase in central venous pressure.

At the time of birth, systolic arterial blood pressure is around 61 mmHg, rising to 139 mmHg at four weeks of age. This change in pressure is associated with a decrease in heart rate, from 240 to 120–125 bpm.

According to recent studies, the vagal nerve does not promote bradycardia in neonates. Therefore, inhibition of the vagus is not an effective means of neonatal resuscitation.

Respiratory system

For the first 3 days of life, stimulation of the genital and umbilical regions induces a breathing reflex.

The respiratory rate of a newborn is 12–18 bpm on day 1, rising to 16–32 bpm at 7 days of age.

Hypoxaemia in the newborn is extremely dangerous, as in 90% of cases it can cause sequelae such as septic shock. The neonate is very susceptible to relative hypoxaemia because of two factors:

- its high metabolic oxygen demand
- the immaturity of receptors in the carotid body, which detect low oxygen levels.

It is extremely important that the neonate's environment is free from irritants, properly oxygenated and that the ambient temperature is correct.

Haematopoietic system

At birth, the neonate has macrocytic red blood cells and increased corpuscular volume. From four weeks of age, mature red blood cells replace foetal red blood cells.

The neonatal haematocrit is 60% higher than in the adult animal. Extramedullary haematopoiesis is commonly observed in the liver of neonates. Due to the possibility of neonatal iso-erythrolysis in the dog and cat, any newborn with signs of lethargy, jaundice and haemoglobinuria should be treated and evaluated aggressively.

Urinary system

The neonatal kidney is morphologically and functionally immature, with nephrogenesis continuing for at least 2 weeks after birth.

The characteristics of the neonatal kidney include:

- low glomerular filtration rate
- low renal plasma flow
- low filtration fraction.

Blood creatinine and urea nitrogen (BUN) values are lower than in the adult (0.4 and 8–10 to 10 mg/dl, respectively), while phosphorus concentrations are high due to rapid skeletal growth.

In the adult dog, the renin–angiotensin–aldosterone system is important for renal autoregulation. However, in the newborn until approximately 6 weeks of age, renal blood flow is directly correlated with arterial pressure and is not affected by angiotensin inhibition.

The kidney of the newborn has a greater density than that of the adult, large irregular vessels, an immature cortical peritubular capillary network and an incomplete sub-endothelial basement membrane.

The oldest and most mature nephrons are in the juxtaglomerular area, whilst in the sub-capsular area nephrons form continuously during the first 2 weeks of life.

Key aspects of the neonate urinary system

- Characteristically, neonate urine has a low specific gravity. Protein, glucose and various amino acids may be present, due to immaturity of the proximal tubule.
- After 3 weeks of age, the proteins in urine and glucose concentrations approach those of the adult dog.
- At 6–8 weeks, urine concentrations can be compared to those of an adult dog.
- Administration of fluid therapy should be performed with care to ensure adequate maintenance of volume without overhydration or oncotic load.
- The daily rate for administration of fluids in neonates is 60–180 ml/kg.
- The potential renal toxicity of certain antimicrobials is 15 times higher in the newborn than in the adult animal. These include penicillin, ampicillin, cephalosporin, fluoroquinolones and aminoglycosides.
- The antimicrobial of choice is Ceftiofur ($C_{19}H_{17}N_5O_7S_3$) at a dose of 2.5 mg/kg/12 hours SC for up to 5 days.

Hepatobiliary system

The hepatobiliary system is functionally immature at birth. Until 42 days of age, the neonate has significantly reduced bile flow and complete lack of secretion of glucagon. In addition, neonate bile contains more sodium chloride, bile acids and bicarbonate than that of the adult.

Despite the relative functional cholestasis in the newborn, serum bile acids can be used to detect hepato-circulatory anomalies in neonates as early as 2 weeks of age.

ALP and GGT are markedly elevated during the first 2 weeks, and moderately elevated until 6 weeks of age. This increase has been attributed to the placenta, colostrum and intestinal activity.

Key aspects of the neonate hepatobiliary system

- Functional cholestasis and atypical hepatic biochemistry are normal.
- Extreme care should be taken when prescribing drugs that require hepatic metabolism or excretion. This is due to a lack of microsomal development and because the enzyme CP450 is inactive between birth and 4–5 months of age.

Gastrointestinal system

The gastrointestinal tract is sterile at birth, with a neutral gastric pH. In addition, gut permeability begins to drop at 10 hours of age. Small intestinal motility starts around day 40. Before this time, it is thought that intestinal transit depends on pressure gradients.

Temperature is crucial to digestion, and an inadequate temperature at the carotid body has a devastating effect on neonatal intestinal motility. A rectal temperature $<35\,^{\circ}C$ heralds paralytic ileus.

A neutral gastric pH alone with increased intestinal permeability means that care must be taken in the administration of oral pharmaceuticals. Normal recommended doses can cause toxicity due to altered absorption.

Eruption of teeth takes place at 2–3 weeks of age, and all teeth should be present by 12 weeks.

Immune system

The foetuses of both dogs and cats are attached via endotheliochorial placentation. However, there are species differences in the percentage of antibodies derived from placental antibody transfer:

- 25% in the cat
- 5–10% in the dog.

Neonatal mortality in puppies is thus 34% higher in the first 3 weeks of life, with septicaemia being the main cause of death.

Resuscitation of the neonate

The highest mortality rate occurs in the first week of life. Prudent veterinary intervention during the antenatal period, birth and post-partum can increase survival by more than 40%.

Optimal breeding has a favourable impact on neonatal survival. This includes adequate management of the birth to reduce stillbirths, parasite control during pregnancy, prevention of infectious diseases and injuries, along with an appropriate environment and optimal nutrition of the mother and newborns.

Even before breeding takes place, appropriate selection of animals and genetic screening helps minimise inherited congenital birth defects that impact neonatal mortality.

Neonatal resuscitation is required when any of the following occurs.

- The mother has been anaesthetised for a surgical procedure.
- The mother rejects the neonates.
- The mother is inexperienced in regard to immediate post-partum care.
- The mother is weak after the birth.

Before starting neonatal resuscitation, always ensure that the neonate is not breathing and does not have a heartbeat. It is dangerous to perform energetic cardiopulmonary resuscitation if the puppy is breathing or has a heartbeat.

Step one: ensure that the airways are open

Actions to be taken are as follows.

- Remove any foetal membranes covering the face.
- Remove fluids from the airways. Use either suction with a paediatric aspirator or a Pasteur pipette or manually, by holding the neonate's head below the chest.
- Use a warm towel to gently, but energetically, dry the neonate. This stimulates breathing and reduce the risk of hypothermia.

Note: Under no circumstances should the neonate be shaken, as this causes **shaken neonate syndrome**. Shaking of the neonate causes significant cerebral trauma, which is potentially lethal; 87% of neonates revived by continuous shaking are affected by neurological changes, seizures, subdural haematoma, subdural haemorrhages and intra-cranial trauma.

Step two: administer oxygen if the neonate is not breathing

For non-breathing neonates, the first step is to start assisted breathing. This must be done with care in order not to over-inflate the lungs or create aerophagia.

Assisted breathing is simply done by cupping the puppy in the palms and gently blowing into the nostrils. Administer two or three breaths in this manner, sufficient to gently inflate the lungs.

If the above does not stimulate effective breathing, ventilatory support is required.

Note: The use of doxapram as a respiratory stimulant does not improve hypoxia associated with hypoventilation, and is therefore not recommended.

To start, administer oxygen via a mask for around one minute. If this has no effect, then initiate positive pressure ventilation. This requires the mask to fit perfectly in order to inflate the lungs (Figure 6.17).

Whilst endotracheal intubation and use of a rebreathing bag is ideal, it is technically difficult given the small size of the patient. In addition, the upper airways are not only small but fragile, making potential trauma likely.

Jen Chung's acupuncture technique is a useful technique to stimulate breathing. Take a small-gauge needle and insert it into the nasolabial fold. Turn the needle until it reaches the cartilage or bone. This stimulates functional neuroreceptors that are present in the neonate at birth.

Step three: perform cardiac massage

Cardiac massage is required to improve systemic perfusion when there is weak or no cardiac output.

To do this, compress the neonate's chest using the thumb and index finger. This is done at a frequency of 80–100 compressions per minute. In addition, provide breathing support every 20 seconds.

If bradycardia persists, then administration of appropriate medication is required, of which epinephrine is the drug of choice for cardiac arrest:

- epinephrine 0.1–0.2 mg/kg or 0.15 ml/kg IV (1:10,000)
- for intra-osseous access, the proximal humerus or femur or proxy-medial tibia should be used.

Cardiac massage should be resumed after administration, until a heartbeat is detectable.

It should be noted that intra-tracheal dosing is not effective in the neonate, and intra-cardiac puncture is traumatic. Venous access is challenging, but the umbilical vein can be used if it has not yet thrombosed. If it has done so, the jugular or cephalic vein is a good alternative.

Other factors affecting neonatal resuscitation

Hypothermia

Neonates suffering from hypothermia do not respond to resuscitation, which means that it is critically important to warm the neonate (**ideal ambient temperature, 36–37°C**).

Puppies and kittens up to four weeks of age lack the ability to self-regulate their body temperature. Therefore, cold neonates must be actively warmed whilst resuscitation attempts continue.

The neonate's cold body should be placed in a bath of **warm water at 36°C** to improve core temperature. Cardiac massage and oxygenation can continue while the neonate remains in the bath. Infrared heat lamps are also useful in raising body temperature (Figure 6.18). However, take care with heated blankets and hot water bottles (Figure 6.19), since if these are too hot the neonate won't move away and will suffer heat burn.

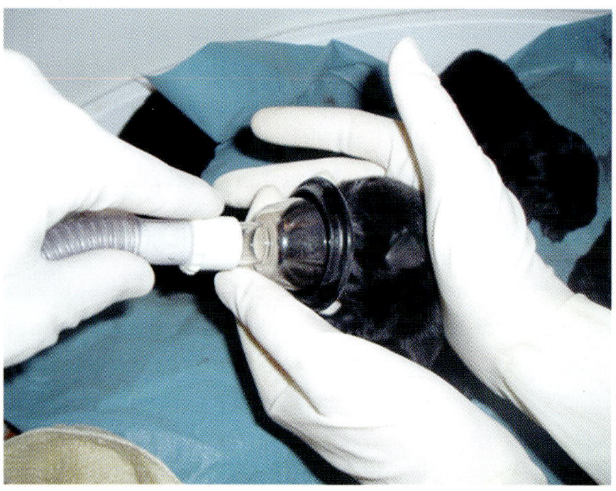

Figure 6.17. Oxygen administration to the neonate using a mask.

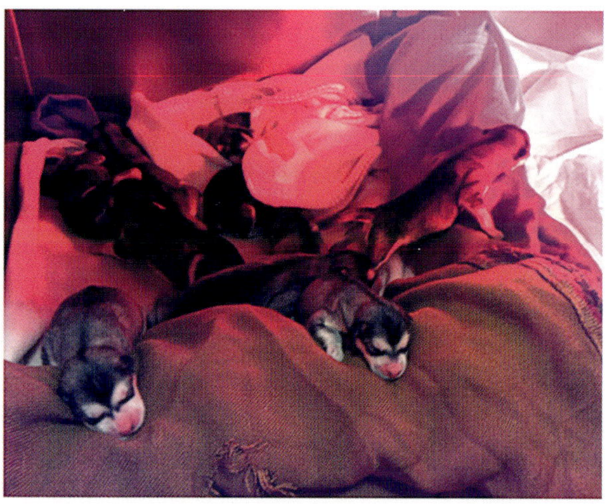

Figure 6.18. Application of heat using an infrared lamp.

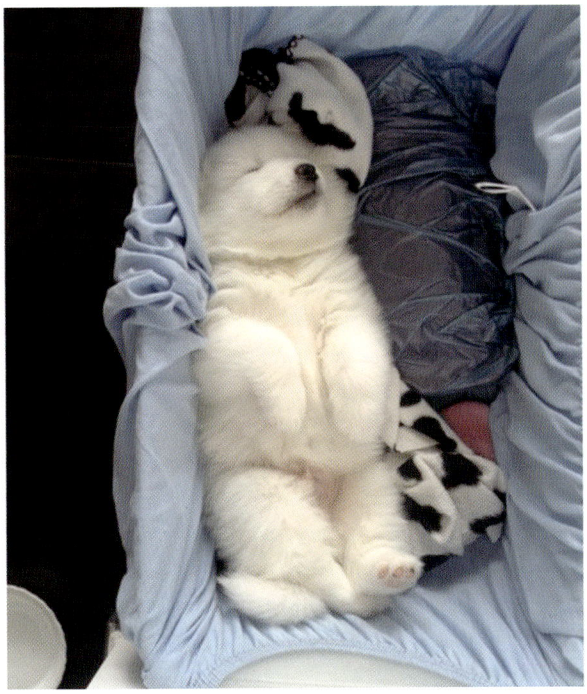

Figure 6.19. Treatment of hypothermia using hot water bottles. The temperature should be gradually increased, never abruptly.

After resuscitation, previously hypothermic neonates should be **warmed slowly** over a period of 30 minutes to avoid peripheral vasodilation and dehydration.

In addition, remember that feeding by stomach tube should be delayed until the neonate is euthermic, as hypothermia causes paralytic ileus.

Hypoglycaemia

Hypoglycaemic neonates respond poorly to resuscitation.

Clinical hypoglycaemia occurs when blood glucose levels fall <40 mg/dl.

Neonates lack glucose reserves and have a low capacity for gluconeogenesis. It is therefore essential to provide energy during resuscitation efforts.

To correct hypoglycaemia, a single dose of parenteral glucose is often sufficient:

- 5–10% dextrose solution: one dose of 2–4 ml/kg IV/IO
- 20% dextrose solution: one dose of 0.5–1 ml/kg IV/IO
- 50% dextrose solution should be used only when applying to mucous membranes, as IV administration can cause phlebitis.

Monitoring of blood glucose levels is required. If multiple doses of dextrose are given; it is advisable to monitor blood glucose levels, since the neonate's regulatory mechanisms are immature.

The neonatal caloric requirements are:

- first week: 133 cal/kg/day
- second week: 155 cal/kg/day
- third week: 175–198 cal/kg/day
- fourth week: 220 cal/kg/day.

The minimum weight gain per day is 10%. Weights should be recorded daily during the first week and then every three days until one month of age.

Dehydration

Neonates are especially vulnerable to dehydration, which can occur rapidly. Water makes up 82% of the neonate's weight, whilst they have a high surface area to weight ratio and physiologically immature kidneys.

Clinical signs:

- cessation of suckling
- continuous moaning
- asthenia
- weight loss
- cooling.

Diagnostic signs:

- persistent skin tenting
- pale mucous membranes
- weight loss.

Treatment

A neonate requires 2 ml of water for every 100 g bodyweight. Options for rehydration include oral, IV and intra-osseous fluids.

Immunity

Neonates are immunologically suppressed, especially during the first 10 days of life. This makes them highly vulnerable to systemic infection of bacterial or viral origin. Indeed, neonatal septicaemia is responsible for 60% of deaths in the first few days of life.

Neonates acquire passive immunity via colostrum. Intestinal absorption of IgG is possible for the first 24 hours after birth, making this a critical period in which to absorb adequate colostrum.

For neonates that have failed to receive colostrum, these can be dosed with the mother's plasma. The dose is split into several treatments and given by mouth at a dose of 0.15 ml/g bodyweight.

Neonatal septicaemia

Factors that predispose to neonatal septicaemia:

- prolonged birth/dystocia
- feeding with substitution formulas

- the use of ampicillin
- stress
- low birth weight
- hypothermia
- hypoglycaemia.

The most common organisms associated with neonatal septicaemia are *E. coli*, *Streptococcus*, *Staphylococcus* and *Klebsiella* spp.

The most common signs of septicaemia are:

- decreased weight gain
- absence of suckling reflex
- haematuria
- persistent diarrhoea
- unusual vocalisations
- abdominal distention
- pain.

Treatment

Septicaemia requires the administration of a third-generation cephalosporin (Ceftiofur sodium). Other factors also play a crucial part such as maintaining body temperature, preventing dehydration and providing adequate nutrition through supplementary feeding.

Hypoxia

Lack of oxygen is the most common cause of death around the time of delivery.

Before birth the lungs are in a state of atelectasis, and it is the neonate's first breath that inflates the lungs. Alveolar collapse after inspiration is prevented by the deposition of lipoprotein surfactants on the alveolar walls. Any circumstance which limits the expansion of the lungs (such as a dystocic birth, long delivery or caesarean section) can compromise the neonate's viability.

The inspiratory reflex for the neonate's first breath is triggered by an increase in CO_2 tension in the umbilical vessels. Delayed delivery may trigger this inspiratory reflex when the puppy is still bathed in fluid, leading to aspiration into the lungs and pneumonia.

Symptoms:

- dyspnoea
- cyanosis
- bradycardia
- maternal rejection.

Examination of the mother and neonates

The neonates are dependent on the mother, and any changes in her health, behaviour or nutritional status will significantly impact the health of the puppies.

A clinical examination of the mother includes assessment of:

- general physical condition
- general nutritional state
- hygiene
- behaviour.

Environmental/habitat assessment:

- clean hygienic conditions: essential for the prevention of infection
- correct environmental temperature and humidity:
  - first week after birth: 30–32°C
  - second week: 25–27°C
  - humidity ~60–65%
- adequate ventilation without draughts
- nesting area: a place of sufficient size to ensure the comfort of the mother and puppies, and prevent overlying due to lack of space.

Neonatal examination

In addition to examining the individual pups, it is important to assess the litter as a whole. This includes:

- observing the general behaviour of the group
- identifying any physical abnormalities compared to the others
- looking for isolated or rejected individuals.

It is usual for neonates to sleep for 80–90% of the time, with the remaining 10–20% spent feeding (Figures 6.20–6.23).

Neonates can present with complex, multi-system symptoms and therefore individual physical examinations should be meticulous, and undertaken in a meticulous manner.

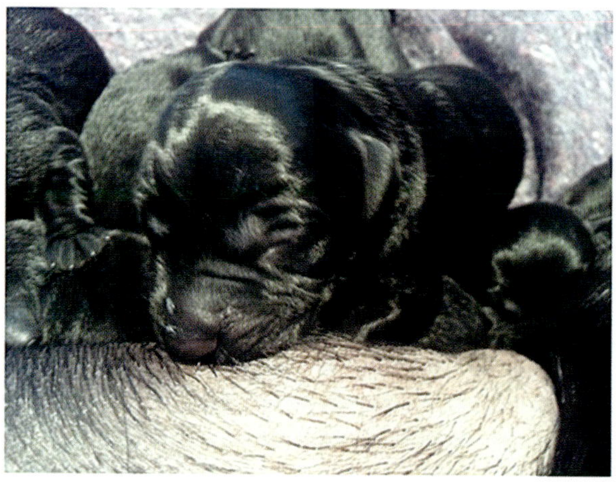

Figure 6.20. Correct position of a puppy while it suckles.

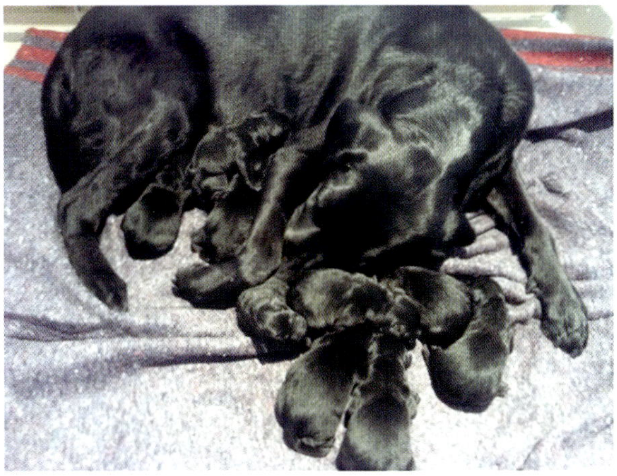

Figure 6.21. Mother placing her puppies.

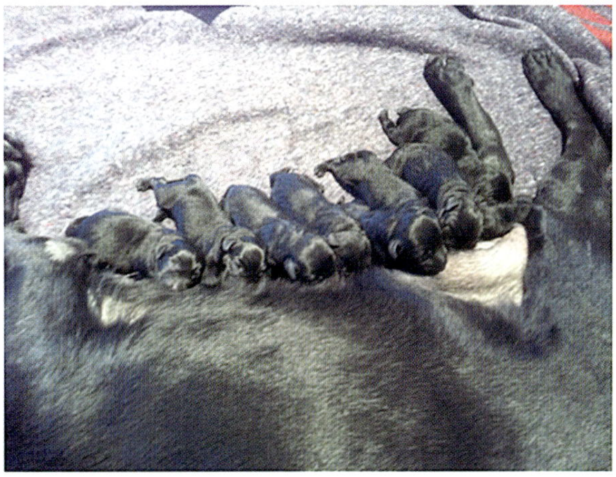

Figure 6.22. All puppies in the litter suckling at the same time.

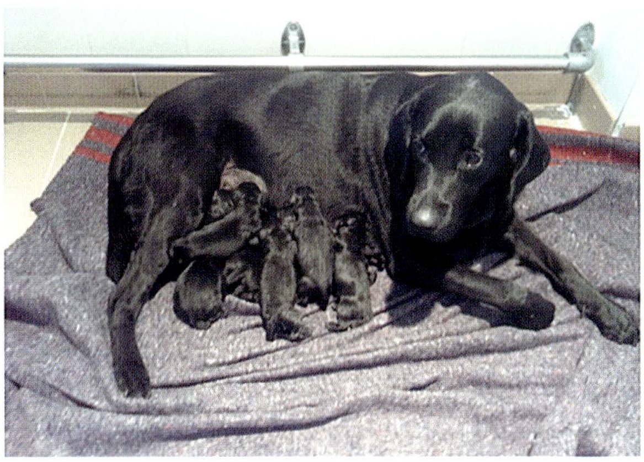

Figure 6.23. Examination of puppies alongside their mother.

The following information on the neonate should be borne in mind.

- Puppies with a birthweight <80 g have a near 100% mortality index.
- The most important causes of weight loss include inadequate nutrition and dehydration.
- Neonates are not able to control their body temperature until around four weeks of age. This can make both hypothermia and hyperthermia a liability, due to poor environment control.
- Primary reflexes are essential for survival, including thermotropism (burrowing reflex), suckling reflex and perineal reflex.
- Normal neonatal heart rate is 200–220 bpm.
- Normal respiratory rate is 15–35 bpm.

Diagnostic approach

A similar diagnostic approach can be used for both neonates and adults. However, take care in interpreting results due to the physiological idiosyncrasies of the neonatal patient.

Commonly used diagnostics include:

- complete blood analysis: haematology and biochemistry
- radiography: factors for interpretation to consider include the low bone density of the neonate, low levels of abdominal fat, high neonatal water content and high respiratory rate
- ultrasound: a valuable and minimally invasive diagnostic tool for the neonate
- video: suckling reflex.

Neonatal pathologies

Congenital pathologies

The incidence of congenital malformations is around 5%.

Those most common factors include:

- cleft lip/palate (Figure 6.24)
- gastrointestinal deformities
- hereditary defects linked to particular bloodlines and breeds
- iatrogenic
- nutritional
- excess vitamin A.

Secondary brain damage

There is a direct correlation between the length of circulatory arrest and the severity of damage to the medulla. Poor blood supply for greater than 10–15 minutes leads to neuronal necrosis of the brainstem.

Hypothermia extends the period of time needed for brain damage to occur, and also shifts the pattern of ischaemic vulnerability from the caudal region to more rostral structures.

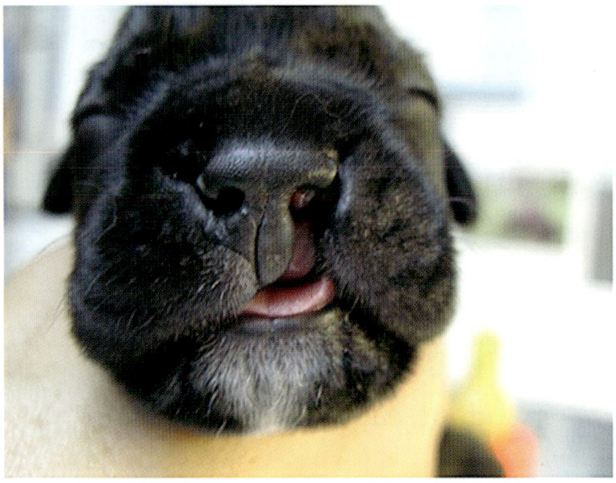

Figure 6.24. Importance of neonatal examination: cleft lip.

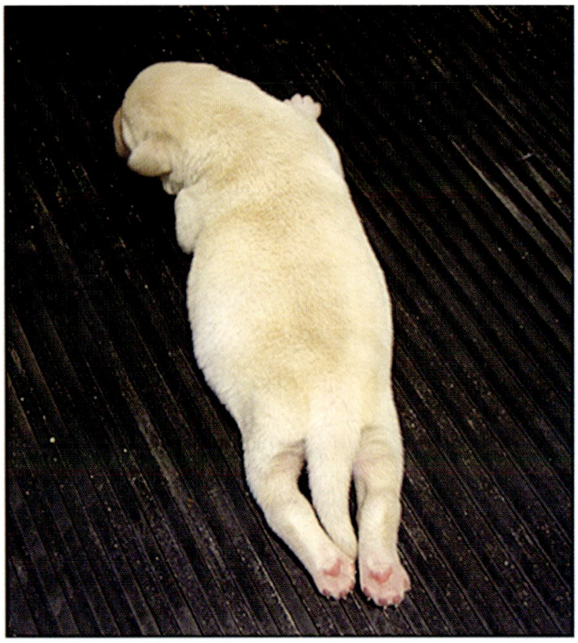

Figure 6.25.

Fading puppy syndrome

This common condition is directly related to the immaturity of the neonate and results in three pathologies:

- hypothermia
- hypoglycaemia
- dehydration.

Fading puppy syndrome is defined as:

> Death from no discernible cause in puppies aged 3–10 days. The puppies are born with no clinically detectable malformations, are of normal birthweight for the breed and demonstrate a normal growth rate. In general, the mother is healthy without complications during pregnancy, birth or post-partum.

Aetiology

The exact aetiology is unknown, but multifactorial. Suspected contributory factors include thymic insufficiency and a phosphatidylcholine deficiency.

Clinical signs

This is a rapidly progressive condition, with death occurring in less than 24 hours. During this period a puppy will stop suckling, become lethargic, moan, enter a coma and die. In addition it will develop symptoms such as hypothermia, hypoglycaemia and dehydration.

Diagnosis is based on clinical examination and the elimination of other causes.

Treatment

Therapy is supportive, with careful maintenance of body temperature, intra-osseous fluid therapy and the administration of glucose.

Toxic milk syndrome

Aetiology

This syndrome causes illness in the neonate due to changes in the mother's milk. Examples of these abnormalities include variations in the milk's components and the presence of high levels of bacteria, viruses, toxins or foreign substances.

This syndrome is linked with dystocia, dirty environmental conditions and inadequate care of the mother. The pathogens most commonly associated with both clinical and subclinical mastitis are *E. coli*, *Staphylococcus* spp. and *Colibacillus*.

Clinical signs

Puppies are most commonly affected at around 3–15 days of age. The larger pups are more likely to be affected as these have ingested the greatest amount of milk.

Affected neonates show signs of:

- pain
- abdominal distention
- tenesmus
- irritated or oedematous anus
- neonatal septicaemia.

Treatment

Neonates should be tube or bottle fed until the mother is fully recovered.

Neonatal isoerythrolysis

Aetiology

This disease is caused by blood group incompatibility between the neonate and antibodies in the mother's colostrum.

The three most common blood groups are A (the most frequent), B and AB. Disease occurs when a kitten of blood group A (or AB, but this is rare) suckles from a type B mother producing colostrum containing anti-A antibodies.

Clinical signs

The symptoms and time course of neonatal isoerythrolysis can vary. The most acute form results in the death of the neonate on day one. Alternatively, at around three days the kitten may develop jaundice, anaemia and haemoglobinuria. Finally, it can be responsible for necrosis of the tail and skin changes, at roughly 20 days of age.

Treatment

Affected neonates should be removed from the mother and given a full blood transfusion.

Prevention

Prevention involves determination of parental blood groups prior to mating to ensure these are compatible.

Swimming puppy syndrome

This syndrome affects pups in the transition phase (1–3 weeks of age). Also known as pancake or frisbee pups, these neonates are often flattened dorsoventrally and can lie only in sternal recumbency. The limbs are rotated externally, with hyperextension of the tarsal and stifle joints. Affected pups are unable to stand or walk.

With adequate physiotherapy, pups can often be rehabilitated. This includes gently manipulating the limbs into the correct position and making walking motions with them. In addition, pups should be supported in lateral recumbency.

The condition is most associated with large pups from small litters. Gaining too much weight too quickly seems to be a factor.

Bibliography

Gestation

Arús, J., Martí, S., Peña, F. and Prats, A. (1998) *Libro de Ponencias Formación Continuada de AVEPA 1.*

Concannon, P.W., England, G., Verstegen III, J. and Linde-Forsberg, C. (2000) Gestación canina: predicción del parto y cronometraje de los acontecimientos de la gestación. In: Concannon, P.W., England, G., Verstegen III, J. and Linde-Forsberg. C. (eds) *Recent Advances in Small Animal Reproduction.* International Veterinary Information Service, Ithaca, NY.

Concannon, P.W., Isaman, I., Frank, D.A., Michel, F.J. and Currie, W.B. (1988) Elevated concentrations of 13,14-dihydro-15-keto-prostaglandin F-2 alpha in maternal plasma during prepartum luteolysis and parturition in dogs (*Canis familiaris*). *Journal of Reproduction and Fertility* 84, 71–77.

Concannon, P.W., McCann, J.P. and Temple, M. (1989) Biology and endocrinology of ovulation, pregnancy and parturition in the dog. *Journal of Reproduction and Fertility* Suppl. 39, 3–25.

Concannon, P.W. et al. (1983) Radiographic diagnosis of canine pregnancy: onset of fetal skeletal radiopacity in relation to times of breeding, preovulatory luteinizing hormone release, and parturition. *American Journal of Veterinary Research* 4, 1506–1511.

Feldman, E.C. and Nelson, R.W. (2007) *Endocrinología y Reproducción Canina y Feline*, 3rd edn. Intermédica, Buenos Aires.

Johnson, C.A. (2008) Pregnancy management in the bitch. *Theriogenology* 70(9), 1412–1417.

Johnston, S.D., Root Kustritz, M.V. and Olson, P.S. (2001) In: *Canine and Feline Theriogenology.* WB Saunders, Philadelphia, PA, pp. 66–104.

Kutzler, M.A., MohAammed, H.O., Lamb, S.V. and Meyers-Wallen, V.N. (2003) Accuracy of canine parturition date prediction from the initial rise in preovulatory progesterone concentration. *Theriogenology* 60(6), 1187–1196.

Luvoni, G.C. and Beccaglia, M. (2006) The prediction of parturition date in canine pregnancy. *Reproduction in Domestic Animals* 41, 27–32.

Verstegenonclin, K. and Verstegen, J. (2008) Endocrinology of pregnancy in the dog: a review. *Theriogenology* 70(3), 291–299.

Zambelli, D. and Prati, F. (2006) Ultrasonography for pregnancy diagnosis and evaluation in queens. *Theriogenology* 66(1), 135–144.

Parturition

Arús, J., Martí, S., Peña, F. and Prats, A. (1998) *Libro de Ponencias Formación Continuada de AVEPA 1.*

Concannon, P.W., England, G., Verstegen III, J. and Linde-Forsberg, C. (2000) Gestación canina: predicción del parto y cronometraje de los acontecimientos de la gestación. In: Concannon, P.W., England, G., Verstegen III, J. and Linde-Forsberg. C. (eds) *Recent Advances in Small Animal Reproduction.* International Veterinary Information Service, Ithaca, NY.

Johnson, C.A. (2008) Pregnancy management in the bitch. *Theriogenology* 70(9), 1412–1417.

Johnston, S.D., Root Kustritz, M.V. and Olson, P.S. (2001) In: *Canine and Feline Theriogenology.* WB Saunders, Philadelphia, PA, pp. 105–128.

Jutkowitz, I.A. (2005) Reproductive emergencies. *Veterinary Clinics of North America Small Animal Practice* 35, 397–420.

Linde-Forsberg, C. and Enroth, A. (2000) Parto. In: Simpson, G.M., England, G.C.W. and Harvey, M.J. (eds) *Manual de reproducción y neonatología en pequeños animales.* JM Sastre Vida (Servicio Universidad), Barcelona, pp. 169–173.

Pretzer, S.D. (2008) Medical management of canine and feline dystocia. *Theriogenology* 70(3), 332–336.

Verstegenonclin, K. and Verstegen, J. (2008) Endocrinology of pregnancy in the dog: a review. *Theriogenology* 70, 291–299.

Infertility

Davidson, A. (2006) Conceptos actuales sobre la esterilidad en la perra. *IVIS* 16(2), 13–21.

Fontbonne, A. (2007) Approach to infertility in the bitch and in the dog. In: *Proceedings of the WSAVA Congress*, Sydney, Australia.

Fontbonne, A. and Maiandain, E. (2007) Infertility in cats. In: *Proceedings of the WSAVA Congress*, Sydney, Australia, 2007.

Johnson, C.A. (2008) High-risk pregnancy and hypoluteoidism in the bitch. *Theriogenology* 70(9), 1424–1430.

Meyers-Wallen, V.N. (2007) Unusual and abnormal canine estrous cycles. *Theriogenology* 68, 1205–1210.

Root Kustritz, M.V. (2005) *Manual de reproducción del perro y el gato*. Multimédia Ediciones Veterinarias, Barcelona, pp. 250–262.

Neonatology

Babbs, C.F. et al. (2009) Neonatal CPR: room at the top–a mathematical study of optimal chest compression frequency versus body size. *Resuscitation* 80(11), 1280–1284.

Bücheler, J. (1999) Fading kitten syndrome and neonatal isoerythrolysis. *Veterinary Clinics of North America Small Animal Practice* 29(4), 853–880.

Davidson, A.P. (2013) *Neonatal Resuscitation: improving the outcome*. Elsevier, St Louis, MO, pp. 897–914.

Lawler, D.F. (2012) Neonatal and pediatric care of the puppy and kitten. *Theriogenology* 70(3), 384–392.

Rickaed, V., Peterson, M. and Kutzler, M. (2011) Birth and the first 24 hours. In: Peterson, M.E. and Kutzler. M. (eds) *Small Animal Pediatrics: the first 12 months of life*. Elsevier-Saunders, St Louis, MO, pp. 11–39.

Tonnessen, R. and Vannuccl, R. (2012) Canine perinatal mortality. *Theriogenology* 77(9), 1788–1801.

Towfighi, J., Borge, K.S., Nodtvedt, A. and Indrebo, A. (2011) Neuropathology of normothermic circulatory arrest in newborn dogs. *Acta Neuropathologica* 93(5), 485–493.

Test

1. **What is progesterone?**
   A) the hormone responsible for anoestrus
   B) the hormone which indicates that ovulation has taken place
   C) the pregnancy hormone
   D) not a hormone
2. **When does birth occur?**
   A) at 65 ± 2 days after the peak of LH
   B) at 67 ± 2 days after the peak of LH
   C) with progesterone levels higher than 2.5 ng/ml
   D) when the rectal temperature rises above 38°C
3. **Nesting in the bitch occurs from approximately what time?**
   A) days 15–17
   B) days 17–20
   C) days 21–23
   D) days 23–25
4. **When does birth occur in the bitch?**
   A) 24–36 hours after progesterone drops below 2.5 ng/ml
   B) when prolactin levels increase
   C) when serum levels of PGF2-alpha drop
   D) 24–36 hours after progesterone drops below 4.5 ng/ml
5. **What happens in the second stage of birth in the dog?**
   A) expulsion contractions occur
   B) myometrial contractions begin
   C) the mother breaks the foetal membranes
   D) the foetus begins to enter the pelvic canal
6. **Is it normal for post-partum vaginal secretions to continue for as long as 3 weeks after birth?**
   A) yes
   B) no
   C) depends on the foetuses which are born
   D) depends on the overall length of the birth

7. What are the main clinical signs of uterine torsion?

A) acute abdominal pain and shock
B) metrorrhagia
C) fever, increased uterine size and dehydration
D) abdominal distension and vulvar discharge

8. When can vaginal prolapse occur?

A) not in pro-oestrus
B) in di-oestrus
C) anoestrus
D) near birth

9. What is the minimum level of progesterone needed to maintain pregnancy in the dog?

A) 5 ng/ml
B) 10 ng/ml
C) Between 1.5 and 3 ng/ml
D) 15 ng/ml

10. During pregnancy, foetal intestines can be seen at what stage?

A) 30 days
B) 30–35 days
C) 59–63 days
D) from day 63 after the peak in LH

11. What happens in the first stage of the birth?

A) expulsion contractions occur
B) the foetus enters the pelvic canal
C) the placentae are expelled
D) regular uterine contractions occur

12. In the protocol for neonatal resuscitation, what is the first thing that we should do?

A) stimulate with heat
B) oxygenate the neonate using a mask or by intubation
C) gently swing the neonate
D) administer pharmacological treatment

13. In the bitch, what is true of inter-oestrus intervals of less than 4 months?

A) bitch is fertile
B) bitch is infertile
C) do not influence fertility
D) show that no hereditary disorders have been detected

14. What might a differential diagnosis of luteal ovarian cysts imply?

A) silent heats or that the heat has gone unnoticed
B) male attraction due to perivulvar vaginitis
C) oestrogen-secreting ovarian tumours
D) cycles with short inter-oestrus interval

15. What is the main clinical sign of sub-involution in areas of placentation?

A) pain upon uterine palpation
B) non-specific uterine secretion during the first week post-partum
C) sanguineous vulvar secretion for more than 6 weeks post-partum
D) purulent vulvar discharge more than six weeks after birth

16. If the neonate is unable to suckle, is bradycardic, dyspnoeic and suffers from convulsions and coma, what is the most likely diagnosis?

A) dehydration
B) cooling
C) hypoglycaemia
D) liver immaturity

Answers on page 286

Clinical case 1

A pregnant dog presents, at day 65 after the peak in LH, with a progesterone level of 2.1 ng/ml and a temperature of 37°C. We perform radiography and see nine perfectly defined spines. We perform an ultrasound and the puppies have an average heart rate of 160 bpm. At the time of the ultrasound the mother has a heart rate of 95 bpm. No contractions have been noted.

1. *What is the diagnosis?*
2. *What is the most appropriate treatment?*

Clinical case 2

We perform an ultrasound on a Labrador 30 days after the peak in LH to confirm that she is pregnant, and we can see six vesicles with a normal heartbeat. The bitch has a history of embryonic resorption.

1. *Which protocol should be followed?*

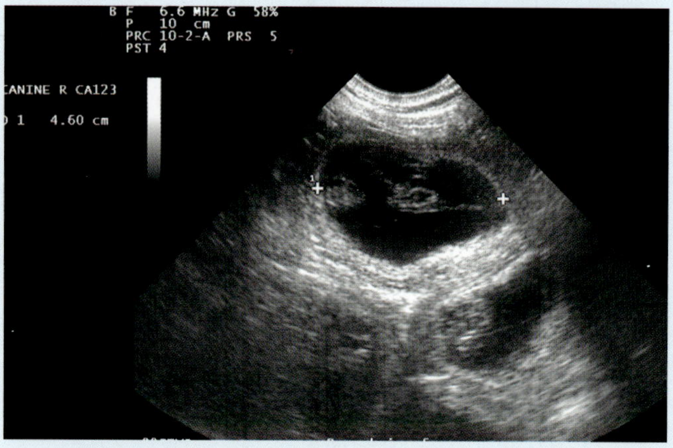

Correct answers

Test

1. B	7. A	13. B
2. A	8. D	14. A
3. C	9. D	15. C
4. A	10. C	16. C
5. A	11. D	
6. A	12. B	

Clinical case 1

1. What is the diagnosis? Foetal distress, as the heart rates of the puppies are less than double that of the mother at the time of the ultrasound.

2. What is the most appropriate treatment option? As progesterone levels are less than 2.5 ng/ml and therefore pulmonary surfactant has been released, the best treatment option is to perform a caesarean as soon as possible.

Clinical case 2

1. Which treatment protocol should be followed? As there is a history of abortion due to resorption, a blood sample should be taken to measure progesterone levels a week after the last mating. If levels are found to be below 15 ng/ml (insufficient to maintain gestation), they should be supplemented with oral progesterone until day 63 after the peak in LH. The recommended dose of progesterone is 0.88mg/kg/d VO.

7

Gastrointestinal disorders

Cristina Pérez Vera

Chapter summary

Gastrointestinal problems are a common reason for pets to visit the vet. However, vomiting and diarrhoea are merely symptoms and not a diagnosis in their own right. Therefore, it is important that the clinician, when presented with a vomiting or diarrhoeic animal, is able to differentiate mild self-limiting disease from conditions which need investigation and more aggressive treatment.

Gastrointestinal disease can be divided into primary disease, where the symptoms reflect the origin of the problem, and secondary disease, where the gut is affected by a disease process elsewhere in the body.

This chapter provides the clinician in practice with a practical grounding in the common causes of vomiting, regurgitation and diarrhoea, including the clinical signs, diagnostic testing and therapy, along with an introduction to endoscopy.

Key learning points

- Differentiating vomiting from regurgitation or dysphagia, and the recommended treatments.
- Understand fluid therapy and the pharmaceutical options for the treatment of vomiting patients.
- Oesophageal disease, the signs and treatment.
- The diagnostic pathway for reaching a definitive diagnosis in cases with intractable diarrhoea.
- Understand the clinical indications for endoscopy: the pros, cons and possible complications.

Vomiting

Definition

Vomiting is an involuntary protective reflex, through which abdominal effort expels material out of the body from the stomach and/or intestine.

There are three phases to the vomiting reflex.

1. **Nausea**: Characterised by changes in behaviour, and tachycardia.
2. **Pre-ejection**: The muscles of the distal oesophageal and cardiac sphincters relax, followed by reverse peristalsis in the intestine.
3. **Expulsion**: Intragastric pressure is elevated by contractions of the abdominal muscles, downward movement of the diaphragm and contractions of the body of the stomach.

Vomiting, whether acute or chronic, is one of the most common clinical signs seen in practice. However, the wide and varied nature of the gastrointestinal and non-gastrointestinal pathologies that cause vomiting can make diagnosis and treatment a challenge (see Table 7.1).

Pathophysiology

The vomiting reflex requires coordination of the following four factors (Figure 7.1).

1. **Visceral receptors.** These receptors are located in the gastrointestinal tract, peritoneum, bile ducts, uterus, prostate and kidneys.
2. **Vagal and sympathetic afferent neurons**
3. **Chemoreceptor trigger zone (CTZ).** Located on the floor of the fourth ventricle, the CTZ reacts to

Table 7.1. Aetiology of vomiting.

Gastrointestinal causes	Non-gastrointestinal causes
Dietary	**Inflammatory or infectious**
Sudden changes	Acute pancreatitis, Prostatitis
Poor-quality food	Pyometra
Excess food	Peritonitis, Septicaemia, Hepatitis, Cholecystitis
Foreign body	Dirofilariosis (cat)
Intolerance	**Endocrine/metabolic**
Dietary allergy	Hyperthyroidism, Hypoadrenocorticism
Inflammatory	Diabetic keto-acidosis, Hypercalcaemia
Gastritis or acute gastroenteritis	**Organic failure**: Hepatic/renal
Acute Haemorrhagic Diarrhoea Syndrome, Pancreatitis	**Central nervous system diseases**
Chronic intestinal inflammation	**Medications**
Infectious	**Allergic reaction**
Viruses	
Canine parvovirus or feline panleukopenia	
Feline leukaemia virus	
Feline infectious peritonitis Feline influenza	
Parasites	
Ancylostoma caninum, Trichuris vulpis	
Coccidia	
Giardia spp.	
Physalloptera	
Ollulanus	
Bacteria	
Salmonella spp.	
Helicobacter spp., *Campylobacter jejuni, Clostridium* spp.	
E. coli	
Yersinia enterocolitica	
Mycosis	
Pythium insidiosum (in endemic areas)	
Histoplasma spp. (in endemic areas)	
Toxic	
Non-steroidal anti-inflammatories	
Antibiotics	
Chemotherapy	

Table 7.1. Continued

Gastrointestinal causes	Non-gastrointestinal causes
Obstructive Foreign body intestinal obstruction Hypertrophy of the pyloric mucosa Granuloma Gastric volvulus and torsion, Trichobezoars Pyloric stenosis Neoplasia	
Other causes Gastrointestinal ulceration, Medications Foreign body Neoplasia Hypoadrenocorticism	

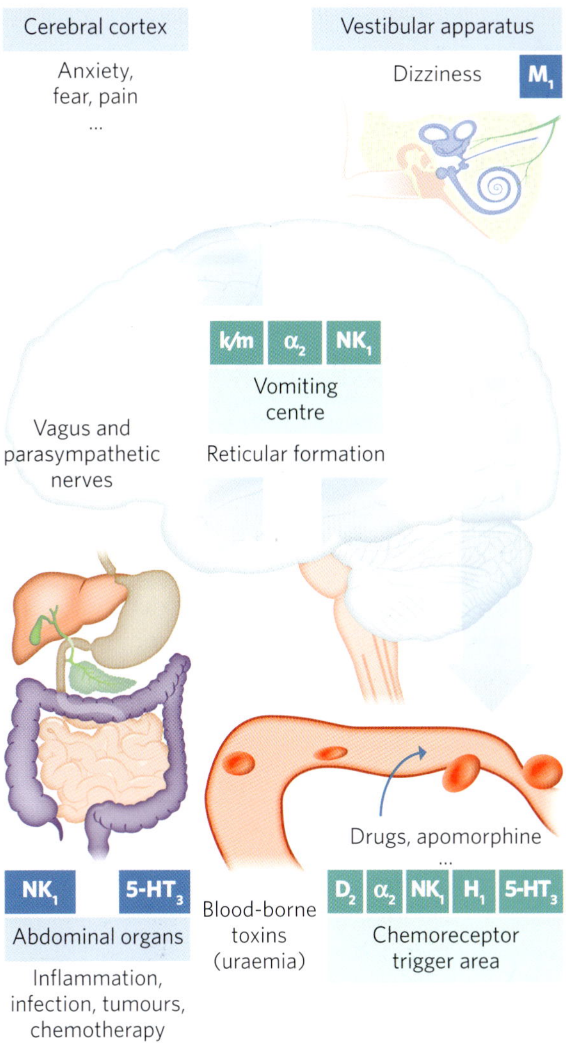

Figure 7.1. Schematic diagram showing the physiopathology of vomiting. Diagram courtesy of J. Gookin, modified. The small squares represent the receptors involved in the vomiting reflex. *Illustration: Elaine Leggett.*

the direct action of haematogenous substances (e.g. uraemia, apomorphine, chemotherapy or drugs) and signals coming from the vomiting centre.

4. **Vomiting centre.** This is located within the reticular formation of the medulla oblongata. It receives vagal and sympathetic neuron information from the CTZ, the vestibular apparatus and the cerebral cortex.

There are two ways the vomiting reflex may be triggered.

- **Humoral pathway**: Toxic haematogenous substances stimulate the CTZ, which then triggers the vomiting centre.
- **Neural pathway**: The vomiting centre is activated by inflammation, infection, malignancy or toxicity.

Vomiting can have serious consequences for the animal, such as **dehydration**, shock, **acid–base imbalances** or **aspiration pneumonia**. In cases of severe vomiting, this also results in **pre-renal azotaemia**, which for patients with pre-existing renal insufficiency can lead to renal failure.

In cases of **severe vomiting** or proximal gastrointestinal obstruction, the most common acid–base imbalance is **metabolic alkalosis**. This is due to the loss of hydrochloric acid from the stomach, along with sodium, potassium and chloride.

Clinical signs

A complete and detailed clinical history is vital to a clinical investigation of vomiting. In the first instance, it is essential to confirm the patient is vomiting, rather than regurgitating (see Table 7.2).

Regurgitation

Definition

Regurgitation is the passive retrograde expulsion of liquid or undigested food from the oesophagus to outside the body.

In the event of acute vomiting, it is important to **differentiate** between self-limiting disease (uncomplicated

Table 7.2. Differences between vomiting and regurgitation.

	Regurgitation	Vomiting
Nausea	No	Yes
Heaving	No	Yes
Appearance of food	Undigested	Variable
Blood	Undigested	Variable
Time since ingestion	Variable	Variable
pH	pH >7	Any
Presence of bile	No	Variable
Abdominal contraction	No	Yes

vomiting) and serious pathology (complicated vomiting).

The following information is helpful.

- *Age and breed*: This can help establish a diagnosis. For example, parasites or parvovirus are more likely in a puppy than an adult (see Table 7.1).
- *Examination and relevant history*: For example, is the patient a puppy or an adult? Is there a possibility of a foreign body? Is the dog vaccinated and de-wormed? Is the dog taking any medications?
- *The nature of the vomiting*: This includes:
- the duration, progression, and severity of the vomiting
- the appearance of the vomit, e.g. food, bile, blood, material with a faecal odour
- type of vomiting, e.g. projectile, intermittent, only in the morning.
- *Other clinical signs*: such as polyuria, polydipsia, coughing, sneezing, diarrhoea, weight loss or gain
- *Environment and diet*: Does the dog scavenge? Does the cat have access to the outdoors?

Physical examination

A thorough, **complete physical examination** is essential. This should include recording the **vital signs** and percentage **dehydration**; and performing **auscultation**, abdominal **palpation** and a **rectal** examination. This not only helps pinpoint areas for investigation with direct respect to vomiting, but can indicate relevant **non-gastrointestinal disease** (e.g. a thyroid nodule in a cat). All abnormal findings should be noted.

First examine the patient from **a distance**. Take note of the animal's body condition, demeanour and posture. Poor body condition can hint at the chronic nature of the problem.

In a case of **acute vomiting** the presence of **fever** suggests a primary non-gastrointestinal problem such as pyometra or pyelonephritis, or a bacterial infection. The latter may be primary (salmonellosis) or secondary (intestinal perforation and peritonitis as a complication of a foreign body, or aspiration pneumonia). It should be noted that pancreatitis rarely causes fever.

The presence of **cranial abdominal pain** can be compatible with pancreatitis, peritonitis, gastrointestinal ulceration (secondary to medicines, a tumour or hypo-adrenocorticism) or a primary non-gastrointestinal process (hepatitis or cholangiohepatitis).

Diagnosis

Laboratory tests

Blood tests (complete blood count, complete biochemistry and blood gas) and **urine tests** help rule out non-gastrointestinal causes and evaluate the severity of the vomiting.

Complete blood count (CBC)

On a CBC particular attention should be paid to dehydration indicators such as **haemoconcentration** and the presence of a **stress leukogram**. A stress leukogram is characterised by neutrophilia, lymphopenia, eosinopenia and potential monocytosis, and its **absence in a sick dog** can be suggestive of **hypo-adrenocorticism**.

Cases of acute Acute Haemorrhagic Diarrhoea Syndrome are typically associated with haemoconcentration and a haematocrit >60%, accompanied by hypo-albuminaemia.

Changes in the haematology, such as **toxic neutrophils** or raised levels of immature neutrophils, are suggestive of severe inflammatory/infectious problems (such as intestinal perforation or acute pancreatitis), whilst **eosinophilia** is suggestive of intestinal parasites, chronic eosinophilic gastroenteritis or hyperadrenocorticism.

Serum biochemistry

Serum biochemistry facilitates the evaluation of the degree of dehydration (as indicated by hyperalbuminaemia, hyperproteinaemia) and any non-gastrointestinal disease (such as kidney or liver failure).

Hyperkalaemia and **hyponatraemia** are typically associated with **hypoadrenocorticism**, although normal electrolyte levels do not rule out this condition. Hyperkalaemia can also occur for reasons other than Cushing's disease, such as renal failure, gastrointestinal parasites and abdominal effusion.

Hypoglycaemia indicates primary disease that is non-gastrointestinal (liver failure), peritonitis or bacterial translocation (such as secondary to Acute Haemorrhagic Diarrhoea Syndrome or parvovirus).

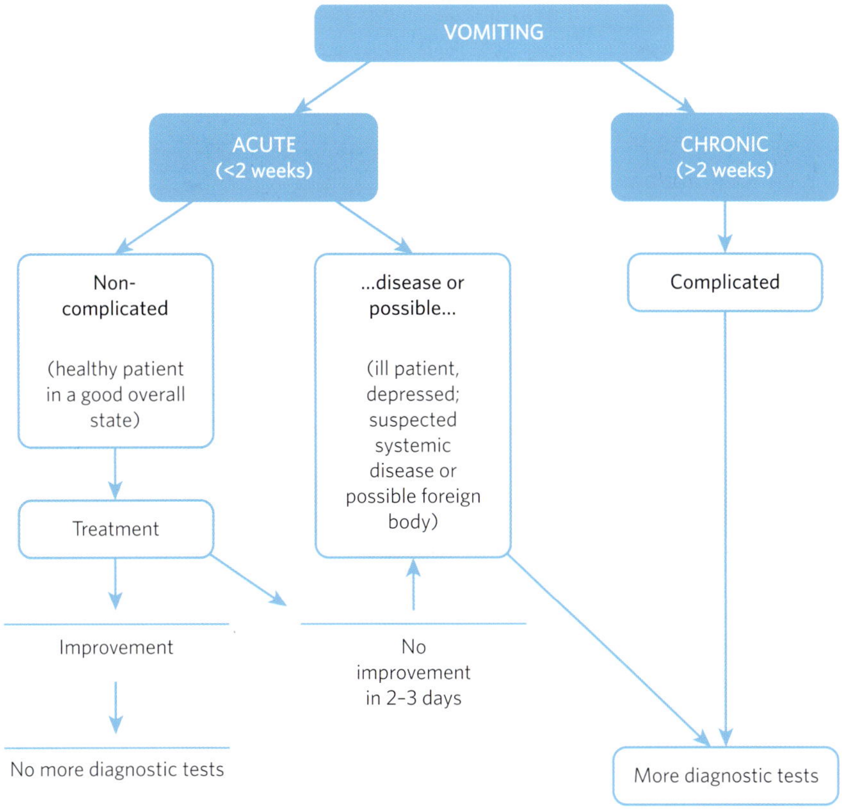

Figure 7.2. Assessment of vomiting.

Urinalysis

Urinalysis is particularly useful when **azotaemia** is present, as it helps differentiate renal disease from secondary problems. A **concentrated urine** confirms the azotaemia as being due to **dehydration**, and should therefore be reassessed once the patient is fully hydrated.

Urinalysis is also insightful into causes of **non-gastrointestinal diseases** such as ketoacidosis in diabetics, pyelonephritis and hepatic problems in cats. It should be noted that in cats, unlike dogs, the presence of bilirubinuria is always abnormal.

In summary

It is advisable to perform diagnostic tests (see Table 7.3) when:

- **Vomiting is severe** or frequent, despite symptomatic treatment.
- The patient presents with symptoms suggestive of **non-gastrointestinal disease**, such as polyuria, oliguria/anuria, purulent vaginal discharge, neurological symptoms or generalised lymphadenopathy.
- There are **abnormalities on physical** examination such as lethargy, fever/hypothermia, pain, abdominal distension, changes in mucous membrane colour or hypovolaemia.
- There is a suspicion of **foreign body** ingestion.

Table 7.3. The diagnostic protocol for vomiting depends on whether it is complicated.

Uncomplicated vomiting	Complicated vomiting
* Complete blood count, biochemistry profile, urinalysis * Stool analysis in the case of diarrhoea or in animals which have not been de-wormed * Occasionally, testing for parvovirus/*Giardia* * Occasionally, abdominal radiography * Symptomatic treatment	* Complete blood count, biochemistry profile, urinalysis * T4/FeLV/FIV testing (cat) * Stool analysis * PLI * Cobalamin, folate, TLI * ACTH-stimulation test (dog), abdominal radiography/ultrasound * Contrast radiography * Endoscopy or exploratory laparotomy

Treatment

Goals for the treatment of vomiting, whether acute or chronic, are:

1. Eliminate the primary cause, if known.
2. Control vomiting.
3. Correct the consequences, such as electrolyte abnormalities, acid–base imbalance and dehydration.

In the case of acute vomiting, the treatment plan includes **gastrointestinal rest** and **supportive therapy**, such as an anti-emetic and fluid therapy.

Fluid therapy

An **individual fluid therapy** plan should be made for dehydrated patients and those that remain hospitalised for ongoing diagnostic tests.

What fluids should be administered?

Vomiting and diarrhoea cause loss of water, sodium, potassium and chlorine, which should be replaced using crystalloid fluids.

- *Lactated Ringers*: Contains small amounts of potassium and lots of sodium, chloride and lactate, the last of these being converted to bicarbonate.
- *Physiological saline (0.9%)*: Does not contain potassium and is acidifying.

If electrolytes levels cannot be measured, a good compromise is to supplement one litre of **lactated Ringers** or saline with **5–10 mEq of potassium chloride**. This is provisional on the absence of azotaemia or suspected hyperkalaemia.

In the presence of moderate to **severe hypalbuminaemia** (i.e. albumin levels <15 g/l), volume expanders such as *Hetastarch* or *Voluven* should be administered at a rate of 20 ml/kg/day, alongside crystalloid therapy.

What fluid rate and volume should be administered?

Daily maintenance requirements for fluid are **40–60 ml/kg/day**. When working out an appropriate fluid rate, other factors need to be corrected including the percentage dehydration estimated fluid losses. For example, for **each vomit** the dog loses approximately **50 ml of fluid**.

Hospitalised patients should be monitored, their **hydration status re-evaluated** periodically and fluid therapy adjusted accordingly every **6–12 hours**. Parameters such as skin elasticity, mucous membrane colour and pulse quality help this assessment.

In the presence of **hypovolaemic shock** a **crystalloid**, such as lactated Ringers, should be administered at a rate appropriate to increase vascular volume and reverse the hypovolaemia.

The recommended rate is to give **a bolus** of one-quarter of the shock volume in **ten minutes**:

- Cats: 10–15 ml/kg
- Dogs: 20 ml/kg.

At the end of this bolus the animal's pulse quality, heart rate and mucous membranes should be reassessed. If necessary, repeat the fluid bolus. If after the second bolus there is still no improvement, and provided there is no bleeding or coagulopathy, it is appropriate to give a **colloid bolus of 10 ml/kg** and monitor the response. Once the hypovolaemia is corrected, a fluid therapy plan for the following 12–24 hours should be outlined.

If the patient is hypo-albuminaemic and receiving colloids, then the total volume of crystalloids should be reduced by 30%.

Anti-emetics

The choice of anti-emetic should be made in consideration of its particular mechanism of action and the physiology of the vomiting reflex. (Figure 7.1). Choose the most appropriate anti-emetic medication based on the aetiology of the vomiting (Table 7.4).

Gastric acid suppressants and antacids

The use of **gastric acid suppressants** is indicated in cases of chronic vomiting or when damage to the gastric mucosa is suspected. The latter includes damage due to medication, a foreign body, pancreatitis or liver disease.

Any defect to the gastric mucosa results in degradation of epithelial cells by hydrochloric acid, bile acids and proteolytic enzymes, which unleash a vicious circle that leads to further mucosal damage.

Although the incidence of gastric ulceration in dogs and cats is unknown, it is known that the most frequent causes of ulceration are the administration of non-steroidal anti-inflammatory drugs, neoplasia and liver disease. Gastric acid production is stimulated by the histamine, gastrin, and acetylcholine hormones. Medicines that decrease the secretion of acid (acid suppressors) help to protect, by various mechanisms, the damaged gastric mucosa (Table 7.5).

It is important not to confuse gastric acid suppressors with antacids, as the latter **do not** decrease acid **production**.

Antihistamines

Famotidine (at a dose of 0.5–1 mg/kg BID) is the strongest antihistamine medication.

Antihistamines such as cimetidine and famotidine help promote mucosal regeneration.

Ranitidine is a prokinetic and does not increase gastric pH, and is therefore not effective as an acid suppressant.

Table 7.4. Anti-emetic drugs most commonly used in cases of vomiting.

Type	Example	Side effects	Contraindications	Dose
Antagonists α2-adrenergic phenothiazines	Chlorpromazine	Sedation, hypotension		0.2–0.4 mg/kg TID SC, IM
Antagonists D2-dopaminergics	Metoclopramide	Extrapyramidal signs, diarrhoea	Gastrointestinal obstruction	0.2–0.4 mg/kg QID PO, SC
H1-histamine antagonists (Not effective on the cat)	Diphenhydramine	Sedation, xerostomia		2–4 mg/kg QID PO, IM
5-HT3 serotonergic antagonists	Ondansetron			0.5–1.0 mg/kg BID PO
	Dolasetron			0.6–1.0 mg/kg BID PO
Anticholinergics	Scopolamine	Tachycardia		0.4 mg/kg
Opioids	Butorphanol	Sedation		0.2–0.4 mg/kg BID IM
NK1 (neurokinin) inhibitors	Maropitant		Animals under 16 weeks of age Cases of liver disease or hypo-albuminemia require extra care	1–2 mg/kg SC, IV, PO

Table 7.5. Gastric acid suppressants and antacids.

Medication	Example	Advantages	Disadvantages
Antihistamines	Ranitidine, Cimetidine, Famotidine	Famotidine is 20 times more potent than cimetidine	Ranitidine is not effective Cimetidine lasts <5 h Cytochrome P450 inhibitors
Proton pump inhibitors	Omeprazole, Pantoprazole	Superior to antihistamines	Cytochrome P450 inhibitors
		Very effective	Delayed effect (3–5 days)
Antacids	Al (OH)³ Mg(OH)² CaCO³ NaHCO³		Do not reduce acid production Rebound effect Chelate other medications Short duration Constipation Not gastroprotective
Sucralfate		Effective in cases of oesophagitis	Chelator Constipation Does not change gastric pH Abdominal pain
Prostaglandin analogue	Misoprostol	Prevents ulcers associated with NSAIDs	Diarrhoea, nausea Contraindicated during pregnancy

Proton pump inhibitors

The strongest **stomach protectors** are proton pump inhibitors (*omeprazole* 0.5–1 mg/kg/12 h), as these block the production of gastric acid almost completely and maintain the pH of the stomach over a longer period of time than other drugs.

Antacids

Antacids are weak bases that help to neutralise gastric acid but, unlike anti-secretory agents, they do not reduce acid production.

Antacids and **sucralfate** are cytoprotective agents that stimulate the production of prostaglandins. Antacids are very effective at neutralising the pH, but have an average half-life of 2–3 hours and can cause a rebound effect (gastric hyperacidity).

Sucralfate is a sucrose sulfate–aluminium complex that adheres to the eroded/ulcerated areas of the gastric mucosa to form a protective barrier.

- Dogs: 0.5 g PO, BID–TID
- Cats: 0.25 g PO, BID–TID.

Sucralfate is recommended if ulceration is suspected in the proximal gastrointestinal region (for example, if melaena or haematemesis is present) or oesophagitis. It should be administered 1–2 hours before or after other medications or food.

Misoprostol is a cytoprotective drug. This cytoprotective effect is due to an increase in bicarbonate secretion, a reduction in pepsin content, an increase in blood flow to the mucosa and an improved regenerative capacity of the mucosa. However, with the exception of aspirin, its ability to prevent ulcers caused by non-steroidal anti-inflammatory drugs (NSAIDs) has not yet been proven in small animals. In addition, it is less effective for the treatment of gastro-duodenal ulceration when compared to antihistamines or proton pump inhibitors.

Acute gastritis

Definition

Acute gastritis is defined as a syndrome characterised by sudden onset vomiting, presumed to be caused by an insult at the level of the gastric mucosa.

Aetiology

In most cases, anamnesis and medical history point to a specific aetiology, although sometimes a definitive cause is not discovered. Possible causes of acute gastritis include:

- **Dietary**: sudden changes in diet, dietary indiscretion, food intolerance or ingestion of food that is 'off'
- **Foreign Body** or **Trichobezoars**
- **Medications and Toxins**: including NSAIDs, antibiotics, cleaning products, plants and heavy metals
- **Non-Gastrointestinal Causes**: systemic diseases such as liver disease, hypo-adrenocorticism or uraemia resulting from renal failure
- **Infection**: parasites, enterotoxicosis.

Clinical signs

The main symptom is vomiting, although depending on the primary aetiology there may also be diarrhoea or signs linked to the primary disease.

Diagnosis

A diagnosis of acute gastritis is made based on the history, clinical pathological findings and a positive response to symptomatic treatment. In the case of acute gastritis, if the initial physical examination and blood tests do not show anomalies, unless a foreign body is suspected it is not necessary to perform diagnostic imaging tests.

Treatment

Treatment is symptomatic and a typical therapeutic plan includes the following.

1. **Gastrointestinal rest for 24 hours**: After 24 hours offer a small amount of easily digestible food. A home-cooked option is boiled rice with chicken or fresh cheese. After this, the normal diet is gradually reintroduced over approximately one week.
2. **Fluid therapy**: In the case of mild dehydration, subcutaneous isotonic, crystalloid fluids are often sufficient to correct dehydration. In contrast, for cases of moderate to severe dehydration, intravenous fluids are necessary to correct the deficit whilst performing further diagnostic tests.

For acute vomition linked to acute gastritis, it is not necessary to administer an anti-emetic. Indeed, to use anti-emetics can make it difficult to monitor clinical improvement. Inappropriate suppression of the vomiting centre can mask an active process, when knowledge of which can indicate the need for further diagnostic tests.

Gastric ulceration

Aetiopathogenesis

Gastric ulceration may be due to gastric or non-gastric processes, or can be idiopathic. Causes of gastric ulceration include:

- **endocrine or metabolic causes**: uraemia, macrocytosis, liver disease, hypo-adrenocorticism in the dog
- **inflammatory causes**: gastritis, pancreatitis
- **neoplasia**: gastric carcinoma, lymphoma, leiomyoma, mastocytoma, gastrinoma, plasmacytoma
- **medications**: NSAIDs, doxycycline, corticosteroids. The combination of NSAIDs and glucocorticoids is highly ulcerogenic
- **gastric hypoperfusion**: sepsis, shock.

The most common cause of gastric ulceration in the dog is the administration of ulcerogenic medications such as NSAIDs, whilst in cats it is systemic mastocytosis.

Gastric ulcers arise when there is a failure in the gastric mucosa's protective mechanism or an excess of harmful substances, in particular stomach acid and pepsin.

1. Diseases that cause an **increase in gastric secretions**, such as renal failure or gastrinoma, are associated with

an increased secretion of gastrin, whilst mastocytomas predispose to gastric ulceration through the release of high levels of histamine.

2. The most common risk factor in the **development of gastric ulcers** is a change in blood flow at the level of the gastric mucosa. For example:
3. a) Ulceration due to **NSAIDs** or glucocorticoids which **reduce local prostaglandin** production, which then reduces local blood flow and the mucosa's regenerative capacity. In addition, it has also been observed that NSAIDs **inhibit angiogenesis** and epithelial proliferation, thus reducing the epithelial protection.
   b) Hypovolaemia, shock, thrombosis and other processes that disrupt gastric perfusion – for example, gastric torsion – also promote ulceration.

Clinical signs

The clinical signs commonly associated with **gastric ulceration** include:

- **anorexia** and **vomiting** (most frequent)
- **haematemesis**
- **melaena** (detectable on rectal examination)
- pale mucous membranes
- abdominal pain
- weakness
- shock.

Diagnosis

The following changes on blood analysis can be indicative of gastric or gastrointestinal ulceration.

CBC

Mild to severe regenerative **anaemia** should be expected. In the case of **acute bleeding** (<3 days) the anaemia may appear **non-regenerative** since bone marrow production has yet to kick in.

If the **bleeding is chronic**, such as linked to long-term arthritis treatment with NSAIDs, then iron deficiency will eventually lead to the development of **non-regenerative anaemia**. The latter is typified by microcytic and hypochromic red blood cells, accompanied by thrombocytosis. Chronic gastrointestinal bleeding is one of the most common causes of anaemia due to **iron deficiency**.

The presence of **eosinophilia** can indicate gastrointestinal parasites, mastocytosis, hypo-adrenocorticism or eosinophilic gastroenteritis.

Gastric perforation can be suspected if the CBC demonstrates a **leucocytosis with left shift** and toxic changes.

Biochemistry

Characteristic of a **gastric ulcer bleed** is **pan-hypoproteinaemia** (hypo-albuminaemia and hypo-globulinaemia) and raised urea, with normal creatinine values due to the intestinal absorption of haemoglobin.

- **Elevated liver enzymes** and **bilirubin** suggest possible **liver disease** or **pancreatitis** as the primary cause of ulceration. However, these will also be raised due to NSAID-induced hepatotoxicity.
- **Hyponatremia with hyperkalaemia**, with or without azotaemia, is highly suggestive of **hypo-adrenocorticism**.

It should be noted that some animals with gastric ulceration will have completely normal blood results.

Other blood tests

In patients with no history of previous treatment with ulcerogenic medications, and where blood analysis and imaging fail to reveal a primary cause of gastric ulceration, **blood gastrin levels** should be measured.

It is important when checking gastrin levels that gastroprotectants are withheld and a fasting sample taken. For animals treated with omeprazole, therapy should be withdrawn for at least one week prior to sampling.

Abdominal ultrasound

Ultrasound examination is useful in the detection of **concurrent disease** (such as gastric or intestinal lymphoma, pancreatitis, pancreatic masses, liver disease and kidney disease), while it also facilitates measurement of the **thickness of the stomach wall**. However, in many cases of gastric ulceration the stomach wall thickness remains normal and therefore ultrasound has low sensitivity with regard to diagnosis of gastric ulceration.

Gastric perforation can be suggested by the presence of **air inside the stomach wall**, free abdominal fluid or hyper-echogenicity of the omentum.

Occult blood in faeces

When **gastrointestinal bleeding** is suspected but there is no melaena, it may be useful to perform an **occult blood test on faeces**. There are three methods used to measure occult blood in stools:

- tests with o-toluidine (for example, **Hematest**), which has the lowest percentage of false positives due to diet; according to one study, it carries a specificity of 92%
- guaiac test for occult blood – for example, **Hemoccult**

- immunoassays for haemoglobin (available in human but not veterinary medicine).

Endoscopy

Endoscopy is the **definitive diagnostic tool** for detection of **gastric ulcer**. However, in cases where the anamnesis, clinical history and analytics are compatible with gastric ulceration, **treatment should be initiated** without necessarily performing an endoscopy.

Endoscopy should be performed when a **concurrent gastric pathology** is suspected, such as a neoplasm, gastritis or foreign body; to confirm the presence of gastric ulceration and examine the oesophagus, or to obtain intestinal biopsies.

When the cause of chronic bleeding is an intestinal mass (for example, a leiomyoma) which goes unnoticed on ultrasound, then balloon endoscopy (which folds the bowel as if it were an accordion) or laparotomy is necessary for a definitive diagnosis.

Treatment

Treatment should be directed at the primary cause of the ulcer, along with managing pain and giving supportive care.

Fluid therapy: Dehydrated or shocked patients should be assessed individually to determine the volume and rate of fluid to be infused.

Anti-emetics: *Metoclopramide, ondansetron* or *maropitant.*

Analgesia. *Buprenorphine* 10–20 mcg/kg IM or IV is a good choice for analgesia to relieve the pain associated with ulceration or a primary process such as pancreatitis.

Reduction of gastric secretions. With *famotidine* (antihistaminic) or *omeprazole*, 1 mg/kg BID. In cases of gastrinoma, the combination of omeprazole and *octreotide* (2–20 mcg/kg SC TID) is an effective treatment to reduce vomiting, gastric secretion and gastrointestinal bleeding in both dogs and humans.

Mucosal protectors: *Misoprostol.* An analogue of prostaglandin PGE2, this agent protects against NSAID-associated gastric ulceration. It is contraindicated in pregnant animals and can cause diarrhoea.

Sucralfate. In dogs, 1 g PO TID.

In the case of a perforating ulcer, or if resection of the stomach is indicated, surgical resection via laparotomy should be used.

Dysphagia and regurgitation

Definitions

Dysphagia refers to difficulty swallowing or alterations in eating.

Regurgitation is the passive retrograde expulsion out of the body of food or liquid from within the oesophagus.

The presence of dysphagia indicates an organic or functional disorder in the pathway taken by the bolus from mouth to stomach.

A patient with an oesophageal problem may present with both dysphagia and regurgitation.

Swallowing is a coordinated process that involves the following anatomical structures: the tongue, the soft and hard palates, pharyngeal muscles, oesophagus and gastro-esophageal junction. For swallowing to occur correctly, besides the requirement for striated muscle and intact neuromuscular transmission, the proper functioning is required of the trigeminal, facial, glossopharyngeal and hypoglossal nerves along with their nuclei, the brainstem and the swallowing centre (located in the reticular formation).

The phases of the swallowing process:

1. oral preparatory phase
2. oral stage
3. pharyngeal phase
4. oesophageal phase.

In most cases the presence of **dysphagia** indicates a problem in the **oropharynx** and/or the **oesophagus**. Dysphagia may be due to a functional, muscular or neurological alteration that affects the swallowing reflex or can be caused by a structural problem – for example, oesophageal stenosis, trauma, foreign body or neoplasm affecting the oropharyngeal or oesophageal areas.

The entirety of the canine oesophagus is composed of skeletal muscle, while the feline oesophagus has smooth muscle in the distal third. These differences are important from a therapeutic viewpoint because prokinetic agents (*metoclopramide, cisapride*) have no effect on the striated musculature in the dog but are effective in the smooth muscle in the cat.

Dysphagia

Classification and aetiology

Dysphagia is classified according to which phase of swallowing is affected.

Oropharyngeal dysphagia

This is the most common type of dysphagia in dogs and cats. The problem may be prehension of food with the lips,teeth or tongue; in moving the food bolus to the base of the tongue; in relaxation of the cricopharyngeal muscles; or the passage of food into the cranial oesophagus.

Aetiology: Common examples include periodontal disease, bone fracture, trauma, stomatitis, gingivitis, myositis, tongue problem, neuropathy of the V, VII or XII cranial nerves, neoplasia, cleft palate, cricopharyngeal or pharyngeal dysfunction.

Oesophageal dysphagia

The oesophageal phase is involuntarily affected due to closure of the proximal sphincter primary and secondary peristaltic contractions.

Aetiology: Mega-oesophagus, stenosis, foreign body, oesophageal diverticulum, granuloma, intra- or extraluminal neoplasia.

Gastro-oesophageal dysphagia

The passage of food is inhibited from the oesophagus into the stomach.

Aetiology: hiatal hernia, gastro-oesophageal intussusception, oesophagitis.

Diagnosis

The diagnostic approach to dysphagia includes steps.

1. **Signalment and clinical history**
   a) Age (puppy or adult), breed, history of trauma, possibility of foreign body, medications. Comprehensive general and neurological physical examination is required to identify the affected phase.
   b) Observe the animal while it eats and drinks. If the problem is in the oral phase, then inspect the mouth under general anaesthesia.
2. **Radiographs** of the thorax and cervical area for a foreign body, mass or mega-oesophagus.
3. **Blood tests:** complete blood count, biochemistry, CK and, if myasthenia gravis is suspected, acetylcholine antibody receptors.
4. **Contrast video fluoroscopy**: to evaluate phases of swallowing and the timing of each phase.
5. **Electromyography**
6. **MRI:** to evaluate myopathies or central nervous system problems
7. **Muscular** biopsy if myopathy is suspected.

Cricopharyngeal dysfunction

Definition

Cricopharyngeal dysfunction involves a problem with the passage of food into the cranial oesophagus.

Aetiology

The most frequent causes of cricopharyngeal dysfunction are:

- cricopharyngeal achalasia
- cricopharyngeal asynchronicity
- neuromuscular disease: myasthenia gravis, hypoadrenocorticism, hypothyroidism.

Clinical signs

Animals with cricopharyngeal dysfunction tend to accumulate food in the pharynx and regurgitate immediately after eating, through the nose or the mouth. They repeatedly try to swallow, which makes them cough and sneeze. The symptoms tend to be worse when the animal drinks water.

Cricopharyngeal achalasia

Definition

Achalasia is defined as a failure of proximal oesophageal sphincter to relax.

Aetiology

Achalasia is usually congenital, with the most frequently affected breeds being the Pug, Dachshund and Cocker Spaniel, but it has also been described in adult animals with hypothyroidism.

Diagnosis

The diagnosis is made by contrast video fluoroscopy, with which real-time images are obtained while the animal swallows liquid barium or food moistened with barium. Video fluoroscopy allows observation of the process of swallowing in detail and measurement of the duration of each stage in relation to the other. In the case of achalasia, cricopharyngeal muscle hypertrophy is also seen.

Treatment

Treatment of achalasia is by myectomy of the cricopharyngeal muscle, either by surgery or laser.

The success of surgical treatment depends on the following factors:

1. confirmation of achalasia using video fluoroscopy
2. adequate pharyngeal function, assessed via video fluoroscopy
3. exclusion of neuropathies, myopathies and neuromuscular diseases
4. experience of the surgeon
5. absence of complications (for example, aspiration pneumonia).

Botox injection (using toxin from *Clostridium botulinum*, which blocks acetylcholine release) has also been described as treatment for cricopharyngeal achalasia, but the effects last only 2–4 months.

Cricopharyngeal asynchrony

Definition

Cricopharyngeal asynchrony refers to a dis-coordination between pharyngeal contraction and relaxation of the sphincter.

Epidemiology

Cricopharyngeal asynchrony is thought to be more common than achalasia. It occurs in animals of all ages and has been most commonly described in the Golden Retriever.

Aetiology

The aetiology of cricopharyngeal asynchrony is unknown, although a neurological origin is suspected.

Treatment

The treatment for cricopharyngeal asynchrony is supportive. Myotomy and myectomy are contraindicated.

Regurgitation

Aetiology

See Table 7.6.

Table 7.6. Aetiology of regurgitation.

Structural problem in oesophagus	Functional problem (dysmotility)
Oesophagitis	
Gastroesophageal reflux	Central neurological problem
Obstruction	Neuropathy
Oesophageal stenosis	Myopathy
Vascular anomaly	Neuromuscular problem
Neoplasia (oesophageal/ peri-oesophageal)	
Oesophageal diverticulum, broncho-oesophageal fistula	
Injury	

Diagnosis

The diagnostic protocol for regurgitation includes:

1. **summary**: age, breed, species
2. **detailed history**: age when clinical signs commenced, recent anaesthetics, medications, possibility of a foreign body
3. **physical examination**: possibility of aspiration pneumonia, complete neurological examination
4. **diagnostic tests**:
    - **laboratory tests**: complete blood count, biochemistry including CK, ACTH-stimulation test, acetylcholine antibody receptors
    - **diagnostic imaging**: thoracic radiographs, contrast radiographs, fluoroscopy, contrast video fluoroscopy
5. **endoscopy.**

Canine mega-oesophagus

Definition

Mega-oesophagus is characterised by a decrease or absence of oesophageal motility that leads to a diffuse dilation of the oesophagus.

Aetiopathogenesis

Mega-oesophagus can be congenital and manifest after weaning, or acquired as a result of process involving a neuromuscular problem. In most cases, however, the aetiology is not found, and it is considered idiopathic.

Mega-oesophagus is hereditary in the Wire-haired Fox Terrier (autosomal recessive) and the Miniature Schnauzer. Given the high incidences in the following breeds, a hereditary factor is suspected: Great Dane, German Shepherd, Labrador, Terranova, Shar Pei and Irish Setter.

The exact pathogenesis of congenital mega-oesophagus is not known, although some studies in puppies show oesophageal motor function to be impaired. Acquired mega-oesophagus can occur in any breed, but is more common in those breeds at risk of congenital mega-oesophagus.

Numerous neuropathologies, myopathies and neuromuscular diseases can cause acquired mega-oesophagus (Table 7.7).

Myasthenia gravis (MG) is an autoimmune disease that affects neuromuscular transmission. It is the most frequent cause of acquired mega-oesophagus in dogs. MG may be focal, such as mega-oesophagus with the absence of other symptoms, or generalised, including weakness, with or without mega-oesophagus.

The gold standard test for the diagnosis of MG is the **serum acetylcholine receptor (AChR) antibody titre**. This test detects 98% of cases with acquired MG. However, in some cases sero-conversion is observed only after 2–3 months. Also, up to 15% of dogs with focal MG test sero-negative. For this reason, many patients diagnosed with idiopathic mega-oesophagus may actually have focal MG.

In the case of **acquired mega-oesophagus** it is important to rule out the possibility of **concurrent hypothyroidism** or **hypo-adrenocorticism**. When an endocrinopathy is present that is then treated, in some cases the mega-oesophagus resolves whilst in others

Table 7.7. Aetiology of acquired mega-oesophagus.

	Acquired mega-oesophagus
Central nervous system problems	Distemper Lesions in the long bone marrow Neoplasia Trauma
Peripheral neuropathy	Polyneuritis Polyradiculoneuritis, Dysautonomia Intoxication Bilateral damage to the vagus nerve
Neuromuscular disease	Myasthenia gravis Botulism Acetylcholinesterase poisoning
Muscular problem	Oesophagitis (lower sphincter) Polymyositis, Dermatomyositis Addison's disease Hypothyroidism
Other	Pyloric stenosis Gastric torsion Thymoma

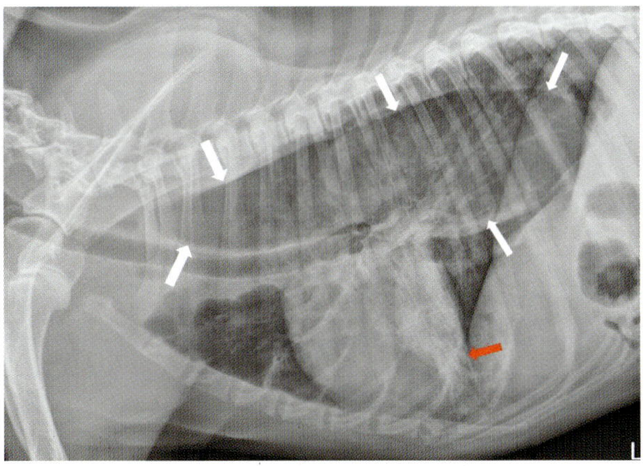

Figure 7.3. Lateral imaging of the thorax showing severe diffuse dilatation of the oesophagus (mega-oesophagus) with an alveolar pattern in the right middle lobe of the lung (aspiration pneumonia secondary to mega-oesophagus).

the mega-oesophagus presents but the clinical signs ease.

Clinical signs

The most frequent clinical signs are regurgitation, dysphagia and ptyalism. Animals with congenital mega-oesophagus are usually the smallest in the litter.

Diagnosis

Mega-oesophagus can generally be confirmed by taking plain thoracic radiographs. In ambiguous cases contrast radiographs or an oesophogram may be necessary to rule out stenosis or a foreign body.

Treatment

In cases of acquired mega-oesophagus it is important to treat the underlying cause, such as correcting hypothyroidism or stabilising hypo-adrenocorticism.

For those patients with idiopathic mega-oesophagus or when mega-oesophagus persists despite treatment, the animal should be fed in the following way.

1. **Feed** in a **vertical position**. To achieve this position the use of a special chair, called the **Bailey chair**, can help. Bailey chairs can be ordered to measure.
2. The dog should remain in the chair for **20–30 minutes** after eating.
3. Some animals respond better to certain types of food than others, e.g. kibble, canned or liquid diets. Trials with different types of food should be carried out to determine which is best for the individual patient. As a general rule, hand-feeding meatballs made from low-fat canned food usually works well.
4. **Multiple meals**, around 3–4 a day, are recommended.
5. Water should also be drunk in a vertical position.

In severe cases, or if the animal is malnourished, it is helpful to place a gastric feeding tube.

Control radiographs are recommended to monitor the progression/resolution of mega-oesophagus or when aspiration pneumonia is suspected. Antibiotic treatment is essential should aspiration pneumonia occur.

Prognosis

Some animals with congenital mega-oesophagus may show improvement over a few months.

Approximately 50% of dogs with acquired idiopathic mega-oesophagus improve with supportive treatment.

The most frequent reasons for euthanasia are recurring episodes of aspiration pneumonia and/or progression of the primary disease.

Oesophagitis

Definition

Oesophagitis is defined as acute or chronic inflammation of the oesophageal mucosa.

Epidemiology

Oesophagitis is seen in cats and dogs of all ages, breeds and in both genders.

Aetiology

Oesophagitis can develop secondary to gastroesophageal reflux, the presence of a foreign body or medications such as tetracycline, clindamycin and alendronate in the cat.

The most common cause of gastroesophageal reflux is relaxation of the oesophageal sphincter under general anaesthesia. It can also occur secondary to a hiatal hernia or persistent vomiting (Figures 7.4–7.6).

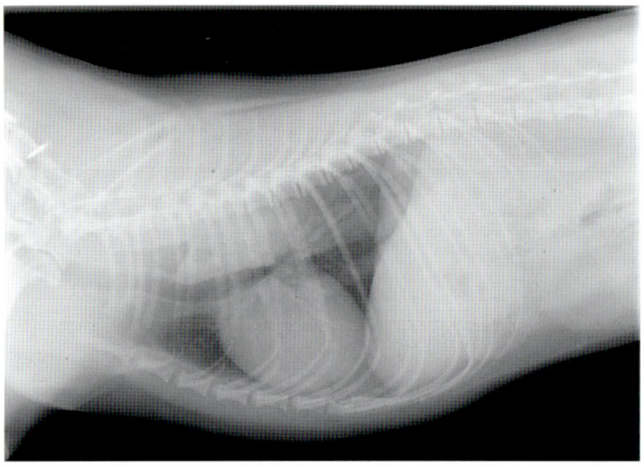

Figure 7.4. Radiography of the thorax demonstrating the presence of a foreign body in the oesophagus.

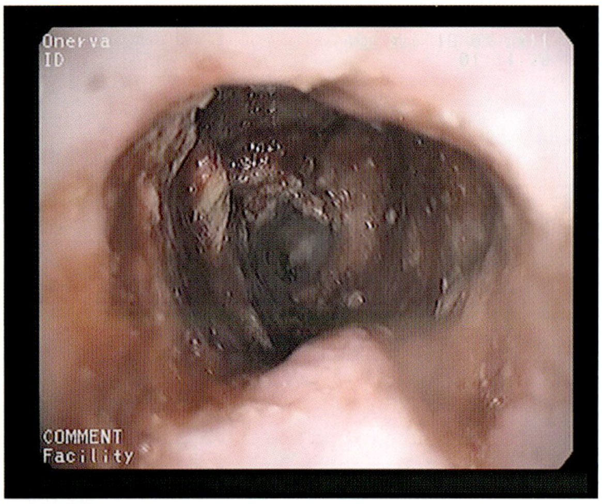

Figure 7.5. Endoscopy. Severe oesophagitis secondary to the presence of a foreign body (bone).

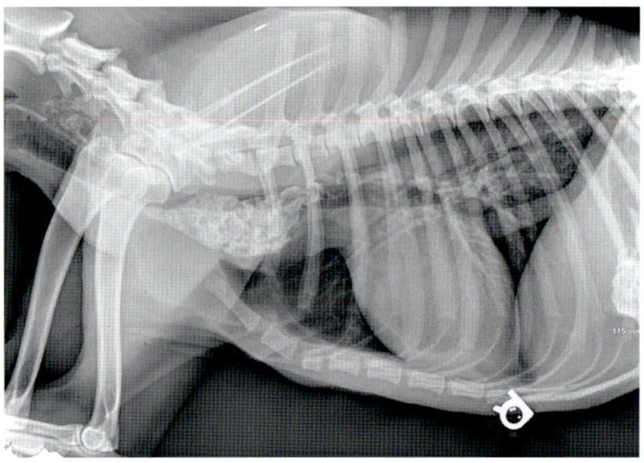

Figure 7.6. Contrast radiographs of a dog with regurgitation and dysphagia 7 days after general anaesthesia for orthopaedic surgery. The radiograph is taken 1 hour after giving a barium feed. A cranial oesophageal stricture can be observed at the base of the heart.

Clinical signs

Animals with moderate to severe oesophagitis may stop eating, regurgitate and show signs of dysphagia or odynophagia (pain upon swallowing, manifested through extension of the neck while swallowing) and ptyalism.

Diagnosis

In the majority of cases a history of recent anaesthesia or the known presence of mega-oesophagus, along with the clinical signs and a good response to treatment, will confirm a suspicion of oesophagitis.

In severe cases, radiographs may show a diffuse area of oesophageal dilation and the diagnosis is then made via endoscopy. This allows visualisation of changes in the texture of the oesophageal mucosa, such as erythema and erosions.

Treatment

The treatment for oesophagitis involves offering small amounts of low-fat food fed at frequent intervals. This stimulates the distal oesophageal sphincter and helps minimise reflux. In addition, dosing with *sucralfate* (0.5–1 g PO TID), will cover and protect the eroded areas from gastric acid.

In moderate cases, in addition to sucralfate, *omeprazole* should be administered (0.5 mg/kg BID) for 2–4 weeks to decrease the acidity of the stomach. Antibiotics are advisable when there is severe ulceration of the mucosa.

Prognosis

In most cases the prognosis is good. However, in severe cases that carry a risk of oesophageal stenosis formation, the prognosis is reserved.

Oesophageal stenosis

Definition

Oesophageal stenosis occurs when circular fibrous tissue forms as a result of a severe oesophagitis, and this results in a narrowing of the oesophageal lumen. In severe cases, the stenosis prevents the passage of the food bolus into the stomach.

Epidemiology

Oesophageal stenosis are more frequent in dogs than in cats, due to the former's less discriminatory eating habits. Stenosis can occur in any part of the oesophagus, but in each individual case this is usually confined to a single area rather than multiple sites.

Aetiology

The two most frequent aetiologies are:

- reflux of stomach acids into the distal oesophagus, especially during **general anaesthesia**
- oesophagitis secondary to a **foreign body**.

Stricture formation leading to stenosis usually occurs 1–3 weeks after the primary insult.

Clinical signs

Animals with **oesophageal stenosis** usually present with **regurgitation**, anorexia and **dysphagia**. These clinical signs are more marked after eating solid food, with water and liquid food being better tolerated.

Diagnosis

Diagnosis is confirmed on contrast radiography using barium, or on endoscopy.

Treatment

Treatment involves breaking down the stenosis with the aid of endoscopy or fluoroscopy, using the **bougienage technique** or **balloon dilation** (Figure 7.7). There are inflatable balloons of varying sizes (up to 20 mm) made from rigid plastic which can withstand a pressure of up to 45 psi, with a manometer connected to facilitate monitoring. Some balloons are introduced through the biopsy channel in the endoscope, while others are advanced using a wire next to the endoscope and placed in the centre of the stenosis.

The position of the balloon is visualised using fluoroscopy or via endoscopy. The balloon is then inflated slowly, controlling the pressure and then left **inflated for 1–2 minutes** at the pressure recommended by the manufacturer, and then deflated. The procedure is **repeated 3–5 times per treatment**. Due to the high recurrence rate, repetition of the procedure is recommended 2–4 times at 2–3-day intervals. Complications of dilatation techniques include bleeding and the risk of perforation.

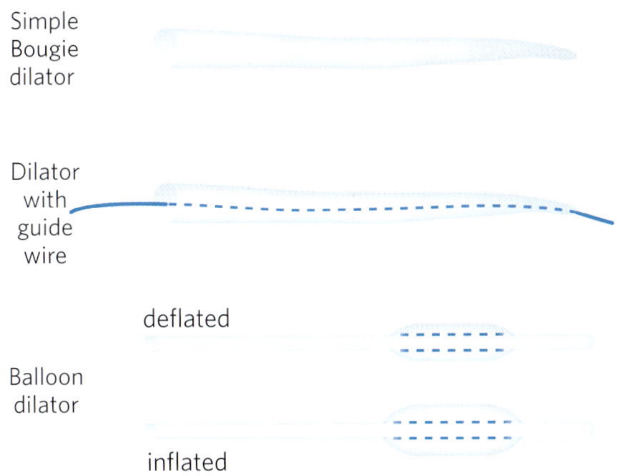

Figure 7.7. Types of dilators available to treat oesophageal stricture. *Illustration: Elaine Leggett.*

Triamcinolone or mitomycin can be injected at the site of the stenosis using endoscopic guidance. However, there are no current studies in veterinary medicine that demonstrate any advantage when compared with dilation without injection.

In recent years, the use of oesophageal stents has been described in animals where stenosis failed to respond to dilation. Once sutured to the oesophageal mucosa (if it is not sutured it rapidly migrates to the stomach), the stent prevents the formation of fibrous tissue.

Another option for palliative treatment in cases of recurring strictures is the placement of a permanent low-profile gastrotomy tube.

Prognosis

Studies indicate a success rate of 77–88% for treatment by dilation. Although the placement of an oesophageal stent has achieved good results in some cases, statistically the success rate is unknown.

Vascular anomalies

Definition

Vascular ring anomalies are congenital malformations of the principal arteries to the heart, which occlude the oesophagus and trachea.

The following anomalies have been described in dogs and cats:

- persistent right aortic arch
- persistent right or left subclavian artery
- persistent right dorsal aorta
- double aortic arch
- left aortic arch and right arterial ligament
- aberrant intercostal arteries.

Epidemiology

The most common vascular ring anomaly in small animals is a **persistent right aortic arch**. Affected animals generally show symptoms from puppyhood, such as **regurgitation** and **delayed growth**, with **aspiration pneumonia** being a frequent complication (Figure 7.8).

Aetiopathogenesis

This is a genetic anomaly and is hereditary in the **German Shepherd**. The Great Dane and Irish Setter also seem over-represented in regard to vascular ring anomalies.

In 95% of cases, as a result of the vascular malformations, a vascular ring forms around the oesophagus. This prevents the normal passage of

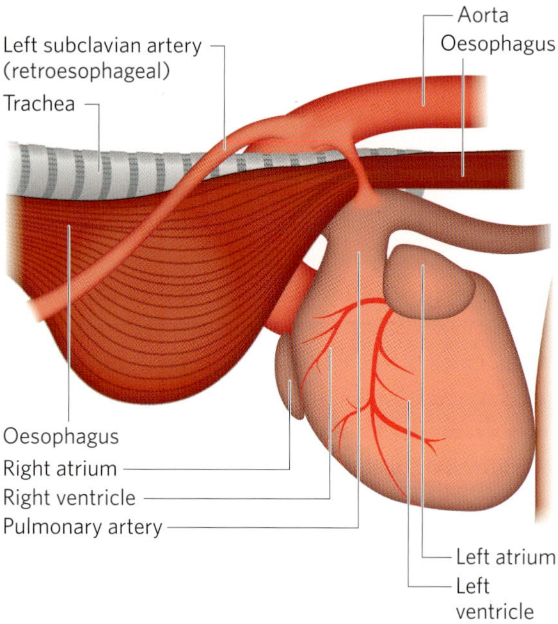

Figure 7.8. Schematic diagram of a persistent right aortic arch. *Illustration: Elaine Leggett.*

food down into the stomach, which results in food retention which then causes an abnormal oesophageal dilation.

Clinical signs

The most common clinical signs include **regurgitation**, which typically starts **after weaning**, weight loss and **delayed growth** (Figure 7.9). Cases that develop aspiration pneumonia as a complication may also be lethargic, pyrexic or dyspnoeic, cough and be exercise intolerant.

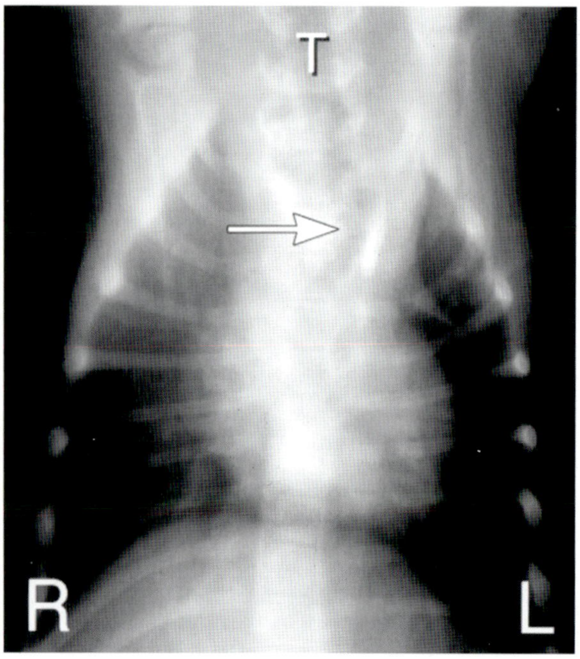

Figure 7.9. Ventrodorsal radiograph of a Golden Retriever puppy with regurgitation. A left deviation of the trachea can be observed (arrow) near the cranial border of the heart. This finding is specific to a persistent right aortic arch (*source: Buchanan JW, JVIM 2004*).

Diagnosis

The diagnosis is based on clinical history and contrast radiographs with barium, which will show a **cranial oesophageal dilatation** at the base of the heart. A study by the University of Philadelphia (USA), observed that moderate **tracheal deviation towards the left** in the chest, in thoracic radiographs without contrast, is typical in animals with a persistent right aortic arch. Focal compression of the trachea was also seen. In these cases, it is not necessary to perform contrast radiographs.

Treatment

Treatment involves thoracotomy to ligate and divide the vascular anomaly.

Prognosis

After surgical correction around 90% of cases improve. However, some patients are left with irreversible oesophageal hypomotility and so their symptoms may persist.

Hiatal hernia

Definition

A hiatal hernia is a protrusion of the stomach through the oesophageal hiatus into the thoracic cavity.

A hiatal hernia is an uncommon cause of chronic vomiting/regurgitation. Hiatal hernias are difficult to diagnose, and once diagnosed, it should be taken into account that they are not always the origin of the animal's clinical signs, since in many cases they do not cause any clinical signs.

Classification

There are two types of hiatal hernia in the dog and cat (Figure 7.10).

- **Sliding**. This is most common. The abdominal portion of the oesophagus and part of the stomach move cranially through the oesophageal hiatus.
- **Paraesophageal**. A part of the stomach herniates towards the mediastinum next to the thoracic oesophagus.

Aetiology

Sliding hiatal hernias can be **congenital** or **acquired**. They have been described in litters of English and French Bulldog puppies, and the Shar Pei (Figure 7.11). In adult animals, a hiatal hernia may be the consequence

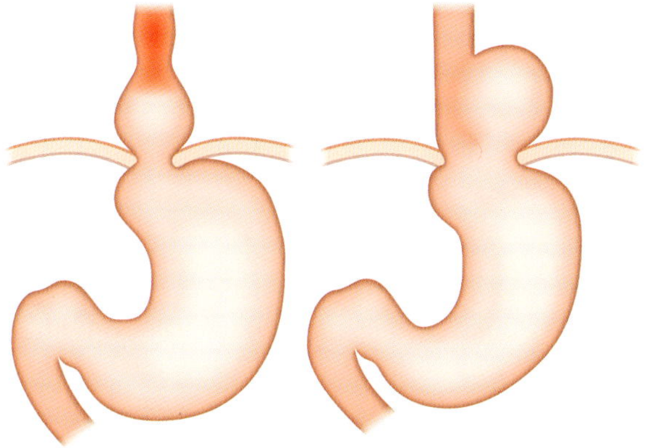

Figure 7.10. Types of hiatal hernia. *Illustration: Elaine Leggett.*

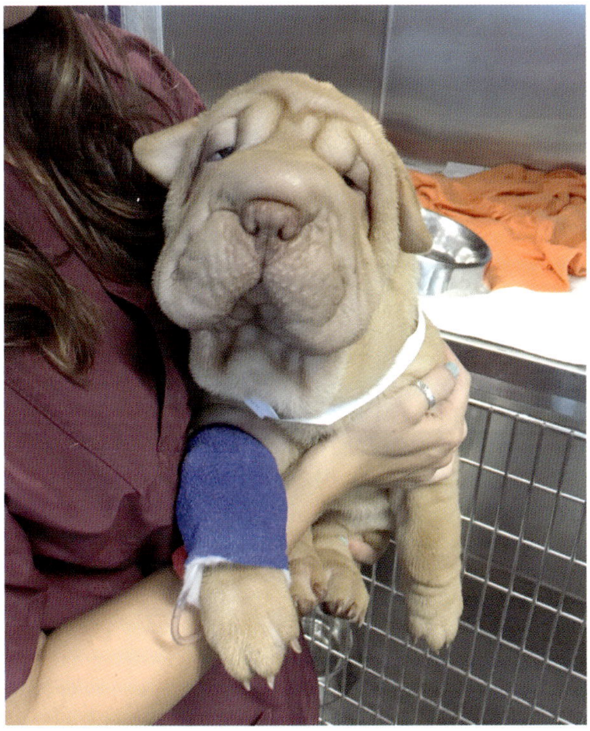

Figure 7.11. Three-month-old Shar Pei puppy with regurgitation.

of a chronic respiratory obstruction, such as laryngeal paralysis or brachiocephalic syndrome.

Clinical signs

Hiatal hernias are not always associated with clinical signs, especially in acquired cases. In congenital forms the clinical signs tend to be more marked and are typically vomiting, regurgitation, hypersalivation, dysphagia, anorexia, weight loss or dyspnoea.

Diagnosis

Thoracic radiographs are useful in the diagnosis of hiatal hernias; however, if the hernia is intermittent then the radiographs may appear normal.

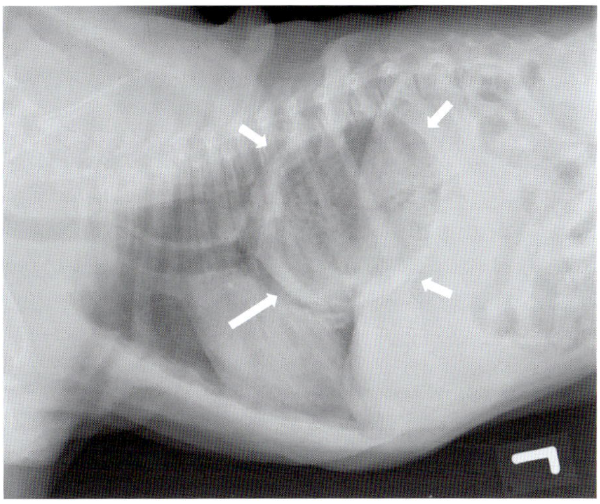

Figure 7.12. Lateral thoracic radiograph showing the presence of a sliding hiatal hernia.

Radiographic findings that typify a hiatal hernia show an intrathoracic soft tissue opacity containing air or dilation of the oesophagus, which can be confused with mega-oesophagus (Figure 7.12).

When a hiatal hernia is suspected but the radiographs are normal, video fluoroscopy will confirm the diagnosis. In cases of intermittent hernia, while fluoroscopy is performed pressure on the abdomen will better demonstrate the herniation.

Alternatively, endoscopy can be used to visualise a hiatal hernia and assess whether oesophagitis is present. Again, applying pressure to the abdomen using a towel encourages the gastric mucosa to protrude into the oesophagus, where it can be seen.

Treatment

When a patient presents with symptoms suggestive of a hiatal hernia, the first option should be conservative medical management with gastric acid suppressants and prokinetics.

Congenital hernias require surgical correction using diaphragmatic plication, oesophagopexy or double gastropexy.

Prognosis

The surgical correction of congenital cases generally carries a good to excellent prognosis.

Diarrhoea

Definition

Diarrhoea is defined as the elimination of stools that are more liquid than normal.

Introduction

Diarrhoea is one of the most commonly presented problems seen in small animal clinics. For young animals in particular, it can be important to reach a diagnosis quickly and start appropriate treatment. However, there are many differential diagnoses for diarrhoea and the condition can be complex, more so even than for vomiting.

The investigatory approach for in animals with chronic small or large intestinal diarrhoea depends on the severity of the clinical signs. Factors that influence decision making include the severity and frequency of the diarrhoea, excessive weight loss, decreased appetite and the presence of hypalbuminaemia, intestinal thickening or mesenteric lymphadenopathy.

The **severity** of the intestinal disease can be **quantified** by determining the **Canine IBD activity index (CIBDAI)**. This takes into account the attitude, activity, appetite, vomiting, stool consistency, frequency of bowel movements and weight loss (Table 7.8). Recording a score on this index facilitates both an initial assessment and the subsequent evaluation of response to therapy.

Table 7.8. Canine IBD activity index (CIBDAI).

CIBDAI	
Activity/ attitude	0 = normal. 1 = slightly reduced. 2 = moderately reduced. 3 = severely reduced.
Appetite	0 = normal. 1 = slightly reduced. 2 = moderately reduced. 3 = severely reduced.
Vomiting	0 = none. 1 = approximately once a week. 2 = 2–3 times a week. 3 = >3 times a week.
Stool consistency	0 = normal. 1 = soft or pasty, or with blood or mucus present. 2 = very soft. 3 = liquid diarrhoea.
Frequency of defaecation	0 = normal. 1 = slightly increased (2–3 times per day). 2 = moderately increased (4–5 times per day). 3 = greatly increased (>5 times per day).
Weight loss	0 = none. 1 = slight (<5%). 2 = moderate (5–10%). 3 = serious (>10%).

The CIBDAI is equal to the sum of the scores of each of the clinical signs. CIBDAI classification:
0–3. Low.
4–5. Slight.
6–8. Moderate.
>9. High.

Classification and aetiology

Diarrhoea can be classified according to:

- **duration**: acute or chronic
- **mechanism:** secretory, osmotic, exudative or mixed
- **anatomy**: small intestinal, large intestinal or mixed origin
- **physiopathology**: allergic, infectious or neoplastic.

Clinical signs

In order to draw up a list of differential diagnoses and minimise the tests required to reach a definitive diagnosis, a complete and **detailed clinical history** is essential. To this end, it is important to collect information about the animal's diet and environment, the frequency of deworming, vaccination (especially relevant in puppies) and the presence of other clinical signs such as a coughing, vomiting, polyuria and polydipsia, weight loss and appetite changes.

Basic parameters to establish are:

1. whether the diarrhoea is acute (<1–2 weeks) or chronic (>2 weeks' duration)
2. whether the diarrhoea is from the small or large intestine or mixed (see Tables 7.9 and 7.10).

Once the history is obtained, a full systematic physical examination should be undertaken.

In cases of acute or severe, chronic diarrhoea the animal may present with **signs of dehydration**, such as prolonged capillary refill time, enopthalmos, delayed skin tenting, tachycardia and cold or dry mucous membranes. For mild, chronic diarrhoea the physical examination is often normal, except for thickened loops of intestine and weight loss.

Table 7.9. Differential diagnosis of small and large intestinal diarrhoea.

	Small intestine	Large intestine
Weight loss	Yes	No (with exceptions)
Frequency	Normal	Increased
Volume	Large quantity	Small quantity
Flatulence	Yes	No
Body condition	Good to bad	Good (with exceptions)
Tenesmus	No	Yes
Presence of blood	Melaena	Haematochezia
Emergency	No	Yes
Mucus	No	Yes

Table 7.10. Aetiological classification of diarrhoea.

Acute diarrhoea		Chronic diarrhoea	
Gastrointestinal aetiology	**Non-gastrointestinal aetiology**	**Small intestine**	**Large intestine**
Infectious Parasites: *Trichuris, Ancylostoma, Uncinaria, Toxocara, Toxascaris, Giardia, Coccidia* Viruses: coronavirus, parvovirus, FeLV, FIV, distemper		Intolerance/dietary allergy Giardiosis, parasites Intestinal bacterial overgrowth Exocrine pancreatic insufficiency	Intolerance/dietary allergy Fibre-responsive diarrhoea Parasites: (*Tritrichomonas foetus* in the cat) Enterotoxicosis due to *Cl. perfringens*
Bacteria: *Salmonella, Clostridia perfringens, Campylobacter jejuni, Yersinia enterocolitica, E. coli*	Acute liver/hepatobiliary disease Acute kidney disease Hypo-adrenocorticism (Addisonian crisis) Acute pancreatitis	Partial obstruction (foreign body, neoplasia) Intestinal lymphangiectasia Neoplasia Chronic intestinal inflammation	Neoplasia Chronic intestinal inflammatory disease Hypo-adrenocorticism (dog)
Non-infectious Dietary: intolerance, allergies, off food, sharp change in diet		Hyperthyroidism (cat)	Granulomatous/histiocytic colitis (entero-invasive *E. coli*)
Idiopathic Acute Haemorrhagic Diarrhoea Syndrome Intussusception, partial obstruction (foreign body) Drugs/toxins		Pythiosis and histoplasmosis (only in endemic areas)	FeLV/FIV Uraemic colitis, Eosinophilic colitis, Histoplasmosis

The **abdomen** should be carefully **palpated** to detect abnormalities such as enlarged intestines that are distended with gas, fluid or ingested content; abdominal masses, organomegaly, foreign bodies or ascites. Rectal palpation should be performed in all cases to detect pain, intraluminal masses, foreign bodies, blood, sublumbar lymphadenopathy or perineal hernia.

Key points: Small intestinal diarrhoea is associated with weight loss, due to the decreased absorption of nutrients. It should be remembered that small intestinal diarrhoea can be due to a primary systemic disease that is non-gastrointestinal, such as hypoadrenocorticism, renal disease, heart disease or feline hyperthyroidism.

Diagnosis

In severe or chronic cases of diarrhoea, **parasitic disease** should always be ruled out. Subsequent to this, take a broad diagnostic view that investigates both gastrointestinal and non-gastrointestinal causes of disease.

An **essential** part of investigation for dogs with diarrhoea (of both large and small intestinal origin) is a **microscopic analysis of faeces**, using a direct smear or faecal flotation technique. Stool examination allows for the identification of eggs, larvae, cysts and adult forms of parasitic disease, which may otherwise be overlooked.

Giardia

Note that routine faecal flotation is **insensitive** for the **identification of** Giardia. Preferred is the **zinc sulfate sediment test**, which has 75% sensitivity on a single test and more than 95% when performed on three samples obtained on consecutive days. The **SNAP Elisa test** for *Giardia* is also sensitive and a good option for detection.

Acute diarrhoea

A **complete blood count** and **biochemistry profile**, along with **stool analysis**, are recommended for the investigation of acute diarrhoea (Table 7.11).

Bacterial causes of acute diarrhoea

With a few exceptions, **primary bacterial** infections are an **infrequent** cause of diarrhoea in dogs and cats. This is because the flora of the intestine prevents colonisation of pathogenic bacteria and promotes a healthy enteric immune system. However, infections linked to

Table 7.11. Differential diagnosis of acute uncomplicated and complicated diarrhoea.

Acute uncomplicated diarrhoea	Acute complicated diarrhoea
Benign cause identified	Complicated cause found
Infrequent/non-severe diarrhoea	Frequent/severe diarrhoea
Animal stable, not dehydrated, normal physical examination	Animal sick, dehydrated or abnormal physical examination
Animal drinking water normally	
Minimum diagnosis	Diagnostic plan
Symptomatic treatment	Aggressive treatment

pathogenic bacteria can pose a diagnostic challenge, as these bacteria can also be a coincidental finding in healthy animals. Their presence in sick animals may be **opportunistic** and secondary to intestinal disease associated with another process.

These pathogenic bacteria include: *Campylobacter*, *Clostridium perfringens* and *Cl. difficile*, *Salmonella spp.*, *Yersinia* and *Escherichia coli*.

Faecal analysis is useful in cases of acute diarrhoea:

- *direct analysis*: This should be performed on fresh samples less than 1 hour old.
- *floatation and centrifugation with zinc sulfate*: For maximum sensitivity (>95%), this test is best performed on three stool samples obtained on different days.
- *tritrichomonas foetus* PCR and/or culture: Indicated for feline cases with large intestinal diarrhoea.
- *faecal culture*: To detect *Salmonella* spp. in cases of fever, haemorrhagic diarrhoea or leucopenia.
- *giardia antigen test*.
- *Elisa SNAP for parvovirus*.

When the physical examination shows significant changes such as fever, melaena, petechiae, azotaemia or suspected sepsis, additional diagnostic tests are indicated, such as radiography or abdominal ultrasound.

Treatment

The majority of cases of acute diarrhoea will **resolve** when the **primary cause** is addressed, such as a sudden change of diet or parasites, and/or with symptomatic treatment.

Appropriate diet

Animals with **acute diarrhoea** benefit from an **easily digestible diet**. Home-made options include boiled rice and chicken, with rice or fresh cheese. This should be given **little and often**. Alternatively, many easily digestible commercial diets are available. Once the diarrhoea is resolved, the patient's regular diet should be gradually reintroduced over the course of several days.

Cases with **mild dehydration** will benefit from the administration of **subcutaneous fluids**. However, when marked dehydration is present then hospitalisation is required, for aggressive **intravenous fluid** therapy. The volume of fluid required is calculated by adding together the patient's maintenance requirements, the percentage dehydration and the volume of fluid lost through sickness and diarrhoea. Potassium supplementation may be necessary, as indicated on blood tests.

Chronic small intestinal diarrhoea

Diagnosis

Screening blood tests

In cases of chronic small intestinal diarrhoea, a complete blood count, biochemistry and urinalysis are often normal, with some exceptions (Figure 7.13).

Eosinophilia

When present, eosinophilia can be indicative of intestinal parasitism, chronic inflammation (IBD) or hypo-adrenocorticism.

Hypoproteinaemia

Pan-hypoproteinaemia refers to the presence of both hypoalbuminaemia and hypoglobulinaemia. When this occurs **without anaemia**, it is suggestive of **protein loss** from the gastrointestinal tract and so-called **protein-losing enteropathy** (Figure 7.14). For dogs with chronic enteropathy, some studies indicate that the presence of hypalbuminaemia is associated with a worse prognosis.

Hyperthyroidism

T4 hormone levels should be measured in adult cats aged 6 years or over with chronic diarrhoea.

FeLV and FIV

Where the history suggests the possibility of FIV or FeLV infection, the status of these viruses should be established.

Exocrine pancreatic insufficiency

In dogs and cats with chronic small intestinal diarrhoea, it is important to rule out exocrine pancreatic insufficiency. This is done by measuring TLI, with

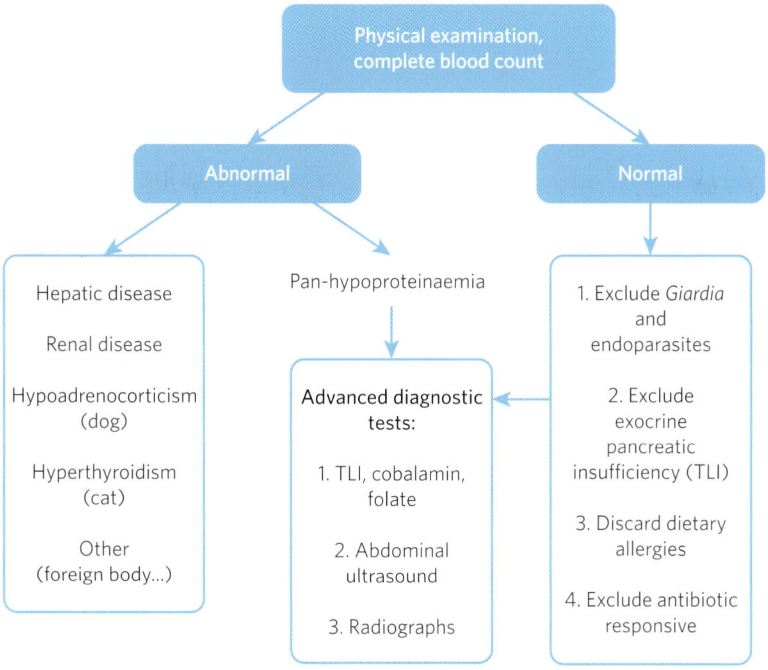

Figure 7.13. Diagnostic approach to chronic small intestinal diarrhoea.

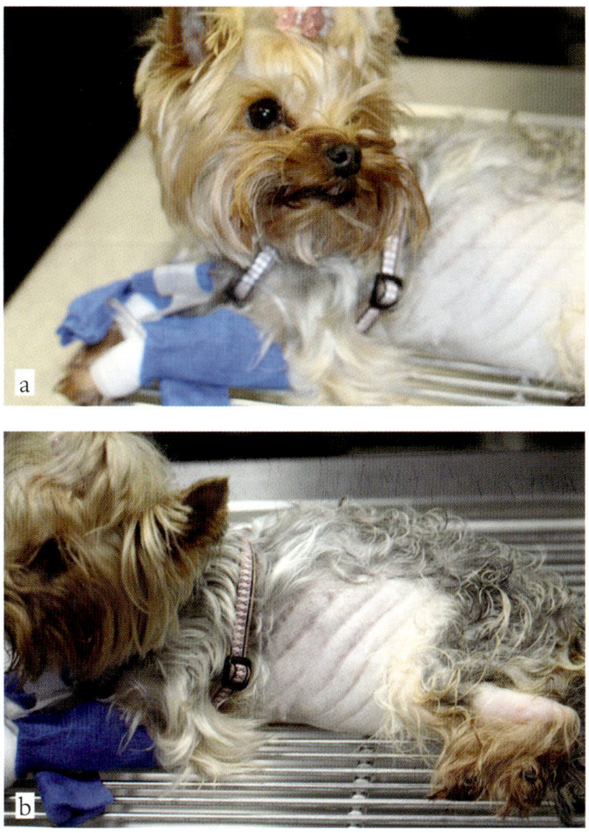

Figure 7.14. A 7-year-old Yorkshire Terrier bitch with protein-losing enteropathy. Severe peripheral oedema can be observed in the image (particularly in the tarsus [b]). The animal presented with abdominal effusion and diarrhoea. After putting it in a bath covered with a grid, the grid left a mark on the skin due to the oedema.

concentrations >5 μg/l indicative of normal exocrine pancreatic function.

Hypocobalaminaemia

In dogs with small intestinal diarrhoea, measurement of circulating concentrations of **cobalamin** and **folate** may give an indirect indication of the location and cause of bowel dysfunction.

Low serum concentrations of cobalamin are observed in dogs with:

- exocrine pancreatic insufficiency
- diffuse ileal disease
- bacterial overgrowth in the small intestine.

Animals with hypocobalaminaemia will benefit from **parenteral supplementation**. However, the interpretation of circulating concentrations of cobalamin in relation to small intestine disease is valid only if TLI levels rule out exocrine pancreatic insufficiency.

Basal cortisol

In dogs with a history of unexplained recurrent gastrointestinal signs such as vomiting, diarrhoea or anorexia, even in the absence of hyperkalaemia or hyponatremia, an ACTH-stimulation test should be performed, or basal cortisol levels should be measured, in order to rule out **hypo-adrenocorticism**, before performing a gastrointestinal biopsy.

Mycosis

In animals from areas where mycosis is endemic in the USA, pythiosis or histoplasmosis should be ruled out, especially if there is chorioretinitis, lymphadenopathy, hyperglobulinaemia or pulmonary changes.

Additional diagnostic tests

Radiography

Abdominal radiographs are often unhelpful in cases of chronic diarrhoea. However, they do facilitate the detection of ascites, help detect the presence of a foreign body and assist in evaluation of abdominal organs such as the prostate, kidneys, liver and spleen.

Ultrasonography

Abdominal ultrasound is always indicated in cases of chronic small intestinal diarrhoea or when there is an abnormality on abdominal palpation such as organomegaly, mass effect or an effusion. Ultrasound also facilitates the targeted harvesting of samples for cytology from abdominal organs and ascitic fluid.

Biopsy

For many conditions, biopsy is required to reach a definitive diagnosis (Table 7.12).

With diffuse intestinal diseases and in animals with hypoproteinaemia, endoscopy allows biopsies to be obtained non-invasively and at low risk. If endoscopy is not possible or obtaining biopsies of other organs is indicated, an exploratory celiotomy should be used.

The pros and cons of gastrointestinal endoscopy should be taken into account.

- Endoscopic biopsies are **restricted to the mucosa**. Surgical biopsies are necessary in patients with focal intestinal lesions in the submucosal or muscular layers where lymphoma is suspected and when endoscopic biopsy does not provide a diagnosis.
- Endoscopically harvested **samples are small** in comparison to surgical biopsies.
- Samples can be obtained only from the **proximal duodenum** and, occasionally, from the distal ileum.

Recent studies have shown that obtaining samples from the ileum, in addition to the duodenum and stomach, increases the sensitivity of the diagnosis in the small intestine, especially in cases of lymphoma. The decision to perform both colonoscopy and gastro-duodenoscopy is dependent on the patient, whilst balancing the advantages and disadvantages of performing two endoscopies as opposed to only a gastro-duodenoscopy or laparotomy.

Once parasitic, foreign body, primary non-gastrointestinal disease, exocrine pancreatic insufficiency and processes that require surgery are excluded, the most common diagnosis are:

- chronic inflammatory bowel disease
- dietary-responsive enteropathy
- lymphangiectasia (Figure 7.15).

Treatment of chronic small intestinal diarrhoea

In mild chronic cases where the patient is in good body condition, and there is no protein-losing enteropathy or hypocobalaminaemia, then feeding a **hypo-allergenic diet** is appropriate. This should be given to the exclusion of all other foods and continued for at least one month. A remission of the diarrhoea is diagnostic of food allergy or dietary intolerance.

If there is no response to diet, then treatment with *metronidazole* (10–15 mg/kg BID) or *tylosin* (8–15 mg/kg

Table 7.12. Advantages and disadvantages of biopsies obtained via endoscopy and exploratory laparotomy.

	Advantages	Disadvantages
Endoscopy	Less invasive, very quick recovery.	Only 1–1.5 m of intestine is examined.
	Visualization of oesophagus, stomach, duodenum and colon.	Superficial biopsies of mucosa, not submucosa, muscular or serosal layers (insensitive in some cases). Biopsy quality depends on the instrument and the endoscopist.
Laparotomy	Allows submucosal, muscular and serosal biopsies and can therefore be used to diagnose disease affecting deeper layers.	More invasive, requires a longer hospitalisation and is painful.
	Allows examination and biopsy of all parts of the intestine. Allows biopsy of other organs and lymph nodes, or placement of a gastric tube.	In the case of hypo-albuminaemia, there is the risk of dehiscence and complications. Biopsies of the large intestine are rarely obtained by this means.

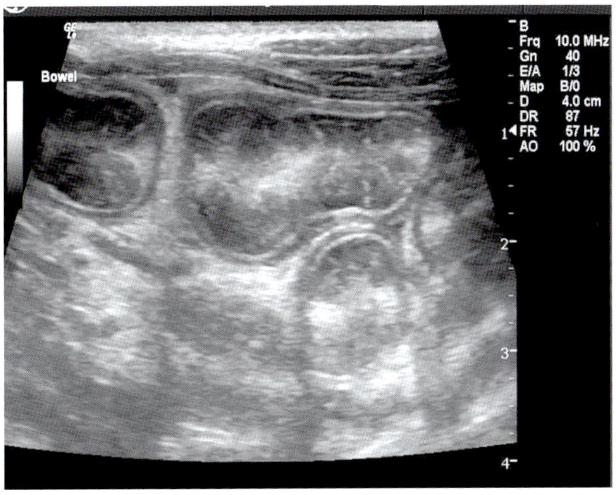

Figure 7.15. Abdominal ultrasound image (longitudinal and transverse sections of the ileum); there are hyper-echogenic striations at the level of the mucosal layer. The definitive diagnosis was intestinal lymphangiectasia and IBD.

TID) is recommended. A good response is suggestive of an antibiotic-responsive enteropathy, and a 4–6-week course of treatment given.

When severe hypocobalaminaemia is present, intestinal biopsies are indicated to establish a definitive diagnosis.

Chronic inflammatory intestinal disease

Definition

Inflammatory bowel disease (IBD) includes a group of enteropathies of uncertain aetiology, which are characterised by infiltration of the gastrointestinal mucosa with inflammatory cells. This cellular infiltrate is composed of lymphocytes, plasma cells, eosinophils, macrophages or a combination thereof.

Aetiopathogenesis

Although the aetiopathogenesis of IBD is not entirely understood, studies indicate the enteric microflora, dietary factors and genetic influence all have a part to play.

Enteric microflora appear to have a role in the initiation and perpetuation of intestinal inflammation in both cats and dogs. Whilst **dietary factors** also seem important in the pathogenesis of IBD, given the improvement shown by many affected individuals on an elimination or hypo-allergenic diet. Finally, there is a strong **genetic predisposition** to the development of IBD as described below:

- lymphoplasmacytic enteritis in the Basenji, German Shepherd and Shar Pei
- eosinophilic enteritis in the Rottweiler
- gluten-sensitive enteropathy in the Irish Setter
- protein-losing enteropathy in the Soft-coated Wheaten Terrier
- lymphangiectasia in the Yorkshire Terrier.

Treatment

Treating chronic IBD can be a challenge because there is often no clear aetiopathogenesis, making it difficult to select the best treatment (Table 7.13).

With IBD the goal of treatment is not necessarily to cure, but to **control the clinical signs** and prevent complications. Indeed, studies show that even with apparently successful treatment, a degree of intestinal inflammation persists.

Possible treatment options include:

- diet
- antibiotics
- immunosuppressant medications
- a combination of the above.

The choice depends upon the severity of the symptoms, histopathology and presence or absence of hypocobalaminaemia or hypoalbuminaemia. In recent years attempts have been made to standardise treatment, using an index of activity (CIBDAI) (see Table 7.8).

Low index of clinical activity

Characterised by normal histopathology and **normal albumin** concentration.

1. Empirical treatment for Giardia and **endoparasites**: *Fenbendazole* 50 mg/kg VPO × 5 days.
2. **Hypo-allergenic diet** with novel or hydrolysed protein. Introduce the diet gradually, over 4–7 days. A good response indicates a diet-responsive enteropathy or food intolerance.
3. **Antibiotic treatment**: *Tylosin* (10–15 mg/kg TID PO) or *metronidazole* (10 mg/kg BID PO). These antibiotics have immunomodulatory properties. A good response is indicative of an antibiotic-responsive protein-losing enteropathy.

Mild to moderate index of clinical activity

Characterised by mild-to-moderate lymphoplasmacytic inflammation on histopathology, and **albumin >2 g/l**.

1. Empirical treatment for Giardia and **endoparasites**: *Fenbendazole* 50 mg/kg PO × 5 days.
2. Offer a **hydrolysed protein diet** for a minimum of 2 weeks.

Table 7.13. Medications used to treat chronic inflammatory bowel disease.

Medication	Mechanism of action	Species	Dose	Adverse effects
Prednisone/ prednisolone	Immunosuppression	Dog/cat	1–2 mg/kg/12 h VO/IV	Polyuria/polydipsia, abdominal distention, iatrogenic HAC, hypercoagulability, infections
Budesonide	Anti-inflammatory	Dog	Small–medium dog: 1 mg Large dog: 2mg	
Azathioprine	Immunosuppression	Dog	2 mg/kg/d or 50 mg/m^2 VO 1–2 weeks, after every 2 days Reduce dose in large dogs	Hepatotoxicity Anorexia Pancreatitis Non-regenerative anaemia takes weeks to take effect
Sulfasalazine	Anti-inflammatory-specific at the level of the large intestine (binds to bacteria in the colon)	Dog	20–40 mg/kg TID for 3 weeks, then 20–40 mg/kg/12 h BID for 3 weeks, after 10–20 mg/kg BID	Anorexia Vomiting Allergic dermatitis Keratoconjunctivitis sicca Not useful in cases of small intestinal IBD
Cyclosporine	Immunosuppression	Dog/cat	5 mg/kg/day	Secondary infections, gingival hyperplasia
Chlorambucil	Immunosuppression	Dog/cat	Dog: 1.5 mg/m^2 every 2 days Cat: 15 mg/m^2 VO then repeat every 3 weeks	Neutropenia Anaemia
Aspirin	Platelet antiaggregant	Dog	0.5 mg/kg/day VO	
Clopidogrel	Platelet antiaggregant	Dog	1-2 mg/kg/day VO	
Metronidazole	Antibiotic, immunomodulator	Dog	15 mg/kg/12 h VO	Hepatotoxicity, vestibular signs
Tylosin	Antibiotic, immunomodulator	Dog	10–15 mg/kg TID VO	
Cobalamin	Vitamin	Dog/cat	<5 kg: 250 mcg SC <10 kg: 400 mcg SC <20 kg: 600 mcg SC <40 kg: 1000 mcg SC <50 kg: 1200 mcg SC >50 kg: 1400 mcg SC	

3. **Antibiotic treatment** for two weeks (tylosin or metronidazole as above). If there is good response, continue for 1 month.
4. **Immunosuppressive treatment** with *glucocorticoids*: 2 mg/kg/day PO for 2–4 weeks (until there is clinical remission) and decrease progressively over 2–3 months.

Or *Budesonide*, a corticosteroid similar to hydroxyprednisolone, has a very high anti-inflammatory activity due to its high affinity to steroid receptors and its hepatic conversion to metabolites with minimal steroid activity. It has fewer systemic effects than the remainder of the corticosteroids. The dose used in small dogs is 1 mg/day, and in large dogs 2 mg/day.

If the response to treatment is poor, consider adding in another immunosuppressant:

- *azathioprine* (only in dogs): 2 mg/kg/day 5 days and then 2 mg/kg every 2 days (consider reducing dose in large dogs, to minimise the risk of toxicity)
- *cyclosporine*: 5 mg/kg/day PO
- *chlorambucil* (in cats): 2-6–2 mg/m2 BID.

If the response to treatment is good, reduce immunosuppression gradually. First reduce the dose of corticosteroids and slowly cease administration, and then finally stop the second immunosuppressant.

Moderate to severe index of clinical activity

Characterised by moderate–severe histopathological changes and **albumin <2.0 g/l**.

1. Empirical treatment for Giardia and **endoparasites**: *Fenbendazole* 50 mg/kg VO × 5 days.
2. Feed a **hydrolysed protein diet**.

3. **Antibiotic treatment** (tylosin or metronidazole) for 2 weeks. If the response is good, continue for 1 month.
4. **Immunosuppressive** treatment with glucocorticoids. If the response to treatment is low, consider adding in another immunosuppressant (azathioprine, cyclosporine, chlorambucil). If there is no response or low intestinal absorption is suspected, consider injectable corticosteroids.
5. Consider treatment with **antithrombotic agents** (*aspirin* 0.5 mg/kg or *clopidogrel* 1 mg/kg/day), since patients with enteropathy due to protein loss are at risk of thromboembolic disease due to the loss of antithrombin-3 in the intestine.
6. In the case of **hypocobalaminaemia**, administer injections of cobalamin once a week for 4 weeks, followed by once a month for 3 months. Then, repeat the measurement of serum cobalamin.

Protein-losing enteropathies

Definition

Protein-losing enteropathy (PLE) is not a diagnosis as such, but a syndrome which means there is a **severe primary intestinal problem** resulting in **malabsorption** of protein in the intestine leading to **pan-hypoproteinaemia**.

Aetiology

- **Inflammatory** causes: lymphoplasmacytic, eosinophilic or granulomatous enteritis.
- **Lymphangiectasia**: primary or associated with portal hypertension due to liver failure or congestive heart failure.
- **Neoplastic** infiltration such as lymphoma.
- **Infectious** causes: Parvovirus, Salmonella, parasites such as pythiosis, ancylostoma, histoplasmosis or severe fungal disease.
- **Structural** problem (intussusception).

Epidemiology

Breeds predisposed to PLE include the Basenji, Lundenhund, Soft-coated Wheaten Terrier, Yorkshire Terrier and Shar Pei.

Clinical signs

Clinical signs are **highly variable**: weight loss (without vomiting or diarrhoea), diarrhoea, vomiting, melaena, **peripheral oedema**, ascites and **pleural effusion** due to low oncotic pressure. With the latter, an animal with PLE can present with dyspnoea as a principal clinical sign. In some cases, there is an aortic thrombosis (and therefore lameness and mono- or paraparesis) due to a state of hypercoagulability associated with the loss of protein at the intestinal level.

Many animals with chronic enteropathy show only weight loss, sometimes with a very good appetite, without any other clinical signs, whilst Yorkshire Terriers with PLE frequently have abdominal or pleural effusion as the sole clinical sign.

Diagnosis

Animals with PLE almost always have **hypoalbuminaemia** and **hypoglobulinaemia**. Exceptionally, these may present with hyperglobulinaemia due either to breed predisposition (for example, the Basenji) or to another systemic process. There is also usually **hypocholesterolaemia** on serum biochemistry, and a complete blood count generally reveals **lymphopenia**.

If there is **pleural or abdominal effusion** the fluid is a **pure transudate**, with very low protein levels and cellularity.

In addition, some animals with PLE, especially Yorkshire Terriers with lymphangiectasia, present with **hypocalcaemia** and **hypomagnesaemia**, which can cause neurological signs. These alterations are associated with malabsorption and failures in vitamin D metabolism and parathyroid hormone (PTH). Therefore, it is important to measure these electrolytes in the Yorkshire Terrier where PLE is suspected.

There is a commercial test that allows confirmation of protein loss in faeces (inhibitor of alpha-1 proteinase inhibitor). However, where the suspicion arises of an enteropathy due to loss of protein, it is important to rule out protein loss at a renal level (with urinalysis with or without urine protein:creatinine ratio) and to exclude liver disease (bile acid stimulation test).

Hypercoagulability-associated PLE has been widely described, although the exact pathogenesis is unknown. It is suspected that the **loss of antithrombin** through the intestine, along with albumin, are just two of the factors that contribute to hypercoagulability.

Very often, animals with PLE have **hypocobalaminaemia**.

Abdominal ultrasound facilitates the detection of abdominal fluid and visualisation of the small intestine.

Finally, the definitive diagnosis of the primary enteropathy depends on obtaining **intestinal biopsies** by endoscopy or laparotomy. Due to hypo-albuminaemia and the risk associated with abdominal surgery, biopsies are usually obtained by endoscopy although the sensitivity required to obtain a diagnosis (especially for neoplasms or lymphangiectasia) is lower than with biopsies obtained by surgery. Endoscopic biopsies must be of high quality and contain the entire thickness of the mucosal layer. In Yorkshire Terriers with PLE, the most common abnormalities on intestinal biopsy are lacteal dilatation, mucosal fibrosis and dilation of the crypts. Lymphoplasmacytic or neutrophilic inflammation can also co-exist.

Treatment

Supportive treatment

Thoracentesis is indicated in the case of dyspnoea, due to the presence of pleural fluid.

In the case of abdominal effusion, abdominocentesis is not necessary unless the distension is causing the animal discomfort.

If the animal is dehydrated due to diarrhoea, the fluids of choice are a combination of crystalloids and a synthetic colloid, to increase oncotic pressure and prevent the progression of the oedema. When an animal presents with **hypocalcaemia**, the concentration of magnesium should be measured, and fluids should be supplemented with *calcium gluconate* (10 mg/kg/h IV) and *magnesium sulfate* (1 mEq/kg/day IV).

Aspirin (0.5 mg/kg/day PO) or *clopidogrel* is recommended to prevent the formation of thrombi, until the primary process is under control.

Where **serum cobalamin levels** are low, supplementation with **subcutaneous vitamin B12** is appropriate. In cases of deficiency of cobalamin, this should be replaced at a dose of 50 µg/kg SC once per week for 6 weeks, then once every 2 weeks for 6 weeks and, after that, once per month for 2–3 months. After this time serum levels should be reassessed. If the intestinal problem persists, cobalamin supplementation may be necessary on an ongoing basis.

In cases of IBD or lymphangiectasia secondary to IBD, a **hypo-allergenic diet** is recommended, preferably with lyophilised proteins and restricted fat (e.g. Hill's Z/D).

In cases of **severe ascites**, loop diuretics (*furosemide* 1.2–2 mg/kg, SC or PO) can help decrease the amount of pleural or abdominal effusion, although it is important to assess hydration and blood volume status on a regular basis, as well as monitor potassium concentrations. Potassium-sparing diuretics (e.g. *spironolactone* at a dose of 2–4 mg/kg PO) can be used in combination with furosemide, to prevent hypokalaemia.

Specific treatment

This depends on the histopathological diagnosis (e.g. neoplasia, lymphangiectasia, chronic intestinal inflammation). It usually includes the use of **immunosuppressants** (*prednisolone* 2–4 mg/kg/day). In refractory cases, a second immunosuppressive is often necessary (*azathioprine, cyclosporine*). In animals in which the side effects of glucocorticoids are intolerable, the use of *budesonide* to substitute prednisolone may be preferable.

Chronic large intestinal diarrhoea

Introduction

For patients with chronic large intestinal diarrhoea, the first tests to perform are stool analysis and rectal cytology, the latter helping in the detection of neoplasia or fungal disease. See Figure 7.16 for a diagnosis algorithm.

The most common infectious causes of chronic large intestinal diarrhoea are:

- clostridial disease
- *tritrichomonas foetus*
- *E. coli.*

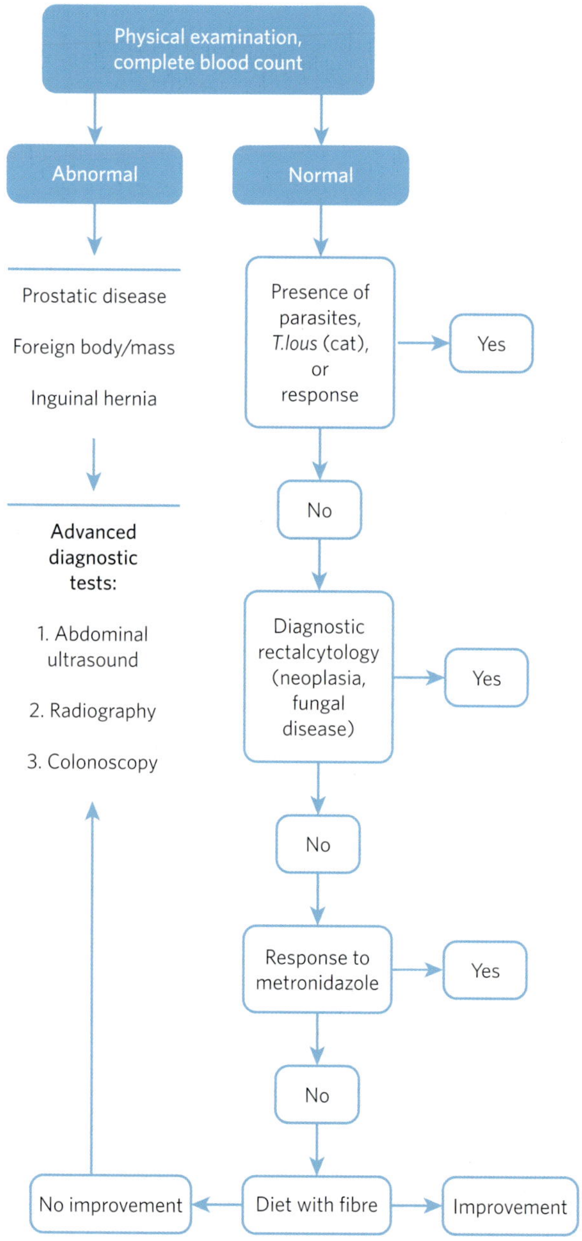

Figure 7.16. Diagnostic approach to chronic diarrhoea of large intestinal origin.

Clostridial disease: overview

Clostridial disease can be hard to diagnose definitively, as *Clostridium perfringens* is a normal part of the intestinal flora and found also in the environment. This means that an anaerobic spore count is not an accurate way of diagnosing active infection.

However, *Cl. perfringens* **types A** and *Cl. difficile* can be pathogenic and cause **endotoxaemia** in dogs.

Cl. perfringens type A is often referred to as **enterotoxigenic** *Cl. perfringens* (**CPE**) because it produces enterotoxins. CPE is associated with nosocomial diarrhoea, haemorrhagic enteritis and acute small or large intestinal diarrhoea.

Cl. difficile produces two important toxins (A and B) and can cause enterocolitis. For diagnosis of enterotoxaemia caused by *Cl. perfringens* or *Cl. difficile*, the presence of toxins can be detected using a specific Elisa test. Treatment is with *metronidazole* at a standard dose.

Tritrichomonas foetus: *overview*

In cats, infection with Tritrichomonas foetus should be ruled out especially in young, pure breed animals. Even in cases where faecal analysis is negative for parasites, the animal should be **de-wormed** with *fenbendazole* (50 mg/kg/day for 3 days). If there is no improvement, a blood test should be performed. In the absence of anomalies, a change to a **high-fibre diet** should be recommended for at least 1 month. Abdominal ultrasound is not as useful as in cases of small intestine diarrhoea, but allows evaluation of the mucosal layer of the colon and whether there is an associated lymphadenopathy. In addition, it allows examination of other organs and non-gastrointestinal disease can be ruled out – for example, prostate disease.

If the diarrhoea does not improve with a high-fibre diet, the next step is to perform a **colonoscopy** and obtain multiple biopsies. Colonoscopy allows evaluation of the descending, transverse and ascending colon, the caecum and ileum. Correct preparation of the patient, by the administration of an enema, is essential to visualise the mucosa.

E. coli: *overview*

In recent years, the aetiology of ulcerative or **granulomatous histiocytic colitis** in the Boxer has been discovered. This type of colitis primarily affects brachiocephalic breeds but can also occur in other breeds. This disease is caused by intramucosal and intracellular invasion of the bowel wall by *E. coli*. Dogs with histiocytic colitis, such as the Boxer, respond to **enrofloxacin**. For a definitive diagnosis of ulcerative colitis caused by enteroinvasive *E. coli*, culture of colonic biopsies and FISH (fluorescent in situ hybridisation) are necessary. When performing a colonoscopy to obtain biopsies, it is advisable to order a kit by which to store the biopsies and send them to a specialised laboratory (for example, Cornell University, USA).

Irritable bowel syndrome (IBS): overview

In some cases of large intestinal diarrhoea, a definitive diagnosis cannot be established. In these cases the existence of IBS, similar to that described in people, is suspected. Symptomatic treatment includes the following.

- A highly digestible, hypo-allergenic diet.
- Fibre supplementation (e.g. psyllium 1–1.5 g/kg/day with food) has a beneficial effect by reducing the colonic inflammatory response.
- Treatment with metronidazole is also effective in many cases.
- Sulfasalazine is used in cases of chronic colitis unresponsive to conventional treatment; the dose is 10–25 mg/kg PO BID or TID (can be raised to 50 mg/kg TID). If there is a response to sulfasalazine, the lowest effective dose should be established. An evaluation of tear production in patients under treatment with sulfasalazine should be performed as this can provoke keratoconjunctivitis sicca.
- In cats, the administration of corticosteroids at immunosuppressive doses is effective in most cases of idiopathic colitis.

Tritrichomonas foetus *infection*

Tritrichomonas foetus can cause chronic large intestinal diarrhoea in the cat.

Aetiology

Tritrichomonas foetus is a single-celled, flagellated, piriform, **parasitic protozoan** (Figure 7.17), and one of the most common infectious aetiologies of **colitis** (large intestinal diarrhoea) in cats. T. foetus infection is considered an emerging disease in cats with diarrhoea. This protozoon is transmitted directly between hosts, and resides mainly in the distal ileum and colon, causing an increase in the permeability of the colonic mucosa and, as a consequence, diarrhoea. In more than 80% of cases the diarrhoea tends to enter spontaneous remission if left untreated. However, almost 60% of these cats will remain infected for more than 2–5 years after diagnosis.

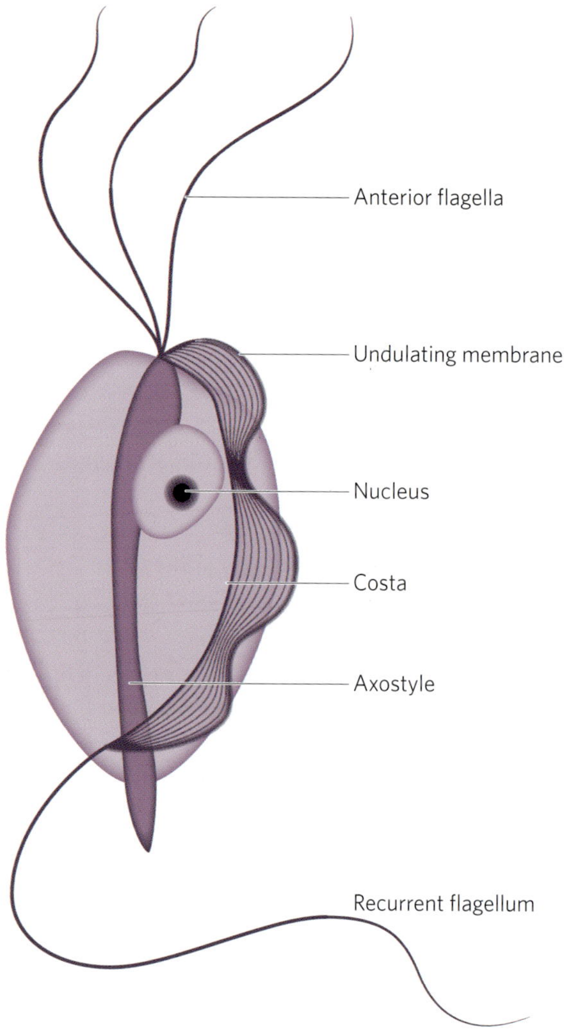

Figure 7.17. Morphology of *T. foetus*. *Illustration: Elaine Leggett.*

Epidemiology

The incidence of this infection in cats is unknown. In a study conducted in the USA, the prevalence of infection by *T. foetus* in purebred cats was 31%. According to other studies, the frequency of infection among cats with or without diarrhoea was 10–15%. This percentage varies depending on the country, the type of study, the cats (with or without diarrhoea, feline colonies or breed) and diagnosis (microscope, culture or PCR).

T. foetus infection mainly affects young purebred animals (Bengal and Siamese, according to a UK study), although it can affect cats of any age. Typically affected cats live in rehoming centres or colonies. There is no gender predisposition. When the diagnosis is made in adult or elderly animals, other concurrent disease such as IBD or neoplasia should be suspected.

Clinical signs

T. foetus mainly causes lymphoplasmacytic colitis with an **increased frequency** of bowel movements, tenesmus, loose stools to **foul-smelling** liquids sometimes accompanied by fresh blood and/or mucus. These signs are usually chronic and intermittent. When the diarrhoea is severe the anus becomes inflamed, causing pain. In some cases there is temporary improvement with antibiotics, followed by recurrence.

Usually there is no weight loss. Cats infected with *T. foetus* tend to have a good appetite and a very good general body condition. On physical examination, the anus may appear red and swollen.

T. foetus should be suspected in young cats with chronic large intestinal diarrhoea, or in those presumptively diagnosed with giardiasis that do not respond to treatment.

Diagnosis

Diagnosis of tritrichomoniasis is made based on the presence of *T. foetus* in faeces by microscopy, culture, PCR or colonic biopsy.

The sample most suitable for diagnostic tests is fresh faeces, which can be obtained using a **rectal probe or swab**. Another option is to obtain a sample by means of a colonic wash using a well-lubricated urinary catheter connected to a 10 ml syringe filled with physiological saline solution.

Under the microscope, *T. foetus* can be confused with *Giardia* spp.; however, the latter has a petal-like appearance and moves like a falling leaf whilst *T. foetus* has an undulating membrane and moves forwards.

- Video: microscopical differences between *T. foetus and Giardia* at http://publication.improveinternational.com.

Important information

- Flotation or sedimentation tests are not useful for diagnosis.
- Refrigeration kills *Tritrichomonas*.
- It is important to use diarrhoeal samples (to be taken into consideration in cats with intermittent diarrhoea).
- There is no single test that is 100% sensitive and specific.

Microscopic examination carries a sensitivity of 2–14%.

Faecal culture is more sensitive than microscopic examination of stools (see biomeddiagnostics.com) (– 55%).

PCR is the most sensitive and specific test (>80%).

Treatment

T. foetus is resistant to all commonly used antiprotozoal medications. **Ronidazole** is currently the only drug with proven efficacy to eliminate *T. foetus* in cats; however, cases of resistance have been reported. Treatment is recommended only in cases where *T. foetus* has been confirmed.

Ronidazole (30 mg/kg/24 h PO for 14 days). At high doses (>40 mg/kg), neurotoxicity (ataxia, tremors) has been described. It is important to warn owners of the risk of toxicity, and to stop treatment if any signs are observed.

Prognosis

The prognosis depends on response to treatment which, according to some studies, can take 6–30 months and depends on how severely the patient is affected. In advanced cases, especially if cirrhosis is present, the prognosis is reserved with an anticipated survival time of less than one month. The presence of hypoalbuminaemia, hypoglycaemia and coagulopathy is associated with a worse prognosis, with a survival time of just one week after diagnosis.

Granulomatous/histiocytic ulcerative colitis

Granulomatous colitis is a cause of chronic large intestinal diarrhoea in the dog.

Definition

Granulomatous colitis (GC), also known as histiocytic ulcerative colitis (HUC), was first described in a colony of **Boxers** in 1965. It is a rare disease with a global distribution that is characterised by **severe large intestinal diarrhoea**, which is accompanied by marked weight loss, anaemia and hypoalbuminaemia.

Aetiopathogenesis

Studies suggest that HUC is the consequence of an excessive **immune-mediated response** towards **commensal intestinal bacteria**. This may be due to genetic factors (a recessive autosomal defect is suspected), which would explain why it affects some breeds in particular, but this has not yet been proven.

The strains of *E. coli* identified in Boxers with colitis are very similar to those in healthy animals, and the number of bacteria in the abdominal contents of dogs with antibiotic-responsive enteropathy is similar to that in dogs with enteropathies responsive to immunosuppression. This suggests that the role of *E. coli* is commensal rather than pathogenic. However, more studies are needed to fully understand the role of *E. coli*.

Epidemiology

HUC typically affects **young** animals (<2 years old), most typically Boxers in the USA, Australia and Europe. It has also been described in other breeds, such as the French Bulldog, and in crossbreed dogs.

Clinical signs

Clinical signs include:

- tenesmus
- increased frequency of defaecation
- pain upon defaecation
- haematochezia
- presence of mucus
- weight loss, which can be severe.

Diagnosis

A definitive diagnosis of HUC is made by colonic biopsy, confirming an infiltration of macrophages (PAS-positive) in the intestinal mucosa. Ulceration of the mucosa and loss of caliciform cells are also typical changes. However, before performing a colonic biopsy it is important to rule out other processes that cause chronic diarrhoea (via blood tests, faecal analysis, abdominal ultrasound).

In affected animals, FISH allows detection of the presence of *E. coli* bacteria the mucosa. It is advisable to perform bacterial culture on at least two or three colonic biopsies and to ask the laboratory to perform an antibiotic sensitivity test.

Treatment

The treatment of choice is *enrofloxacin* (5 mg/kg/12 h PO for a minimum of 8 weeks), although resistant cases of *E. coli* have been described and are associated with a worse prognosis and may require euthanasia.

Although damage to the cartilage has not been described in animals treated with fluoroquinolones, when dosed for prolonged periods it is advisable to give glycosaminoglycans and chondroitin sulfate alongside.

A poor response to treatment is almost always due to enrofloxacin resistance. Therefore, the empirical use of enrofloxacin is not recommended in animals with suspected colitis without having obtained a previous diagnosis of granulomatous colitis with *E. coli* colonisation.

Principles of gastrointestinal endoscopy

Introduction

Endoscopy is a useful, non-invasive method for evaluation of the gastrointestinal mucosa and the detection of foreign bodies, ulcers, neoplasms and localised inflammatory changes. Chronic gastroenteric signs such as chronic diarrhoea, vomiting and weight loss are the most frequent reasons for performing an endoscopy and obtaining biopsies in the dog and cat.

Endoscopy is not only a diagnostic tool but also a therapeutic one – it allows the extraction of foreign bodies, treatment of oesophageal or rectal strictures and the placement of feeding tubes (for example, the placement of a PEG (percutaneous endoscopic gastrotomy) tube for percutaneous endoscopic gastrotomy).

This technique can be performed in both the anterior digestive tract (oesophago-gastro-duodenoscopy) and the posterior region (recto-colonoscopy), either with a flexible fibre-optic endoscope or one with electronic video.

A flexible endoscope is preferable to a rigid one for exploration of the proximal gastrointestinal tract, due to the manoeuvres required for this procedure. For the exploration of the descending colon, a rigid endoscope is adequate.

Materials required

Fibre-endoscopes. Endoscopes in which light and images are transmitted by optical fibres. Visualisation is through the eyepiece.

Video endoscopes. Endoscopes that capture images through magnetic impulses. Visualisation is on a monitor, which facilitates exploration and allows several people to view the images simultaneously.

There is no single optimal device for all endoscopic procedures and for all species. However, a multi-functional endoscope that can be used for gastroscopy, colonoscopy and bronchoscopy in animals of different sizes has the following features: a small-diameter video endoscope (<10 mm), movement of the end in four directions and a channel to work through/biopsy >2.8 mm in diameter and 125 cm in length.

An endoscopy tower has:

- a high-resolution monitor
- a light source
- an aspiration system
- air for inflation
- water
- auxiliary tools such as biopsy forceps, brush for scrapings, rat-tooth forceps, three-hook clamps and polypectomy handles (in addition to dilatation catheters with balloons and needles for cytology, it is important that the outer diameter of these is slightly smaller than the biopsy channel and length slightly greater – for example, if the channel measures 2.0 mm, forceps should be 1.8 mm and 50 cm longer).

Diagnostic indications

- regurgitation, suspected oesophagitis, stricture or foreign body
- haematemesis or melaena, iron-deficiency anaemia
- haematochezia, dyschezia, tenesmus
- chronic vomiting or diarrhoea
- protein-losing enteropathy
- weight loss with normal appetite
- to obtain samples (biopsies).

Obtaining biopsies

- Indicated in all cases in which gastrointestinal disease is suspected.
- Sampling of both normal and abnormal tissue.
- Crocodile or oval forceps can be used. Forceps with a central needle help in obtaining biopsies especially when the clamp is not totally perpendicular to the tissue.
- The more perpendicular the forceps to the tissue, the better the sample that can be obtained.
- Deflating the stomach to reduce luminal tension makes it easier to obtain samples.
- A minimum of seven to eight good-quality samples should be obtained from the stomach and six from the intestine (10–15 if they are of sub-optimal quality).
- It is important to handle the samples carefully and place them in the cassettes and the formaldehyde container as soon as possible.

Therapeutic indications

- foreign body extraction
- treatment of stenosis in the oesophagus and colon
- placement of PEG tube.

Procedure

The two golden rules in all endoscopic examinations are:

1. do not advance without visibility
2. when in doubt, go back.

Limitations

The findings of gastrointestinal endoscopy should be interpreted alongside information obtained in the history, physical examination and the results of blood and imaging tests.

- Endoscopy does not allow exploration of the entire small intestine (unless a double-balloon endoscope is used, which seals the intestine).
- Endoscopy allows for superficial biopsies of the mucosa, but not of the submucosal or muscular layers. In cases where the inflammatory or neoplastic process is located in the deeper layers, the sensitivity of endoscopy is low and only full-thickness biopsy (via laparotomy) allows a diagnosis to be made.
- The sensitivity of endoscopy for the diagnosis of digestive diseases depends on biopsy quality and size. The better the quality, the fewer samples are necessary to obtain a histopathological diagnosis; on the other hand, if the biopsies are small and of poor quality, more samples are needed. The quality of the biopsies, in turn, depends on the equipment and the operator performing the endoscopy.
- Endoscopy alone does not provide information on the function of the gastrointestinal tract.
- The diagnostic value is proportional to the experience of the clinician, and to the quality of the endoscope and auxiliary tools.

Complications

Endoscopy is considered a safe and low-risk procedure compared to a surgical procedure, and can generally be performed without complications. Even so, the owners of the animal should be informed of possible complications, such as:

- those associated with general anaesthesia
- perforation – for example, in cases of deep gastric ulcer or friable neoplasia
- bleeding; however, this is rare, unless the animal has a problem with coagulation or is thrombocytopenic
- bradycardia due to increased vagal tone
- aspiration pneumonia.

Gastro-duodenoscopy

Preparation of the animal

- The animal should be fasted for 12–24 hours but, in cases of emergency such as retrieval of a foreign body, this is not necessary.
- Place the animal in left lateral recumbency.
- Use mouth clamp to protect the endoscope.
- Administer general anaesthesia and always use endotracheal intubation in order to ensure ventilation and protect the respiratory tract.
- Monitor heart rate and rhythm, blood pressure, CO_2 level and oxygen saturation. This is to prevent and minimise the complications associated with anaesthesia.
- Examine the oral cavity to identify foreign bodies, fistulae or other injuries.

Preparation of equipment

Ensure that the endoscope works correctly, including that it moves in all directions and that the suction and water aspiration functions are working.

- Check the focus and clean the lens if necessary.
- Adjust the white balance.
- Prepare all other necessary material (biopsy forceps, biopsy cassettes, formaldehyde, gauze, 25 G needle to deposit the samples in the cassette).
- Always wear gloves.

Procedure

A gastro-duodenoscopic examination can take between 20 minutes and 1 hour depending on the clinician's experience.

Firstly, carefully insert the tip of the endoscope into the animal's mouth, passing it down into oesophagus. As the endoscope is advanced through the oesophagus and stomach, examine the mucosa for abnormalities such as foreign bodies, inflammation, ulcers or masses. If there is an assistant, they can create circular pressure around the oesophagus with their hands, which helps with air distension and oesophageal visualisation. The normal oesophagus is pale pink and bright. The small blood vessels of the submucosa are easily seen. Images and videos should be taken, not only of any abnormalities but also of normal structures.

To improve the examination of the gastric mucosa, suction out any gastrointestinal secretions. There are then two options: examine the stomach first and then the duodenum, or examine the duodenum first and then back off and perform the examination of the stomach. Many people prefer the latter, and examine the duodenum first and then back up into the stomach. This is advantageous, because the former distends the stomach with air, which closes the pylorus and makes the passage of the endoscope into the duodenum more difficult.

In order to facilitate the advance of the endoscope through the pylorus and into the duodenum, it is advisable to first suck the air out of the stomach. If the endoscope has a diameter >9.0–9.5 mm, entry into the small dog or cat will be difficult. An endoscope in which the tip can move in four directions also facilitates entry into the duodenum. If the pylorus is open, entry to the duodenum is relatively easy with practice and experience. If it is especially difficult to pass through the pylorus, biopsy forceps can be used as a guide by insertion through the pylorus into the proximal duodenum.

However, advance carefully because there is a risk of puncturing the duodenum.

Harvest at least six stomach biopsies and ten small intestinal biopsies. The best biopsies are obtained directing the instrument at a 90° angle (perpendicular) to the surface of the mucosa at the duodenal flexures.

At the end of the endoscopic procedure, the air in the stomach and any secretions in the oesophagus should be suctioned to minimise the risk of aspiration pneumonia.

Figures 7.18–7.36 show endoscopic images of the digestive tract, from the oesophagus to the duodenum.

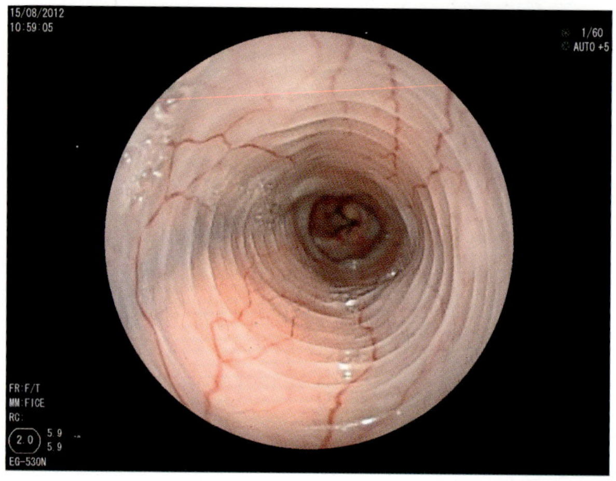

Figure 7.18. Feline oesophagus with characteristic transverse folds.

Colonoscopy

Patient preparation

The key to successful colonoscopy lies in patient preparation.

To perform a recto-colonoscopy the animal should be hospitalised for two to three days and fasted for 48–72 hours (without restriction of water consumption) and several enemas performed.

Ways to clean the large intestine and facilitate endoscopic exploration

1. Cathartic solutions with electrolytes (for example, *Goytely®*) to promote osmotic diarrhoea (30 ml/kg/6 h for 24 h). Placement of a naso-esophageal tube is recommended for ease of administration. It has been shown in the dog that this method produces better colonic preparation than multiple enemas.
2. The day before endoscopy, give four doses of *Osmoprep®* tablets (1 g/3 kg every 4–6 h). It is recommended to administer intravenous fluids during this treatment.
3. *Bisacodyl* or senna laxatives. Dosage: one 5 mg tablet in cats and small dogs; one to three 5 mg tablets in medium or large dogs. Do not break the tablets.
4. Perform three rectal enemas (20 ml/kg) starting the day before the procedure, and a final enema on the day of the endoscopy. The final enema should provide a reflux of clean water without faecal matter and should be administered at least 12 h before the intervention, to facilitate evacuation and minimise hyperaemia of the mucosa caused by the device.

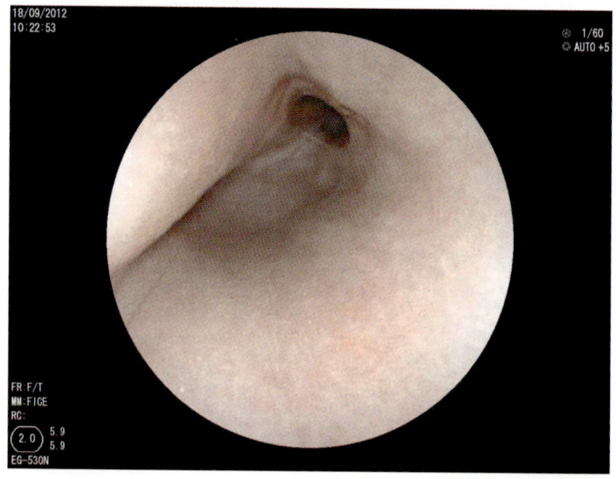

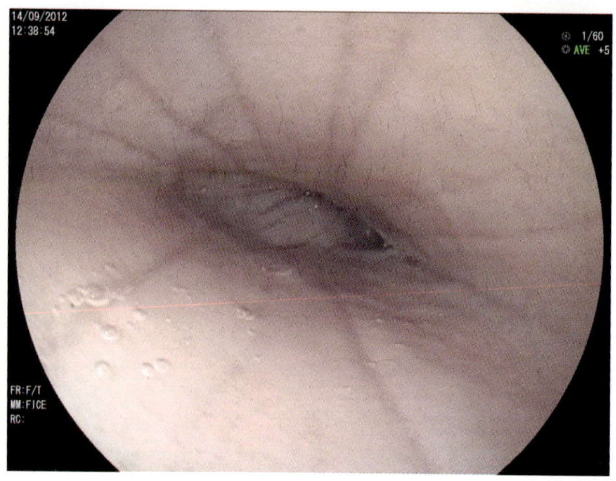

Figures 7.19 and 7.20. Normal canine oesophagus.

Procedure

The animal should be anaesthetised and positioned in left lateral recumbency. Before beginning the endoscopy, perform digital palpation of the anus and rectum (sometimes foreign bodies, neoplasms and stenosis can be detected ahead of performing the endoscopy). Generously lubricate the end of the endoscope and advance slowly through the anus to the colon. The colon is inflated with air to expand the rectum and facilitate the advance of the endoscope and improve visualisation. If there is an assistant, they can close the anus

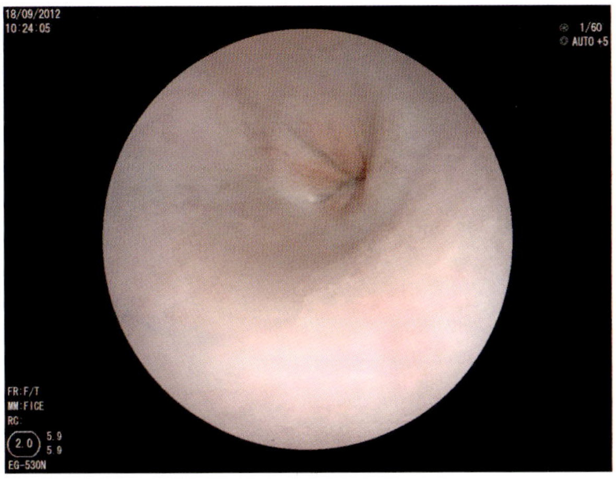

Figure 7.21. Distal oesophageal sphincter.

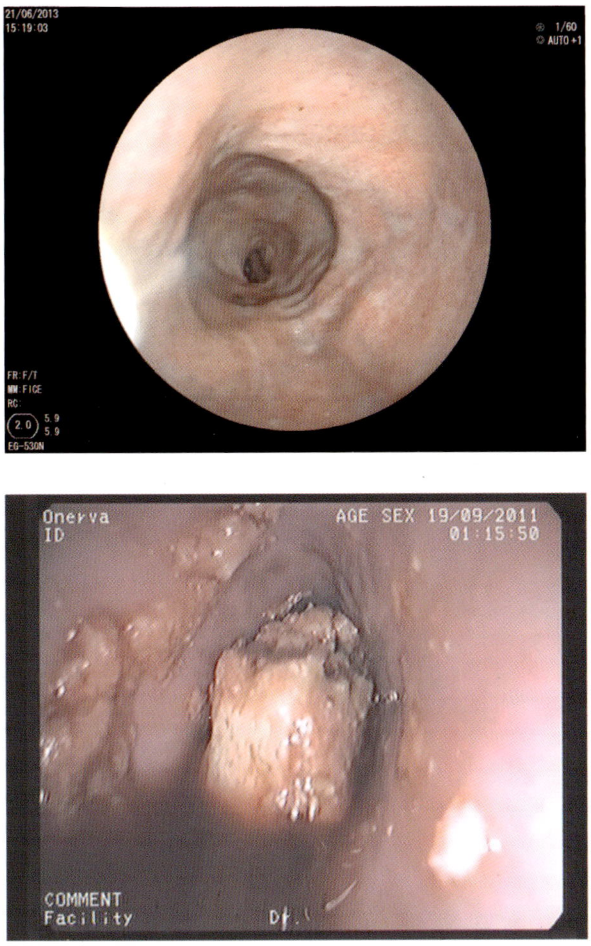

Figures 7.22 and 7.23. Oesophageal foreign body (bone). In this case, endoscopy was carried out 5 days after ingestion.

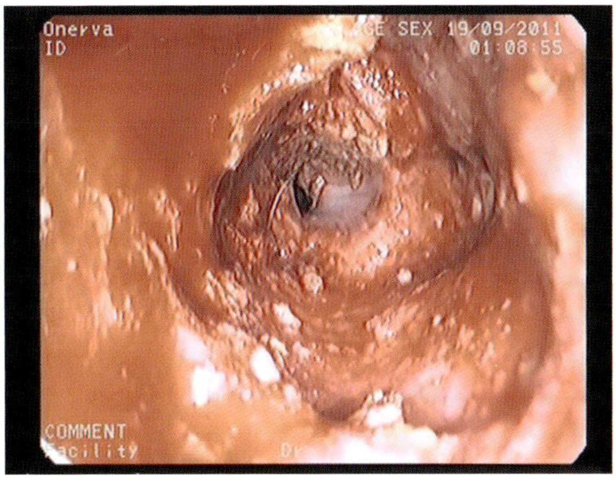

Figure 7.24. Moderate to servere diffuse oesophagitis.

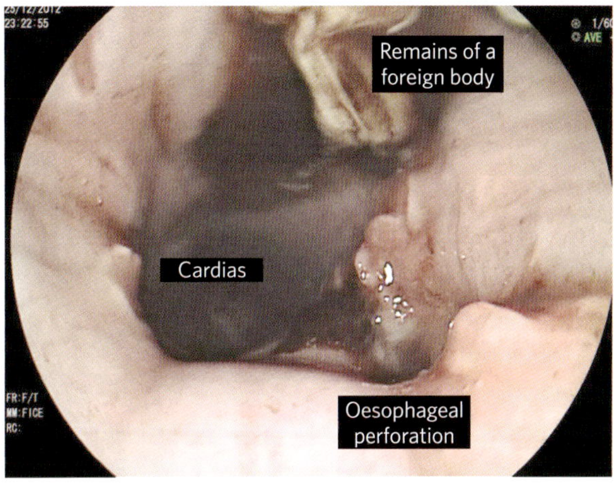

Figure 7.25. Oesophageal perforation due to a foreign body (bone). At the end, the distal oesophageal sphincter can be seen. The perforation is on the right-hand side of the image.

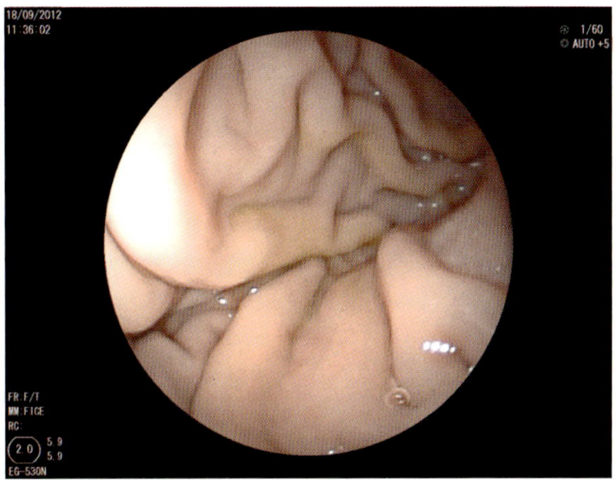

Figure 7.26. Stomach: gastric folds.

with the fingers around the endoscope to allow better distention of the colon. The lumen should always be visible and the endoscope should move easily. The normal mucosa of the colon is pale pink, soft and shiny. The blood vessels of the submucosa are visible throughout the entire length. In addition, lymphoid follicles of approximately 1–3 mm in the rectum and the caecum are visible.

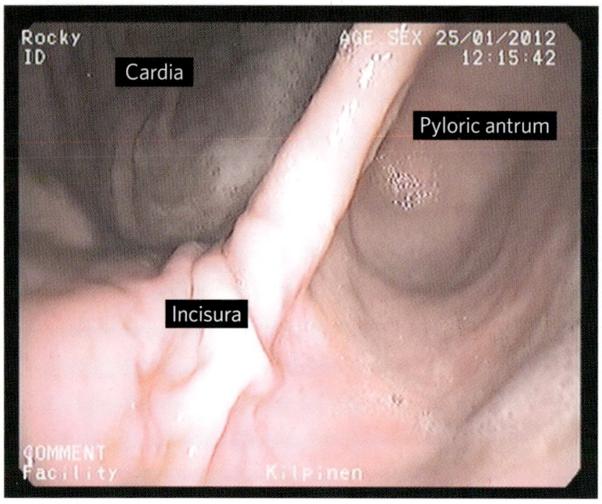

Figure 7.27. Retroverted stomach: in the centre of the image is the angular incisure; to the right, the pyloric antrum and to the left, the cardia. By means of a complete 180° flexion of the steerable end of the endoscope, the tip is retroverted over the antrum and reveals the angle and totality of the lesser curvature when the endoscope is removed. It is preferable to perform this manoeuvre of complete retroversion after having examined the duodenum, in order to avoid excessive insufflation during the introduction.

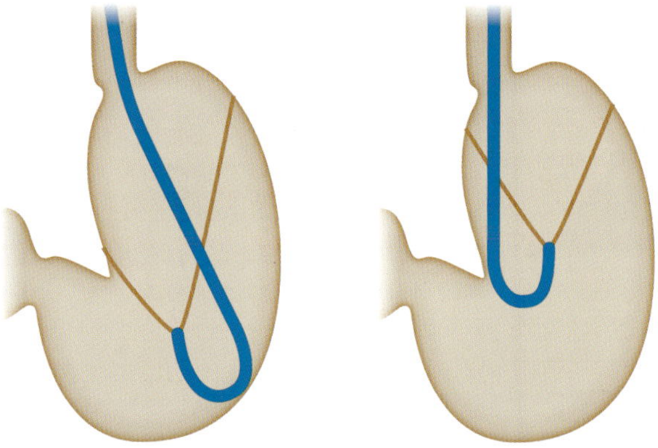

Figure 7.28. Diagram of how to obtain the image in reverse. *Illustration: Elaine Leggett.*

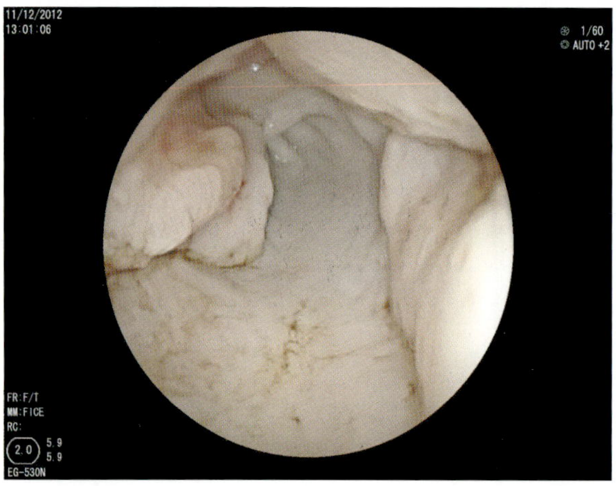

Figure 7.29. Gastric lymphoma: the mucosa has a nodular appearance (left side of the image). In the background is the pyloric antrum.

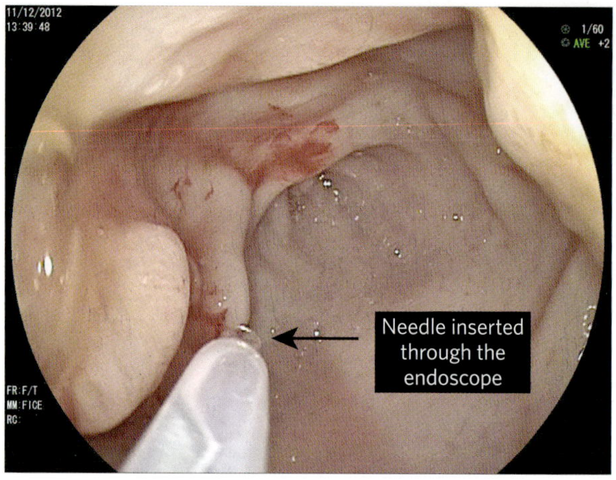

Figure 7.30. Gastric lymphoma in the pyloric antral area. The nodules were very firm, making it difficult to obtain biopsies. Needle cytology by endoscopy (in the image) was diagnostic.

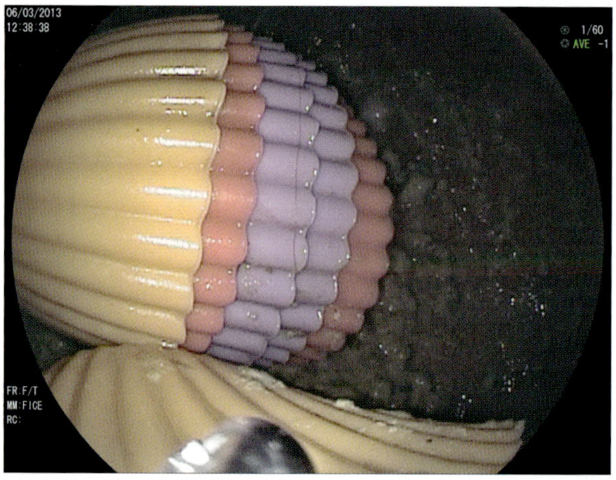

Figure 7.31. Gastric foreign body (moulds for muffins).

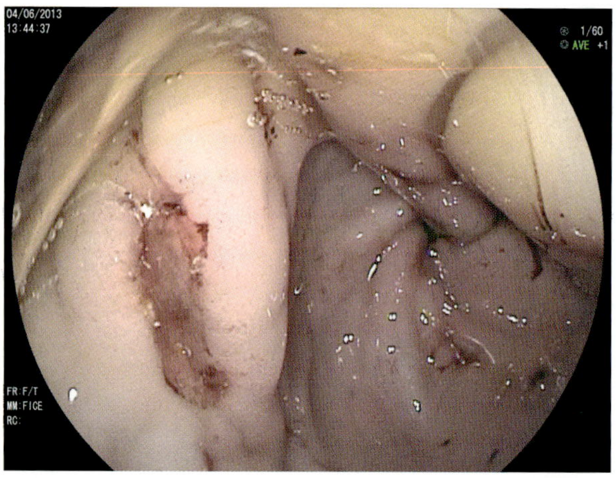

Figure 7.32. Gastric ulcer on the lesser curvature of the stomach.

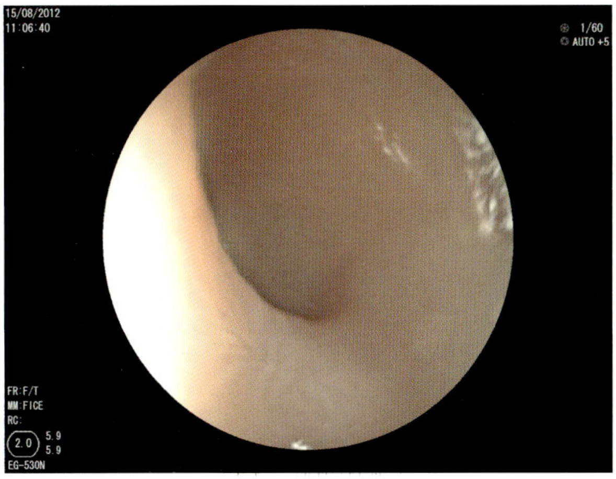

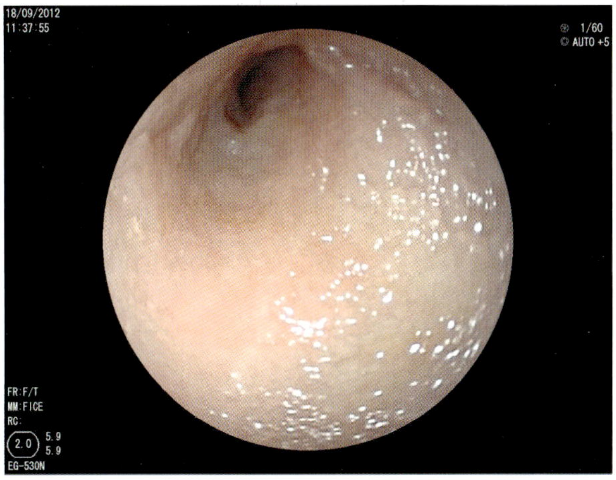

Figures 7.33 and 7.34. Normal duodenum.

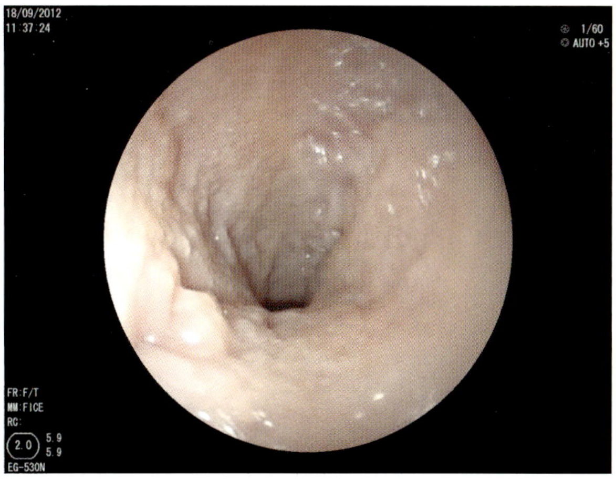

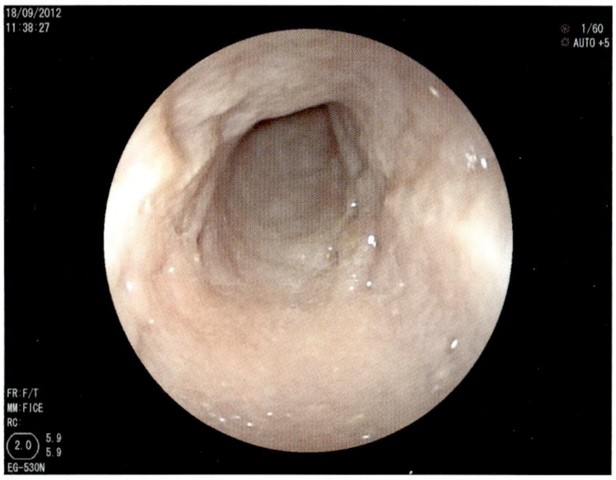

Figures 7.35 and 7.36. Proximal duodenum. A change in coloration (pallor, oedema) and mucosal texture is observed. The histopathological diagnosis was moderate lymphoplasmacytic inflammation.

Once the transverse colon is reached, the ileo-colic and caeco-colic sphincters can be identified. In some animals, the endoscope may reach the ileum. If there is a considerable resistance, blind biopsies can be obtained (monitor the pressure exerted, as there is a risk of perforation).

Normally 10–20 biopsies of the colon/ileum are obtained, independent of the appearance of the mucosa (Figures 7.37, 7.38).

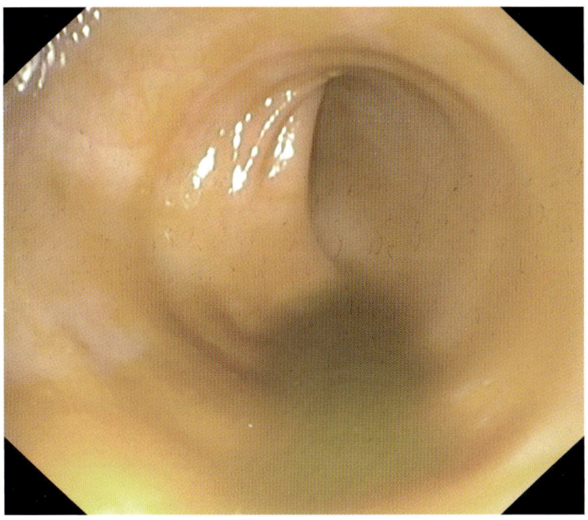

Figure 7.37. Colon, splenic flexure.

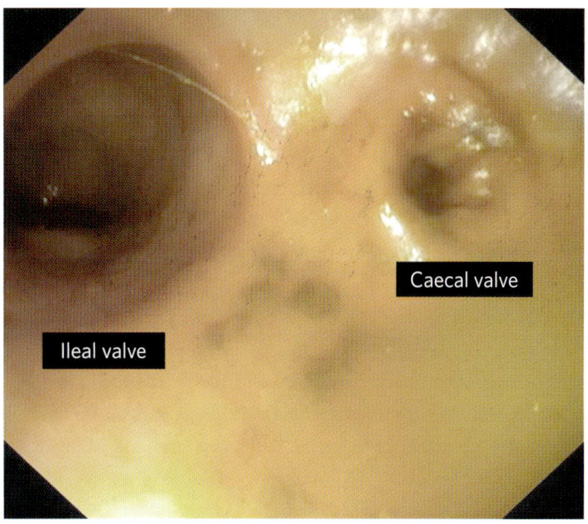

Figure 7.38. Colonoscopy.

Bibliography

Gastrointestinal disorders

Allenspach, K., Rüfenacht, S., Sauter, S., Gröne, A., Steffan, J., Strehlau, G. et al. (2006) Pharmacokinetics and clinical efficacy of cyclosporine treatment of dogs with steroid-refractory inflammatory bowel disease. *Journal of Veterinary Internal Medicine* 20(2), 29–44.

Allenspach, K., Wieland, B., Gröne, A. and Gaschen, F. (2007) Chronic enteropathies in dogs: evaluation of risk factors for negative outcome. *Journal of Veterinary Internal Medicine* 21, 700–708.

Benchaoui, H.A., Siedek, E.M., de la Puente-Redondo, V.A., Tilt, N., Rowan, T.G. and Clemence, R.G. (2007) Efficacy of maropitant for preventing vomiting associated with motion sickness in dogs. *Veterinary Record* 161, 444–447.

Boothe, D.M. Gastrointestinal pharmacology (1999) *Veterinary Clinics of North America Small Animal Practice* 29(2), 343–376.

Cook, A.K., Gilson, S.D., Fischer, W.D. and Kass, P.H. (1992) Effect of diet on results obtained by use of two commercial test kits for detection of occult blood in feces of dog. *American Journal of Veterinary Research* 53(10), 1 749–1.

Craven, M., Simpson, J.W., Ridyard, A.E. and Chandler, M.L. Canine inflammatory bowel disease: retrospective analysis of diagnosis and outcome in 80 cases (1995–2002) (2004). *Journal of Small Animal Practice* 45, 336–342.

deNovo, R.C. (2003) Diseases of the stomach. In: Tams, T.R. (ed). *Handbook of Small Animal Gastroenterology*, 2nd edition. WB Saunders Co., Philadelphia, PA, pp. 159–194.

Fox, L.E., Rosenthal, R.C., Twedt, D.C., Dubielzig, R.R., MacEwen, E.G. and Grauer, G.F. (1990) Plasmahistamine and gastrin concentrations in 17 dogs with mast cell tumors. *Veterinary Internal Medicine* 4, 242–246.

German, A.J., Day, M.J., Ruaux, C.G., Steiner, J.M., Williams, D.A. and Hall, E.J. (2003) Comparison of direct and indirect tests for small intestinal bacterial overgrowth and antibiotic-responsive diarrhoea in dogs. *Journal of Veterinary Internal Medicine* 17(1), 33–43.

Gionchetti, P., Rizzello, F., Lammers, K.M., Morselli, C., Sollazzi, L., Davies, S. et al. (2006) Antibiotics and probiotics in treatment of inflammatory bowel disease. *World Journal of Gastroenterology* 12, 3306–3313.

Guilford, W.G. (1996) Idiopathic inflammatory bowel diseases. In: Strombeck, D.R., Williams, D.A. and Meyer, D.J. (eds). *Strombeck's Small Animal Gastroenterology*, 3th edn. Guilford WG, Center SA, pp. 451–486.

Guilford, W.G., Jones, B.R., Markwell, P.J., Arthur, D.G., Collett, M.G. and Harte, J.G. (2001) Food sensitivity in cats with chronic idiopathic gastrointestinal problems. *Journal of Veterinary Internal Medicine* 15, 7–13.

Janeczko, S., Atwater, D., Bogel, E., Greiter-Wilke, A., Gerold, A., Baum-Gart, M. et al. (2008) The relationship of mucosal bacteria to duodenal histopathology, cytokine mRNA, and clinical disease activity in cats with IBD. *Veterinary Microbiology* 128, 178–193.

Jergens, A., Crandell, J.M., Evans, R., Ackermann, M., Miles, K.G. and Wang, C. (2010) A clinical index of disease activity in cats with chronic enteropathy. *Journal of Veterinary Internal Medicine* 24, 1027–1033.

Jergens, A.E., Schreiner, C.A., Frank de Niyo, Y., Ahrens, F.E., Eckersall, P.D. et al. (2003) A scoring index for disease activity in canine inflammatory bowel disease. *Journal of Veterinary Internal Medicine* 17, 291–297.

Liptak, J.M., Hunt, G.B., Barrs, V.R., Foster, S.F., Tisdall, P.L., O'Brien, C.R. et al. (2002) Gastroduodenal ulceration in cats: eight cases and a review of the literature. *Journal of Feline Medicine and Surgery* 4, 27–42.

Marks, S.L., Laflamme, D.P. and McAloose, D. (2002) Dietary trial using a commercial hypoallergenic diet containing hydrolyzed protein for dogs with inflammatory bowel disease. *Veterinary Therapeutics* 3, 109–118.

Penninck, D., Matz, M. and Tidwell, A. (1997) Ultrasonography of gastric ulceration in the dog. *Veterinary Radiology and Ultrasound* 38, 308–312.

Pollard, R.E., Marks, S.L., Davidson, A. and Hornof, W.J. (2000) Quantitative videofluoroscopic evaluation of pharyngeal function in the dog. *Veterinary Radiology and Ultrasound* 41(5), 409–412.

Ramsey, D.S., Kincaid, K., Watkins, J.A., Boucher, J.F., Conder, G.A., Eagleson, J.S. et al. (2008) Safety and efficacy of injectable and oral maropitant, a selective neurokinin 1 receptor antagonist, in a randomized clinical trial for treatment of vomiting in dogs. *Journal of Veterinary Pharmacology and Therapeutics* 31(6), 538–543.

Schurig, J.E., Florczyk, A.P., Rose, W.C. and Bradner, W.T. (1982) Antiemetic activity of butorphanol against cisplatin-induced emesis in ferrets and dogs. *Cancer Treatment Reports* 66, 1831–1835.

Swidsinski, A., Ladhoff, A., Pernthaler, A., Swidsinski, S., Loening-Baucke, V., Ortner, M. et al. (2002) Mucosal flora in inflammatory bowel disease. *Gastroenterology* 122, 44–54.

Twedt, D.C. (2004) Vomiting. In: Ettinger, S. and Feldman, E.C. (eds) *Textbook of Veterinary Internal Medicine*, 6th edn. WB Saunders Co, Philadelphia, PA, pp. 132.

Washabau, R.J., Day, M.J., Willard, M.D., Hall, E.J., Jergens, A.E., Mansell, J. et al., WSAVA International Gastrointestinal Standardization Group (2010) Endoscopic, biopsy, and histopathologic guidelines for the evaluation of gastrointestinal inflammation in companion animals. *Journal of Veterinary Internal Medicine* 24, 10–26 (Erratum in Journal of *Veterinary Internal Medicine* 2010 24, 796.)

Washabau, R.J. and Elie, M.S. (1995) Antiemetic therapy. In: Bonagura, J.D. (ed.) *Kirk's Current Veterinary Therapy XII: Small Animal Practice*. WB Saunders Co, Philadelphia, PA, pp. 679–684.

Washabau, R.J. and Hall, J.A. (1997) Diagnosis and management of gastrointestinal motility disorders in dogs and cats. *Compendium of Continuing Education for the Practising Veterinarian* 721–737.

Watrous, B.J. (1983) Clinical presentation and diagnosis of dysphagia. *Veterinary Clinics of North America Small Animal Practice* 13(3), 437–459.

Westermarck, E., Skrzypczak, T., Harmoinen, J., Steiner, J.M., Ruaux, C.G., Williams, D.A. et al. (2005) Tylosin-responsive chronic diarrhoea in dogs. *Journal of Veterinary Internal Medicine* 2005 19(2), 177–186.

Willard, M.D., Jergens, A.E., Duncan, R.B., Leib, M.S., McCracken, M.D., deNovo, R.C. et al. (2002) Inter observer variation among histopathologic evaluations of intestinal tissues from dogs and cats. *Journal of the American Veterinary Medical Association* 220(8), 1177–1182.

Winslet, M.C., Allan, A., Poxon, V., Youngs, D. and Keighley, M.R. (1994) Fecal diversion for Crohn's colitis: a model to study the role of the fecal stream in the inflammatory process. *Gut*

Gastrointestinal Endoscopy

Goutal-Landry, C.M., Mansell, J., Ryan, K.A. and Gaschen, F.P. (2013) Effect of endoscopic forceps on quality of duodenal mucosal biopsy in healthy dogs. *Journal of Veterinary Internal Medicine* 27, 456–461.

Leib, M.S., Baechtel, M.S. and Monroe, W.E. (2004) Complications associated with 355 flexible colonoscopic procedures in dogs. *Journal of Veterinary Internal Medicine* 18(5), 642.

Mansell, J. and Willard, M.D. (2003) Biopsy of the gastrointestinal tract. *Veterinary Clinics of North America Small Animal Practice* 33(5), 1099–1116.

Procoli, F., Motskula, P.F., Keyte, S.V., Priestnall, S. and Allenspach, K. (2013) Comparison of histopathologic findings in duodenal and ileal endoscopic biopsies in dogs with chronic small intestinal enteropathies. *Journal of Veterinary Internal Medicine* 27, 268–274.

Rychlik, A., Nieradka, R., Kander, M., Depta, A., Nowicki, M. and Sarti, K. (2007) Usefulness of endoscopic examination for the diagnosis of inflammatory bowel disease in the dog. *Polish Journal of Veterinary Science* 10(2), 113–118.

Washabau, R.J., Day, M.J., Willard, M.D., Hall, E.J., Jergens, A.E., Mansell, J. et al. (2010) Endoscopic, biopsy, and histopathologic guidelines for the evaluation of gastrointestinal inflammation in companion animals. *Journal of Veterinary Internal Medicine* 24, 10–26.

Willard, M.D. (2001) Colonoscopy, proctoscopy, and ileoscopy. *Veterinary Clinics of North America Small Animal Practice* 31(4), 657–669.

Willard, M.D., Lovering, S., Cohen, N. and Weeks, B.R. (2001) Quality of tissue specimens obtained endoscopically from the duodenum of dogs and cats. *Journal of the American Veterinary Medical Association* 219, 474–479.

Willard, M.D., Mansell, J., Fosgate, G.T., Gualtieri, M., Olivero, D., Lecoindre, P. et al. (2008) Effect of sample quality on the sensitivity of endoscopic biopsy for detecting gastric and duodenal lesions in dogs and cats. *Journal of Veterinary Internal Medicine* 22, 1084–1089.

Test

1. What is the difference between vomiting and regurgitation?

A) Vomiting occurs hours after eating, while regurgitation always occurs immediately after food or liquid intake
B) There is no undigested food in vomit
C) Abdominal contractions occur during vomiting, while regurgitation is a passive act
D) The pH of the food is alkaline in case of regurgitation and acid in the case of vomiting

2. Which of the following signs characterises small intestinal diarrhoea?

A) Weight loss
B) Haematochezia
C) Low-volume but high-frequency diarrhoea
D) Mucus

3. Rocco, a 2-month-old, un-neutered male mongrel, vomits and has haemorrhagic liquid diarrhoea for 24 hours. Rocco was vaccinated 2 weeks ago. On physical examination the animal is in compensated shock, is 7-8% dehydrated and has pain on abdominal palpation. The complete blood count shows mild–moderate leucopenia and blood biochemistry is normal. A test for parvovirus is negative. What is the most likely differential diagnosis?

A) Parvovirus
B) Giardiasis
C) Foreign body
D) Distemper

4. Laika, a 4-year-old mongrel, was anaesthetised 10 days ago for an ovariohysterectomy. She has been regurgitating non-stop for 3 days and is very lethargic today. Physical examination: heart rate 130 bpm, respiratory rate 78 bpm, mucous membrane colour pink and pale, temperature 40.1°C. There is no abdominal pain or dehydration. Based on the physical examination, what tests would you perform?

A) Thoracic radiography
B) Endoscopy of the oesophagus
C) Complete blood count
D) Abdominal ultrasound

5. Which of the following medications is a treatment option for giardiasis?

A) Amoxycillin/clavulanic acid
B) Praziquantel
C) Fenbendazole
D) Losartan

6. Lilly, an 8-year-old Golden Retriever, has been regurgitating for weeks. No signs of mega-oesophagus can be seen on thoracic radiography. What is the next step to rule out mega-oesophagus?

A) Perform an endoscopy
B) Measure anti-acetylcholine receptor antibodies
C) Perform contrast radiograph (giving Lilly kibbles or tinned food with barium)
D) Perform a thoracic CT

7. Luna, a 4-year-old un-neutered Poodle, has been vomiting and lethargic for 2 days. She has not eaten anything since yesterday and is very apathetic. On physical examination there is mild dehydration and cranial abdominal pain. We perform a blood–gas analysis and emergency blood test (normal values in parentheses):

- pH 7.4 (7.3–7.46)
- pCO_2 39.1 (30.8–42.8)
- HCO^{3-} 22.5 (18.8–25.6)
- SBE –1 (–0.2–3.4)
- Na^+ 127 (145–154)
- K^+ 6.2 (4.1–5.3)
- Cl^- 105 (105–116)
- Creatinine 1.7 (0.5–1.2)
- HTC 57 (39–52)
- TP 68 (55–75)

What is the most likely diagnosis?

A) Pyometra
B) Urinary obstruction
C) Intestinal foreign body
D) Hypo-adrenocorticism

8. A 3-year-old Persian cat has had chronic diarrhoea for 2 months. The owner tells us that the stools smell very bad and are very small. It is been de-wormed several times with no sign of improvement. The other cats (3 others) at home are healthy. On physical examination the body condition is good. The anus is moderately irritated. Blood tests are normal. Faecal analysis is negative. What infectious disease should we rule out?

A) Feline panleukopenia
B) *Tritrichomonas foetus* infection
C) Campylobacteriosis
D) Toxoplasmosis

9. Why is metoclopramide not an effective anti-emetic at a central level in cats?

A) Due to its extrapyramidal side effects
B) Because cats have fewer dopaminergic receptors
C) Because it does not cross the blood–brain barrier
D) Because cats have fewer serotonergic receptors

10. Which of the following drugs is most effective as a gastric protector?

A) Omeprazole
B) Ranitidine
C) Famotidine
D) Cimetidine

11. Which breed has a genetic predisposition to a persistent right aortic arch?

A) Yorkshire Terrier
B) Miniature Schnauzer
C) German Shepherd
D) Giant Poodle

12. Darko is a 9-year-old Boston Terrier who presents with diarrhoea which started 4 days ago. The owner explains that they think he is constipated because he tries to defaecate but fails. Yesterday he vomited once. On physical examination body condition is good. On rectal examination no faeces are palpated in the rectum and mucus is seen on the glove. Where would you place the origin of Darko's diarrhoea?

A) Large intestine
B) Duodenum
C) Ileum
D) Mixed origin

13. What breed of dog has a predisposition to congenital hiatal hernia?

A) German Shepherd
B) Border Collie
C) Great Dane
D) Shar Pei

14. Minnie, a 15-year-old cat, vomits intermittently for 2 months. She has lost a lot of weight. Blood tests and abdominal ultrasound are normal. T4 concentration is normal. The owner has changed to a hypo-allergenic diet without any signs of improvement. What test would you recommend?

A) Intestinal biopsy
B) TLI
C) TSH
D) ACTH stimulation

15. Yago, a 3-year-old Boxer, has chronic diarrhoea, which is characterised by frequent and painful tenesmus and defaecation. Blood tests and three stool analyses are normal. He has lost a lot of weight and responded to neither a hypo-allergenic diet nor metronidazole. What would you recommend?

A) Abdominal ultrasound
B) Colonoscopy, intestinal biopsy and bacterial culture of the biopsy
C) Measurement of cobalamin concentration
D) Treatment with prednisone

16. Lula, a 6-year-old German Shepherd dog, has not eaten for 2 days and is very lethargic. She has been treated with meloxicam for the last two months. The blood analysis shows 26% haematocrit (40–55) with microcytosis and hypochromia, hypalbuminaemia and hyperglobulinaemia. Creatinine is normal but urea is high. What is the most likely cause of the pan-hypoproteinaemia?

A) Neoplasia
B) IBD
C) Azotaemia
D) Chronic GI bleeding

Answers on page 326

Clinical case

A 12 kg dog which vomits 2–3 times a day and presents with 7% dehydration and needs to be rehydrated within 12 hours.

1. Calculate the total quantity of fluids that should be administered.
2. What would be the case if the dog was suffering from hypo-albuminaemia?

Correct answers

Test

1. C	7. D	13. D
2. A	8. B	14. A
3. A	9. B	15. B
4. A	10. A	16. D
5. C	11. C	
6. C	12. A	

Clinical case

1. **Calculate the total volume of fluids which should be administered.**

   Daily requirements:

   60 ml/kg/d x 12 kg = 720 ml/d.

   720 ml/24 h = 30 ml/h.

   Rehydration:

   0.07 x 12 kg x 1 000 ml/kg= 840 ml.

   840 ml/12 h rehydration = 70 ml/h.

   Daily losses:

   50 ml/vomit x 3 vomits/day = 150 ml/d.

   150 ml/24 h = 6.2 ml/h.

   Total fluids for administration:

   30 ml/h + 70 ml/h + 6.2 ml/h = 106.2 ml/h.

2. **What would be the case if the dog was suffering from hypoalbuminaemia**

   If this dog had hypoalbuminaemia, instead of administering 106.2 ml/h, 74.3 ml/h should be administered.

8

Hepatobiliary and exocrine pancreas disorders

Cristina Pérez Vera

Chapter summary

Hepatobiliary disease represents a range of conditions commonly seen in first opinion practice. However, whilst raised liver enzymes may raise a suspicion of liver disease, the clinician must differentiate a primary hepatic problem from liver involvement in its reactive capacity to disease processes elsewhere in the body.

Take the example of a dog admitted for dental attention. Their pre-anaesthetic blood panel shows moderately elevated liver enzymes. The clinician must then assess the possible cause, the significance of the changes, and decide if the procedure should go ahead. Factors such as the patient's breed and age add another layer of complexity as these are relevant to the underlying predispositions to hepatobiliary disease.

Unfortunately, finding the answer in a case of suspected hepatobiliary disease is not necessarily straightforward. A screening blood panel is merely the initial step for an investigation that may ultimately require a liver biopsy to reach a definitive diagnosis.

Indeed, the propensity to hepatobiliary disease differs in the cat and dog. There are species variations in predisposition to hepatobiliary disease, whilst in most cases the symptoms are non-specific, such as sickness and diarrhoea. All of which can make it a challenge for the clinician to reach an accurate definitive diagnosis.

Key learning points

- Appreciate species-specific differences with regards to hepatobiliary disease.
- Differentiate between primary hepatic disease and secondary, reactive disease processes.
- Understand the clinical pathology of common hepatobiliary diseases of the dog and cat.
- Be aware of the possible complications arising as a result of hepatobiliary disease.
- The optimal treatment of commonly occurring liver and biliary problems of the cat and dog.

Hepatobiliary disorders

Introduction

The **liver** performs many unique and vital functions such as the **metabolism of carbohydrates, lipids, and proteins**; aiding **fat digestion**; **detoxification** of endogenous and exogenous substances; storage of vitamins and glycogen; and the **synthesis of coagulation factors.**

Elevation of liver enzymes, with or without jaundice, is a frequent reason for concern in small animals. However, differentiating between a **primary hepatobiliary** problem and secondary **reactive disease** can be difficult, especially without the invaluable information supplied by a liver biopsy. In addition, hepatobiliary disease tends to be **species specific**, with different pathologies predominating in dogs and cats.

However, the general characteristics of liver disease can be described as follows.

- The **clinical signs** are often vague and **non-specific.**
- A **normal blood panel** does not rule out liver disease. The results should always be interpreted in the light of the clinical history and a physical examination.
- The liver has a **large functional reserve** capacity. This means that by the time the animal becomes **symptomatic**, the disease process is already **well advanced**.
- Once the liver's functional reserve is exceeded, symptoms such as jaundice, hepatic encephalopathy, coagulopathies, oedema, and hypoglycaemia may develop.

Differences between cats and dogs

Location of the inflammation

In the cat, hepatobiliary disease is classified as inflammatory or non-inflammatory. In feline patients, **inflammation** most commonly **affects the biliary system**, whilst in **dogs** it is the **liver parenchyma** that is affected. As a consequence, cats with liver disease are often jaundiced but rarely present with micro hepatitis due to cirrhosis.

Anatomy of the bile duct

Another important difference between the two species is how the bile duct drains into the duodenum. In **80% of cats** the pancreas drains into the duodenum through a **single (pancreatic) duct**, where the bile duct joins the pancreatic duct before reaching the superior duodenal papilla, whereas in dogs, the pancreatic and bile ducts enter the duodenum separately.

About 20% of cats have an accessory pancreatic duct, which predisposes them to triaditis. **Triaditis = cholangitis + pancreatitis + inflammatory bowel disease (IBD).**

Metabolic variations

Cats are poorly equipped to metabolize toxic drugs, due to a **low level** of the enzyme **glucuronyl transferase**. Cats are also more susceptible to **hepatic lipidosis** than dogs, because of a high requirement for the amino acid arginine in the urea cycle.

The presence of **bilirubinuria** is **always significant in the cat**. Conversely, it may be normal in the dog, especially in males.

Clinical signs

The clinician should start the consultation with a complete clinical history, with the following information being especially relevant:

- age
- species
- breed (Table 8.1)
- diet
- FIV/FeLV status (cat)
- are the signs suggestive of acute or chronic disease?
- behavioural signs suggestive of hepatic encephalopathy
  - irritability
  - aggression
  - disorientation
  - ptyalism (cat)
- medications, especially those which may be hepatotoxic
- vaccination status (with relevance to leptospirosis and adenovirus)
- deworming
- recent travel
- access to plants, mushrooms, chewing gum, or medicines
- are other animals in the litter/household affected?

As previously mentioned, the clinical signs of hepatobiliary disease are generally non-specific and can be:

- **gastrointestinal**: anorexia, vomiting, diarrhoea
- **urinary**: polyuria, polydipsia
- **neurological**: lethargy, depression.

Table 8.1. Breeds with predisposition to hepatobiliary diseases.

Vascular abnormalities		**Amyloidosis**	
Dogs	**Cats**	**Dogs**	**Cats**
Cairn Terrier Australian Cattle Dog Dachshund Golden Retriever Irish Wolfhound Maltese Miniature Schnauzer	Himalayan Persian	Shar Pei	Siamese Abyssinian
Liver disease caused by copper accumulation		**Chronic hepatitis**	
Dogs	**Cats**	**Dogs**	**Cats**
Bedlington Terrier Dalmatian Skye Terrier West Highland White Terrier Labrador Retriever	Siamese	Cocker Spaniel (English and American) Doberman Pinscher Poodle	

Specific signs of liver disease include:

- **hepatic encephalopathy**: blindness, coma, stupor, and seizures
- in addition, in cats:
  - ptyalism
  - jaundice
  - coagulopathies.

The findings on a physical examination are varied and non-specific. Of particular relevance to hepatobiliary disease are:

- **vital signs**: e.g. fever
- **mucous membranes**: icteric mucosae
- **abdominal palpation**: ascites, hepatomegaly
- **neurological exam:** hepatic encephalopathy.

Diagnosis

For all cases of suspected hepatobiliary disease, the basic laboratory tests include a **complete blood count**, **biochemistry** profile, and **urine analysis** (Figure 8.1). Also, in cats older than 6 years of age, measurement of **T4** is recommended, since hyperthyroidism can

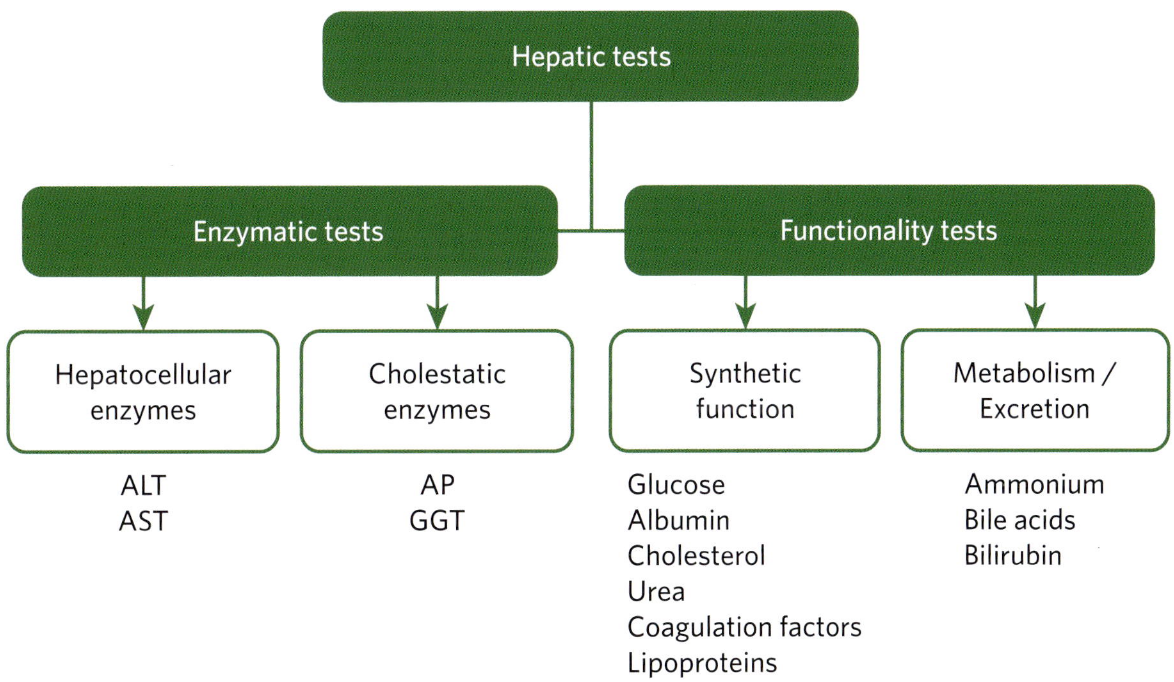

Figure 8.1. Hepatic laboratory tests.

cause elevation of liver enzymes. These tests help to assess the presence of a liver-specific disease or a reactive process, and establish if other organs are affected.

Blood tests: complete blood count

Changes in a complete blood count may include:

- abnormalities in the morphology and size of erythrocytes:
  - **microcytosis**: due to abnormal transport of iron in the liver
  - **target cells**
  - **poikilocytes**: due to alterations in the red blood cell membrane lipoproteins
  - **anaemia**: due to gastrointestinal bleeding, oxidation, or chronic disease
- **thrombocytopenia**: caused by concurrent disease or thrombopoietin deficiency as this is synthesized in the liver.

Should a puppy have microcytosis or hypochromia, with or without the anaemia, then the possibility of a portosystemic shunt should be investigated.

Blood tests: blood biochemistry

Blood biochemistry may indicate the presence of elevated levels of liver enzymes, but this does not differentiate primary liver disease from a reactive condition. Inflammation of the pancreas or intestine can trigger raised liver enzymes due to the liver's proximity to these organs. Other causes of raised liver enzymes in the absence of hepatic pathology include non-hepatic disease (such as dental disease) and medications such as phenobarbital or glucocorticoids (Table 8.2).

It is important to know that the numerical elevation of an enzyme level has no prognostic value, and the pattern of elevation over time is not always linked with the progression of the primary problem. For example, in chronic hepatitis or cirrhosis, once the disease process is advanced and less functional tissue is present, the levels of liver enzymes will drop.

Alanine transaminase (ALT) was formerly known as glutamic-pyruvic transaminase (GPT). **ALT** and aspartate aminotransferase (**AST**) are **hepatocellular enzymes**. ALT is found in the cytosol of liver cells, and is released into the bloodstream when these are damaged or inflamed. However, ALT can also be raised in cases of muscle damage.

Table 8.2. Non-hepatic processes which can cause elevation of liver enzymes.

Cause		AP	GGT	ALT	AST
Drugs	Corticosteroids (dog)	↑↑↑	↑↑	↑	↑
	Anticonvulsants (dog)	↑	↑	↑	
Endocrine diseases	Hyperadrenocorticism (dog)	↑↑↑	↑↑	↑	↑
	Diabetes mellitus	↑			
	Hypothyroidism (dog)	↑			
	Hyperthyroidism (cat)	↑		↑	
Hypoxia/hypotension	Congestive heart failure	↑		↑↑	↑
	Severe acute anaemia				
	Status epilepticus				
	Severe hypotension				
Muscular diseases	Myopathies			↑	↑↑↑
	Trauma				
	Malignant hyperthermia				
Neoplasms	Adenocarcinoma	↑		↑	↑
	Sarcoma				
	Hepatic metastasis				
Bony changes	Growth	↑			
	Osteosarcoma				
	Osteomyelitis				
	Panosteitis				
Other causes	Systemic infections	↑		↑	↑
	Gestation (cats)	↑			
	Young animals	↑			
	Gastroenteritis			↑	↑
	Pancreatitis	↑	↑	↑	↑
	Haemolysis				↑

Note: ALT, alanine transaminase; AP, alkaline phosphatase; AST, aspartate aminotransferase; GGT, gamma glutamyl transpeptidase.

The half-life of ALT is 2.5 days in the dog and 6 hours in the cat. Thus elevated levels in the **cat** are especially significant as a sign of **active damage**.

Aspartate aminotransferase (**AST**) is present in liver cell cytoplasm and also in hepatocyte mitochondria. It is a more sensitive, but less specific, indicator of liver damage than ALT.

Elevation of AST can be indicative of severe **hepatocellular** damage, **muscle injury**, or **haemolysis**. For example, a marked elevation of AST is frequently to be found in cases with haemolytic anaemia.

The half-life of AST is 22 hours in the dog and 77 minutes in the cat.

Alkaline phosphatase (**AP**) **and gamma glutamyl transpeptidase** (**GGT**) are both enzymes that indicate cholestasis.

AP elevation is **not specific to liver disease**, especially in the dog. AP is present in the membranes of other tissues, such as **bone**, and its release is induced by corticosteroids (which does not occur in the cat). GGT may also increase due to treatment with anticonvulsants and glucocorticoids.

The half-life of AP is 70 hours in the dog and 6 hours in the cat.

Cats have lower concentrations of AP and GGT, and the average half-life is shorter than in dogs. Therefore, any elevation in these enzymes is considered a sign of significant liver disease in the cat.

Albumin, glucose, urea, and cholesterol are specific indicators of hepatic disease, but they are not very sensitive. Likewise, liver disease cannot be ruled out on the basis of normal biochemistry.

Figure 8.2 outlines the approach to take in patients with elevated liver enzymes.

Urinalysis

Animals with liver disease often present with **polyuria/polydipsia** due to multifactorial causes.

It is important to evaluate whether the animal has a **urinary infection** (described in 30% of cases of portosystemic shunt) and to perform an examination of **urinary sediment** (ammonium urate crystals). The presence of urate crystals in the urinalysis of a puppy with clinical signs (delayed growth, neurological signs) should raise suspicions of a portosystemic shunt.

The presence of **bilirubin in urine** is **normal in dogs**, especially in male dogs; this is due to a lower reabsorption threshold and the presence of renal enzymes that metabolize bilirubin. But **bilirubinuria** is an **abnormal finding in cats**.

The presence of **glycosuria, without hyperglycaemia**, in an animal with elevated liver enzymes, indicates a **kidney problem** or tubular or glomerular damage. This can occur in cases of intoxication with non-steroidal anti-inflammatory drugs (NSAIDs) and also in cases of leptospirosis, since this disease can affect the liver and/or kidney, causing a generalized tubular failure.

When the initial analysis points towards a hepatobiliary problem, the next step is to perform **liver function**

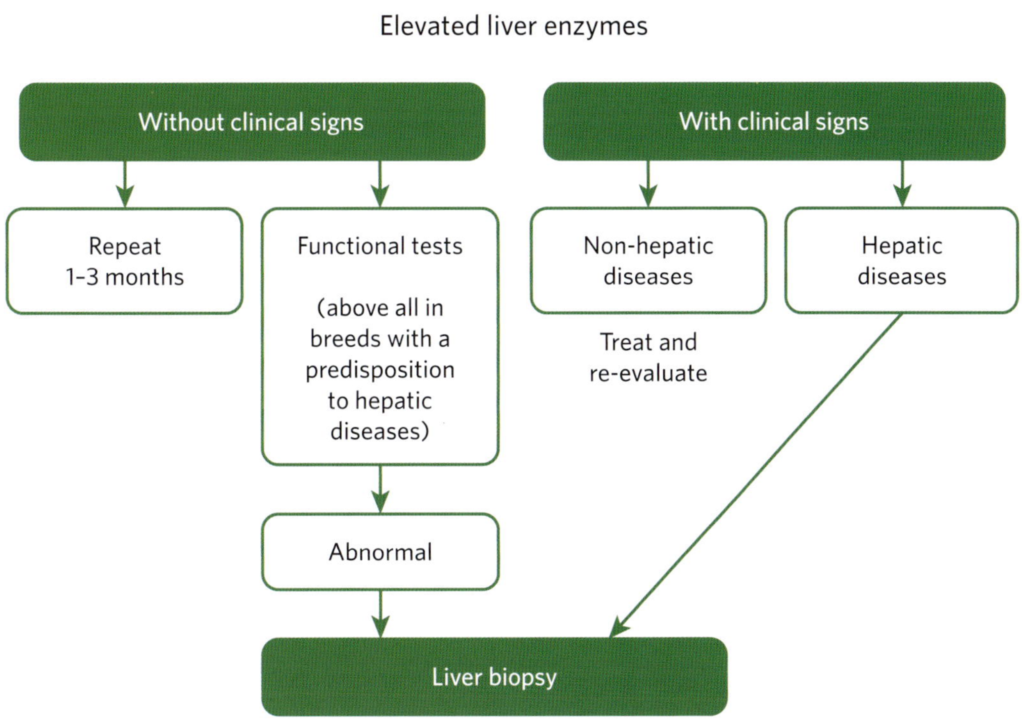

Figure 8.2. How to approach elevated liver enzymes.

tests and **imaging**. In many cases, a **liver biopsy** is necessary to reach a definitive diagnosis.

Function tests

Bile acids

Bile acids are synthesized **exclusively in the liver** from cholesterol. Once conjugated with taurine or glycine, they are **secreted in bile** and stored in the gall bladder. When the gall bladder contracts after eating, bile acids are transported to the intestine and 95% are reabsorbed in the distal ileum (facilitated by the enterohepatic circulation). An **alteration** at any point of the **enterohepatic circulation** in the liver, gall bladder, or common bile duct will lead to an **increased level of bile acids in the blood**.

In the absence of anaemia, the elevation of bilirubin indicates a problem with the enterohepatic circulation. Therefore, in cases of hyperbilirubinaemia without anaemia, measurement of bile acids is not necessary.

Test features:

- **Not sensitive:** 60–70%, except in cases of vascular anomalies and cirrhosis, where it is almost 100%. To maximize the sensitivity of the test, bile acids are measured on an empty stomach and again 2 hours after eating. If bile acids are high in the first sample, the second measurement is not necessary.
- **Highly specific:** 95–100% in hepatobiliary disease; therefore it is the ideal test to evaluate liver function.

Test limitations:

- The degree of bile acid elevation **does not differentiate** one disease from another.
- The degree of elevation has **no prognostic value**. Increases or decreases in bile acid levels do not correlate with the severity of the primary disease.
- Values may vary over time, without implying an improvement or worsening of the primary disease.

Ammonium

Ammonium is produced by **intestinal bacteria in the colon** and **detoxified in the liver**, where it is transformed into urea (Figure 8.3). An **increase in ammonium** levels is indicative of a **vascular anomaly**, a loss of more than 70% of hepatic parenchyma, or congenital alterations of urea cycle metabolism.

Test features:

- This test must be run immediately after obtaining the sample.
- **Very sensitive** for the detection of vascular anomalies. Hyperammonaemia is 100% sensitive for the detection of a portosystemic shunt, with 80% sensitivity in cases of acquired shunts secondary to chronic hepatic pathologies.

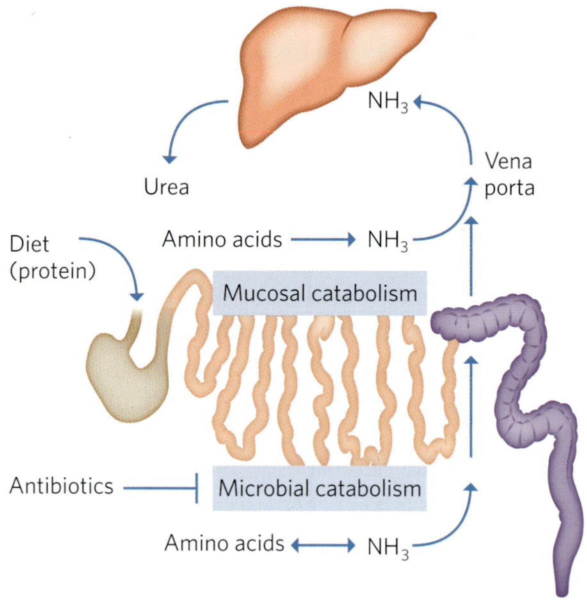

Figure 8.3. Production of ammonium and its metabolism in the liver, giving rise to urea.

Transient hyperammonaemia has also been described in Irish Wolfhound puppies, with spontaneous correction at 3–4 months. It has also been found to occur in dogs and cats with arginine and cobalamin deficiency.

An advantage of measuring ammonium, as opposed to bile acids, is that the result is not influenced by the presence of gall bladder disease. Thus **raised ammonium levels** are more specific for **liver function impairment due to a shunt** than increased levels of bile acids (Figure 8.4).

Bilirubin

A **rise in bilirubin** is associated with **liver failure**, but with **low specificity**. Raised bilirubin levels can come about through haemolysis (pre-hepatic), decreased liver function (hepatic) or cholestasis, pancreatitis, or gall bladder problems (post-hepatic). It can also be elevated due to sepsis and its associated multifactorial causes (Figure 8.5).

Coagulation tests

In addition to **synthesizing coagulation factors**, the liver takes part in the metabolism of the products and factors activated during fibrinolysis. Therefore, prothrombin (PT) and activated partial thromboplastin (APTT) times should be evaluated, especially before performing an invasive procedure such as liver biopsy.

Cholestatic diseases such as hepatic lipidosis and cholangiohepatitis are usually associated with

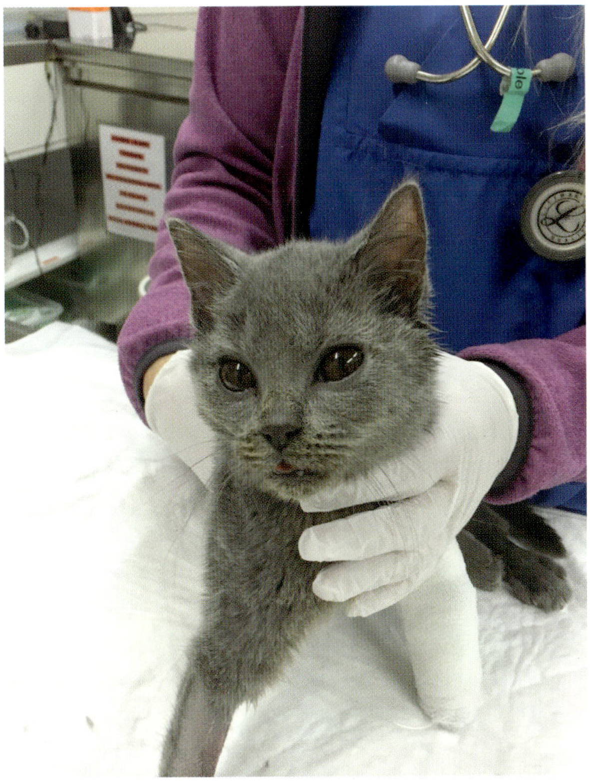

Figure 8.4. A 4-month-old cat with hepatic encephalopathy due to a portosystemic shunt. The cat presented with blindness, intermittent changes in behaviour and stupors. On physical examination, the eyes were a dark copper colour. The ammonium concentration was 250 mmol/l (<30 mmol/l).

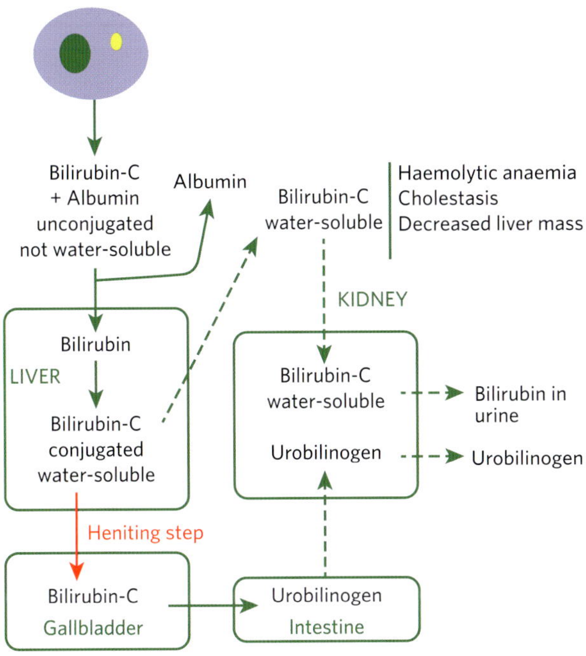

Figure 8.5. Degradation of haemoglobin and formation of bilirubin.

hypo-coagulability and, consequently, **prolonged coagulation times**. Approximately 50–75% of dogs and cats with hepatobiliary disease have prolonged PT and APTT times.

Vitamin K deficiency is multifactorial and can be associated with hepatobiliary disease. For example, it can arise due to a lack of bile acids in the intestine or a low intake of vitamin K in anorexic animals. The most frequent finding in cases of vitamin K deficiency (due to liver disease or cholestasis) is a **prolongation of PT**, since coagulation factor VII is the factor with the shortest half-life. Vitamin K is a cofactor in carboxylation and activation of factors II, VII, XI, X, and protein C.

The best test to evaluate overall haemostasis is thromboelastography or thromboelastometry, although the availability of these tests is limited outside universities. Animals with severe prolongation of coagulation times (>1.5 times greater than reference values) have a higher risk of bleeding. However, it has been observed that coagulation times do not necessarily correlate with the risk of bleeding.

In fact, fibrinogen levels better predict the risk of bleeding. **Liver biopsy is contraindicated** in animals with **fibrinogen levels less than 50%** of the reference value.

Diagnostic imaging

Abdominal radiographs may be useful to evaluate the position, shape, margins, and size of the liver.

Ultrasound is more sensitive and allows the liver to be assessed more fully for size, echogenicity, the presence of masses, and abnormal vascularization. A scan also enables assessment of the biliary structures (gall bladder and bile ducts), the pancreas, and the rest of the abdomen for lymphadenopathy, neoplasms, and ascites. The procedure has the advantage of facilitating ultrasound-guided aspiration of the liver, ascitic fluid, and gall bladder or an **echo-guided tru-cut biopsy**. Therefore, in any animal where hepatobiliary disease is suspected, an abdominal ultrasound scan is advisable.

However, a normal appearance does not exclude liver pathology. To diagnose or rule out a shunt (congenital or acquired), the following techniques are useful.

- **Colorectal scintigraphy**. This non-invasive test helps evaluate the presence of a shunt. In normal animals, the technetium is transported from the colon to the portal system and the liver. In animals with shunts, most of the technetium bypasses the liver and goes directly to the heart. The shunt fraction compares the activity of the liver with that of the heart. In animals with shunts it is >60%, although there is wide variability.
- **Ultrasound-guided trans-splenic scintigraphy**. This test allows the number of shunts and their locations to be determined.

- **Computed tomography (CT) and magnetic resonance imaging (MRI)**. These non-invasive tests provide more detailed anatomical information. They are performed under anaesthesia or sedation and allow the clinician to find the anatomical location of the shunt and to differentiate between intra- and extrahepatic shunts.
  - CT angiography allows detailed evaluation of venous anatomy.
  - In MRI, the use of a contrast agent is not necessary. The sensitivity and specificity of MRI for the diagnosis of portosystemic shunts are 80% and 100% respectively.

Abdominocentesis and abdominal fluid analysis

When **ascitic fluid** is present, a sample should be obtained and analysed for **urine specific gravity (USG), total protein content, nucleated cells,** and **cytological examination**. This can help to obtain a diagnosis in cases of biliary peritonitis or carcinomatosis. Knowing whether the fluid is a transudate, exudate, or haemorrhage also helps to prioritize the differential diagnoses. Analysis can also confirm or rule out the need to perform surgery, for example in cases of septic peritonitis.

Other tests

In cats where hepatobiliary disease is suspected, testing for **FeLV** and **FIV** along with **T4** should be considered.

Liver biopsy

Once extrahepatic diseases have been ruled out, a **liver biopsy** is essential to obtain a **definitive diagnosis**. Biopsy is of prognostic value, and when performed after treatment it facilitates an assessment of the response to treatment.

The main **indications** for liver biopsy are as follows.

- **Persistent elevation of hepatocellular enzymes** (such as ALT) or cholestasis markers once other possible causes have been ruled out.
- **Persistent hyperbilirubinaemia** or altered hepatic function tests.
- **Alterations in liver size** or changes of hepatic parenchyma on ultrasound exam.
- To **identify** the type of hepatic mass or nodule.
- Sequential evaluation of **disease progression**, when the prognostic information obtained is of use.
- Sequential evaluation of the **response to treatment**, when superior to other methods.

Contraindications for liver biopsy include **cystic lesions** and a **high risk of bleeding**. The latter is indicated by severe prolongation of coagulation times, marked thrombocytopenia, or severe hyperfibrinogenaemia.

There are several methods of obtaining a biopsy sample, which all have advantages and disadvantages. These are described below. The most appropriate method should be chosen according to the size of the liver, the differential diagnoses, and overall state of the animal.

Fine-needle aspiration for cytology

- Advantages:
  - no need for anaesthesia
  - cheap and easy
  - low risk
  - sensitive for diagnosis of vacuolar liver disease, inflammation, lymphoma, and hepatic lipidosis, although the cytological diagnosis of hepatic lipidosis does not exclude other processes.
- Disadvantages:
  - imprecise: in general, fine-needle aspirate cytology has a low correlation with biopsy samples (30%)
  - does not provide information on fibrosis, severity, location, cholestasis, necrosis, coexistence of vascular or other problems.

Ultrasound-guided biopsy or tru-cut

- Advantages:
  - non-invasive
  - requires deep sedation or general anaesthesia
  - provides deeper biopsies yielding information about hepatic architecture.
- Disadvantages:
  - more expensive than cytology (but less expensive than laparoscopy)
  - higher risk of bleeding
  - biopsy sample sizes are small
  - difficult to perform in cases of fibrosis or micro hepatitis
  - results have a correlation of 50–60% with the final diagnosis.

Laparoscopy

- Advantages:
  - allows visualization of the liver
  - allows larger biopsy samples to be obtained
  - low risk of bleeding
  - a brief intervention when performed by an experienced surgeon.
- Disadvantages:
  - cost of the necessary equipment

- requires general anaesthesia
- should be performed by experienced personnel
- the samples obtained are superficial.

Laparotomy

- Advantages:
  - allows excellent visualization of the liver
  - provides good sized biopsies
  - allows other biopsy samples to be obtained and/or placement of a feeding tube
  - facilitates control of bleeding
  - allows biopsies from other organs to be obtained and aspiration of the gall bladder.
- Disadvantages:
  - more invasive and painful than other tests
  - requires a longer anaesthetic than laparoscopy
  - more expensive than other tests.

For more information, see the video on laparoscopy at http://publication.improveinternational.com

Treatment of hepatobiliary diseases

Nutrition

A balanced diet is essential. Protein restriction is only indicated in patients showing signs of hepatic encephalopathy.

Dietary recommendations for patients with hepatic disease

Adapted from Rutgers and Biourge, Die Ernährung von Hunden mit Lebererkrankungen.

Source of nutrients

Foods should have high palatability and energy density (110–130 kcal/kg PV 0.75). Provide several small meals distributed throughout the day in order to:

- increase total food intake
- ensure intake of energy and nutrients
- avoid exceeding the metabolic capacity of the liver.

Fat

The ideal diet is food with a normal fat content, where 30–50% of the energy is supplied by fat. An excessive intake of fatty foods can result in severe cholestasis, hyperlipidaemia, or vacuolar liver disease.

Carbohydrates

Carbohydrate should provide no more than 45% of the diet's energy content.

Protein

- Offer high quality, highly digestible proteins.
- **Avoid protein restriction**. Protein should provide at least 14% of the energy content, preferably more than 20% as this aids tissue repair.
- Adjust protein intake depending on body condition and serum albumin levels.

Fibre

Soluble fibre should be offered in moderate amounts, as this can reduce absorption of ammonium from the gut.

Vitamins and minerals

Patients with hepatobiliary disease have a **heightened need for B-complex vitamins**.

- The antioxidant properties of vitamin E can reduce damage by free radicals.
- Reduced sodium content is beneficial when oedema or ascites are present.
- Potassium supplementation can be beneficial.
- Reduced consumption of copper is recommended.

Additional antioxidants

The following are recommended:

- high zinc content (greater than 43 mg/1000 kcal) to decrease intestinal absorption of copper
- high levels of vitamin E (dosage 10–100 iu/kg)
- supplementation with vitamin C
- added taurine.

Dietary modifications in the presence of complications

Hepatic encephalopathy

- Restrict protein intake to a minimum of 2.1 g/kg/day.
- Use parallel measures to reduce the impact of protein metabolism:
  - provide non-protein sources of energy
  - lactulose 0.25–0.5 ml/kg/8 h PO
  - metronidazole 7.5 mg/kg/12 h PO
  - increase the amount of soluble fibre in the diet
  - change the source of proteins to vegetables and/or milk.

Ascites

The following are recommended:

- food with a low sodium content (<0.5 g Na/1000 kcal)
- diuretics (spironolactone 1.2 mg/kg/12 h)
- furosemide 2–4 mg/kg/8–12 h PO.

Antioxidants

S-Adenosylmethionine (SAM-e)

SAM-e provides methionine for the synthesis of glutathione, which protects against oxidative damage. SAM-e should be administered on an empty stomach.

Dosage: 20 mg/kg PO (coated tablets).

Silibinin/silymarin (milk thistle)

Prevents and helps the liver **recover from insult caused by certain toxins** (*Amanita* mushrooms). It has antioxidant, anti-inflammatory, and antifibrotic properties, in addition to promoting regeneration.

Dosage: 20–50 mg/kg/24 h PO.

Ursodeoxycholic acid (USDA)

USDA **protects against the harmful effects of hydrophobic bile acids** in the liver, bile, and blood. It is also a cytoprotectant, at the level of hepatocellular membranes and possibly also at the blood–brain barrier. USDA is immunomodulatory and promotes bile flow, which helps the elimination of biliary toxins.

Dosage: 15 mg/kg/12 h PO.

Copper reduction

1. **Reduce copper** intake with a low copper diet.
2. **Zinc supplementation** as this reduces the intestinal absorption of copper.

   Dosage: 5–10 mg/kg/12 h elemental zinc PO (30 minutes before eating). Do not use zinc and chelators at the same time.

3. **Chelators** are indicated when the amount of copper exceeds 1500 µg/mg liver.

   Dosage: D-penicillamine 15 mg/kg PO BID, 30 minutes before eating, for at least 6 months.

Immunomodulation

Useful drugs for immunomodulation include:

- prednisone/prednisolone
- azathioprine
- cyclosporine.

Vitamin K

Prophylactic administration of vitamin K is recommended empirically in animals with **prolongation of coagulation times**, especially those with cholestatic diseases such as hepatic lipidosis, and when liver biopsy is planned. In cases of vitamin K deficiency, coagulation times are usually normalized after parenteral vitamin administration.

Dosage: vitamin K 1–2 mg/kg/day SC, for 3–4 days.

Fresh frozen plasma

In animals with evidence of active bleeding due to a coagulopathy associated with liver pathology, the treatment of choice is fresh frozen plasma because of its coagulation factors.

Liver disease in the dog

Chronic hepatitis

Introduction

Reaching a definitive diagnosis can be a challenge in the face of suspected hepatic or hepatobiliary disease. Often it is not possible to make that diagnosis based solely on history, clinical signs, and blood work, because imaging and invasive tests such as biopsies are required.

In general, dogs with **elevated liver enzymes** are more likely to have secondary or **reactive disease**, rather than a primary liver problem. But differentiating between primary and secondary liver diseases, such as those caused by endocrinopathy, medication, intestinal disease, and pancreatic problems, may require extensive investigation. Table 8.3 lists hepatocellular and post-hepatic or biliary diseases in the dog.

Aetiology

Chronic hepatitis is **not uncommon** in the dog, but because of the liver's large reserve capacity it often goes **undetected**. By the time clinical disease becomes evident, it is often too late to identify the inciting or primary cause. A list of possible causes is shown in Table 8.4.

Epidemiology

Certain types of chronic hepatitis are associated with **specific dog breeds**. Therefore, when drawing up a list of differential diagnosis, the patient's breed and age should be taken into consideration (see Table 8.4).

The following breeds are linked with an increased risk of hepatitis: Doberman Pinscher, Labrador Retriever, Skye Terrier, Springer Spaniel, West Highland White Terrier, Cocker Spaniel, and Scottish Terrier (see Table 8.4).

Table 8.3. Classification of liver diseases in the dog.

Hepatocellular diseases	Post-hepatic or biliary diseases
Acute hepatitis (drugs, toxins, canine adenoviruses 1, leptospirosis, bacterial cholangiohepatitis, abscesses) Chronic hepatitis (hereditary, drugs, chronic idiopathic hepatitis, hepatitis due to copper accumulation) Lobular dissecting hepatitis Vascular anomalies (portosystemic shunts, arteriovenous fistula) Vacuolar liver disease Neoplasia (primary or secondary) Vacuolar liver disease, hepatic lipidosis Mycoses	Cholangitis Biliary neoplasia Biliary mucocele Extrahepatic obstruction (cholelithiasis, neoplasia) Pancreatic abscess, pancreatitis Neoplasia

Table 8.4. Possible aetiologies of chronic canine hepatitis.

Known cause	Unknown causes
Hepatitis due to copper accumulation Breed associated hepatitis: • Doberman Pinscher • Skye Terrier • West Highland White Terrier • Labrador Retriever • Cocker Spaniel • Maltese Leptospirosis Infectious canine hepatitis virus Hepatitis associated with medications	Idiopathic hepatitis Lobular dissecting hepatitis Idiopathic cirrhosis Breeds with high prevalence of chronic hepatitis / cirrhosis: • Doberman Pinscher • Kerry Blue Skye Terrier • West Highland White Terrier • Labrador Retriever • Cocker Spaniel • Beagle • German Shepherd • Bernese Mountain Dog • Giant Poodle • Bedlington Terrier

Clinical signs

The clinical signs of chronic hepatitis are **non-specific** and can include diarrhoea, icterus, and coagulopathy. In some cases, for example in young Labrador Retrievers, the patient is often asymptomatic with the only finding being persistently elevated ALT.

Diagnosis

The large functional reserve of the liver means that apparently well animals that raise a suspicion of hepatitis should be worked up. An **early diagnosis** by means of a **liver biopsy** is recommended.

By the time clinical signs are present, it is often too late to delay progression or reverse the process. As disease progresses the dog may develop **liver failure**, reflected in a blood panel with hypalbuminaemia, hyperbilirubinaemia, elevated bile acids, hypoammonaemia, and coagulopathies.

Treatment

Chronic canine idiopathic hepatitis is a cyclic process whereby **inflammation leads to fibrosis** and loss of functional liver tissue. In the majority of cases there is no effective treatment and therapy consists of **supportive care** and minimizing the clinical signs.

Treatment of hepatic encephalopathy

Treatment aims to reduce the absorption of ammonium from the intestine.

- **A highly digestible diet** containing **high quality protein** which is low in minerals. Mild to moderate protein restriction is advisable, since severe protein restriction results in undesirable catabolism.
- **Lactulose:** This is an osmotic laxative which reduces the pH of the colon and thereby **minimizes the absorption of ammonium**. Lactulose can be given *per rectum* in collapsed patients that are unable to swallow.
- **Antibiotics:** Metronidazole or neomycin will reduce the population of ammonium-producing bacteria in the gut. Dosage: metronidazole 7.5 mg/kg/12 h.

Antioxidants/choleretics

- ursodeoxycholic acid
- SAM-e.

Ascites

In cases of severe ascites, use spironolactone 2–4 mg/kg BID in combination with furosemide.

Stomach protectors

- omeprazole 0.5–1.0 mg/kg PO SID
- famotidine 0.5–1.0 mg/kg PO SID or BID.

Anti-inflammatory drugs

In the only study of more than 100 dogs with chronic hepatitis, **glucocorticoid** administration appears to be **beneficial.** Dosage: prednisolone 1 mg/kg/day with a reducing dose over time.

The use of cyclosporine also appears helpful to bring about a clinical improvement and decrease hepatic inflammation.

Prognosis

The prognosis for patients with chronic hepatitis is variable. The outlook depends on the patient's state and response to therapy, with **survival times of 6–30 months** according to studies. In advanced cases and those with cirrhosis the prognosis, at less than one month, is guarded. In addition, the presence of hypoalbuminaemia, hypoglycaemia, and coagulopathy is associated with the worst prognosis, a survival time of less than one week (Strombeck study).

Leptospirosis

Aetiology

Leptospirosis is caused by infection with **spirochete bacteria** from the genus *Leptospira*. *Leptospira* are highly mobile, elongated, Gram-negative bacteria, wound in a helical shape. There are more than 20 species of *Leptospira*, for example, *Leptospira interrogans* serovar *Australis*.

Epidemiology

Leptospirosis is a **zoonotic disease** with a worldwide distribution. It can affect most mammals, with several species acting as reservoirs, for example small rodents, cows, and pigs. Clinical disease is **common in dogs**, but rare in the cat; but both dogs and cats can excrete *Leptospira* in their urine.

Leptospira can **survive for several months** in water and moist soil. Leptospirosis is a **seasonal** disease, with cases most likely to occur during the rainy season and floods. The organism is inactivated by freezing or dehydration, so infection is less likely in extreme weather conditions.

Those most at risk of acquiring infection are **young animals** in contact with standing water or in waterlogged conditions. However, cases have been diagnosed in dogs that live in apartments; therefore it should be remembered that leptospirosis can infect any dog regardless of breed, age, or lifestyle.

Based on the latest epidemiological studies, the serogroups that most commonly affect dogs living in Europe are: *Icterohaemorrhagiae*, *Grippotyphosa*, *Australis*, *Sejroe*, and *Canicola*.

The risk of disease can vary within a country, depending on regional environment and climatic conditions. In Spain, leptospirosis is diagnosed occasionally, especially in temperate or hot climates with abundant water such as Catalonia, Aragon, Asturias, and river deltas, whilst in the rest of Spain the incidence is lower.

Aetiopathogenesis

Reservoir hosts contract leptospirosis, through their mucous membranes or a skin lesion, by direct contact with urine, blood, or saliva from infected animals. Alternatively, they become infected indirectly by contact with contaminated soil, food, or water.

Based on experimental studies, the **incubation time** for clinical disease is around **5–7 days**. Once infected, animals excrete *Leptospira* in their urine for weeks to months afterwards, hence posing an infection risk to others, including humans.

Leptospira can penetrate damaged and intact skin, and mucous membranes. The *Leptospira* invade endothelial cells causing vasculitis, inflammation, and haemorrhage. They are able to replicate in many organs, including the kidneys, liver, spleen, central nervous system, eyes, and genital tract.

Clinical signs

Clinical signs are highly variable, with disease severity ranging from **mild to severe**, or even fatal. In adapted species (rodents, cows, pigs) the animal is usually asymptomatic; however, for incidental hosts (humans, dogs) the clinical signs can be severe and very serious.

Animals with leptospirosis may manifest **external bleeding** (epistaxis, haematuria, haemoptysis) due to failures in primary and/or secondary haemostasis, and they often have **generalized pain** that is difficult to locate.

Affected dogs often have a history of contact with standing water and are unvaccinated. In the early stages of active disease the **symptoms can be vague** and include lethargy, vomiting, diarrhoea, anorexia, and polydipsia.

The majority of infected dogs suffer **renal and hepatic failure**, with 30% of cases having only one organ affected. In recent years, especially in Europe, a **haemorrhagic pulmonary syndrome** associated with *Leptospira* has been described. This is characterized by intra-alveolar haemorrhage, causing haemoptysis and respiratory failure. The mortality rate in dogs with respiratory failure is 70%.

Diagnosis

In most cases blood tests demonstrate **thrombocytopenia**, anaemia, azotaemia, and elevated cholestatic liver enzymes (AP usually higher than ALT). Typical urinalysis shows **isosthenuria**, with glycosuria and proteinuria.

In cases with acute renal failure, the presence of thrombocytopenia, especially accompanied by **glycosuria with normoglycaemia**, is suggestive of leptospirosis.

Definitive diagnosis is obtained by **culture of the urine** or blood. However, culture of *Leptospira* is difficult and can take up to 6 months, and it is not currently available in Europe. Dark field microscopy has low sensitivity and specificity.

Serological tests

- **Microscopic agglutination test** (MAT) **with live antigens** is the most widely used test. Several serum dilutions are made and agglutination observed *in vitro* with live *Leptospira*. The presence of antibodies against a serovar suggests exposure to a serovar in the corresponding serogroup, not necessarily the serovar analysed. Measurement of antibodies with **paired serum samples** (1–2 weeks apart) is recommended to demonstrate seroconversion.
- **Enzyme-linked immunosorbent assay** (**ELISA**) for the detection of IgG to *Icterohaemorrhagiae*, *Canicola*, *Pomona*, and *Grippotyphosa* serovars. This test has recently been marketed in Europe. The advantage of this test is that results can be obtained in just a few minutes. However, it has little specificity (animals vaccinated in the last 4–5 months can appear as positive) or sensitivity. For the moment, sufficient information does not exist to recommend this test.
- **Polymerase chain reaction** (**PCR**) to detect the presence of *Leptospira* DNA in blood, urine, or tissues. To maximize sensitivity, sending blood and urine to the laboratory is recommended. Results are interpreted as follows.
  - Positive PCR in blood confirms leptospiraemia.
  - Positive PCR in urine indicates that the animal eliminates *Leptospira* in the urine (this can be an infected and asymptomatic animal, or a patient ill with leptospirosis).
  - Negative PCR does not rule out infection, since the life cycle of leptospiraemia is short, and the elimination of *Leptospira* in urine can be intermittent. Recent studies show that animals with leptospirosis that have been treated with antibiotics can give negative results.

Treatment

Treatment consists of a combination of **antibiotics** and **supportive care**.

Antibiotics

The recommended treatment is **doxycycline** 5 mg/kg/12 h PO or 10 mg/kg/24 h for 15 days. In the case of gastrointestinal signs or anorexia, a penicillin derivative should be administered parenterally (e.g. **ampicillin** at 20–30 mg/kg/6–8 h IV, penicillin G 25,000–40,000 IU/kg/6–8 h, or amoxicillin 20–30 mg/kg/6–8 h IV).

Any **other dogs that live with the infected dog** should be treated with doxycycline at a dose of 5 mg/kg/12 h or 10 mg/kg/24 h PO for 2 weeks.

Supportive treatment

The objectives of supportive treatment are as follows, to:

- correct dehydration, electrolyte changes, and acid–base disorders with fluid therapy
- treat systemic hypertension
- manage gastrointestinal complications with antiemetics and stomach protectors
- provide the necessary nutrients
- provide analgesia with buprenorphine.

It is important to avoid over-hydration in animals with oliguria or anuria. Although many animals with mild to moderate azotaemia respond to medical treatment, **haemodialysis** is necessary in some cases of severe renal failure (Figure 8.6). Indications for haemodialysis include when there is oliguria or anuria with hyperkalaemia or severe over-hydration that does not respond to medical treatment. Studies show that performing haemodialysis early increases survival rates and reduces hospitalization time in dogs with leptospirosis and severe renal failure.

Prevention

Leptospirosis has been diagnosed in dogs vaccinated with the bivalent *Icterohaemorrhagiae* and *Canicola* vaccine. Therefore, **bivalent vaccines do not provide enough protection** against the pathogenic serovars that usually infect dogs. Recently, new vaccines have become available in Europe which contain serovars of the serogroups *Icterohaemorrhagiae*, *Canicola*, *Grippophytosis*, and also *Bratislava*.

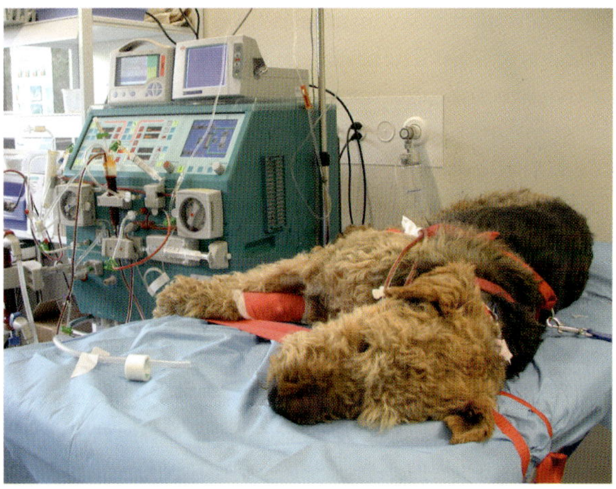

Figure 8.6. Treatment using haemodialysis in a dog with acute renal failure due to leptospirosis. University of Bern, Switzerland. Image courtesy of A. Schweighauser.

Since leptospirosis is a widespread disease and the risk of reaction to the vaccine is minimal, vaccination with quadrivalent vaccines is recommended in all dogs that have outside access to a garden or park. After an initial course of vaccinations (2 injections 3–4 weeks apart depending on the manufacturers' recommendations), **annual revaccination** is recommended especially in those animals at risk of contracting leptospirosis. The latter include dogs exposed to stagnant water, lakes, rivers, infected pets, or wild animals.

Liver disease due to toxic damage

The liver is a key organ for the metabolism of drugs and toxins. There is a large range of substances that can damage the liver, due to intrinsic or idiosyncratic reactions. The consequences of toxic damage vary from survival of the hepatocyte to apoptosis or necrosis. From the clinicopathological point of view, **toxic liver disease** can be very **difficult to differentiate** from other hepatic processes which cause **hepatocellular necrosis**. Therefore, a complete history is key to diagnosis.

Aetiopathogenesis

Intrinsic toxicity, due to medication for example, usually causes liver necrosis without inflammation and is:

- dose dependent
- predictable
- high incidence.

An example is paracetamol.

Idiosyncratic toxicity is due to immune-mediated mechanisms and is:

- not dose dependent
- unpredictable
- difficult to reproduce.

Examples are carprofen, phenobarbital in dogs, and diazepam in the cat.

Clinical signs

Toxic liver disease can be zonal or can affect all hepatic lobes. Typical histopathological findings include **hepatic necrosis** and degeneration, with or without cholestasis (Table 8.5).

In the clinical history, it is vital to collect information about:

- access to hepatotoxic medicines
- ingestion of homemade food
- access to mushrooms

Table 8.5. Histological patterns and biochemical changes characteristic of hepatotoxic drugs commonly used in small animals.

Drugs	Species	Histological findings	Enzymatic pattern
Paracetamol	Dog	Zonal necrosis	ALT↑↑
Halothane	Cat	Zonal necrosis	ALT↑↑
Sulphonamides	Dog	Toxic hepatitis	ALT↑↑
Tetracyclines	Dog	Microvesicular steatosis	ALT, AP
Amiodarone	Dog	Phospholipidosis	ALT↑
Azathioprine	Dog Cat	Veno-occlusive disease	ALT↑↑ (dose dependent)
Phenobarbital	Dog	Cirrhosis, vacuolar nodular liver disease associated with hepatocutaneous syndrome	↑↑AP
Phenobarbital	Cat	Panlobular hepatocellular necrosis	ALT/AST/CK↑ Then AP and GGT

Note: ALT, alanine transaminase; AP, alkaline phosphatase; AST, aspartate aminotransferase; CK, creatine kinase; GGT, gamma glutamyl transpeptidase.

- the existence of palm trees in the house, or other plants
- access to xylitol, commonly found in toothpaste, chewing gum, sweets, and cakes.

Clinical signs are variable: from non-specific vomiting, diarrhoea, or weakness, to jaundice and severe hepatic failure.

Diagnosis

The diagnosis is made based on the clinical history, symptoms, and clinicopathological changes.

Treatment

In mild cases, **stopping administration** of the toxic substance is sufficient. Severe cases require hospitalization and supportive treatment.

- **Rehydration** with crystalloids plus electrolyte and glucose supplementation where necessary. Colloids may be required in cases of moderate to severe hypalbuminaemia.
- Glutathione precursors (SAM-e).
- N-acetylcysteine 140 mg/kg diluted in NaCl, slow administration IV. Then 70 mg/kg/6 h, 5–8 doses in total.
- Provide symptomatic treatment with antiemetics and gastroprotectants.

Toxic liver disease associated with aflatoxins

Aetiopathogenesis

Aflatoxins are food **toxins found in grains** and are considered unavoidable. They originate from *Aspergillus flavus* and *Aspergillus parasiticus*. They are very **heat resistant**, with aflatoxin B1, 2, M1, 2ID. Aflatoxin B1 being **carcinogenic, teratogenic**, and the most toxic. The animals most susceptible to these toxins are dogs and poultry.

Dog food is routinely tested for the presence of aflatoxins. Therefore, the risk of poisoning by aflatoxins is very low in animals that only eat commercial dog food. However, cases of feed contamination with aflatoxin have been described.

Clinical signs

Although aflatoxicosis is usually a **chronic intoxication**, the clinical signs are acute and non-specific, including as **melena** and **haematochezia**. These animals may also be **jaundiced**.

Diagnosis

The biochemical profile is non-specific but may include the following.

- **Coagulopathy** as reflected by thrombocytopenia and extended PT (prothrombin time)/APTT (activated partial prothrombin time).
- **Elevation of bilirubin** greater than that of ALT, AP, or AST (the latter being only moderately raised).

The diagnosis is made based on the clinical signs and food analysis, along with liver biopsy, or at post-mortem. To identify aflatoxins in vomit, the latter has to be frozen. The urine sediment is useful, as in the case of *Amanita* mushroom poisoning.

Treatment of Aflatoxicosis

There is **no antidote** and treatment is largely supportive care including:

- fluid therapy
- vitamin K, plasma
- gastroprotectants and antiemetics
- SAM-e or NAC (N-acetyl cysteine) until liver enzymes return to normal.

Table 8.6. Mechanism of action and clinicopathological changes associated with the most frequent hepatotoxins in dogs and cats.

	Cicad Plant	Amanita	Aflatoxins	Xyloitol	Carprofen	Diazepam
Toxin	Cicasin ↑-methylamino-alanine Neurotoxin The whole plant is toxic	α-Amanitin (1 mushroom can be lethal)	Aflatoxin B1	Xyloitol	Carprofen Idiosyncratic reaction	Oral diazepam converted to an unidentified reactive metabolite, 50% metabolized to desmethyldiazepam Idiosyncratic reaction
Affected organs	Liver Gastrointestinal Nervous system	Liver Intestine Kidney	Liver Kidney	Pancreatic B cells Liver	Liver above all Kidney Gastrointestinal	Liver
Clinical signs	First 24 h: gastrointestinal, neurological signs	Severe gastroenteritis for the first 6–12 h Liver and kidney failure in 36–48 h	Variable, depending on the amount ingested Normally after ingesting toxins for >1 month	Liver Pancreatic B cells	First signs at 5–30 daysLabrador Retrievers (over-represented) take longer to manifest signs (>2 weeks)	Signs which appear in the first 7 days: anorexia, sedation, jaundice
Biochemistry	24–48 h: ↑ ALT / AST in 1/2 animals ↑ Bilirubin in 1/2 animals Thrombocytopenia in 30%	Hypoglycaemia Coagulopathy	Jaundice, ALT	30 min–1 h: hypoglycaemia 9–72 h: liver failure	↑ ALT/AST Renal toxicity in 2/3 of animals (proteinuria, glucosuria)	Hypoglycaemia, ↑ ALT and especially bilirubin.
Histopathology	Acute centrolobular necrosis with neutrophilic inflammation	Pan-lobular hepatocellular necrosis, tubular necrosis	Diffuse lipid hepatocellular vacuolation, portal fibrosis, biliary hyperplasia In chronic cases, fibrosis	Periacinar/midzone to diffuse necrosis	Necrosis, secondary cholestasis, fibrosis, minimal inflammation	Massive acute necrosis with centrilobular distribution

Definitive diagnostic tests	History	Detection of alpha-amanitin using ELISA on vomit	ELISA/HPLC	History and compatible signs	Histopathology, history, breed and time for appearance of clinical signs	Histopathology, exposure to medications
Antidote	Administration of activated charcoal	Activated charcoal Silibinin 50 mg/kg IV 5 h and 24 h after ingestion	N-acetylcysteine, SAM-e	No antidote exists Activated charcoal does not work	Stop treatment	Stop treatment, Silymarin is effective for the first 24 h after ingestion
Prognosis	Degree of elevation of AST associated with prognosis	Elevation of PT and creatinine associated with a poor prognosis	Granular cylinders in urinalysis predicts 100% mortality	Excellent when there is no hepatic failure. If there is, reserved.	Very good prognosis in Labradors, 50% in other breeds. The dose does not affect prognosis	Serious. Most cats die in the first 5 days

Note: ALT, alanine transaminase; AP, alkaline phosphatase; APTT, activated partial thromboplastin time; AST, aspartate aminotransferase; CK, creatine kinase; ELISA, enzyme-linked immunosorbent assay; GGT, gamma glutamyl transpeptidase; HPLC, high-performance liquid chromatography; PT, prothrombin time.

Prognosis
The prognosis is reserved to poor, with a mortality rate greater than 60%.

Toxic liver disease associated with xylitol poisoning

Xylitol is a **sweetener** widely found in candy, chewing gum, chocolate, toothpaste, pastries, and other human products.

Aetiopathogenesis
Xylitol is **rapidly absorbed** after ingestion and its mechanisms of action include causing oxidative damage and a decrease in adenosine triphosphate (ATP).

In non-primates, xylitol produces a **dose-dependent release of insulin** six times more potent than that produced by glucose, causing wide-ranging damage that is dose related:

- hypoglycaemia at a dose of 0.15 g/kg
- hepatic necrosis at a dose of 0.5 g/kg
- vomiting, depression, weakness, and hypoglycaemic seizures at a dose of 1 g/kg.

Clinical signs
Symptoms appear between 30 minutes to 12 hours after ingestion.

Diagnosis
Laboratory findings include:

- hypokalaemia and hypophosphatemia
- raised ALT within 4 hours of ingestion (the elevation of ALT and AST are much higher than for AP)
- coagulopathy, with signs such as epistaxis, melena, and petechiae
- thrombocytopenia
- increased TP/APTT.

Treatment
There is no antidote for xylitol poisoning. Activated charcoal is not recommended since the rapid rate at which xylitol is absorbed renders it ineffective.

The following treatments are advisable:

- **induce emesis** (<30 min): apomorphine 0.03 mg/kg IV or IM
- monitor glucose, electrolytes, and liver parameters at 12, 24, and 48 hours
- **IV dextrose** in cases of hypoglycaemia
- plasma in the case of coagulopathy
- fluid therapy with the addition of glucose
- SAM-e or Denosyl 20 mg/kg/day PO
- N-acetylcysteine.

Hepatopathy due to copper accumulation – primary

Aetiopathogenesis
This hepatopathy is the result of **copper accumulation** in the centrolobular area. It is an **autosomal recessive, hereditary** disease, commonly associated with the **Bedlington Terrier.** It has also been described in the West Highland White Terrier, Doberman, Labrador, and Dalmatian.

The gene responsible is COMMD1, which affects the biliary elimination of excess copper. The build-up of copper in the liver causes oxidative stress, damage to hepatocytes, chronic hepatitis, and finally, cirrhosis.

Clinical signs
The clinical signs may only appear in late stage disease, when the copper accumulation is already severe. Thus chronic disease often presents in an acute form with jaundice, ascites, or signs associated with **hepatic encephalopathy**.

Many dogs with this condition are healthy, with the only biochemical abnormality being elevated ALT. In some cases functional tests, such as a bile acid stimulation test, may also be normal.

Diagnosis
Elevated ALT is a non-specific sign, and abdominal ultrasound may be normal. The definitive diagnosis is made on **liver biopsy** with the **quantification of copper levels**. This can be either semi-quantitative (via rhodamine or rubeanic acid staining) or quantitative. Copper levels above 2000 Cu/g are consistent with copper hepatopathy, with value over 1000 makes the condition likely.

Treatment
Treatment involves the administration of D-penicillamine 10–15 mg/kg/12 h PO, over a minimum of 4 months. Recent studies in Labradors with copper-related liver disease show a diet low in copper reduces hepatic copper levels.

Hepatopathy due to copper accumulation – secondary

Aetiopathogenesis
Cholestasis may lead to an accumulation of copper in the periportal areas of the liver with an associated hepatopathy.

Congenital portosystemic shunt

Definition

A portosystemic shunt (PSS) refers to a vascular communication between the portal and systemic circulation. Congenital shunts appear as a result of abnormal embryonic development, which causes the persistence of vessels communicating between the portal vessels and the systemic circulation. These shunts can be **intra-** or **extrahepatic**. Acquired shunts can occur due to **portal hypertension**, for example, due to chronic liver disease.

Epidemiology

Portosystemic shunts are the most frequent congenital anomaly of the canine hepatobiliary system, with a reported incidence of 0.18%. **Small breeds** carry a higher risk of PSS, with the Miniature Schnauzer, Yorkshire Terrier, and Maltese Terrier being over-represented. **Extrahepatic shunts** represent around **two-thirds of cases**, with **intrahepatic shunts** being most common in **medium to large breeds.**

Physiopathology

The presence of a PSS reduces the liver's capacity to detoxify blood and results in encephalopathy. The diversion of portal blood from the liver causes multiple toxic substances (ammonium, mercaptans, fatty acids, and neurotransmitters) to remain in circulation. The resulting **hepatic encephalopathy** is characterized by behavioural changes, depression, seizures, ptyalism, and blindness. The symptoms are often worse after eating.

A reduced blood supply to the liver deprives the organ of oxygen, nutrients, and hepatotrophic factors. In turn, this can cause severe hepatic atrophy, resulting in a small liver size.

A large number of animals with shunts have ammonium biurate crystals and urate stones in the bladder, due to their inability to convert ammonium to urea.

Clinical signs

Animals with portosystemic shunts usually have a small stature due to delayed growth.

The main reasons for initial presentation tend to be either **polyuria/polydipsia** or **neurological** symptoms. The latter are due to hepatic encephalopathy linked to high ammonium and bile acid concentrations. These signs include:

- ptyalism
- mental dullness
- tremors
- circling
- head pressing
- ataxia
- seizures
- loss of consciousness.

Approximately 30% of PSS cases have associated urinary tract infections or urolithiasis. This is due to the presence of ammonium biurate and urate crystals in the urine. This can lead to signs such as:

- haematuria
- dysuria
- pollakiuria
- haematuria
- stranguria.

Diagnosis

In around 72% of cases, haematology shows non-specific changes, such as microcytosis with or without anaemia.

Common changes in **biochemistry** include:

- hypoalbuminaemia
- hypoproteinaemia
- decrease in urea
- hypocholesterolaemia
- hypoglycaemia
- variable elevation of liver enzymes.

Specific tests may demonstrate raised levels of bile acid and ammonium.

Urinalysis may show:

- hyposthenuria
- crystalluria (ammonium biurate), with or without bacterial cystitis.

Abdominal ultrasound facilitates evaluation of the liver's size and vascularization, along with checking the urinary system for uroliths. The sensitivity for finding shunts is variable and depends on the experience of the person performing the ultrasound. Before surgery, a detailed assessment of the shunt by CT, MRI, or portovenography is necessary.

Treatment

The treatment of choice is surgical attenuation. But in some cases a conservative medical treatment is chosen, due to the cost of surgery or when intrahepatic shunts are present.

Medical treatment

Medical treatment aims to reduce or control the clinical signs associated with encephalopathy ahead of surgical

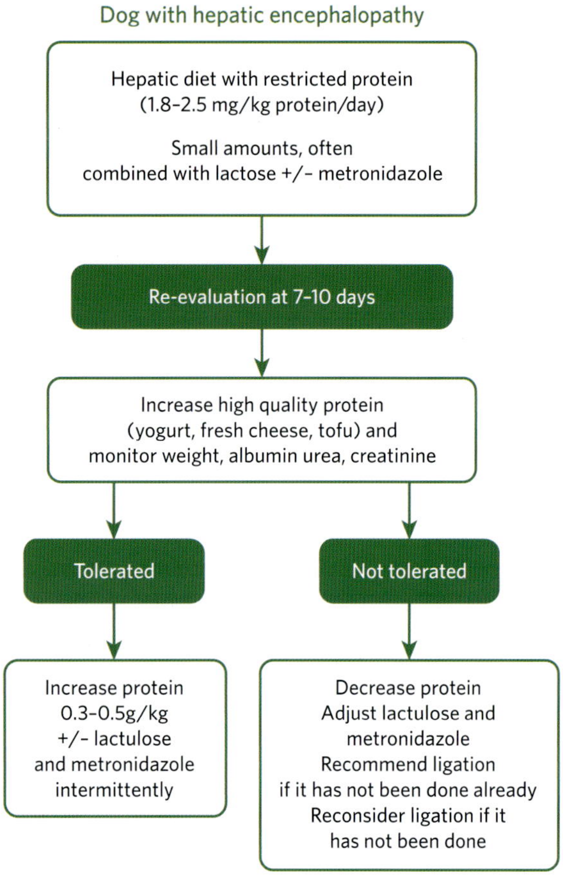

Figure 8.7. Diagram of dietary and medical interventions to treat hepatic encephalopathy in dogs (based on the University of Cornell, USA protocol).

correction of the shunt (Figure 8.7). Long-term medical treatment is a very good option for intrahepatic shunts or when, for economic reasons, the owner chooses not to opt for surgery. Although more studies are needed to establish a long-term prognosis with certainty, it is possible for an animal to live for many years with medical treatment.

Medical treatment consists of the following.

- **Low protein hepatic diet** or renal diet, to control hepatic encephalopathy. After surgical correction of the shunt, or when the animal has improved, the amount of protein in the diet should be gradually increased.
- **Lactulose:** This helps to reduce the production and absorption of ammonium in the colon. The dose is 0.5 ml/kg PO 3–4 times/day. The dose should be adjusted depending on the side effects; for example, if diarrhoea follows as a side effect the dose should be lowered.
- **Lactulose enema:** In cases of acute encephalopathy, in which the animal cannot safely swallow oral lactulose, the treatment of choice is a lactulose enema. A Foley urinary catheter with a balloon is introduced into the colon, a dilution of lactulose is prepared (3 parts lactulose and 7 parts saline), a dose of 1–10 ml/kg is administered, and the balloon is inflated and left for 20–30 minutes.
- **Gastric protectants** (omeprazole, famotidine): These are used to prevent gastrointestinal haemorrhages, which are very common in animals with liver disease and an important source of protein loss, which can exacerbate the signs of encephalopathy.
- **Antibiotics:** Metronidazole (7.5 mg/kg/12 h) or neomycin (10–20 mg/kg 3 times/day). They help reduce the number of ammonium-producing bacteria and are part of the treatment for hepatic encephalopathy, especially when oral lactulose is not sufficient.

Surgical treatment

Several methods exist for the surgical occlusion of shunts (Figures 8.8 and 8.9):

- ameroid ring
- cellophane band
- hydraulic occluders
- ligature with sutures
- minimally invasive endovascular techniques.

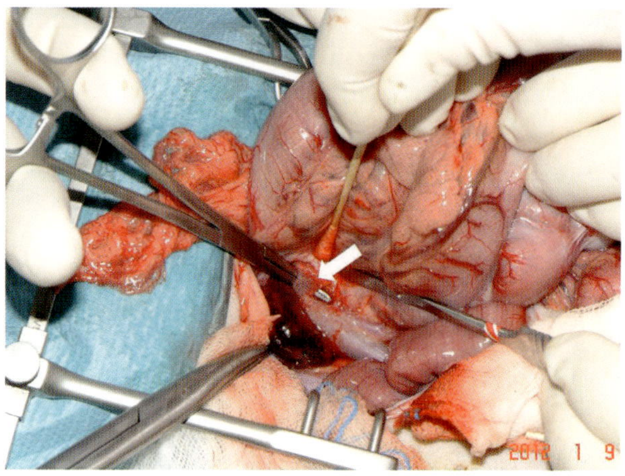

Figure 8.8. Intraoperative image of a dog with a portosystemic shunt (in the centre of the image).

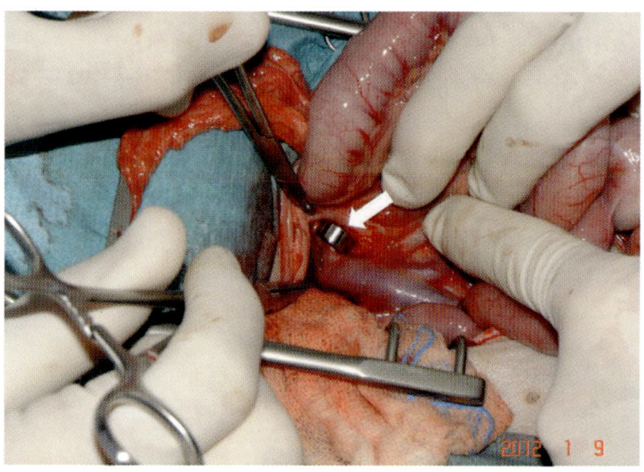

Figure 8.9. After placement of an ameroid ring.

The choice of one method over another depends on the experience and preference of the surgeon. Neutering of affected animals is recommended.

In general, all methods that gradually occlude the shunt are preferred and effective. The success rates using the ameroid ring and the cellophane band are similar. If the shunt closes too early, the liver may form collateral shunts.

Despite the many studies looking at this, it is not known why the majority of animals respond very well to surgical treatment but others do not. Due to the variety of animals, breeds, and methods used and types of study carried out (retrospective and prospective), it is difficult to compare results (Table 8.7).

Postoperative complications include:

- refractory hypoglycaemia (44%)
- portal hypertension and ascites (up to 14% of animals after ligation)
- gastrointestinal bleeding
- convulsions: to avoid this, it is advisable to start administering levetiracetam prior to surgery.

Prognosis

The studies so far have shown a more favourable long-term prognosis for animals that receive surgical treatment (good to excellent prognosis: 94% of extrahepatic shunts and 80% of intrahepatic shunts) than for those who receive medical treatment (good prognosis: 30%).

Animals that cannot be stabilized with medical treatment prior to surgery have a very poor prognosis. Mortality associated with surgery ranges from 2 to 30%.

Hypoplasia of the portal vein

Initially called hepatic microvascular dysplasia, portal vein hypoplasia is **a malformation of the microscopic portal circulation.** There is a decrease in size of the intrahepatic portal veins which causes hypoperfusion in the liver.

The histological changes are similar to those of a portosystemic shunt, with the loss or reduction of the portal vein, atrophy of the hepatic sinusoids, hyperplasia and twisting of the hepatic arterioles, and hepatocellular atrophy. There may or may not be portal hypertension.

Epidemiology

This condition is recorded in the Cairn Terrier, Yorkshire Terrier, and Maltese.

Clinical signs

Clinical signs are variable, and can range from asymptomatic to typical manifestations of a portosystemic shunt.

Diagnosis

Blood tests show a variable elevation of liver enzymes, and raised bile acids are observed. An abdominal ultrasound is usually normal. A definitive diagnosis is made with a liver biopsy.

Treatment

Treatment is symptomatic and supportive.

Hypoplasia with hypertension (non-cirrhotic portal hypertension)

Epidemiology

This condition is described in **young, large-breed** dogs and commonly presents in young dogs less than 2.5 years old.

Clinical signs

The clinical signs are similar to those of a shunt, including gastrointestinal symptoms and hepatic encephalopathy.

Table 8.7. Comparison of the surgical methods available for shunts.

Method	Study	Number of cases and type of shunt	Healing (%)	Mortality rate (%)	Neurological signs (%)
Ameroid ring	Mehl et al, 2005	168 dogs (extrahepatic)	81	7.1	4.8
		11 (intrahepatic)	57	9	9
Cellophane band	Hunt et al, 2004	95 dogs (extrahepatic)	87	3	9
		11 dogs (intrahepatic)	71	27	9
		5 cats (extrahepatic)	60	0	20
	Cabassu et al, 2011	9 cats (extrahepatic)	56	23	23
Hydraulic occluder	Adin et al, 2006	10 dogs (intrahepatic)	50	0	0
Embolization with coil	Bussador et al, 2007	6 dogs (intra- and extrahepatic)	83	0	0
Amplatzer	Hogan et al, 2011	6 dogs (extrahepatic)	83	0	0

Diagnosis

Blood tests usually show liver failure, with severe elevation of bile acids. On ultrasound, micro hepatitis and abdominal effusion as well as acquired shunts may be visible.

The diagnosis is made by histology of a liver biopsy, with the same findings as in dogs with portosystemic shunts.

Treatment

Treatment consists of sodium restriction and supportive treatment.

Prognosis

Although the symptoms, tests, and ultrasound can point towards a reserved prognosis, the prognosis is often favourable.

Biliary mucocele

Definition

A biliary mucocele is described as an enlarged gall bladder containing viscous mucoid material. The change in bile consistency is usually the result of biliary obstruction or peritonitis. A mucocele is the most frequent cause of gall bladder perforation in the dog.

On ultrasound the gall bladder appears to have a number of immobile grooves, giving it an appearance reminiscent of a kiwi fruit or cart wheel.

Epidemiology

This is an emerging disease that has been diagnosed more frequently in recent years. Any dog of any age and breed can have a mucocele, although the condition is more frequent in adult animals (>10 years old).

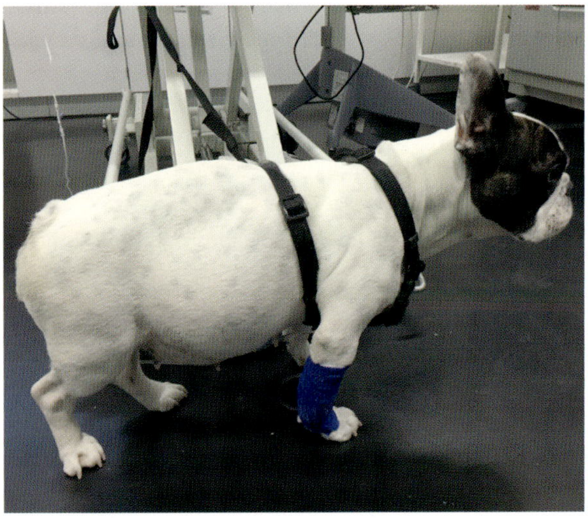

Figure 8.10. A 5-year-old French Bulldog with severe abdominal effusion associated with non-cirrhotic portal hypertension.

Aetiopathogenesis

The exact mechanism by which a biliary mucocele forms is not known, nor how **bile** becomes **thicker** than normal. However, several risk factors have been described.

- **Breed:** Shelties (Shetland Sheepdogs) have a genetic predisposition for biliary mucocele formation. In one study, it was observed that Shelties with a biliary mucocele had a mutation in the hepatobiliary transporter gene ABCB4. However, a second study with a larger sample size did not find any correspondence between this mutation and the presence of biliary mucoceles. Other breeds in which this condition is described include Cocker Spaniel, Bichon Frise, Poodle, West Highland White Terrier, Dachshund, and German Shepherd as well as mongrels.
- **Age:** 11 years (3–17) without sex predilection.
- **Concurrent endocrine pathology:** Hyperadrenocorticism (20%), hypothyroidism (12–14%), diabetes mellitus (6%).
- **Hyperlipidaemia.**

In a recent retrospective study (2015), the relationship between the appearance of a biliary mucocele and the use of certain medications was investigated. It was observed that Sheltie dogs exposed to imidacloprid were at a nine times higher risk of developing a biliary mucocele in comparison with Shelties that had not been treated with this antiparasitic agent. Further studies are needed to clarify whether imidacloprid is a predisposing factor to the formation of biliary mucocele in the dog.

Clinical signs

Animals with a biliary mucocele usually present with **non-specific signs** such as vomiting, anorexia, lethargy, jaundice, abdominal pain, and fever. In some cases the animals may be asymptomatic.

Diagnosis

Most animals show changes in biochemistry (hyperbilirubinaemia, elevation of AP and GGT), but some are completely asymptomatic and the mucocele may be an incidental finding on abdominal ultrasound.

Diagnosis is made by abdominal ultrasound (Figure 8.11), which also allows evaluation of the bile ducts and the gall bladder wall, as well as detection of ascites and collection of fluid for analysis.

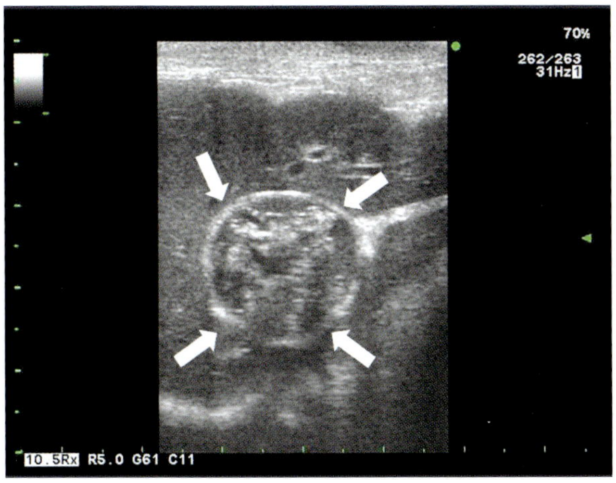

Figure 8.11. Abdominal ultrasound. Biliary mucocele (arrows).

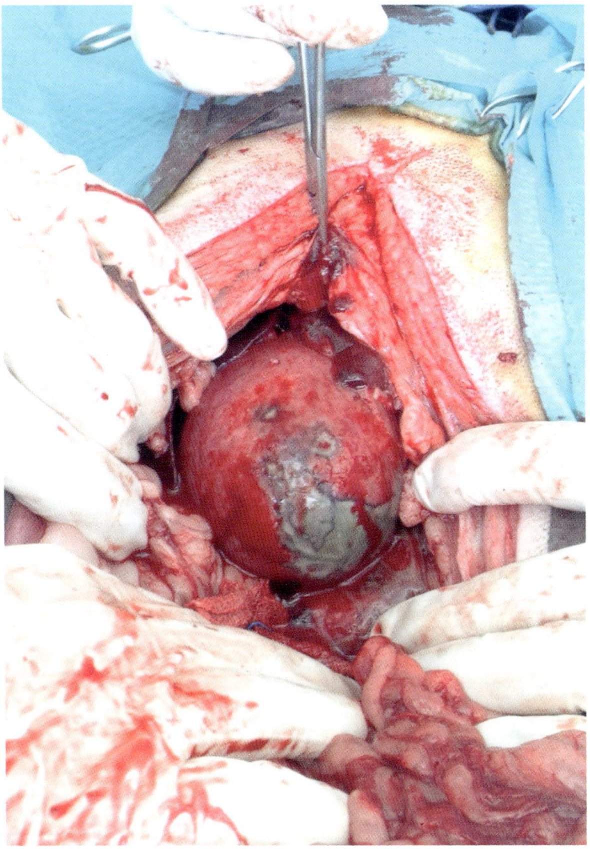

Figure 8.12. Intraoperative image of a dog with biliary mucocele and necrosis of the gall bladder.

Treatment

Dogs with mucoceles can be treated medically with **ursodeoxycholic acid**, a **low-fat diet** and periodic ultrasound monitoring. However, the treatment of choice is a **cholecystectomy** (Figure 8.12), especially if the animal shows clinical signs associated with the condition.

Prognosis

The prognosis after cholecystectomy and postoperative recovery is excellent, especially if liver enzymes normalize. There is a 20% mortality rate associated with cholecystectomy.

Liver disease in the cat

Classification

Those diseases of the liver most frequently occurring in cats are:

- **reactive liver** disease (25%):
  - feline infectious peritonitis (FIP), hyperthyroidism, medications.
- **non-inflammatory** diseases (50%):
  - hepatic lipidosis (50%)
  - neoplasia (lymphoma 7%)
  - intoxications
  - portosystemic shunt
  - polycystic disease.
- **inflammatory** diseases:
  - cholangitis–cholangiohepatitis complex (25%).

Hepatic lipidosis

Definition

Hepatic lipidosis is a **metabolic disorder** in which the rate of **lipid accumulation** in the hepatic parenchyma exceeds its rate of utilization or degradation. Triglycerides displace more than half of the hepatocellular cytosol, and when more than 75% of hepatocytes are infiltrated, this results in impaired liver function.

Aetiology

Hepatic lipidosis is a syndrome caused by an increase in catabolism as a **result of anorexia**.

The catabolic state results in a decrease in the insulin/glucagon ratio, which stimulates hormone-sensitive lipase. This in turn promotes the release of circulating fatty acids, which go to the liver for metabolism. But due to the deficiency (as a result of anorexia) of essential amino acids for the urea cycle and synthesis of apoproteins, fatty acids accumulate in the liver (Figures 8.13 and 8.14).

Hepatic lipidosis was considered an idiopathic syndrome, since its aetiology was rarely identified, but nowadays it is recognized that in 85% of cases there are one or **multiple underlying processes** that cause loss of appetite and weight loss. Among these causes are other hepatic disorders (cholangitis), pancreatitis, inflammatory bowel disease (IBD), endocrine problems (diabetes mellitus, hyperthyroidism), neoplasms, and kidney disease.

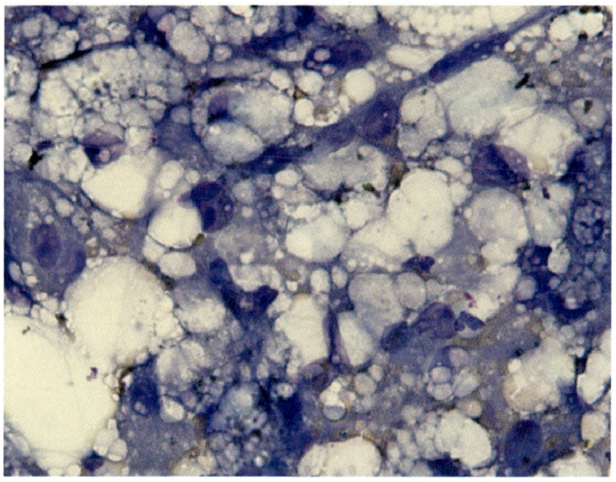

Figure 8.13. Fine-needle aspirate of the liver of a cat with hepatic lipidosis. Numerous cytoplasmic vacuoles are observed within the hepatocytes.

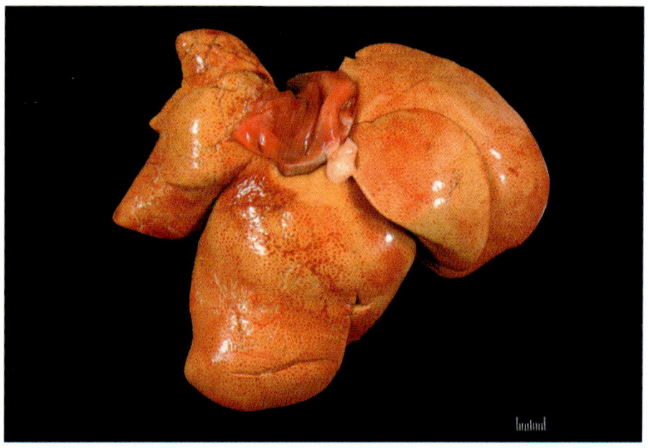

Figure 8.14. Liver with hepatic lipidosis: post-mortem image.

Hepatic lipidosis can develop over variable periods of time, from a few days to weeks after the cat stops eating. Described risk factors include:

- obesity
- protein restriction
- taurine, arginine, and carnitine deficiencies.

Clinical signs

Cats with hepatic lipidosis can present with non-specific clinical signs (anorexia, vomiting, lethargy, and depression), often linked with **significant weight loss** (40–50% of their body weight) in a short period of time. In cases of hepatic encephalopathy, symptoms include ptyalism, blindness, and stupor. Physical examination usually shows dehydration, poor coat condition, and hepatomegaly. The mucous membranes are often visibly icteric.

Diagnosis

Clinical history

Cats with hepatic lipidosis have a history of rapid weight loss over a short time, anorexia, and jaundice.

Physical examination

Typical physical findings include poor body condition, jaundice, hepatomegaly, and pytalism.

Abdominal palpation is often not painful and **abdominal effusion is uncommon**. Indeed, the presence of ascitic fluid indicates the following.

- The animal does not have hepatic lipidosis but another process that causes ascites.
- The animal has lipidosis secondary to a process associated with ascites (e.g. pancreatitis, lymphocytic cholangiohepatitis, neoplasia, FIP, heart failure).

Blood tests

A blood profile for hepatic lipidosis is similar to other liver pathologies, but there are small differences that raise suspicion of hepatic lipidosis:

- mild, non-regenerative anaemia
- absence of a marked leucocytosis and band neutrophils
- poikilocytosis and Heinz bodies on a blood smear, due to oxidation and precipitation of haemoglobin.

During hospitalization, some cats with lipidosis develop severe anaemia, requiring a blood transfusion.

Biochemistry

- AP is significantly raised, from 3 to 29 times the reference value
- GGT, ALT, and AST may be normal or slightly elevated
- elevated bilirubin levels
- elevated ammonium
- low blood albumin levels and urea
- changes associated with anorexia or vomiting, such as hypokalaemia, hyponatraemia, hypophosphatemia, and hypochloraemia.

A moderate to marked rise in AP with normal or slightly elevated GGT, ALT, and AST is typical of hepatic lipidosis. Other processes causing hepatic inflammation, such as cholangitis, are associated with high levels of ALT and GGT, but only mild increases in AP.

Coagulation profiles

Coagulation times may or may not be increased. In cases where coagulation times are prolonged, vitamin K should be administered and invasive procedures delayed. The latter includes fine-needle aspiration of the liver and the placement of feeding tubes.

Many cats with hepatic lipidosis may have pancreatitis. In some studies, almost 50% of cats with hepatic lipidosis have elevated feline pancreatic lipase (fPLI) serum values, even without evidence of abdominal pain or changes on ultrasound.

Abdominal ultrasound

A fatty liver will be enlarged, with increased ultrasound echogenicity. An ultrasound exam also enables the clinician to check for the presence of other liver pathologies, such as masses/tumours or biliary processes, which may be the primary cause of the hepatic lipidosis.

Liver biopsy

Ultrasound-guided **fine-needle aspiration** is a simple and safe technique to confirm a diagnosis of hepatic lipidosis. However, fine-needle aspiration can miss other concurrent processes of significance, such as neoplasia or inflammation. Thus, in cases where the diagnosis is not clear, liver biopsy (with the addition of duodenal biopsy) is advisable.

Treatment

Treatment of hepatic lipidosis has the following aims.

1. Eliminate or reverse the primary process that triggered the hepatic lipidosis.
2. Correct systemic complications arising from hepatic dysfunction.
3. Encourage hepatic regeneration.

Treatment of hepatic lipidosis includes the following.

- **Fluid therapy**: Crystalloids with supplementary potassium chloride are used to correct electrolyte and acid–base imbalances. B vitamins can also be added at a rate of 2–4 ml/500 ml of crystalloid fluid.
- **Vitamin K:** Three doses at 0.5–1.5 mg/kg/12 h SC.
- **Manage vomiting and nausea** using:
  - metoclopramide CRI 0.01–0.02 mg/kg/h
  - ondansetron 0.1–0.2 mg/kg/6–12 h
  - Cerenia (maropitant) 1 mg/kg IV SID.
- **Gastroprotectants** such as:
  - omeprazole 0.5–1.5 mg/kg PO SID
  - famotidine 0.1–1.0 mg/kg PO SID–BID.
- **Other supportive treatments.**
  - In cases of pancreatitis or concurrent disease causing abdominal pain, analgesia with buprenorphine 0.006–0.02 mg/kg IV, IM, SC TID is recommended.
  - Also, L-carnitine 250 mg/kg PO SID promotes the oxidation of fatty acids.
  - In cases of hepatic encephalopathy, use lactulose, SAM-e/Denosyl 20 mg/kg PO BID. This is a natural metabolite of hepatocytes that restores glutathione deficits, with antioxidant, antiapoptotic, and choleretic effects.
  - Vitamin B12: 250 μg SC, in cases of deficiency due to concurrent intestinal disease.
- **Nutritional support:** Nutrition is the only curative treatment. It must be of high quality, low in carbohydrates, and contain essential amino acids (arginine, taurine, and carnitine). Protein restriction is contraindicated.

The majority of cats with hepatic lipidosis lack appetite due to nausea and hepatic encephalopathy. The best way to provide the necessary nutritional support is through an enteral feeding tube, since this allows control of the calories and is less stressful than assisted feeding.

Feeding tubes

There are several different options for feeding tubes, depending on the needs of the individual patient.

When choosing the type of feeding tube, the following should be considered:

- the primary disease
- whether the patient can tolerate general anaesthesia
- serum albumin levels
- whether supported feeding may be necessary in the short (a few days), intermediate (weeks), or long term (months).

The pros and cons of naso-oesophageal vs. oesophagostomy tubes are summarized below.

Naso-oesophageal feeding tube

These are passed through the nose with the distal end sitting in the distal oesophagus (Figure 8.15).

Advantages: These are easy to place, inexpensive, and sedation is not required for placement. After checking that the tube is correctly positioned with thoracic

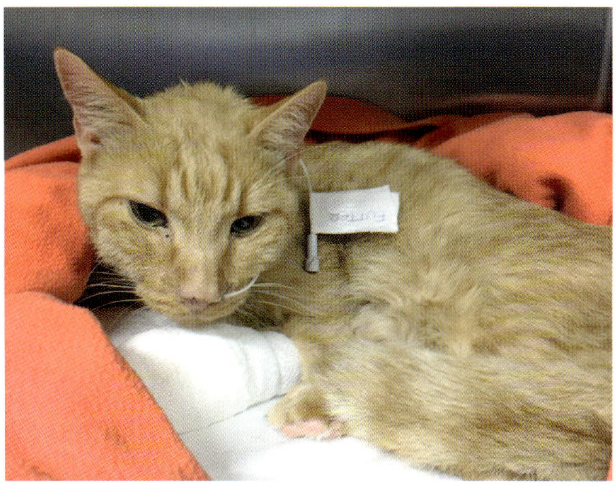

Figure 8.15. Cat with naso-oesophageal feeding tube.

radiography, it can be used immediately. The tube can be used continuously if vomiting persists or there is hypomotility. But it can also be used intermittently if the patient has some appetite.

Disadvantages: The tube should be changed once a week; and due to its small diameter, dietary options are limited. In some animals it causes discomfort, as evidenced by sneezing or epistaxis, although this is not normally significant in the cat.

Oesophagostomy tube

Advantages: Placement is easy, with few associated complications. The tube's diameter is wider than that of a naso-oesophageal tube, meaning there are more dietary options for feeding. The tube can be used 24 hours after placement, and left *in situ* for weeks to months (Figure 8.16).

Disadvantages: Placement requires a short general anaesthesia (10–15 minutes). Sometimes the edges of the stoma can become infected.

How to calculate the calorific needs of each cat

The objective is to provide enough calories to cover daily requirements.

Resting energy requirements (RER):

- animals <2 kg: RER (kcal) = (70 × weight) + 0.75
- animals >2 kg: RER (kcal) = (30 × weight) + 70

The initial percentage of RER offered is affected by how long the patient has been anorexic. In general, to reduce the risk of **refeeding syndrome**, in cats with lipidosis 25–30% of the RER is administered on day one, 50% on day two, and this is then slowly increased to 100% as long as the cat tolerates feeding.

Refeeding syndrome is frequently seen in humans when food is reintroduced after a prolonged period of malnutrition. It is characterized by a rapid release of insulin, causing severe electrolyte changes such as hypokalaemia, hypophosphatemia, and hypomagnesaemia.

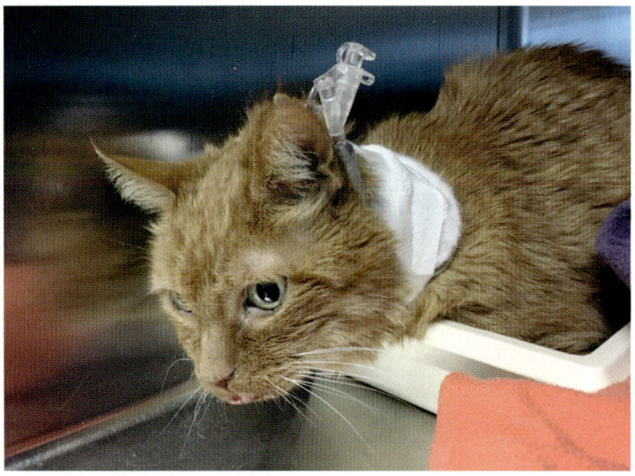

Figure 8.16. Cat with oesophagostomy tube.

Prognosis

The prognosis is guarded and varies according to the nature of the primary disease. However, with aggressive treatment, survival rates can reach 60–70%. But this may necessitate hospitalization for upwards of a week and continued tube feeding for several weeks.

Cholangitis

Since **hepatic parenchyma is rarely affected** in the cat, the term cholangitis is more appropriate than cholangiohepatitis. There are three histological forms of cholangitis:

- neutrophilic
- lymphocytic
- chronic – associated with trematodes.

Neutrophilic cholangitis

Definition and aetiopathogenesis

Neutrophilic cholangitis is an **ascending bacterial infection** of the biliary tract that originates in the small intestine and can ascend to the pancreas through the pancreatic duct. For this reason, IBD is present in a high percentage of cases (83% in some studies), and pancreatitis may result in up to 50% of them, leading to so-called triaditis.

Epidemiology

Neutrophilic cholangitis affects cats of any age, but it is diagnosed more frequently in middle to old aged cats.

Clinical signs

In acute cases the clinical signs include fever, anorexia, vomiting, icterus, and abdominal pain. The condition can become chronic (chronic neutrophilic cholangitis).

Diagnosis

In the early stages, bilirubin levels or liver enzymes may not be significantly elevated. Abdominal ultrasound often shows thickening of the wall of the gall bladder and a dilated bile duct. A definitive diagnosis requires **cytology** and **bacterial culture** (aerobic and anaerobic) of the bile.

In chronic neutrophilic cholangitis cases, a common finding is hyperglobulinaemia, and ultrasound usually shows chronic changes in the pancreas, as well as cholecystitis and dilation of the bile ducts.

Treatment

Antibiotics

Ideally, the antibiotic is selected according to **biliary culture**, and it should be administered for between **1 and 3 months**. A study of liver and bile cultures in dogs and cats determined that up to 40% of the bile samples were resistant to amoxicillin. Therefore, if culture is not possible, the administration of a broad-spectrum antibiotic or a combination of two antibiotics is recommended:

- amoxicillin–clavulanic acid 20 mg/kg/12 h + metronidazole 7.5 mg/kg/12 h
- fluoroquinolones 5–10 mg/kg/d + metronidazole 7.5 mg/kg/12 h.

Supportive treatment

This includes:

- fluid therapy, as determined by the hydration status of the patient
- ursodeoxycholic acid 10–15 mg/kg/d PO
- vitamin K 1–2 mg/kg PO (with food) or SC, until clinical resolution
- SAM-e
- antiemetics, gastroprotectants
- parenteral vitamin B12 in case of deficiency.

Biliary obstruction

In some severe cases, there may be biliary obstruction due to thickening of the bile or **cholelithiasis**. In these cases, **catheterization of the bile duct** (using endoscopy), the placement of stents (requires adequate equipment and experience), or surgery (cholecystectomy and/or catheterization of the common bile duct) are necessary.

Prognosis

The prognosis depends on the severity of the clinical signs and accompanying metabolic alterations, and especially on concurrent diseases.

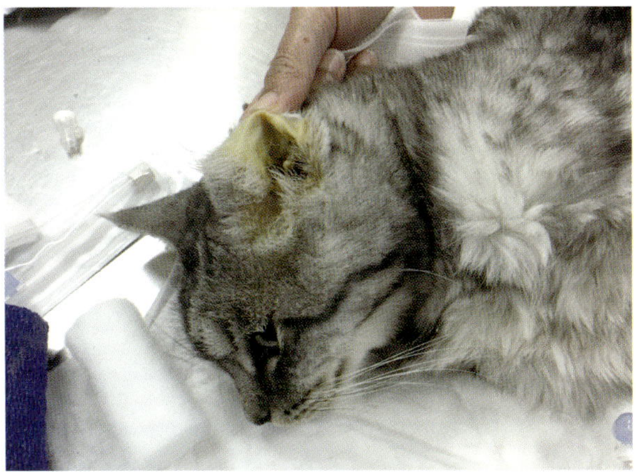

Figure 8.17. Cat with jaundice due to neutrophilic cholangitis.

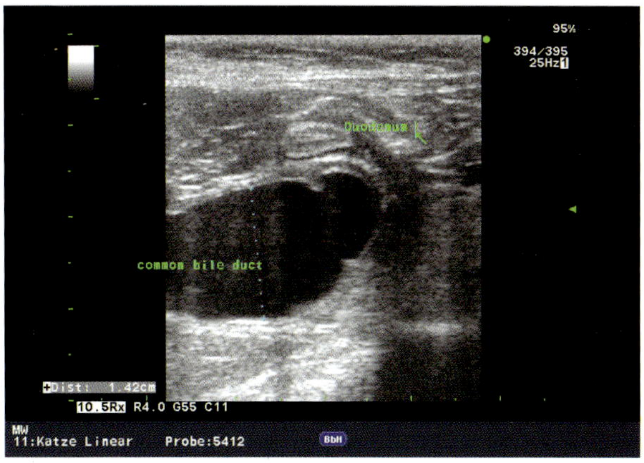

Figure 8.18. Ultrasound image of a cat with obstruction of the bile duct. A general dilation of the common bile duct at the level of the duodenal papilla is observed.

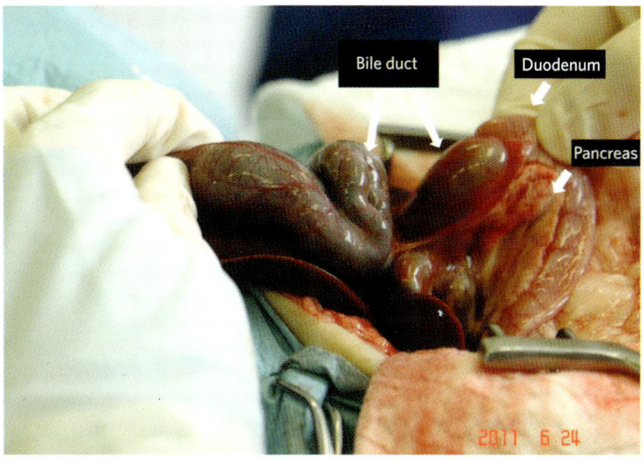

Figure 8.19. Intraoperative image of a cat with necrotizing neutrophilic cholangitis and biliary obstruction secondary to thickening of bile. On laparotomy, a massive dilation of the bile duct was found at the level of the papilla in addition to a mucocele. A cholecystectomy was performed and a stent placed in the bile duct.

Lymphocytic cholangitis

Aetiopathogenesis

The aetiology of lymphocytic cholangitis is unknown, although it is suspected to have an **immune-mediated** origin.

Clinical signs

Cats with lymphocytic cholangitis are **typically young**, with Persians being at a higher risk than other breeds. The clinical signs are usually chronic.

Cats with lymphocytic cholangitis, unlike those with neutrophilic cholangitis, are usually clinically stable, but have jaundice and weight loss. If the disease progresses to the point of biliary cirrhosis, then portal hypertension may lead to the development of ascites.

Diagnosis

Blood tests show elevation of liver enzymes and hyperbilirubinaemia. Coagulation times may be extended.

Analysis of abdominal fluid shows it is typically high in proteins, which can be confused with FIP. Definitive diagnosis is possible with histopathology, as characterized by:

- periportal lymphocytic infiltration
- portal fibrosis
- proliferation of the bile ducts.

Treatment

- prednisolone 1–2 mg/kg/12h PO. Once clinical signs have subsided, reduce doses over 6–12 weeks to 1 mg/kg/48 h
- other immunosuppressants:
  - methotrexate 0.13 mg/cat/8–12 h PO for three doses, given every 7–10 days
  - chlorambucil 2–4 mg/cat PO every 1–3 weeks
  - cyclosporine 2 mg/kg/12 h PO
- supportive treatment (ursodeoxycholic acid, SAM-e).

Prognosis

In general, animals with lymphocytic cholangitis usually respond to treatment, although there are currently few studies that have evaluated the long-term prognosis. The presence of ascites is associated with a worse prognosis. It is important to explain to the owner that, even if the cat improves clinically with treatment, there is the possibility of relapse and that the animal needs treatment for life.

Chonic cholangitis associated with trematodes

Aetiology

This condition is caused by infection with species of the Opisthorchiidae family.

Epidemiology

Endemic areas are in North and South America, China, Japan, India, and Northern Europe.

Aetiopathogeneis

Cats become infected by eating raw fish infected with Opisthorchiidae. The trematodes migrate from the duodenum to the liver through the bile ducts.

Clinical signs

Infected cats may be asymptomatic or have anorexia, vomiting, abdominal pain, and jaundice.

Diagnosis

Diagnosis is made by liver biopsy or cholecystocentesis.

Treatment

Treatment consists of praziquantel 30 mg/kg/24 h PO for 5–10 days.

Disease of the exocrine pancreas

Introduction

The **exocrine pancreas** is the principal source of **digestive enzymes** that act in the lumen of the **small intestine**. It is made up of compound tubular acinar glands that synthesize and excrete enzymes such as amylase and lipase, along with inactive proenzymes and zymogens of digestive enzymes (trypsinogen and chymotrypsinogen) essential for the digestion of proteins, triglycerides, and complex carbohydrates. These then drain into the proximal duodenum via a system of ducts. Between the acini is connective tissue laced with capillaries and nerve endings.

The exocrine pancreas also secretes other essential substances, such as a **large amount of bicarbonate**, which buffers gastric acid, and intrinsic factor necessary for the absorption of cobalamin in the ileum.

Pancreatitis

Pancreatitis is an **underdiagnosed condition** in small animals, especially in cats.

Classification

Pancreatitis can be divided into three types.

- **Acute:** This is characterized by neutrophilic inflammation, interstitial oedema, and necrosis of mesenteric fat. In general it is a **reversible process**, unless it develops into acute necrotizing pancreatitis.
- **Acute necrotizing:** This is characterized by pancreatic necrosis and generates multi-organ failure. It is an uncommon form of pancreatitis and carries a poor prognosis.
- **Chronic:** This is characterized by **irreversible histological changes**; there is more fibrosis than inflammation (which is typically lymphocytic, with macrophages and eosinophils). Other histological changes include cystic dilation and lobulation.

Epidemiology

Although the incidence of clinical pancreatitis is unknown, a recent study investigated the presence of pancreatitis in cats at post-mortem by histopathological examination, and found **pancreatic inflammation present in up to 67% of cats**. Pancreatitis is therefore suspected to be underdiagnosed in cats.

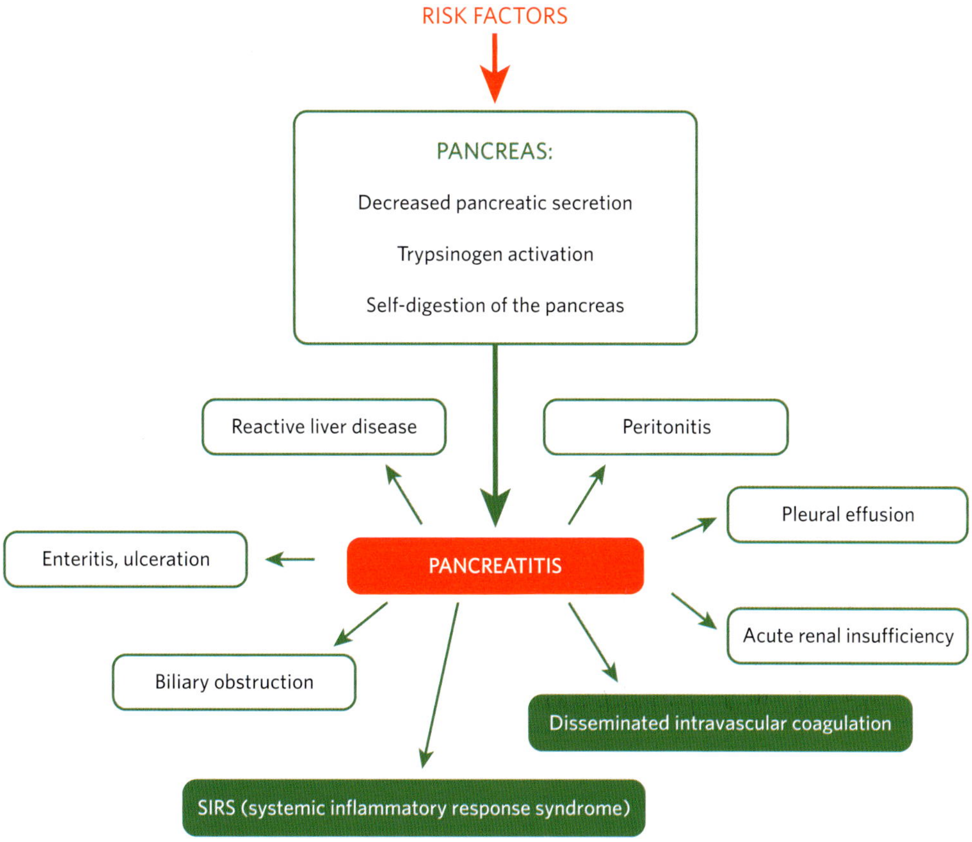

Figure 8.20. Pathophysiology of acute pancreatitis.

Aetiopathogenesis

Risk factors and/or triggers in the dog include:

- medications: potassium bromide, azathioprine, furosemide, corticosteroids
- diet: food high in fat, dietary indiscretion
- recent anaesthesia
- hyperlipidaemia (familial in Miniature Schnauzers),
- endocrine related disease: diabetes mellitus, hypothyroidism, hyperadrenocorticism
- hypercalcaemia
- abdominal trauma

In cats, the precipitating factors are generally unknown although some studies suggest:

- **breed** predisposition: Siamese (over-represented in some studies)
- **infectious** causes: toxoplasma, FIP, herpesvirus, calicivirus
- **hypotension**, hypoperfusion, which is why it is important to keep the pancreas well perfused, especially during anaesthesia
- **triaditis**, IBD, cholangitis
- **hypercalcaemia.**

Clinical signs

The symptoms are variable and depend on the severity of the inflammation, which can be:

- mild pancreatitis, sometimes subclinical
- severe pancreatitis.

Symptoms observed in a retrospective study in 70 dogs were:

- anorexia (91%)
- vomiting (90%)
- abdominal pain (58%)
- diarrhoea (33%).

In the cat, the symptoms are even more non-specific:

- anorexia (80%)
- vomiting (50%)
- jaundice (40%)
- abdominal pain (20%).

In two-thirds of cases other diseases are present, such as cholangitis, IBD, or triaditis. There may also be uncontrolled diabetes or signs of exocrine pancreatic insufficiency; and in severe cases there may be hypotension, shock, multi-organ failure, and disseminated intravascular coagulation (DIC).

Diagnosis

The owners should be asked about possible triggers such as diet, medicines, and other diseases.

Tests should rule out diseases which cause similar symptoms and require surgery such as:

- septic peritonitis
- intestinal obstruction
- pyometra.

Diseases that require specific treatment should also be ruled out, including:

- diabetic ketoacidosis and other metabolic causes
- liver disease
- kidney disease.

Complete blood count

This usually shows non-specific changes.

- Lipaemia.
- Leucocytosis (mild to severe), with or without toxic neutrophils.
- Disseminated coagulation with typical signs such as schistocytes and thrombocytopenia.
- Coagulation times may be extended. It is advisable to measure the coagulation times to assess the severity of pancreatitis and the prognosis, and to decide whether the administration of fresh plasma is indicated.
- Anaemia and high levels of urea, without elevation of creatinine. This is compatible with gastrointestinal bleeding, which is a frequent complication of acute pancreatitis.

Biochemistry

Typical findings include the following.

- Elevated liver enzymes (ALT, AP).
- Hyperbilirubinaemia, usually mild. In cases of extrahepatic biliary obstruction, the bilirubin concentration may be very high.
- Hypocalcaemia of multifactorial origin.
- C-reactive protein: In acute pancreatitis, it is usually very high (>100). A normal concentration of C-reactive protein almost always rules out acute pancreatitis.
- Hypoalbuminaemia: This is also multifactorial. As it is an acute phase protein, it may be due to abdominal effusion or gastrointestinal bleeding.

Lipase and amylase

These are synthesized in the gastrointestinal mucosa and excreted by the kidney. They are affected by corticosteroids. They have low sensitivity and specificity for pancreatitis at just 50%.

Trypsin-like immunoreactivity (TLI)

This measures trypsinogen and trypsin levels. In cases of pancreatitis it rises quickly and decreases rapidly to normal levels. However, it has good specificity for exocrine pancreatic insufficiency.

Pancreatic lipase

In both dogs and cats, according to different studies, pancreatitis is unlikely if the result of this test is negative.

Canine pancreatic lipase (cPLI)

- pancreatitis: >400 μg/l (healthy animals: <200 μg/l)
- both qualitative (ELISA) and quantitative (good correlation)
- sensitivity: 21–88%
- specificity: 80–97%.

Feline pancreatic lipase (fPLI)

This is the best of the tests currently available for pancreatitis. It has:

- variable sensitivity: 60–100%
- very high specificity: 91%.

Abdominal ultrasound

- sensitivity: 24–67%
- specificity: 73%.

In many cases the findings are normal. However, possible findings include:

- peritoneal effusion
- changes in peripancreatic fat
- dilation of the bile ducts.

Abdominal fluid analysis

In cases of acute pancreatitis, it is common to find variable amounts of abdominal fluid. The latter is usually an exudate or modified neutrophilic transudate, indicating non-septic peritonitis.

A recent study in dogs with pancreatitis found that cPLI >500 in abdominal fluid is 100% sensitive for the diagnosis of acute pancreatitis. Its specificity is 94%.

Pancreatic biopsy

This is considered the gold standard method of diagnosis. However, biopsy does have important limitations.

- In many cases the animal is not stable enough to withstand general anaesthesia.
- The inflammation may not be homogeneous, so histopathology may not be diagnostic.

Treatment of acute pancreatitis

The objectives of the treatment must be the following.

1. Identify and eliminate risk factors or causes.
2. Maintain normovolaemia with the use of fluid therapy.
3. Correct electrolyte / acid–base disorders.
4. Provide necessary calories through nutrition. Enteral is preferable to parenteral.
   A) In **dogs a low-fat diet.**
   B) In cats the impact of diet is unknown.
   C) If IBD is suspected then a **hypoallergenic diet** is recommended.
   D) Food can be supplemented with pancreatic enzymes and vitamin B12.
5. Treat complications such as anorexia, vomiting, abdominal pain, hypocalcaemia, DIC, arrhythmias, pleural effusion, or lung oedema.
   A) Antiemetics.
   B) Gastroprotectants.
   C) Analgesia.
   D) Plasma – recommended when DIC is present.
   E) NB: Antibiotics are not necessary, but they are recommended in cases where other infectious diseases are suspected such as cholangitis in the cat, or sepsis.

Exocrine pancreatic insufficiency

Definition

Exocrine pancreatic insufficiency (EPI) occurs when the exocrine pancreas does not produce or secrete sufficient digestive enzymes. As a consequence, there is a failure of assimilation of nutrients at the intestinal level resulting in malabsorption and malnutrition.

Aetiopathogenesis

The most common cause of EPI in dogs is pancreatic acinar atrophy, followed by chronic pancreatitis. This is in contrast to cats and humans, where chronic pancreatitis is the most common inciting cause. Pancreatic or extra-pancreatic tumours that obstruct the pancreatic duct can also cause EPI.

Clinical signs

The following factors should be considered.

- Dogs:
  - hereditary in the German Shepherd and Long-haired Collie
  - common in the Cavalier King Charles Spaniel, Chow, and English Setter
  - clinical signs develop by 1–3 years of age, or just 5 months in the English Setter.
- Cats:
  - no breed predisposition to EPI
  - clinical signs can develop at any age
  - chronic diarrhoea in cats with diabetes should raise a suspicion of EPI.

Clinical signs appear when 90% of exocrine function is lost, by which time the process is irreversible.

The most common clinical signs are:

- **weight loss** despite a good appetite; indeed, some patients are polyphagic
- **bulky stools,** diarrhoea, steatorrhea, and flatulence; in cats, soft stools are more common than diarrhoea
- vomiting
- unkempt, dry coat
- behavioural changes due to abdominal discomfort.

Diagnosis

Screening blood tests are usually unremarkable, except for occasional hypocholesteraemia.

Trypsin-like immunoreactivity

The TLI test is species specific. It measures the levels of trypsinogen released from the pancreas into the blood stream. With acute pancreatitis levels rise, due to release of trypsinogen from damaged cells. Low levels indicate an insufficiency of production or release, and EPI (Table 8.8).

Trypsinogen is excreted by the kidneys; therefore when azotaemia is present, extra care is needed when interpreting TLI test results.

- Dogs:
  - normal: 5.7–45.2 μg/l
  - diagnostic: ≤2.5 μg/l (100% sensitivity/specificity).
- Cats:
  - normal: 5.7–45.2 μg/l
  - probable diagnosis: ≤8 μg/l.

In cases of suspected EPI, measurement of cobalamin and folate concentrations is recommended (Table 8.8). Cobalamin deficiency can be corrected with a supplement of parenteral vitamin B12.

Table 8.8. Laboratory findings in different pathologies.

Process	Folate	Cobalamin	TLI
Exocrine pancreatic insufficiency (EPI)	↑	↓	↓
Small intestinal bacterial overgrowth (SIBO)	↑	↓	N
Proximal small intestinal disease	↓	N	N
Distal small intestinal disease	N	↓	N
Diffuse intestinal disease	↓	↓	N

Note: TLI, trypsin-like immunoreactivity.

Classic laboratory findings indicative of EPI are:

- low TLI
- low cobalamin
- high folate
- the rest of the analysis is usually normal.

Treatment

The treatment requires life-long supplementation of pancreatic enzymes.

Enzyme supplements are available in a variety of formulations (tablets, capsules, and powder). A recent study shows that dogs with EPI gain more weight if they take **coated tablets.** However, there are animals that improve clinically when the enzymes are administered in powder form, which is also the case in humans.

As a side effect, oral bleeding has been described in the dog, which resolves when the dose is reduced. Once the symptoms improve, an attempt should be made to lower the dose.

- Dog: 1 spoonful/10 kg.

In some cases, despite the addition of enzyme supplements, the absorption of fat is not normalized. This is due to the pH of the stomach destroying the enzyme before it can act. In such cases, the administration of a **once daily dose of omeprazole** increases the pH of the stomach, improving the effectiveness of the supplement. This is common practice in humans.

A highly digestible, low-fat food is not necessary, and only recommended for refractory cases where enzyme supplementation does not resolve the symptoms. In some cases **cobalamin deficiency** may complicate the picture, in which case parenteral supplementation becomes necessary. However, the majority of patients do respond to enzyme replacement therapy once a formulation (coated tablets vs. powder) is found that best suits them.

Dosage:

- In dogs, depending on weight:
  - <5 kg: 250 μg
  - 5–10 kg: 400 μg
  - 10–20 kg: 600 μg
  - 20–30 kg: 800 μg
  - 30–40 kg: 1000 μg
  - 40–50 kg: 1200 μg
  - >50 kg: 1500 μg.
- In cats: 250 μg SC once a week for 6 weeks, then once a month for 2 months. After this a repeated measurement of the vitamin B12 concentration is recommended.

Patients with EPI that do not respond to a change in the type of preparation or brand may well have an undiagnosed concurrent problem. Of these, chronic intestinal inflammation (IBD) or bacterial overgrowth are most common, and usually respond to treatment with metronidazole 15 mg/kg/12 h PO.

Stool consistency should normalize 3–4 days after starting therapy, and the patient should be reweighed at 2–4 weeks and subsequently monitored once or twice a year.

Prognosis

EPI is associated with an irreversible loss of pancreatic acinar tissue. However, with appropriate treatment and monitoring, animals with EPI improve clinically, gain weight, and can have a very good quality of life.

Bibliography

Batt, R.M. (1993) Exocrine pancreatic insufficiency. *The Veterinary Clinics of North America. Small Animal Practice* 23, 595–608.

Bunch, S.E. (1995) Specific and symptomatic medical management of diseases of the liver. In: Ettinger, S.J. (ed.) *Textbook of Veterinary Internal Medicine*. WB Saunders Co, Philadelphia, PA, pp. 1358–1371.

Bunch, S.E., Johnson, S.E. and Cullen, J.M. (2001) Idiopathic noncirrhotic portal hypertension in dogs: 33 cases (1982–1998). *Journal of the American Veterinary Medical Association* 218, 392–399.

Center, S.A. (2005) Feline hepatic lipidosis. *The Veterinary Clinics of North America. Small Animal Practice* 35, 225–269.

Christiansen, J.S., Hottinger, H.A., Allen, L., Phillips, L. and Aronson, L.R. (2000) Hepatic microvascular dysplasia in dogs: a retrospective study of 24 cases (1987–1995). *Journal of the American Animal Hospital Association* 36, 385–389.

Gookin, J.L., Correa, M.T., Peters, A., Malueg, A., Mathews, K.G., Cullen, J. and Seiler, G. (2015) Association of gall bladder mucocele histologic diagnosis with selected drug use in dogs: a matched case-control study. *Journal of Veterinary Internal Medicine* 29, 1464–1472.

Johnson, S.E. (1995) Diseases of the liver. In: Ettinger, S.J. (ed.) *Textbook of Veterinary Internal Medicine*. WB Saunders Co, Philadelphia, PA, pp. 1313–1357.

Lecoindre P., et al. (2009) Vacuolar Hepatopathy in Scottish Terriers: Clinical, Biochemical, Ultrasonographic and Histological Findings in 13 Cases. *Proceedings of the 19th European Congress of Veterinary Internal Medicine for Companion Animals Annual Congress, Porto*.

MacPhail, C.M., Lappin, M.R., Meyer, D.J., Smith, S.G., Webster, C.R. and Armstrong, P.J. (1998) Hepatocellular toxicosis associated with administration of carprofen in 21 dogs. *Journal of the American Veterinary Medical Association* 212, 1895–1901.

Meier, R.F. and Beglinger, C. (2006) Nutrition in pancreatic diseases. *Best Practice & Research. Clinical Gastroenterology* 20, 507–529.

Qin, H.L., Su, Z.D., Hu, L.G., Ding, Z.X. and Lin, Q.T. (2007) Effect of parenteral and early intrajejunal nutrition on pancreatic digestive enzyme synthesis, storage and discharge in dog models of acute pancreatitis. *World Journal of Gastroenterology* 13, 1123–1128.

Rand, J.S., Best, S.J. and Mathew, K.A. (1987) Portosystemic vascular shunts in a family of American Cocker spaniels. *Journal of the American Animal Hospital Association* 24, 266–272.

Rothuizen, J. (2006) Cholangitis in cats—a review. *Proceedings of the 31st World Small Animal Congress, Prague, Czech Republic*.

Schermerhorn, T., Center, S.A., Dykes, N.L., Rowland, P.H., Yeager, A.E., Erb, H.N., Oberhansley, K. and Bonda, M. (1996) Characterization of hepatoportal microvascular dysplasia in a kindred of Cairn terriers. *Journal of Veterinary Internal Medicine* 10, 219–230.

Schuller, S., Francey, T., Hartmann, K., Hugonnard, M., Kohn, B., Nally, J.E. and Sykes, J. (2015) European consensus statement on leptospirosis in dogs and cats. *The Journal of Small Animal Practice* 56, 159–179.

Sherding, R.G. (2000) Feline jaundice. *Journal of Feline Medicine and Surgery* 2, 165–169.

Test

1. The liver performs vital functions. Which of the following is a function of the liver?
A) The liver produces bile acids, which are responsible for the breakdown of carbohydrates and proteins in the diet.
B) The liver maintains euglycaemia: it is responsible for gluconeogenesis, glycogenolysis, and glycogen storage.
C) The liver synthesizes erythropoietin.
D) The liver produces ammonium and urea.

2. What is the most common clinical sign in cats with hepatic encephalopathy?
A) convulsions
B) aggressiveness
C) excessive salivation
D) horizontal nystagmus.

3. Which of the following factors can predispose dogs to developing pancreatitis?
A) NSAIDs
B) recent anaesthesia
C) cyclosporine
D) high protein diet.

4. Noir is a 6-year-old castrated male cat who has been anorexic and weak for a few days. On physical examination he is found to be jaundiced. On blood tests haematocrit is 15%, total protein 70 g/dl, and on biochemistry liver enzymes are normal but bilirubin is higher than normal. What is the most likely diagnosis?
A) haemolytic anaemia
B) hepatic lipidosis
C) hepatic neoplasia
D) cholangitis.

5. What is the most common aetiology of vacuolar liver disease in dogs?
A) idiopathic vacuolar liver disease
B) excess of corticosteroids
C) obesity
D) hepatocellular carcinoma.

6. Which endocrine disease can predispose the appearance of a biliary mucocele?
A) hypoadrenocorticism
B) hyperthyroidism

C) hypothyroidism
D) acromegaly.

7. Toby, a 2-year-old mongrel, weighing 6 kg, presents with jaundice, fever, polyuria, and polydipsia and has been vomiting for 48 hours. Tests reveal elevated liver enzymes, hyperbilirubinaemia, and azotaemia. The urinalysis shows glycosuria. What is the likely diagnosis?
A) leptospirosis
B) pancreatitis
C) *Amanita phalloides* poisoning
D) amyloidosis.

8. Milú, a 4-month-old Yorkshire Terrier, presents with delayed growth and depression. A portosystemic shunt is suspected. What are we likely to find on Milú's complete blood count?
A) leucopenia
B) thrombocytosis
C) hypochromic microcytosis
D) polychromatophilia.

9. Milú's blood biochemistry reveals slightly increased liver enzymes and low urea. Glucose, albumin, and cholesterol are normal. The ammonium is high. An abdominal ultrasound is performed and no vascular anomalies are found. Which of the following is true?
A) The most likely diagnosis is hypoplasia of the portal vein.
B) We should repeat the ultrasound in 2 weeks' time.
C) The next step is to perform other imaging tests: portography, trans-splenic scintigraphy, or CT.
D) We should measure bile acids to confirm the presence of a shunt.

10. With reference to the different methods of obtaining a liver biopsy, what is an advantage of the echo-guided biopsy/tru-cut technique?
A) It poses a lower risk of bleeding.
B) It allows deeper samples to be obtained.
C) It facilitates high quality biopsies compared to other methods.
D) It is especially useful when the liver is small.

11. Mulan is an 8-year-old common European cat that has been anorexic for a week. He has lost a lot of weight and is jaundiced. On physical examination he is found to have hepatomegaly. Blood tests show hyperbilirubinaemia and raised AP. On abdominal ultrasound the liver is hyperechogenic and the bile ducts are normal. What is the best treatment for Mulan?
A) low protein diet
B) amoxicillin/clavulanate
C) low carbohydrate diet with high quality protein
D) metronidazole and lactulose.

12. A castrated male German Shepherd dog is referred due to a possible hepatopathy. On physical examination there is abdominal pain and fever. Blood tests show leucocytosis with a left shift and elevation of liver enzymes and C-reactive protein. Abdominal ultrasound shows changes in the gall bladder and hepatic parenchyma that suggest a cholangiohepatitis. Which bacteria are the most frequent cause of bacterial cholangiohepatitis?
A) *Streptococcus*
B) *Bartonella*
C) *Escherichia coli*
D) mycobacteria.

13. In which breed has a genetic mutation responsible for copper liver disease been described?
A) Labrador Retriever
B) Yorkshire Terrier
C) Cocker Spaniel
D) Bedlington Terrier.

14. In relation to the liver enzyme AP, which of these statements is true?
A) The half-life is shorter in cats (3 hours) than in dogs (3 days).
B) In the dog there is also an isoenzyme associated with lung disease.

C) Elevated AP, with normal GGT, is a typical finding in cats with cholangitis.
D) If the cat has been treated with corticosteroids over various days, AP enzymes will appear elevated on blood tests.

15. How can we differentiate liver disease from post-hepatic disease?

A) In hepatic disease, blood levels of albumin, glucose, cholesterol, and urea are always reduced.
B) Bile acids will only be elevated in post-hepatic disease.
C) By ultrasound: in the case of an extrahepatic problem, the ultrasound will show changes in the gall bladder, bile ducts, and pancreas.
D) If ammonium is normal, then it is almost certain that the problem is extrahepatic.

16. Which of the following findings is more common in cats with lymphocytic cholangitis than in cats with neutrophilic cholangitis?

A) fever
B) ascites
C) leucocytosis with a left shift
D) hepatic encephalopathy.

Answers on page 362

Clinical case

Linda, a 7-year-old Miniature Schnauzer bitch, has been vomiting for 2 days and is very apathetic. The physical examination shows the following:

- weight: 5.7 kg
- temperature: 38.4°C
- pulse: 160
- respiratory rate: 38
- attitude: depressed
- mucous membranes: pink, capillary filling time <2
- pain: 3/4
- lymph nodes within normal limits
- dehydration: 7
- cardiorespiratory: tachycardia, palpable femoral pulse; normal pulmonary and cardiac auscultation
- gastrointestinal/urogenital: pain on cranial abdominal palpation
- musculoskeletal: normal, symmetrical musculature.

1. What is on the list of Linda's problems?

2. Please update the problem list taking the blood tests into account.

Complete blood count

Parameter	Results	Normal range
Erythrocytes	8 × 106/µl	5-11 × 10^6/µl
Haematocrit	40%	32–48%
Haemoglobin	10 g/dl	8–15 g/dl
VCM	40 fl	39–50 fl
HCM	14 pg	13–18 pg
CMHC	32 g/dl	30–35 g/dl
Leukocytes	25 × 10^3/µl	5.5–19.5 × 10^3/µl
Neutrophils segmented	22.3 × 10^3/µl	2.7–6.9 × 10^3/µl
Bands	2800	
Lymphocytes	0.1 × 10^3/µl	0.4–5 × 10^3/µl
Monocytes	0.6 × 10^3/µl	0–0.8 × 10^3/µl
Eosinophils	0	0–0.8 × 10^3/µl
Platelets	450 × 10^3/µl	200–500 × 10^3/µl

Note: CMHC; HCM; VCM.

Serum biochemistry

Parameter	Results	Normal range
Total protein	7.3 mg/dl	5.5–8.2 mg/dl
Albumin	3.6 g/dl	3–4 g/dl
Globulin	3.7 g/dl	3–4 g/dl
Glucose	140 mg/dl	63–140 mg/dl
Alkaline phosphatase	450 U/l	15–96 U/l
Alanine transaminase	180 U/l	27–127 U/l
Bilirubin	4.6 mg/dl	0–0.4 mg/dl
Cholesterol	510 mg/dl	73–265 mg/dl
Urea	30 mg/dl	17–35 mg/dl
Creatinine	1.8 mg/dl	0.8–2.3 mg/dl
Ca	11 mg/dl	8.2–11.5 mg/dl
K	3.8 mmol/l	4–5.5 mmol/l
Na	134 mmol/l	130–140 mmol/l
P	6 mg/dl	3.4–8.5 mg/dl

3. **Taking the blood test into account, what kind of problem is most likely?**
   A) pre-hepatic
   B) hepatic
   C) post-hepatic.
4. **Abdominal ultrasound shows a biliary mucocele with dilation of the bile duct. The omentum is hyperechogenic around the gall bladder and there is a minimal amount of abdominal fluid between the hepatic lobes. What would you recommend?**
   A) Perform laparotomy and cholecystectomy.
   B) Measure T4 and perform an ACTH stimulation test.
   C) Perform an ultrasound-guided aspiration of the bile, to rule out bacterial cholecystitis, and treat with antibiotics.
5. **Owing to the presence of a mucocele and the suspicion of peritonitis, the aforementioned tests were performed, biopsy and culture (aerobic and anaerobic) of the gall bladder and bile, and abdominal fluid analysis (non-septic neutrophilic inflammation). A surgical intervention was performed. Two days later, liver enzymes and bilirubin had decreased by 50% but were still high. Linda recovered very well from the surgery and was discharged. What treatment was she discharged with?**
6. **Which pathologies should be ruled out at a later stage, and when?**

Correct answers

Test

1. B	7. A	13. D
2. C	8. C	14. A
3. B	9. C	15. C
4. A	10. B	16. B
5. B	11. C	
6. C	12. C	

Clinical case

1. **What is on the list of Linda's problems?**
   1. Abdominal pain.
   2. Acute vomiting
   3. Tachycardia
   4. 7% dehydration.

2. Please update the problem list taking the blood tests into account.

1. Abdominal pain.
2. Acute vomiting
3. Tachycardia
4. 7% dehydration.
5. Moderate leukocytosis with a left shift.
6. Hyperbilirubinaemia.
7. Elevation of AP and ALT enzymes.

3. Taking the blood test into account, what kind of problem is most likely?

C. Posthepatic

Blood tests show a marked elevation of the AP enzyme compared to the ALT enzyme, suggesting a problem with cholestasis.

Elevation of cholesterol is frequently associated with either an intrahepatic or extrahepatic cholestastic problem, (for example, a common bile duct or gallbladder problem).

Albumin, urea and glucose are within normal limits.

Although we cannot rule out a liver problem, it is most likely diagnosis is that it is extrahepatic cholestasis.

Taking the leucocytosis with a left shift and the abdominal pain that the animal presents with into account, the differential diagnoses are:

– Cholangiohepatitis / bacterial cholecystitis.
– Biliary obstruction (due to cholelithiasis, biliary mucocele or neoplasia).
– Pancreatitis / pancreatic neoplasia.

4. Abdominal ultrasound shows a biliary mucocele with dilation of the bile duct. The omentum is hyperechogenic around the gallbladder and there is a minimal amount of abdominal fluid between hepatic lobes. What would you recommend?

A. Laparotomy and cholecystectomy.

5. Due to the presence of a mucocele and the suspicion of peritonitis, the aforementioned tests were performed, biopsy and culture (aerobic and anaerobic) of the gallbladder and bile, and abdominal fluid analysis (non-septic neutrophilic inflammation). A surgical intervention was performed. Two days later, liver enzymes and bilirubin had decreased by 50% but were still high. Linda recovered very well from the surgery and was discharged. What treatment was she discharged with?

1. Analgesia (tramadol 3-5 mg / kg / 8 h VO).
2. S-adenosylmethionine (Denamarin 30 mg ½ tablet per day VO).
3. Ursodeoxycholic acid (10-15 mg / kg / 24 h VO).
4. Antibiotics (amoxicillin-clavulanic acid and metronidazole 7.5 mg / kg / 12 h) whilst waiting for the results of the culture.
5. Omeprazole (0.5 mg / kg BID VO).

6. What pathologies should be ruled out at a later stage? When?

At a later date, at least a couple of weeks after the animal has recovered from surgery, the physical examination and blood tests should be repeated. If there are changes compatible with hypothyroidism or hyperadrenocorticism, these two endocrinopathies should be ruled out.

Index